Diagnosis and Treatment of Cardiac Arrhythmias

Diagnosis and Treatment of Cardiac Arrhythmias

Editor: Joe Tyler

AMERICAN
MEDICAL PUBLISHERS
www.americanmedicalpublishers.com

AMERICAN
MEDICAL PUBLISHERS
www.americanmedicalpublishers.com

Cataloging-in-Publication Data

Diagnosis and treatment of cardiac arrhythmias / edited by Joe Tyler.
p. cm.
Includes bibliographical references and index.
ISBN 979-8-88740-057-0
1. Arrhythmia. 2. Arrhythmia--Diagnosis. 3. Arrhythmia--Treatment.
4. Heart--Diseases. 5. Heart beat. I. Tyler, Joe.
RC685.A65 D53 2023
616.128--dc23

American Medical Publishers,
41 Flatbush Avenue,
1st Floor, New York,
NY 11217, USA

ISBN 979-8-88740-057-0 (Hardback)

Contents

Preface

In my initial years as a student, I used to run to the library at every possible instance to grab a book and learn something new. Books were my primary source of knowledge and I would not have come such a long way without all that I learnt from them. Thus, when I was approached to edit this book; I became understandably nostalgic. It was an absolute honor to be considered worthy of guiding the current generation as well as those to come. I put all my knowledge and hard work into making this book most beneficial for its readers.

Cardiac arrhythmias refer to the irregularities in the heartbeat. A person in this condition may experience either tachycardia, where heart rate reaches more than 100 beats per minute, or bradycardia, where heart rate reaches 60 beats per minute. Some common symptoms of cardiac arrhythmias are palpitations, dizziness, chest pain, fatigue, blurry vision and sweating. The diagnosis of cardiac arrhythmias includes electrocardiogram tests, stress test, echocardiogram test, cardiac catheterization, etc. Various treatment options available for arrhythmia include invasive therapies, electrical devices, medications, lifestyle changes and surgery. Catheter ablation and electrical cardioversion are some of the invasive therapies that are utilized for eliminating and treating irregular heart rhythms. Pulmonary vein isolation is a type of ablation, which targets those areas which cause atrial fibrillation. Various devices like implantable cardioverter-defibrillator (ICD) and permanent pacemaker can be used to treat arrhythmias. This book outlines the diagnosis and treatment of cardiac arrhythmias in detail. It will also provide interesting topics for research which interested readers can take up. Students, researchers, experts and all associated with the study and treatment of these disease will benefit alike from this book.

I wish to thank my publisher for supporting me at every step. I would also like to thank all the authors who have contributed their researches in this book. I hope this book will be a valuable contribution to the progress of the field.

Editor

1

Role of sinoatrial node architecture in maintaining a balanced source-sink relationship and synchronous cardiac pacemaking

Sathya D. Unudurthi[1,2], Roseanne M. Wolf[3] and Thomas J. Hund[1,2,4]*

[1] Department of Biomedical Engineering, College of Engineering, The Ohio State University, Columbus, OH, USA
[2] The Dorothy M. Davis Heart and Lung Research Institute, The Ohio State University Wexner Medical Center, Columbus, OH, USA
[3] Department of Mathematics, The University of Dubuque, Dubuque, IA, USA
[4] Division of Cardiovascular Medicine, Department of Internal Medicine, The Ohio State University Wexner Medical Center, Columbus, OH, USA

Correspondence:
Thomas J. Hund, The Dorothy M. Davis Heart and Lung Research Institute, The Ohio State University Wexner Medical Center, 473 W. 12th Avenue, Columbus, OH 43210, USA
e-mail: thomas.hund@osumc.edu

Normal heart rhythm (sinus rhythm) depends on regular activity of the sinoatrial node (SAN), a heterogeneous collection of specialized myocytes in the right atrium. SAN cells, in general, possess a unique electrophysiological profile that promotes spontaneous electrical activity (automaticity). However, while automaticity is required for normal pacemaking, it is not necessarily sufficient. Less appreciated is the importance of the elaborate structure of the SAN complex for proper pacemaker function. Here, we review the important structural features of the SAN with a focus on how these elements help manage a precarious balance between electrical charge generated by the SAN ("source") and the charge needed to excite the surrounding atrial tissue ("sink"). We also discuss how compromised "source-sink" balance due, for example to fibrosis, may promote SAN dysfunction, characterized by slow and/or asynchronous pacemaker activity and even failure, in the setting of cardiovascular disease (e.g., heart failure, atrial fibrillation). Finally, we discuss implications of the "source-sink" balance in the SAN complex for cell and gene therapies aimed at creating a biological pacemaker as replacement or bridge to conventional electronic pacemakers.

Keywords: sinoatrial node, automaticity, pacemaking, source-sink relationship, intercellular coupling, sick sinus syndrome, arrhythmia

INTRODUCTION

The sinoatrial node (SAN), located in the right atrium, serves as the primary site for initiation of the normal heartbeat (sinus rhythm) (**Figure 1**). Together with the cardiac conduction system [the atrioventricular node (AVN) and the His–Purkinje system], the SAN is responsible for orchestrating the precise sequence of electrical events underlying the normal heart rhythm. This sequence begins with generation of the electrical impulse in the SAN, which then spreads rapidly through the atria and to the AVN. AVN conduction is slow, thereby introducing a delay between atrial and ventricular systole to facilitate filling of the ventricles before they contract. The AVN also serves as a secondary pacemaker in the event of SAN failure (e.g., due to aging, cardiovascular disease). After exiting the AVN, the impulse propagates rapidly through the His-Purkinje system, comprised of a common bundle (the bundle of His), and left and right bundle branches that give rise to a network of terminal Purkinje fibers which simultaneously communicate the impulse to the ventricular muscle at multiple discrete locations (Purkinje-muscle junctions). The His–Purkinje system supports rapid conduction with action potential (AP) propagation velocities up to ten-fold higher than in the ventricular mass to ensure synchronous activation of the ventricular muscle (Boyett, 2009). This sequence of electrical events is essential for normal heart function and depends on a number of distinguishing cell and tissue properties shared by each component of the pacemaker and conduction system. First and foremost, cells in the pacemaker and conduction system possess the defining characteristic of automaticity, an ability to generate an action potential in the absence of an external stimulus. Automaticity is required for cardiac pacemaking and depends on a unique ion channel expression profile conducive to spontaneous AP generation. Second, and the major focus of this review, aside from active cell membrane properties (e.g., voltage-gated ion channel activity), tissue structure and cell-to-cell communication are tightly controlled in these tissues to handle the unique energetic demands placed on them during the excitation cycle. Specifically, these tissues are designed to balance the supply of depolarizing current generated by activating cells ("sources") with the demand of downstream quiescent cells ("sinks"). Source-sink relationships are important throughout the heart, but tissues in the pacemaker and conduction system, in particular, have evolved elaborate structures/properties to facilitate activation of a large tissue mass by a relatively small number of cells (e.g., atrial activation by the sinoatrial node; ventricular activation by His-Purkinje fibers). The goal of this review is to discuss mechanisms important for regulation of cardiac pacemaking with a specific focus on the role of passive tissue properties.

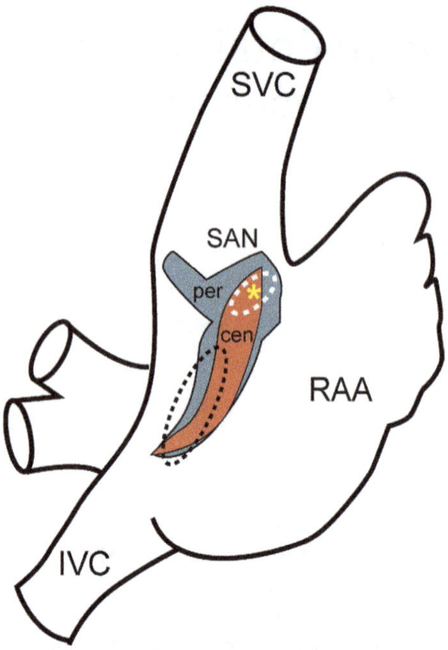

FIGURE 1 | Sinoatrial node anatomy. Schematic diagram of the right atrium showing approximate location and extent of rabbit sinoatrial node determined by computer three-dimensional reconstruction (red, central SAN region; blue, peripheral SAN region; yellow asterisk, leading pacemaker site) compared to previous estimates from the human based on anatomy and function (white dashed line, SAN; black dashed line, ectopic atrial region) (Talano et al., 1978; Dobrzynski et al., 2005). (SVC, superior vena cava; IVC, inferior vena cava; RAA, right atrial appendage).

THE SINOATRIAL NODE

SINOATRIAL NODE ANATOMY

The SAN was discovered over a century ago by Arthur Keith and Martin Flack as an anatomically defined tissue at the junction of the superior vena cava and right atria (Keith and Flack, 1907). For decades following this discovery, the SAN was defined as a compact unifocal region surrounded by secondary extranodal atrial pacemakers that could randomly compete with the leading pacemaker site in the SAN. Today, the SAN is recognized to be a distributed and heterogeneous complex adjacent to the crista terminalis with distinct regions defined by unique electrophysiological and structural properties (**Figure 1**) (Boineau et al., 1980, 1988; Dobrzynski et al., 2005, 2007; Fedorov et al., 2012). In larger animals, including the human, the node is functionally isolated with the exception of well-defined exit pathways that allow for communication between the SAN and atrial tissue (Fedorov et al., 2009, 2010, 2012; Nikolaidou et al., 2012). The anatomical basis of this insulation has been attributed to surrounding connective tissue, which insulates the pacemaker's automaticity from the hyperpolarizing electrical activity of the atrial myocardium. Other reports describe nodal/atrial interdigitations without a fibrous border that rely upon delicate spatial control of gap junction coupling (Ten Velde et al., 1995; Sanchez-Quintana et al., 2005). A distinguishing feature of SAN found in multiple species is the presence of a centrally located artery around which the SAN cells are organized (Sanchez-Quintana et al., 2005).

SINOATRIAL NODE CELL MORPHOLOGY

The sinoatrial node is a collection of weakly coupled, heterogeneous cells, including pacemaker cells as well as non-pacemaker cells such as atrial myocytes, adipocytes and fibroblasts. Within the node, pacemaker cells vary by size and electrophysiological properties and may be divided into three major classes: (1) "Elongated spindle shaped cells," which range up to 80 μm in length and have a faintly striated cell body with one or more nuclei; (2) "Spindle cells," which have a similar shape to that of elongated spindle cells, but are shorter in length, extending up to 40 μm and are predominantly mono-nucleated; and (3) "Spider cells" have irregularly shaped branches with blunt ends (Verheijck et al., 1998) (**Figure 2**). A gradual transition has been observed in AP properties from the central area toward the SAN periphery (Kodama and Boyett, 1985). One of the possible reasons for this transition has been attributed to the arrangement and distribution of nodal cells in SAN node, although there is some debate about the exact underlying cellular distribution (Zhang et al., 2001; Dobrzynski et al., 2005; Oren and Clancy, 2010) (**Figure 2**). Regardless, it is clear that heterogeneity is the rule as none of the described cell types have been found exclusively in a specific SAN area. In rabbit, for example, a uniform distribution of the three major pacemaker cell types has been observed in the central SAN area. In the crista terminalis region, atrial cells are the predominant cell type (63 ± 18%), with a subpopulation of pacemaker cells, most of which are elongated spindle nodal cells. The septal area of SAN is mostly composed of atrial cells (88 ± 19%) and all the four types of SAN cells have an almost uniform presence in this region (Verheijck et al., 1998). Despite the diversity in morphology and electrophysiology within the SAN region, there are important unifying active membrane properties of these cells that are essential for normal pacemaking.

SINOATRIAL NODE CELL ACTIVE MEMBRANE PROPERTIES

SAN cell automaticity depends on an electrophysiological profile that is distinct from that in atrial or ventricular cells (Mangoni and Nargeot, 2008). First and foremost, while APs from ventricular and atrial cells possess a stable rest potential, the SAN AP lacks a stable rest potential due in large part to lack of the inward rectifier K^+ channel I_{K1} (**Figure 3**). Instead the SAN AP reaches a maximum diastolic potential (~-60 mV) followed by a spontaneous depolarization phase that eventually reaches threshold to generate another AP. Pacemaking depends on tight regulation of this spontaneous depolarization phase, which results from the coordinated effort of multiple ion channels/transporters/exchangers. Among the important currents contributing to diastolic depolarization is the hyperpolarization-activated "funny" current (I_f) (due primarily to *HCN4* in SAN cells), with permeability to both Na^+ and K^+ and biophysical properties that make it a depolarizing current during diastole. I_f activates as the membrane potential approaches its max diastolic value and helps to spontaneously depolarize the membrane. At the same time, a low level of Ca^{2+} release from sarcoplasmic reticulum ryanodine receptor Ca^{2+} release channels likely promotes a depolarizing

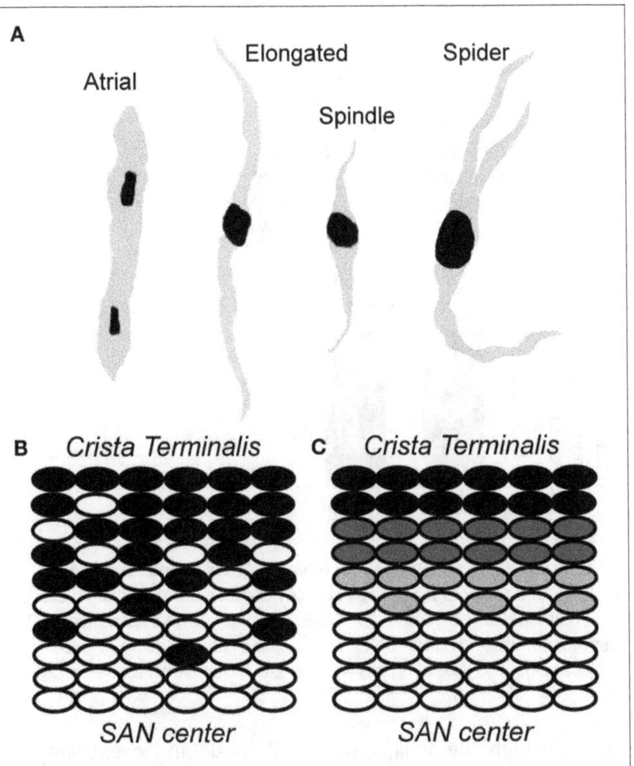

FIGURE 2 | Sinoatrial node is a heterogeneous collection of morphologically and electrophysiologically distinct myocytes. (A) A schematic representation of cells found in the sinoatrial node region, including relatively large "elongated" spindle shaped cells, "spindle" cells that are similar in shape to that of elongated spindle cells with a shorter length, and irregularly shaped "spider" cells. **(B,C)** Two different models have been proposed to account for transition from typical/central SAN (white ovals) to atrial (black ovals) cells: **(C)** a gradual transition of intermediate cells (gray) from SAN center to crista terminalis; and **(B)** "mosaic" model involving gradually decreasing ratio of SAN to atrial cell densities from SAN center to crista terminalis (Verheijck et al., 1998).

current via the Na^+/Ca^{2+} exchanger (Lakatta et al., 2010). Once the membrane potential reaches about −50 mV, transient or T-type Ca^{+2} channels (namely, $Ca_v3.1$, $Ca_v3.2$, and $Ca_v3.3$) open, allowing for Ca^{2+} entry into the cell and further depolarization of the cell membrane. As the membrane potential approaches −40 mV, L-type Ca^{2+} channels (first $Ca_v1.3$, then $Ca_v1.2$ at slightly less negative potentials) activate, giving rise to the SAN cell upstroke, which is much slower than that in atrial or ventricular myocytes due to the low levels of voltage-gated Na^+ channel (Na_v) expressed in SAN cells (orders or magnitude smaller than Na_v in ventricular myocytes). Although Na_v does not have the prominent role in the SAN AP upstroke, Na_v expression in SAN (and surrounding atrial) tissue is important for source-sink balance and pacemaking (discussed more below), such that Na_v deficiency is often associated with bradycardia and/or defects in the pacemaker and conduction system (Benson et al., 2003; Veldkamp et al., 2003; Makiyama et al., 2005). SAN AP repolarization is promoted by the activities of several classes of voltage-gated K^+ channels. The transient outward K^+ current (I_{to}), carried by $K_v1.4$, $K_v4.2$, and $K_v4.3$, is responsible for the early phase of SAN AP repolarization, while delayed-rectifier K^+ currents ultrarapid (I_{Kur}, $K_v1.5$), rapid (I_{Kr}, ERG), and slow (I_{Ks}, K_vLQT1) K^+ currents control late repolarization and the maximal diastolic potential (especially I_{Kr}). Other K^+ currents (e.g., $I_{K,ATP}$, $I_{K,Ach}$) are important for dynamic response of SAN excitability to parasympathetic, metabolic factors. While steady-state rest is never achieved in the normal SAN, the activities of these K^+ channels together with inactivation of L-type Ca^{2+} channels allows the membrane to reset for the next spontaneous action potential.

SOURCE-SINK RELATIONSHIPS IN HEART

While the ionic events described in the previous section are essential for SAN cell automaticity, cardiac pacemaking is, in fact, an emergent property of a heterogeneous, coupled system of both spontaneously active and quiescent cells (**Figure 3**). Therefore, a complete analysis of pacemaking accounts for not only events at the single cell level but also those tissue-level factors that will shape the emergent behavior. In particular, to understand the behavior of the intact SAN, it is helpful to reflect on the delicate electrical source-sink relationships that exist in the SAN region (Nikolaidou et al., 2012). Throughout the heart, successful propagation of the action potential depends on a cell first receiving electrical current from neighboring excited cells and then, once excited, sending current downstream to neighboring quiescent cells. Thus, every cell will both give charge to ("source") and take charge from ("sink") surrounding tissue at different times in their activation cycle. Propagation will be successful as long as the active sources can generate enough current to satisfy local sinks. Alternatively, if the sink overwhelms the source, propagation will fail. Tissue structure and electrical coupling have a huge influence on source-sink relationships, and can tip the balance for or against successful propagation at critical junctures (Joyner et al., 1991; Rohr et al., 1997; Shaw and Rudy, 1997). The concept of safety factor has been introduced to quantify the balance between sources and sinks in ventricular and atrial tissue (Delgado et al., 1990; Shaw and Rudy, 1997; Kleber and Rudy, 2004; Boyle and Vigmond, 2010). Briefly, safety factor is the ratio of how much charge a cell generates to the charge threshold for activation. A safety factor greater than one is indicative of safe conduction with an appropriate balance between source and sink, while a safety factor less than one is indicative of a source-sink mismatch with high susceptibility to conduction failure. Experimental and modeling studies have shown that safety factor tends to be low for propagation that occurs from a smaller cell to a larger cell and/or from a relatively small number of cells to a larger number of cells (Fast and Kleber, 1995; Rohr et al., 1997; Wang and Rudy, 2000), conditions that are highly relevant for the SAN complex. It is known that the atrium places a considerable electrical load on the SAN (Kirchhof et al., 1987). How, then, does the heart manage robust pacemaking under these unsafe conditions? The complete answer to this question cannot be understood without considering the SAN architecture itself.

SINOATRIAL NODE STRUCTURE AND SOURCE-SINK BALANCE

Perhaps the most important structural features for managing source-sink balance in SAN region are conduction barriers found

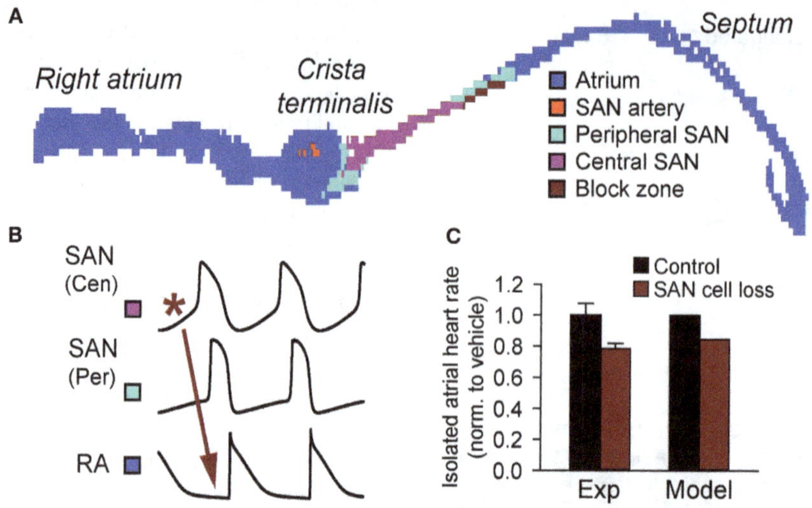

FIGURE 3 | Importance of source-sink balance in the intact sinoatrial node complex. (A) A two-dimensional histologically reconstructed mathematical model of the intact sinoatrial node based on immunohistological data (Dobrzynski et al., 2005; Butters et al., 2010) identifying the distribution of cells throughout the right atrium (adapted from Luo et al., 2013). **(B)** Normal activation initiates in the central SAN region, spreads through the SAN periphery, and finally to the right atrium. **(C)** Cell loss slows activation of the right atrium in both experiment (19% cell loss induced by streptozotocin (STZ) treatment and assessed by TUNEL staining) and computer simulations (Replacement of 19% of SAN cells with inexcitable elements) (Luo et al., 2013).

between the SAN and surrounding atrial tissue (Fedorov et al., 2012; Nikolaidou et al., 2012). In large animals (e.g., canine and human), where the SAN is embedded in a relatively thick, three-dimensional atrial wall, layers of connective tissue isolate much of the SAN from the atrial myocardium (Fedorov et al., 2012; Nikolaidou et al., 2012). In smaller animals, the atrial wall is much thinner (practically two-dimensional) reducing the load on the SAN. However, even in this environment, a discrete region of conduction block ("block zone") prevents direct activation of the interatrial septum and likely consists of fibrous, connective, and/or fatty tissue (Fedorov et al., 2012; Nikolaidou et al., 2012) (**Figure 3**). Thus, in both large and small animals well-defined non-conducting regions help reduce electrical loading of the SAN and preserve a sustainable source-sink balance.

Another important way source-sink balance is maintained in the SAN region is through electrical coupling between cells. Specifically, electrical coupling is poor in the SAN relative to that in the surrounding atrial myocardium due to preferential expression of gap junctions containing low conductance connexins (Connexin45) (Boyett et al., 2006; Dobrzynski et al., 2007). Modeling and experimental studies have demonstrated a somewhat counter-intuitive relationship between electrical coupling and safety factor, with uncoupling decreasing conduction velocity while increasing safety over a wide range (Shaw and Rudy, 1997; Rohr et al., 1998; Kleber and Saffitz, 2014). Partial uncoupling of SAN cells from neighboring cells prevents these cells from becoming overwhelmed by demand, in essence reducing the apparent size of the atrium (Joyner and Van Capelle, 1986; Watanabe et al., 1995). Importantly, experimental and modeling studies have shown that successful entrainment of atrial activation by the SAN requires only a low degree of coupling between SAN and atrial cells (Cai et al., 1994; Joyner et al., 1998). Once the electrical impulse emerges from the SAN, it can then propagate safely through the atria, into the AV node and eventually into the His-Purkinje system. Another region where a similar potential mismatch is observed is at the Purkinje muscle junction where the terminal Purkinje fibers couple to the ventricular mass. In fact, uncoupling has been shown to improve conduction across the Purkinje muscle junction (Morley et al., 2005). Aside from influencing safety for propagation, the degree of electrical coupling may also affect the dynamics of SAN cell spontaneous activation, with potential implications for synchronization of pacemaker activity (Glynn et al., 2014).

Finally, multiple experimental and modeling studies have demonstrated the importance of a gradient in membrane properties from the central to peripheral SAN region for normal pacemaking (Boyett et al., 2000; Zhang et al., 2007; Inada et al., 2014). Contributing to this gradient is the observed relationship between SAN cell size (or membrane capacitance) and densities of multiple ion currents, including voltage-gated Na^+ and Ca^{2+} currents, as well as transient outward K^+ current (I_{to}), rapid and slow delayed rectifier K^+ currents (I_{Kr}, I_{Ks}) and funny current (I_f). Mathematical modeling has shown that, in particular, increased expression of the voltage-gated Na^+ channel in the SAN periphery is necessary to support excitation of the atria by the SAN (Zhang et al., 2007).

Mounting experimental and modeling data support the notion that defects in SAN tissue architecture may tip the source-sink balance in a negative direction and promote sinus node dysfunction (Thery et al., 1977; Sanders et al., 2004; Dobrzynski et al., 2007; Fedorov et al., 2012; Nikolaidou et al., 2012). In fact, it has been known for almost 40 years that SAN structural changes (e.g., SAN cell loss and fibrosis) with aging is associated with sinus node dysfunction (Thery et al., 1977). Alterations in the normal gradient of electrophysiological properties in the SAN complex has been proposed as an additional mechanism for slowing of pacemaking with aging (Alings and Bouman, 1993). Besides the normal aging process, cardiovascular disease (e.g., heart failure) has also been shown to produce dramatic electrophysiological and structural remodeling in the atrium (Sanders et al., 2004; Dobrzynski et al., 2007). Increased expression of adenosine receptors within the SAN region together with increased fibrosis have recently been linked to loss of synchrony and sinus node dysfunction in a canine heart failure model (Lou et al., 2014). At the same time, experimental and modeling work has found that chronic angiotensin infusion (heart failure condition) in the mouse results in CaMKII-induced apoptosis resulting in SAN cell loss, which disrupts the normal source-sink balance leading to sinoatrial node dysfunction (Swaminathan et al., 2011) (**Figure 3**). A similar relationship between cell loss and sinus node dysfunction has been observed in a mouse model of diabetes and in ankyrin-B syndrome (Luo et al., 2013; Wolf et al., 2013).

IMPLICATIONS OF SOURCE-SINK RELATIONSHIP FOR THERAPY

Studies from multiple groups have focused on development of a biological pacemaker as a replacement or bridge to traditional implantable electronic devices (reviewed in Cho and Marban, 2010; Rosen et al., 2011; Munshi and Olson, 2014; Rosen, 2014). These efforts are motivated by the limitations of electronic pacemakers, which include risk for infection (affecting ~2% of patients Rosen, 2014), lead fracture, and/or lack of autonomic responsiveness. Approaches include gene- and cell-based therapies to induce pacemaker activity from cells/regions that normally are quiescent (Miake et al., 2002; Bucchi et al., 2006; Tse et al., 2006; Zhang et al., 2011; Boink et al., 2012; Hu et al., 2014). Results have been mixed with reports of successful induction of physiologic heart rate using biological pacemaker in large animal models (Boink et al., 2013; Hu et al., 2014). Important limitations to these studies include both the magnitude and duration of the response to the intervention. For example, a recent gene therapy study used the transcription factor T-box 18 to reprogram right ventricular myocytes into pacemaker cells in a porcine heart block model *in vivo* (Hu et al., 2014). While authors reported a restored heart rate between 75 and 80 bpm in the T-box 18 transduced animals, there is some question about the exact mechanism as the adenoviral vector alone (GFP) also partially rescued heart rate (~65 bpm). Furthermore, heart rate effects in both the T-box 18 and GFP groups were transient and began to decline at time points greater than 11 days after injection (Hu et al., 2014; Rosen, 2014). While these biological approaches are compelling, the question is can we solve this challenging problem without considering the structure of the natural cardiac pacemaker? Is there a way to increase the efficacy of biological pacemakers by implanting/reprogramming them in supportive structures? Can we find a way to repair the natural pacemaker itself? New gene and cell-based therapies that address some of these questions may help fulfill the promise of an effective biological pacemaker.

CONCLUSIONS

The SAN is an intricately designed structure tailored to support robust pacemaking, from the molecular composition of SAN cells to their spatial arrangement and connectivity to other cells. While cardiac pacemaking depends on the automaticity of the individual myocyte, architectural factors at the tissue level are also essential for robust pacemaking. This architecture involves a distinct SAN anatomy, a unique pattern of intercellular coupling, and gradients in electrophysiological profiles that help manage a very delicate source-sink balance, due to a very small number of cells having responsibility for activating a much larger number of cells. Importantly, structural remodeling of the SAN pacemaker complex is commonly associated with sinus node dysfunction (e.g., with aging, atrial fibrillation or heart failure). A major challenge going forward is to determine whether/how we can tune SAN architecture and the associated source-sink relationship for therapeutic benefit.

ACKNOWLEDGMENTS

This work was supported by National Institutes of Health (NIH) (grant number HL114893 to Thomas J. Hund) and James S. McDonnell Foundation (to Thomas J. Hund).

REFERENCES

Alings, A. M., and Bouman, L. N. (1993). Electrophysiology of the ageing rabbit and cat sinoatrial node–a comparative study. *Eur. Heart J.* 14, 1278–1288. doi: 10.1093/eurheartj/14.9.1278

Benson, D. W., Wang, D. W., Dyment, M., Knilans, T. K., Fish, F. A., Strieper, M. J., et al. (2003). Congenital sick sinus syndrome caused by recessive mutations in the cardiac sodium channel gene (SCN5A). *J. Clin. Invest.* 112, 1019–1028. doi: 10.1172/JCI200318062

Boineau, J. P., Canavan, T. E., Schuessler, R. B., Cain, M. E., Corr, P. B., and Cox, J. L. (1988). Demonstration of a widely distributed atrial pacemaker complex in the human heart. *Circulation* 77, 1221–1237. doi: 10.1161/01.CIR.77.6.1221

Boineau, J. P., Schuessler, R. B., Hackel, D. B., Miller, C. B., Brockus, C. W., and Wylds, A. C. (1980). Widespread distribution and rate differentiation of the atrial pacemaker complex. *Am. J. Physiol.* 239, H406–H415.

Boink, G. J., Duan, L., Nearing, B. D., Shlapakova, I. N., Sosunov, E. A., Anyukhovsky, E. P., et al. (2013). HCN2/SkM1 gene transfer into canine left bundle branch induces stable, autonomically responsive biological pacing at physiological heart rates. *J. Am. Coll. Cardiol.* 61, 1192–1201. doi: 10.1016/j.jacc.2012.12.031

Boink, G. J., Nearing, B. D., Shlapakova, I. N., Duan, L., Kryukova, Y., Bobkov, Y., et al. (2012). Ca^{2+}-stimulated adenylyl cyclase AC1 generates efficient biological pacing as single gene therapy and in combination with HCN2. *Circulation* 126, 528–536. doi: 10.1161/CIRCULATIONAHA.111.083584

Boyett, M. R. (2009). "And the beat goes on." The cardiac conduction system: the wiring system of the heart. *Exp. Physiol.* 94, 1035–1049. doi: 10.1113/expphysiol.2009.046920

Boyett, M. R., Honjo, H., and Kodama, I. (2000). The sinoatrial node, a heterogeneous pacemaker structure. *Cardiovasc. Res.* 47, 658–687. doi: 10.1016/S0008-6363(00)00135-8

Boyett, M. R., Inada, S., Yoo, S., Li, J., Liu, J., Tellez, J., et al. (2006). Connexins in the sinoatrial and atrioventricular nodes. *Adv. Cardiol.* 42, 175–197. doi: 10.1159/000092569

Boyle, P. M., and Vigmond, E. J. (2010). An intuitive safety factor for cardiac propagation. *Biophys. J.* 98, L57–L59. doi: 10.1016/j.bpj.2010.03.018

Bucchi, A., Plotnikov, A. N., Shlapakova, I., Danilo, P. Jr., Kryukova, Y., Qu, J., et al. (2006). Wild-type and mutant HCN channels in a tandem biological-electronic cardiac pacemaker. *Circulation* 114, 992–999. doi: 10.1161/CIRCULATIONAHA.106.617613

Butters, T. D., Aslanidi, O. V., Inada, S., Boyett, M. R., Hancox, J. C., Lei, M., et al. (2010). Mechanistic links between Na+ channel (SCN5A) mutations and impaired cardiac pacemaking in sick sinus syndrome. *Circ. Res.* 107, 126–137. doi: 10.1161/CIRCRESAHA.110.219949

Cai, D., Winslow, R. L., and Noble, D. (1994). Effects of gap junction conductance on dynamics of sinoatrial node cells: two-cell and large-scale network models. *IEEE Trans. Biomed. Eng.* 41, 217–231. doi: 10.1109/10.284940

Cho, H. C., and Marban, E. (2010). Biological therapies for cardiac arrhythmias: can genes and cells replace drugs and devices? *Circ. Res.* 106, 674–685. doi: 10.1161/CIRCRESAHA.109.212936

Delgado, C., Steinhaus, B., Delmar, M., Chialvo, D. R., and Jalife, J. (1990). Directional differences in excitability and margin of safety for propagation in sheep ventricular epicardial muscle. *Circ. Res.* 67, 97–110. doi: 10.1161/01.RES.67.1.97

Dobrzynski, H., Boyett, M. R., and Anderson, R. H. (2007). New insights into pacemaker activity: promoting understanding of sick sinus syndrome. *Circulation* 115, 1921–1932. doi: 10.1161/CIRCULATIONAHA.106.616011

Dobrzynski, H., Li, J., Tellez, J., Greener, I. D., Nikolski, V. P., Wright, S. E., et al. (2005). Computer three-dimensional reconstruction of the sinoatrial node. *Circulation* 111, 846–854. doi: 10.1161/01.CIR.0000152100.04087.DB

Fast, V. G., and Kleber, A. G. (1995). Block of impulse propagation at an abrupt tissue expansion: evaluation of the critical strand diameter in 2- and 3-dimensional computer models. *Cardiovasc. Res.* 30, 449–459. doi: 10.1016/S0008-6363(95)00071-2

Fedorov, V. V., Glukhov, A. V., and Chang, R. (2012). Conduction barriers and pathways of the sinoatrial pacemaker complex: their role in normal rhythm and atrial arrhythmias. *Am. J. Physiol. Heart Circ. Physiol.* 302, H1773–H1783. doi: 10.1152/ajpheart.00892.2011

Fedorov, V. V., Glukhov, A. V., Chang, R., Kostecki, G., Aferol, H., Hucker, W. J., et al. (2010). Optical mapping of the isolated coronary-perfused human sinus node. *J. Am. Coll. Cardiol.* 56, 1386–1394. doi: 10.1016/j.jacc.2010.03.098

Fedorov, V. V., Schuessler, R. B., Hemphill, M., Ambrosi, C. M., Chang, R., Voloshina, A. S., et al. (2009). Structural and functional evidence for discrete exit pathways that connect the canine sinoatrial node and atria. *Circ. Res.* 104, 915–923. doi: 10.1161/CIRCRESAHA.108.193193

Glynn, P., Onal, B., and Hund, T. J. (2014). Cycle length restitution in sinoatrial node cells: a theory for understanding spontaneous action potential dynamics. *PLoS ONE* 9:e89049. doi: 10.1371/journal.pone.0089049

Hu, Y. F., Dawkins, J. F., Cho, H. C., Marban, E., and Cingolani, E. (2014). Biological pacemaker created by minimally invasive somatic reprogramming in pigs with complete heart block. *Sci. Transl. Med.* 6, 245ra294. doi: 10.1126/scitranslmed.3008681

Inada, S., Zhang, H., Tellez, J. O., Shibata, N., Nakazawa, K., Kamiya, K., et al. (2014). Importance of gradients in membrane properties and electrical coupling in sinoatrial node pacing. *PLoS ONE* 9:e94565. doi: 10.1371/journal.pone.0094565

Joyner, R. W., Kumar, R., Golod, D. A., Wilders, R., Jongsma, H. J., Verheijck, E. E., et al. (1998). Electrical interactions between a rabbit atrial cell and a nodal cell model. *Am. J. Physiol.* 274, H2152–H2162.

Joyner, R. W., Sugiura, H., and Tan, R. C. (1991). Unidirectional block between isolated rabbit ventricular cells coupled by a variable resistance. *Biophys. J.* 60, 1038–1045. doi: 10.1016/S0006-3495(91)82141-5

Joyner, R. W., and Van Capelle, F. J. (1986). Propagation through electrically coupled cells. How a small SA node drives a large atrium. *Biophys. J.* 50, 1157–1164. doi: 10.1016/S0006-3495(86)83559-7

Keith, A., and Flack, M. (1907). The form and nature of the muscular connections between the primary divisions of the vertebrate heart. *J. Anat. Physiol.* 41, 172–189.

Kirchhof, C. J., Bonke, F. I., Allessie, M. A., and Lammers, W. J. (1987). The influence of the atrial myocardium on impulse formation in the rabbit sinus node. *Pflugers Arch.* 410, 198–203. doi: 10.1007/BF00581916

Kleber, A. G., and Rudy, Y. (2004). Basic mechanisms of cardiac impulse propagation and associated arrhythmias. *Physiol. Rev.* 84, 431–488. doi: 10.1152/physrev.00025.2003

Kleber, A. G., and Saffitz, J. E. (2014). Role of the intercalated disc in cardiac propagation and arrhythmogenesis. *Front. Physiol.* 5:404. doi: 10.3389/fphys.2014.00404

Kodama, I., and Boyett, M. R. (1985). Regional differences in the electrical activity of the rabbit sinus node. *Pflugers Arch.* 404, 214–226. doi: 10.1007/BF00581242

Lakatta, E. G., Maltsev, V. A., and Vinogradova, T. M. (2010). A coupled SYSTEM of intracellular Ca^{2+} clocks and surface membrane voltage clocks controls the timekeeping mechanism of the heart's pacemaker. *Circ. Res.* 106, 659–673. doi: 10.1161/CIRCRESAHA.109.206078

Lou, Q., Hansen, B. J., Fedorenko, O., Csepe, T. A., Kalyanasundaram, A., Li, N., et al. (2014). Upregulation of adenosine A1 receptors facilitates sinoatrial node dysfunction in chronic canine heart failure by exacerbating nodal conduction abnormalities revealed by novel dual-sided intramural optical mapping. *Circulation* 130, 315–324. doi: 10.1161/CIRCULATIONAHA.113.007086

Luo, M., Guan, X., Di, L., Kutschke, W., Gao, Z., Yang, J., et al. (2013). Diabetes increases mortality after myocardial infarction by oxidizing CaMKII. *J. Clin. Invest.* 123, 1262–1274. doi: 10.1172/JCI65268

Makiyama, T., Akao, M., Tsuji, K., Doi, T., Ohno, S., Takenaka, K., et al. (2005). High risk for bradyarrhythmic complications in patients with Brugada syndrome caused by SCN5A gene mutations. *J. Am. Coll. Cardiol.* 46, 2100–2106. doi: 10.1016/j.jacc.2005.08.043

Mangoni, M. E., and Nargeot, J. (2008). Genesis and regulation of the heart automaticity. *Physiol. Rev.* 88, 919–982. doi: 10.1152/physrev.00018.2007

Miake, J., Marban, E., and Nuss, H. B. (2002). Biological pacemaker created by gene transfer. *Nature* 419, 132–133. doi: 10.1038/419132b

Morley, G. E., Danik, S. B., Bernstein, S., Sun, Y., Rosner, G., Gutstein, D. E., et al. (2005). Reduced intercellular coupling leads to paradoxical propagation across the Purkinje-ventricular junction and aberrant myocardial activation. *Proc. Natl. Acad. Sci. U.S.A.* 102, 4126–4129. doi: 10.1073/pnas.0500881102

Munshi, N. V., and Olson, E. N. (2014). Translational medicine. improving cardiac rhythm with a biological pacemaker. *Science* 345, 268–269. doi: 10.1126/science.1257976

Nikolaidou, T., Aslanidi, O. V., Zhang, H., and Efimov, I. R. (2012). Structure-function relationship in the sinus and atrioventricular nodes. *Pediatr. Cardiol.* 33, 890–899. doi: 10.1007/s00246-012-0249-0

Oren, R. V., and Clancy, C. E. (2010). Determinants of heterogeneity, excitation and conduction in the sinoatrial node: a model study. *PLoS Comput. Biol.* 6:e1001041. doi: 10.1371/journal.pcbi.1001041

Rohr, S., Kucera, J. P., Fast, V. G., and Kleber, A. G. (1997). Paradoxical improvement of impulse conduction in cardiac tissue by partial cellular uncoupling. *Science* 275, 841–844. doi: 10.1126/science.275.5301.841

Rohr, S., Kucera, J. P., and Kleber, A. G. (1998). Slow conduction in cardiac tissue, I: effects of a reduction of excitability versus a reduction of electrical coupling on microconduction. *Circ. Res.* 83, 781–794. doi: 10.1161/01.RES.83.8.781

Rosen, M. R. (2014). Gene therapy and biological pacing. *N. Engl. J. Med.* 371, 1158–1159. doi: 10.1056/NEJMcibr1408897

Rosen, M. R., Robinson, R. B., Brink, P. R., and Cohen, I. S. (2011). The road to biological pacing. *Nat. Rev. Cardiol.* 8, 656–666. doi: 10.1038/nrcardio.2011.120

Sanchez-Quintana, D., Cabrera, J. A., Farre, J., Climent, V., Anderson, R. H., and Ho, S. Y. (2005). Sinus node revisited in the era of electroanatomical mapping and catheter ablation. *Heart* 91, 189–194. doi: 10.1136/hrt.2003.031542

Sanders, P., Kistler, P. M., Morton, J. B., Spence, S. J., and Kalman, J. M. (2004). Remodeling of sinus node function in patients with congestive heart failure: reduction in sinus node reserve. *Circulation* 110, 897–903. doi: 10.1161/01.CIR.0000139336.69955.AB

Shaw, R. M., and Rudy, Y. (1997). Ionic mechanisms of propagation in cardiac tissue. Roles of the sodium and L-type calcium currents during reduced excitability and decreased gap junction coupling. *Circ. Res.* 81, 727–741. doi: 10.1161/01.RES.81.5.727

Swaminathan, P. D., Purohit, A., Soni, S., Voigt, N., Singh, M. V., Glukhov, A. V., et al. (2011). Oxidized CaMKII causes sinus node dysfunction in mice. *J. Clin. Invest.* 121, 3277–3288. doi: 10.1172/JCI57833

Talano, J. V., Euler, D., Randall, W. C., Eshaghy, B., Loeb, H. S., and Gunnar, R. M. (1978). Sinus node dysfunction. An overview with emphasis on autonomic and pharmacologic consideration. *Am. J. Med.* 64, 773–781. doi: 10.1016/0002-9343(78)90516-8

Ten Velde, I., De Jonge, B., Verheijck, E. E., Van Kempen, M. J., Analbers, L., Gros, D., et al. (1995). Spatial distribution of connexin43, the major cardiac gap junction protein, visualizes the cellular network for impulse propagation from sinoatrial node to atrium. *Circ. Res.* 76, 802–811. doi: 10.1161/01.RES.76.5.802

Thery, C., Gosselin, B., Lekieffre, J., and Warembourg, H. (1977). Pathology of sinoatrial node. Correlations with electrocardiographic findings in 111 patients. *Am. Heart J.* 93, 735–740. doi: 10.1016/S0002-8703(77)80070-7

Tse, H. F., Xue, T., Lau, C. P., Siu, C. W., Wang, K., Zhang, Q. Y., et al. (2006). Bioartificial sinus node constructed via *in vivo* gene transfer of an engineered pacemaker HCN Channel reduces the dependence on electronic pacemaker in a sick-sinus syndrome model. *Circulation* 114, 1000–1011. doi: 10.1161/CIRCULATIONAHA.106.615385

Veldkamp, M. W., Wilders, R., Baartscheer, A., Zegers, J. G., Bezzina, C. R., and Wilde, A. A. (2003). Contribution of sodium channel mutations to bradycardia and sinus node dysfunction in LQT3 families. *Circ. Res.* 92, 976–983. doi: 10.1161/01.RES.0000069689.09869.A8

Verheijck, E. E., Wessels, A., Van Ginneken, A. C., Bourier, J., Markman, M. W., Vermeulen, J. L., et al. (1998). Distribution of atrial and nodal cells within the rabbit sinoatrial node: models of sinoatrial transition. *Circulation* 97, 1623–1631. doi: 10.1161/01.CIR.97.16.1623

Wang, Y., and Rudy, Y. (2000). Action potential propagation in inhomogeneous cardiac tissue: safety factor considerations and ionic mechanism. *Am. J. Physiol. Heart Circ. Physiol.* 278, H1019–H1029.

Watanabe, E. I., Honjo, H., Anno, T., Boyett, M. R., Kodama, I., and Toyama, J. (1995). Modulation of pacemaker activity of sinoatrial node cells by electrical load imposed by an atrial cell model. *Am. J. Physiol.* 269, H1735–H1742.

Wolf, R. M., Glynn, P., Hashemi, S., Zarei, K., Mitchell, C. C., Anderson, M. E., et al. (2013). Atrial fibrillation and sinus node dysfunction in human ankyrin-B syndrome: a computational analysis. *Am. J. Physiol. Heart Circ. Physiol.* H1253–H1266. doi: 10.1152/ajpheart.00734.2012

Zhang, H., Holden, A. V., and Boyett, M. R. (2001). Gradient model versus mosaic model of the sinoatrial node. *Circulation* 103, 584–588. doi: 10.1161/01.CIR.103.4.584

Zhang, H., Lau, D. H., Shlapakova, I. N., Zhao, X., Danilo, P., Robinson, R. B., et al. (2011). Implantation of sinoatrial node cells into canine right ventricle: biological pacing appears limited by the substrate. *Cell Transplant.* 20, 1907–1914. doi: 10.3727/096368911X565038

Zhang, H., Zhao, Y., Lei, M., Dobrzynski, H., Liu, J. H., Holden, A. V., et al. (2007). Computational evaluation of the roles of Na^+ current, I_{Na}, and cell death in cardiac pacemaking and driving. *Am. J. Physiol. Heart Circ. Physiol.* 292, H165–H174. doi: 10.1152/ajpheart.01101.2005

2

Exploring susceptibility to atrial and ventricular arrhythmias resulting from remodeling of the passive electrical properties in the heart: A simulation approach

Natalia A. Trayanova *, Patrick M. Boyle, Hermenegild J. Arevalo and Sohail Zahid

Department of Biomedical Engineering, Institute for Computational Medicine, Johns Hopkins University, Baltimore, MD, USA

Correspondence:
Natalia A. Trayanova, Department of Biomedical Engineering, Institute for Computational Medicine, Johns Hopkins University, 3400 N Charles St., 316 Hackerman Hall, Baltimore, MD 21218, USA
e-mail: ntrayanova@jhu.edu

Under diseased conditions, remodeling of the cardiac tissue properties ("passive properties") takes place; these are aspects of electrophysiological behavior that are not associated with active ion transport across cell membranes. Remodeling of the passive electrophysiological properties most often results from structural remodeling, such as gap junction down-regulation and lateralization, fibrotic growth infiltrating the myocardium, or the development of an infarct scar. Such structural remodeling renders atrial or ventricular tissue as a major substrate for arrhythmias. The current review focuses on these aspects of cardiac arrhythmogenesis. Due to the inherent complexity of cardiac arrhythmias, computer simulations have provided means to elucidate interactions pertinent to this spatial scale. Here we review the current state-of-the-art in modeling atrial and ventricular arrhythmogenesis as arising from the disease-induced changes in the passive tissue properties, as well as the contributions these modeling studies have made to our understanding of the mechanisms of arrhythmias in the heart. Because of the rapid advance of structural imaging methodologies in cardiac electrophysiology, we chose to present studies that have used such imaging methodologies to construct geometrically realistic models of cardiac tissue, or the organ itself, where the regional remodeling properties of the myocardium can be represented in a realistic way. We emphasize how the acquired knowledge can be used to pave the way for clinical applications of cardiac organ modeling under the conditions of structural remodeling.

Keywords: arrhythmia, computer modeling, structural remodeling, fibrosis, infarct

INTRODUCTION

Computer modeling has emerged as a powerful platform for the investigation of lethal heart rhythm disorders. Biophysically detailed simulations can explain experimental observations and help reveal how organ-scale arrhythmogenic phenomena (ectopic heartbeats, conduction failure, electrical turbulence, etc.) emerge from pathological effects at the tissue, cell, and protein levels. The development of this extensive "virtual heart" methodology (Noble, 2002; Vigmond et al., 2009; Gurev et al., 2011; Trayanova, 2011; Winslow et al., 2012) builds upon a strong foundation of research that seeks to use experiments and simulation to quantitatively characterize the action potential response of cardiac cells to electrical stimuli. Recent advancements in single-cell action potential modeling have produced building blocks for constructing models of the atria (Courtemanche et al., 1998; Nygren et al., 1998; Grandi et al., 2011), the ventricles (Ten Tusscher and Panfilov, 2006; Fink et al., 2008; Grandi et al., 2010; O'Hara et al., 2011), and the cardiac conduction system (Stewart et al., 2009; Aslanidi et al., 2010; Sampson et al., 2010; Li and Rudy, 2011; Vaidyanathan et al., 2013) with unprecedented levels of biophysical detail and accuracy. Such developments have helped to fuel the exciting progress made in simulating cardiac electrical behavior at the organ level (Moreno et al., 2011; Tandri et al., 2011; Trayanova et al., 2012; Boyle et al., 2013, 2014; Hu et al., 2014; Trayanova and Boyle, 2014; Clayton and Bishop, in press). Emergent, integrative behaviors in the heart result not only from complex interactions within a specific level but also from feed-forward and feedback interactions that connect a broad range of hierarchical levels of biological organization.

Several recent reviews have been written on our current understanding the mechanisms of atrial and ventricular mechanisms from an integrative interactions perspective (Janse, 2004; Rubart and Zipes, 2005; Jacquemet et al., 2008; Rudy et al., 2008; Plank et al., 2008b; Fishman et al., 2010; Dossel et al., 2012; John et al., 2012; Trayanova, 2012, 2014; Chen et al., 2014; Heijman et al., 2014), often derived from computer simulations, however, most of these focus on how remodeling in the active electrophysiological properties of the diseased heart contributes to the increased propensity to arrhythmias. One aspect of cardiac tissue behavior that has received less attention is the contribution, to the initiation and maintenance of arrhythmias, of the changes in the "passive" tissue properties that take place in the diseased heart. Under "passive" we refer to the aspects of electrophysiological behavior that are not associated with active ion transport across cell membranes; these include current flow in the intra- and extracellular domains of cardiac tissue and the aspects of tissue composition and structure that determine the direction and magnitude of these currents. Under diseased conditions, remodeling of the passive tissue properties takes place, most often resulting from structural remodeling such as gap junction down-regulation and lateralization, fibrotic growth infiltrating the myocardium, or the development of an infarct scar. Such structural remodeling renders atrial, or ventricular tissue as a major substrate for arrhythmias. The current review focuses on these aspects of cardiac arrhythmogenesis.

However, because of this inherent complexity of cardiac arrhythmias, it is often difficult to dissect the contributions of individual players, and to elucidate interactions at a particular spatial scale. Computer simulations of cardiac electrophysiology have provided this ability. In this article, we review the current state-of-the-art in modeling atrial and ventricular arrhythmogenesis as arising from the disease-induced changes in the passive tissue properties, as well as the contributions these modeling studies have made to our understanding of the mechanisms of arrhythmias in the heart. Because of the rapid advance of structural imaging methodologies in cardiac electrophysiology, we chose to present studies that have used such imaging methodologies to construct geometrically realistic structural models of cardiac tissue, or the organ itself, where the regional remodeling properties of the myocardium can be represented also in a realistic way. We emphasize how the acquired knowledge can be used to pave the way for clinical applications of cardiac organ modeling under the conditions of structural changes. This review does not intend to be exhaustive on the subject, but to provide examples of how computer modeling could be instrumental in understanding arrhythmogenesis as it arises from disease remodeling at the various levels of biological and structural organization of the heart.

OVERVIEW OF METHODOLOGY FOR SIMULATING ARRHYTHMOGENESIS AND REPRESENTING THE REMODELING IN THE PASSIVE PROPERTIES OF THE MYOCARDIUM

Computer modeling of arrhythmogenesis has made enormous progress over the last decade, enabling the simulation of electrical function in cardiac tissue as well as in the entire organ. A schematic of the current state-of-the-art general approach to 3D multi-scale (from the molecule to the organ) arrhythmia modeling (atrial or ventricular) is shown in **Figure 1A**. Ionic exchanges across cell membranes, via ionic channels, pumps, and exchangers, represented by an action potential ionic model comprising of numerous ordinary differential and algebraic equations, drive current flow in the tissue. In the multi-scale atrial or ventricular model, propagation of the wave of action potential is simulated by solving (Vigmond et al., 2002, 2003; Plank et al., 2008b) a reaction-diffusion partial differential equation describing current flow through tissue composed of myocytes that are electrically connected via low-resistance gap junctions. Cardiac tissue has orthotropic passive electrical conductivities that arise from the cellular organization of the myocardium (cardiac muscle) into fibers and laminar sheets. Global conductivity values in the atrial or ventricular model are obtained by combining fiber and sheet organization with myocyte-specific local conductivity values.

Local fiber directions are typically mapped based on histological sectioning information (Nielsen et al., 1991; Vetter and McCulloch, 1998), or on diffusion tensor (DT) magnetic resonance imaging (MRI) (Helm et al., 2005), sometimes using an atlas heart (Vadakkumpadan et al., 2012). **Figure 1B**, left panel presents fiber orientation, as reconstructed from DTMR images, in the canine ventricles shown in **Figure 1A**. In cases where neither histological nor DTMR imaging information is available, rule-based approaches have been used to assign fiber orientation consistent with measurements, either manually or using a semi-automatic rule-based approach (Krueger et al., 2011; Bayer et al., 2012; Dossel et al., 2012). This particularly applies to atrial fiber orientation (**Figure 1B**, right panel) since DT imaging of the thin atrial walls does not provide reliable information about atrial fiber architecture.

The passive electrical properties of the myocardium (**Figure 1A**) can be regionally remodeled in disease, with the regional change originating from several major sources: (1) changes in gap junction resistance between cells resulting in changes in conductivity values; (2) deposition of collagen forming either local resistive barriers between fibers or replacing myocytes (interstitial or replacement fibrosis; in the atria, it is a hallmark of the aging tissue); (3) formation of an infarction scar in the ventricles as a result of ischemic cardiac disease; and (4) abnormal proliferation, under diseased conditions, of non-myocyte cells, such as myofibroblasts, which may or may not interact with the cardiomyocytes electrically.

Multi-scale models of arrhythmias are typically modular, allowing the use of any cellular ionic models, of different species and with different levels of biophysical detail. Furthermore, solutions are executed on user-specified organ geometries, which can be idealized, or anatomically-accurate, the latter either representing averaged geometries obtained from histological sectioning (Nielsen et al., 1991; Vetter and McCulloch, 1998), or individual hearts' (atria and/or ventricles) geometry, and structure (Bishop et al., 2010; Vadakkumpadan et al., 2010). Using MRI data for model geometry is essential in represent individual hearts' structural remodeling in the passive tissue properties, such as ventricular infarction or atrial fibrosis. **Figure 2A** presents the generation of the geometry/ structure of a whole-heart model of canine infarction from high-resolution *ex-vivo* MRI scans, where a level set method was applied to the MRI image stack to separate the myocardium from the surrounding suspension media. The infarct was segmented out into the two infarct zones, scar and the electrically-remodeled border zone, also termed gray zone (GZ) based on it appearance in the MRI scans; to do so the combined information from both the DTMRI, and the structural MRI scans was used (via the calculation of fractional anisotropy, **Figure 2A**). The resulting infarct segmentation revealed strands of GZ tissue penetrating the electrically inert scar tissue (segmentation panel, **Figure 2A**). The reconstructed whole heart canine model is shown in **Figure 2A** with the locations of different remodeling regions combined with the organ geometry information.

Clinical MRI scans with a contrast agent (late gadolinum enhancement, LGE, MRI) can also be used to visualize the structural remodeling in atria and ventricles (Nazarian et al., 2005; Assomull et al., 2006; Oakes et al., 2009; Roes et al., 2009;

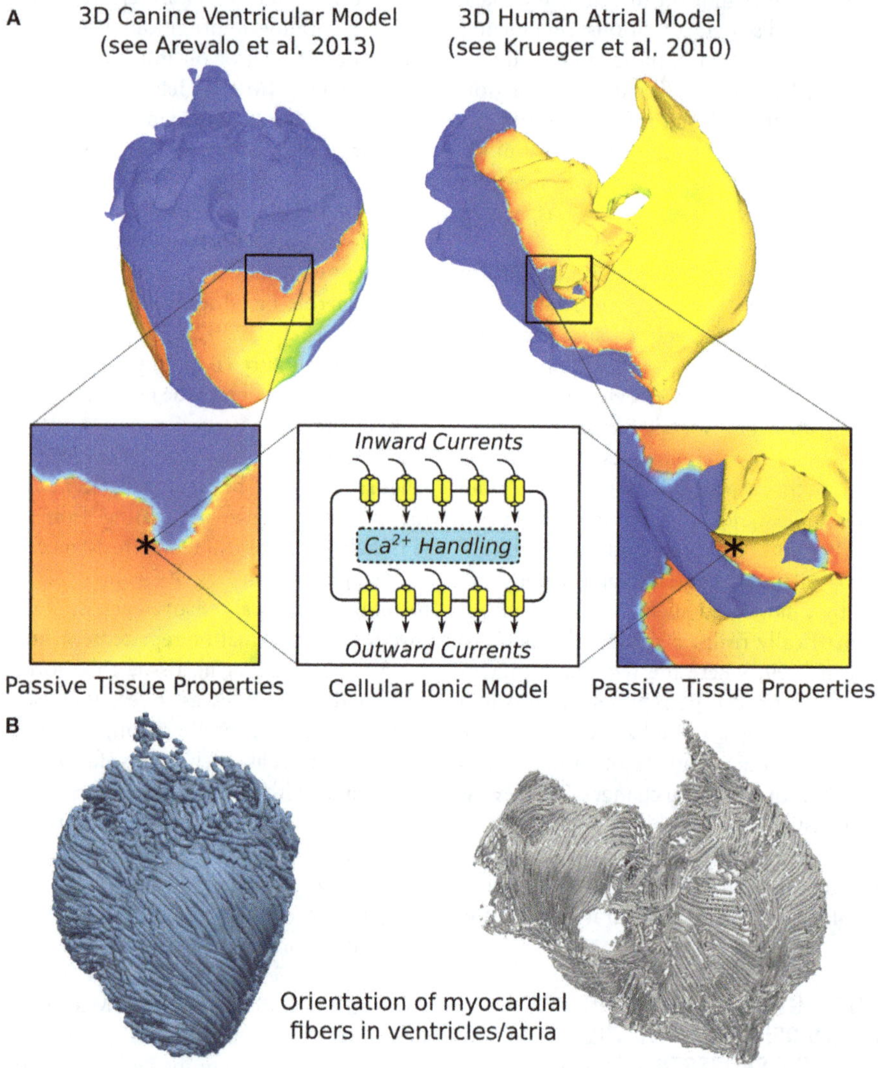

FIGURE 1 | Overall approach to image-based modeling of cardiac electrophysiology. (A) The multiscale aspect of cardiac electrophysiological models. Passive electrical coupling of cardiac cells mediates the tissue-scale propagation of bioelectric impulses that originate at the membrane level (action potentials). *indicates representative points in ventricular and atrial tissue models. 3D geometrical models are reconstructed from images of a canine heart (left), as in Arevalo et al. (2013), and human patient atria (right), as in Krueger et al. (2011). **(B)** Schematics showing the orientation of myocardial fibers in the ventricular and atrial models. Left panel modified with permission from Arevalo et al. (2013).

Akoum et al., 2011). **Figure 2B** presents ventricular model generation from clinical LGE-MRI images, as described in a recent paper (Prakosa et al., 2014). Finally, **Figure 2C** illustrates structural changes in a patient atrium, as reconstructed from clinical LGE-MRI scans, and described in detail in the original papers (McDowell et al., 2012, 2013) It has to be noted, however, that the segmentation of the LGE MRI fibrotic regions and even segmentation of the geometry of the thin atria from clinical MRI is fraught with uncertainty and an area of intense image-processing research.

Figure 2B, right-most panel, demonstrates how the images can be used to examine susceptibility to arrhythmias of the substrate and specifically, the role of structural remodeling (and thus remodeling in the passive electrical properties). It shows the generation of a reentrant arrhythmia in the infracted patient ventricles. Numerical approaches for simulating the electrical behavior of the heart have been described in detail in previous publications, some of which offer comprehensive reviews on the subject (Rodriguez and Trayanova, 2003; Jacquemet et al., 2008; Plank et al., 2008b; Trayanova, 2011; Dossel et al., 2012).

FIBROTIC REMODELING IN THE ATRIA AND ITS CONTRIBUTION TO ATRIAL FIBRILLATION

Structural remodeling, and specifically fibrosis, has been associated with the persistent/permanent version of atrial fibrillation (AF) (Burstein and Nattel, 2008; Yue et al., 2011). Fibrotic remodeling of atrial tissue involves processes that occur in parallel across multiple scales: at the membrane level, gap junction

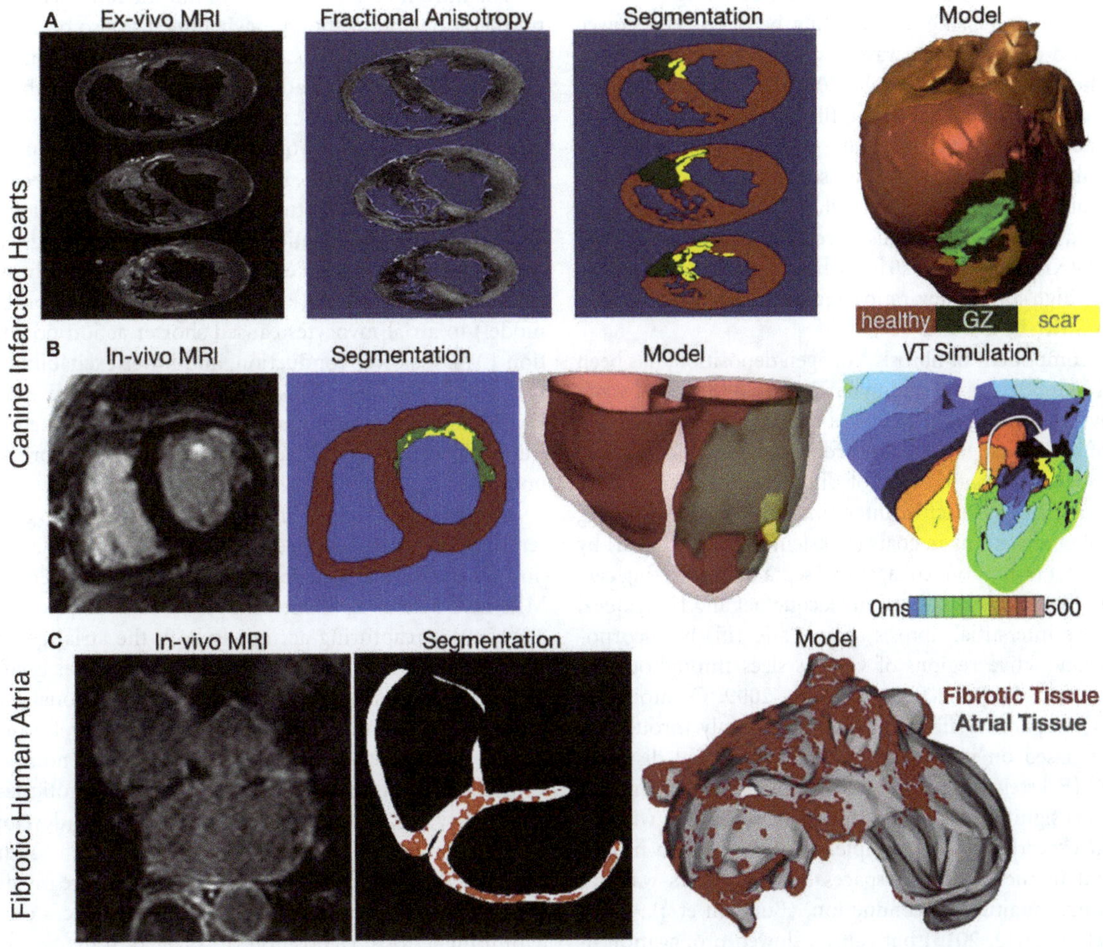

FIGURE 2 | Constructing image-based models of the ventricles from an infarcted canine heart (A,B) and the fibrotic atria of a human patient with AF. (A) Reconstruction from an *ex-vivo* MRI scan of an infarcted canine heart. Fractional anisotropy (FA) maps as calculated from the DT-MRI, brighter color corresponds with higher FA value. The images are segmented into healthy myocardium, gray zone (GZ), and scar, to reconstruct an image-based model of the infracted canine heart (right-most panel). Modified with permission from Arevalo et al. (2013). **(B)** Construction of a patient-specific ventricular model of arrhythmia from a clinical MR scan. Shown are images of an infarcted patient heart before ablation (treatment) and the corresponding segmentation: healthy (red), GZ (green), or scar (yellow). An image of the three-dimensional geometric model of the patient heart rendered with the epicardium and the infarct border zone semitransparent is shown in the third panel. The right-most panel presents *in silico* activation map of arrhythmia, revealing reentry on the left ventricular endocardium. The color code in the bottom right shows electrical activation time. Modified with permission from Winslow et al. (2012). **(C)** A model of the fibrotic human atria generated from a patient LGE-MRI scan (top left) following segmentation (top right) into normal and fibrotic tissue (fibrotic lesions in red). With permission from McDowell et al. (2012).

remodeling due to connexin 43 (Cx43) protein downregulation/hypophosphorylation, and lateralization (Kostin et al., 2002; Burstein et al., 2009), at the cellular level, fibroblast proliferation and phenotype switching (Rohr, 2009; Yue et al., 2011), and at the tissue level, the deposition of excess collagen (Xu et al., 2004; Burstein and Nattel, 2008), both from reactive interstitial fibrosis separating muscle bundles, and from reparative fibrosis replacing dead cardiomyocytes, both interfering with electric continuity and slowing conduction (Xu et al., 2004; Iwasaki et al., 2011). Thus, structural remodeling, combined with remodeling at the ion channel level, gives rise to complex interactions at the organ level, setting the stage for AF initiation and maintenance in the fibrotic atria.

Models of the fibrotic atria have accounted for different aspects of fibrotic remodeling, in an attempt to elucidate the mechanisms leading to altered conduction and those responsible for the drivers and organization of permanent AF. The simplest model representation of atrial structural remodeling was based on the assumption that a component of structural remodeling, gap junction remodeling (Cx43 downregulation/hypophosphorylation, and lateralization), occurs throughout the atria in a uniform fashion. Two such studies have been conducted thus far: one assumed that the coupling strength between computational cells was decreased (Cx43 downregulation/hypophosphorylation only) (Krogh-Madsen et al., 2012), while the other modeled increased anisotropy throughout the LA (representing both aspects of Cx43 remodeling) (Plank et al.,

2008a). One of these simulation studies showed (Krogh-Madsen et al., 2012) that decreasing the coupling between cells slowed conduction and decreased the wavelength, further perpetuating AF. The other study (Plank et al., 2008a) demonstrated that increased anisotropy throughout the fibrotic human LV was an additional mechanism for the breakup of PV ectopic waves into multiple reentrant circuits; higher anisotropy ratios resulted in sustained reentrant activity even though the ectopic focus was no longer present. Similar conclusions were obtained from a human atrial model (Krueger et al., 2014) where the locations of the fibrotic (i.e., high-anisotropy-ratio) regions were implemented from patient MRI-LGE scans.

The next component of fibrosis, collagen deposition, has been represented in models as insulating barriers, and in several ways: (i) by removing randomly the electrical connections between two 2D layers of atrial tissue, the endocardial and the epicardial, in order to model an increased level of dissociation between these two layers (a form of reactive interstitial fibrosis), mimicking experimental observations in goats (Eckstein et al., 2011); (ii) by introducing a set of random collagenous septa disconnecting cardiac fibers in the transverse direction (Jacquemet and Henriquez, 2009) (reactive interstitial fibrosis again); and (iii) by incorporating non-conductive regions of various sizes throughout the tissue (Tanaka et al., 2007; Burstein et al., 2009; Comtois and Nattel, 2011) (reparative fibrosis), either randomly throughout the atria, or based on imaging data. Endo-epicardial dissociation resulted (Eckstein et al., 2011) in a number of AF reentrant waves that was significantly higher than that in the case without dissociation, exacerbating AF complexity. The increase in collagen content in the interstitial spaces between fibers was not found to affect longitudinal conduction, (Burstein et al., 2009; McDowell et al., 2012, 2013) but caused slowed propagation in transverse direction, with the degree of slowing dependent of the length of the collagenous septa (Jacquemet and Henriquez, 2009).

Atrial models incorporating transverse collagen deposition (Tanaka et al., 2007; Burstein et al., 2009; Comtois and Nattel, 2011) (as in reparative fibrosis) have highlighted the significant interruption and disarray in atrial conduction patterns caused by it. Importantly, collagen deposition rather than connexin-43 (Cx43) remodeling was found to be the major factor in atrial conduction disturbances under HF conditions (Burstein et al., 2009) (**Figure 3A**). Furthermore, it was established that not only the total amount, but also the specific spatial distribution of collagen deposition (e.g., as generated by a stochastic algorithm) governed the occurrences of conduction block (Comtois and Nattel, 2011). To evaluate the consequences of HF remodeling (ionic and structural) on AF dynamics in the posterior left atrium (LA), Tanaka et al. (Tanaka et al., 2007) used 2D models of transmural posterior LA sections generated from histological data; patchy distributions of collagen were also reconstructed from that data. Simulations demonstrated that whether the mechanism sustaining AF was reentrant or focal, fibrous patches of large size were the major factor responsible for the different dynamics of AF waves in failing vs. control hearts; they anchored reentrant circuits and impaired wave propagation to generate delays and signal fractionation (**Figure 3B**).

The third major component of fibrotic remodeling, fibroblast proliferation and phenotype switching, has also been represented in computational models of the atria, particularly in view of the fact that fibroblasts, in addition to being part of the structural remodeling of the atria, can also exert electrophysiological influences on neighboring myocytes, possibly either through electrical coupling (Camelliti et al., 2004), or via paracrine effects (Pedrotty et al., 2009). The first study to explicitly incorporate fibroblast presence as a representation of fibrotic remodeling was the 2D atrial model by Ashihara et al. (2012). Within the fibrotic region, coupling of fibroblasts (kinetics governed by a fibroblast ionic model) to atrial myocytes caused shorter action potential duration (APD), slower conduction, and lower excitability as well as spiral wave breakups. This effect was exacerbated when fibroblast density increased (**Figure 4A**). Interestingly, when fibroblasts were substituted by collagen in the model, wave breakups were not observed.

All three elements of fibrotic remodeling (gap-junction remodeling, collagen deposition, and myofibroblast proliferation), were combined together in the LA model generated from MRI-LGE data of a patient with permanent AF (McDowell et al., 2012, 2013), capturing accurately both the atrial geometry and the distribution of fibrotic lesions. The model was used to examine the mechanisms for AF initiation by pulmonary vein (PV) ectopic stimulation. The study found that for fibrotic lesions typical of human remodeled atria under the conditions of persistent AF, gap junction remodeling in the fibrotic lesions was a necessary but not sufficient condition for the development of AF following a PV ectopic beat. The sufficient condition was myofibroblast proliferation in these lesions, where myofibroblasts exerted either electrotonic, or paracrine influences on myocytes within the lesions. Deposition of collagen in the lesions assisted the myofibroblasts' paracrine, or electrotonic effects by additionally shortening APD there (**Figure 4B**). The electrophysiological representation of fibrotic remodeling in the human atrial models remains, however, controversial because of the lack of sufficient experimental data.

ISCHEMIC CARDIOMYOPATHY REMODELING IN THE VENTRICLES AND ITS CONTRIBUTION TO VENTRICULAR TACHYCARDIA

Understanding ventricular arrhythmia mechanisms for a variety of diseases involving regional changes in the passive electrical properties has been aided, to a significant degree, by models and simulations. For instance, models representing regional ischemia (Tice et al., 2007; Jie et al., 2008, 2010; Jie and Trayanova, 2010) characterized the substrate for ischemia phase 1B arrhythmias by examining how the interplay between different degrees of hyperkalemia in the surviving layers, and the level of cellular uncoupling between these and the mid-myocardium layers (i.e., change in the passive properties of the myocardium) combine with the specific geometry of the ischemic zone in the ventricles to result in reentrant arrhythmias.

Ischemic cardiomyopathy (i.e., infarct-related) VT is the most frequent clinical ventricular arrhythmia, present in 64% of patients with ventricular rhythm disorder and in 89% of patients with sudden cardiac death (Stevenson et al., 1985). Recently, the

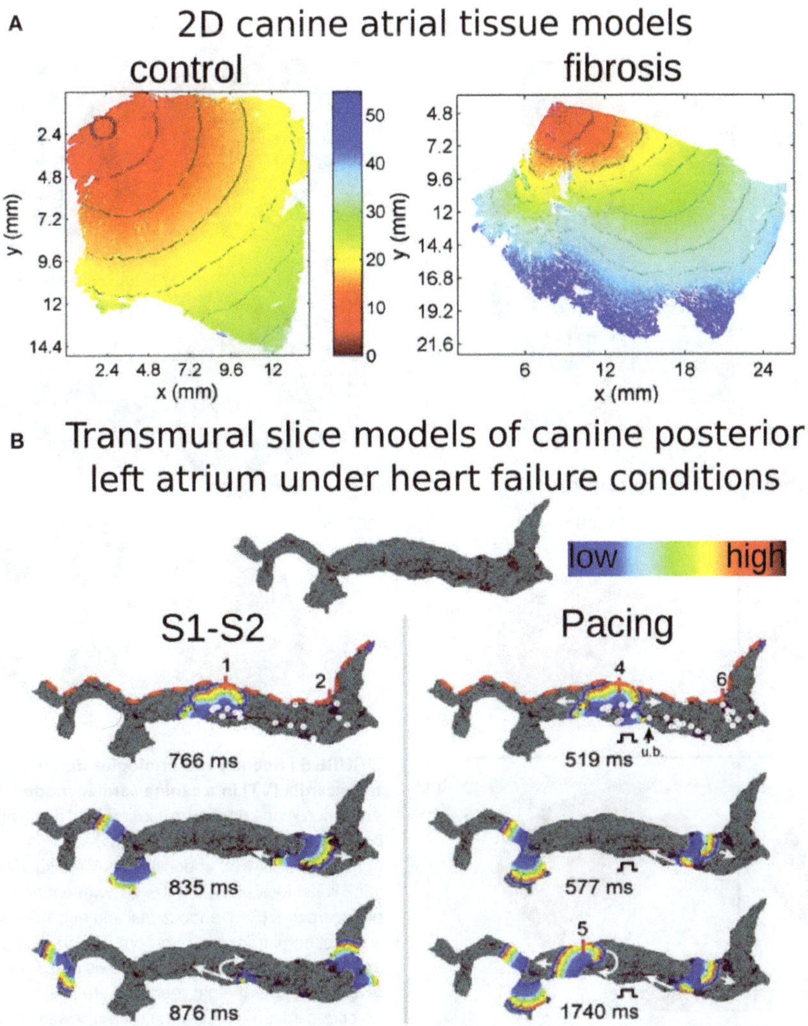

FIGURE 3 | Modeling fibrosis as regions of collagen presence. Collagen is represented as an insulator. **(A)** Simulations of propagation in models of 2D tissue sections of canine atrium (control, left, and fibrosis, right). With permission from Burstein et al. (2009). **(B)** Simulations in models of a transmural slice of canine posterior LA under HF conditions; the top of the slice (red dashed lines) corresponds to the epicardial surface. Snapshots at several timeframes for cross-field stimulation (left), and pacing at a frequency of 6 Hz (right), as well as endocardial time-space plots. Colors indicate transmembrane voltage from low (blue) to high (red). The site of unidirectional block (ub). is indicated by a black arrow. White circles on the upper voltage maps indicate sites of wavebreak. With permission from Tanaka et al. (2007).

peri-infarct (border) zone surrounding the necrotic scar, also known as GZs, as indicated above, based on its appearance as a region of intermediate intensity in the LGE-MRI scans, has been shown to correlate with post-MI mortality (Yan et al., 2006), clinical VT (Roes et al., 2009), and VT inducibility (Schmidt et al., 2007). Histological studies have shown these GZ regions to be a heterogeneous mix of viable myocardium and necrotic scar (Arheden et al., 2000). Animal experimental evidence has implicated the GZ as the arrhythmogenic substrate in myocardial infarction (MI) (Estner et al., 2011); Ashikaga et al. demonstrated that in infarcted swine hearts, reentrant circuits were anchored to strands of viable myocardium positioned over intramural scars (Ashikaga et al., 2007).

A recent swine heart study (Ng et al., 2012) demonstrated the feasibility of using simulations to predict the existence of VT circuits. In another study (Pop et al., 2011), a correspondence between *in vivo* electroanatomical and *in silico* voltage maps was demonstrated using a model of infarcted pig ventricles reconstructed from *ex vivo* MRI, and DTMRI data. Their simulations in two infarcted hearts successfully predicted the VT-inducibility consistent with the *in vivo* electrophysiological studies.

A clinically significant question is how infarct-related VTs relate to the specific GZ distribution and size in the ventricles. Addressing this question would provide an impetus to the development of improved criteria for stratifying arrhythmia risk in post-MI patients. A recent study (Arevalo et al., 2013) took this concept further and examined the role of infarct-related GZ extent in arrhythmogenesis, establishing that a minimum volume of remodeled tissue is needed for VT maintenance and demonstrating that the organizing center of infarct-related VT is located

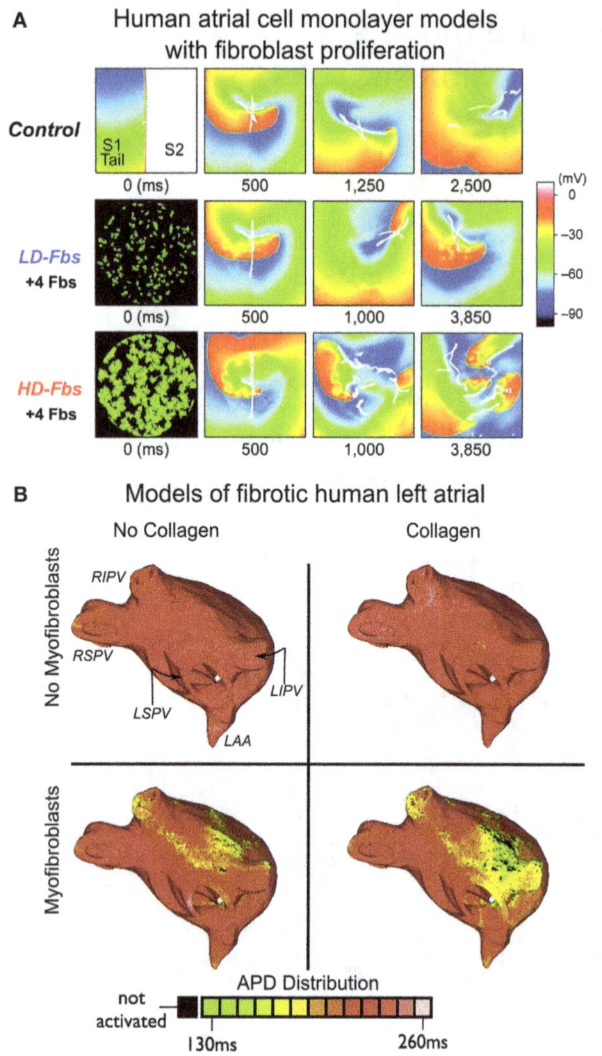

FIGURE 4 | Modeling fibroblast proliferation in the regions of fibrosis. **(A)** Effect of myocyte-fibroblast coupling (modeled as in Maleckar et al., 2009a) on spiral wave behavior in a human atrial cell monolayer model of size 4.5 × 4.5 cm. Top, control case without fibroblasts. Middle and bottom, models of low-density and high-density fibroblast proliferation (LD-Fbs and HD-Fbs) in a central circular region of the sheet. In the LD-Fbs, and HD-Fbs models, atrial myocytes (100 pF), each connecting to 4 fibroblasts (6.3 pF) within the Fb-Area, account for 12.5% and 50.0% of that area, respectively. With permission from Ashihara et al. (2012). **(B)** Maps of action potential duration (APD) in four human atrial models (same atrial geometry). Fibrotic lesions are modeled with (bottom row), and without (top row) myofibroblast infiltration (and coupling to myocytes), as well as with (right column), and without (left column) diffuse collagen deposition for both sets of maps. Myofibroblasts in the fibrotic regions were coupled to atrial myocytes as described in Maleckar et al. (2009a) and Maleckar et al. (2009b). Anatomical landmarks in upper-left sub-panel: right inferior, right superior, left inferior, and left superior pulmonary veins (RIPV, RSPV, LIPV, LSPV, respectively); left atrial appendage (LAA). With permission from McDowell et al. (2013).

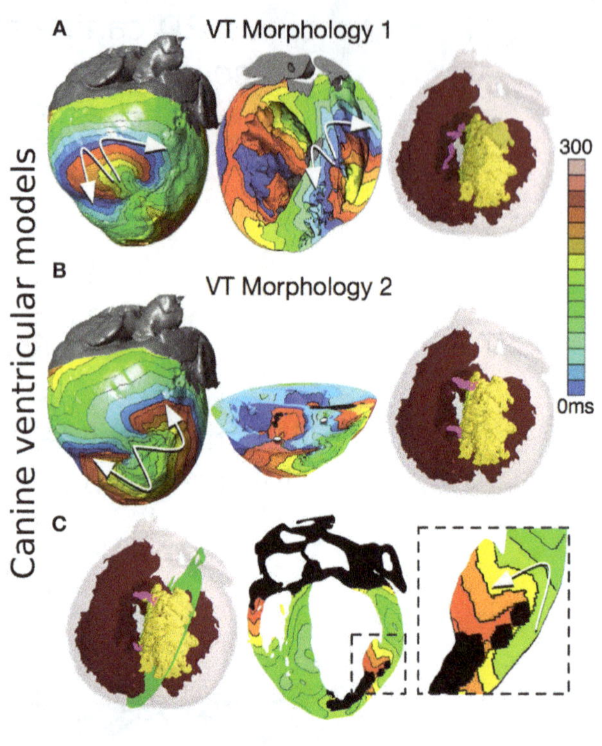

FIGURE 5 | Reentry morphologies during post-infarction ventricular tachycardia (VT) in a canine cardiac model. **(A)** VT morphology 1: Activation maps on the epicardium and in a long-axis cross-section of the ventricles, revealing figure-of-eight reentries on the epicardium, and on the right ventricular (RV) endocardium. VT is sustained by two I-type filaments (pink lines) located within the GZ with endpoints on the epicardium and RV endocardium. (Red: endocardial and epicardial surfaces, Yellow: scar surface, semi-transparent green: GZ) **(B)** VT morphology 2: Activation maps on the epicardium and in a short-axis cross-section of the ventricles, revealing figure-of-eight reentry on the epicardium, and two breakthroughs on endocardium (white dots). Reentry was organized around two I-type filaments with endpoints on the epicardium and scar (pink lines). **(C)** Activation map showing an apparent reentry around a scar distal from filaments. The overall VT morphology is similar to VT morphology 2 in Panel **B**. With permission from Arevalo et al. (2013).

within the border zone, regardless of the pacing site from which VT is induced. An example of simulations of infarct-related VT using an MRI-based canine heart model (see **Figure 1**) is presented in **Figure 5**; the model incorporated experimental data on electrophysiological remodeling in GZ. Programmed stimulation from the endocardial surface in this model revealed conduction slowing in the GZ, giving rise to VT inducibility, and reentrant circuit morphology consistent with experimental data. There are two distinct VT morphologies in this infracted canine heart. The first VT morphology was a figure-of-eight pattern on the epicardium and right ventricular (RV) endocardium (**Figure 5A**). For this VT morphology, the reentry revolved around two I-type filaments (organizing centers of reentrant activity) with endpoints at the epicardium and RV endocardium (**Figure 5A**, pink lines). The filaments were fully contained within the GZ and the endpoints remained in the same locations for the duration of the VT. The second VT morphology was a figure-of-eight reentry on the epicardium, had a direction of rotation (chirality) opposite to that of the first VT morphology, and was manifested as breakthroughs on the LV, and RV endocardial surfaces (**Figure 5B**). This was due to the reentrant activity being organized around two I-type filaments with endpoints at the epicardium and the infarct scar (**Figure 5B**, pink lines). Since the filaments did not extend to the endocardium, no rotational activity was observed there. Both filaments were stably located within the GZ throughout the duration of the simulation. The intramural behavior of the reentrant circuits associated with the second VT morphology is presented in **Figure 5C**. Overall, the simulation results demonstrated that the organizing center of infarct-related VT is located within the GZ, regardless of the pacing site from which VT is induced. This result has important implications for ablation of infarct-related VT; it indicates that patient-specific simulations of VT could provide guidance for VT ablation in patients. Such simulation guidance could have a major clinical impact in predicting the optimal targets for catheter ablation of infarct-related VT in individual patient hearts.

Another recent study (Ashikaga et al., 2013) was the first attempt to take this concept to the clinic. **Figure 6A** presents a schematic how computer simulation prediction of the optimal VT ablation targets could be used in lieu of invasive electroanatomical mapping of the ventricles. **Figure 6B** presents comparisons between simulation-guided and standard electrophysiological approaches for identifying ablation targets in two patients with

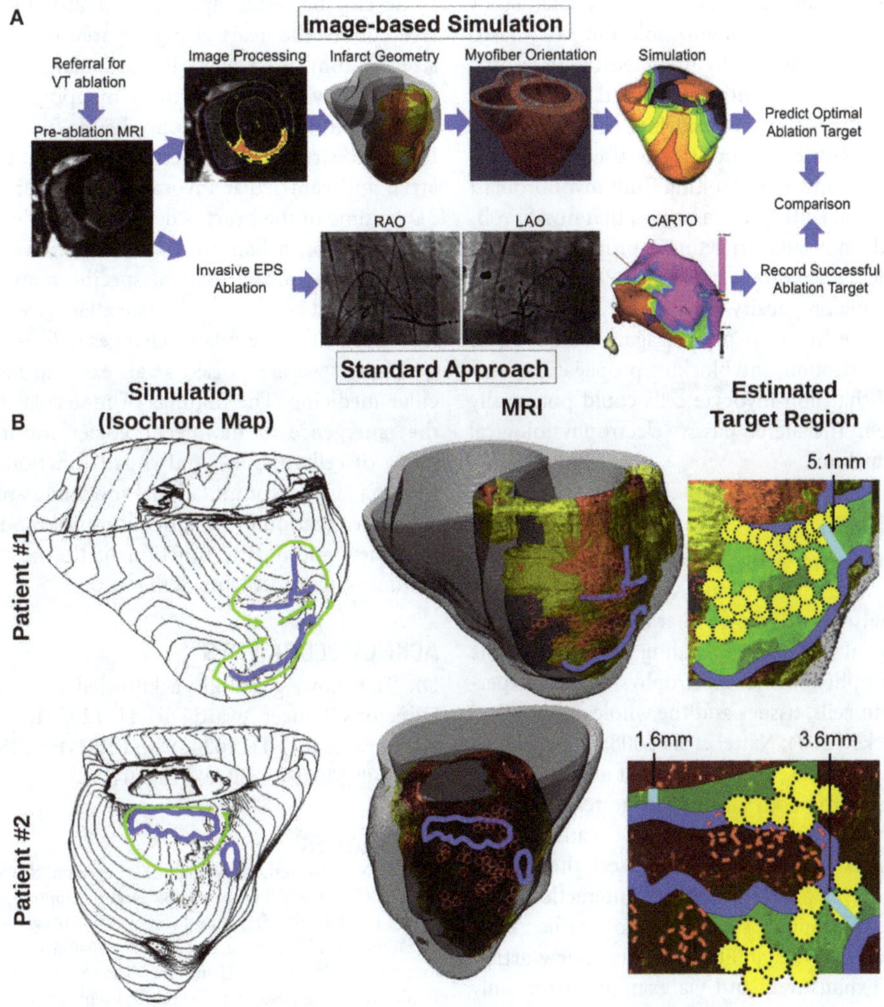

FIGURE 6 | (A) Proposed simulation-guided approach for determining the ablation targets of infarct-related ventricular tachycardia. The patients referred for ventricular tachycardia (VT) ablation undergo pre-ablation MRI, which was processed to provide the heart and infarct geometry (scar: red; GZ: yellow). These geometrical data were incorporated into a model of VT to estimate potential target regions. This method is alternative to an invasive electrophysiology study (EPS), and ablation ["Standard Approach"; by using biplane X-ray fluoroscopy and electroanatomical mapping (CARTO)]. LAO—left anterior oblique; RAO—right anterior oblique. **(B)** Comparison between simulation-guided and standard electrophysiological approaches for identifying endocardial ablation targets in two patients with infarct-related ventricular tachycardias (VTs). Left column: propagation pathways (green) and lines of conduction block (blue) are overlaid over VT activation maps simulated in image-based patient heart models. Middle column: preablation infarct geometry (infarct scar: orange, border zone: yellow, and non-infarcted: gray) along with ablation lesions delivered by the standard approach (red circles), and conduction block lines as calculated from ventricular simulations. Right column: optimal ablation zones (green shading) predicted by simulations, with narrowest isthmuses indicated (cyan); in both cases, only a fraction of the ablation sites from the standard approach were within the predicted optimal LV endocardial ablation zone (yellow circles). Modified with permission from Ashikaga et al. (2013).

infarct-related VTs. The results of the study demonstrated that that non-invasive simulation prediction of optimal targets for ablation of infarct-related VT could result in lesions that are much smaller than those executed in the clinic that successfully terminated VT (**Figure 6B**, right columns).

Simulation studies of ventricular arrhythmogenesis have recently begun to incorporate the role of cells other than myocytes in creating the arrhythmogenic substrate. Similar to the conditions under atrial fibrosis, differentiating fibroblasts, called myofibroblasts, have been reported to possibly play a role in the electrophysiological behavior of the scar, and GZ. Coupling to myofibroblasts in the region of infarct could affect cardiomyocyte electrophysiology, as demonstrated by simulation results (Maleckar et al., 2009a; Ashihara et al., 2012). A later study (McDowell et al., 2011) employed a high-resolution MRI-based computational model of the chronically infarcted rabbit ventricles, which was previously used (Rantner et al., 2012) to explore the role of infarct-related structural remodeling in vulnerability to electric shocks. The ventricular model was used to characterize the arrhythmogenic substrate resulting from myofibroblast infiltration (McDowell et al., 2011). It was found that myofibroblasts at low densities do not alter arrhythmia propensity, while at intermediate densities, myofibroblasts cause APD shortening, and exacerbate arrhythmia propensity. Interestingly, at high densities, myofibroblasts were found to protect against arrhythmia by causing resting depolarization, and blocking propagation. This study clearly indicated that non-myocyte cells could potentially have an important role in the altered passive electrophysiological properties of the myocardium.

CONCLUDING COMMENTS

The mechanisms that govern arrhythmia initiation and persistence in the heart, in both atria and ventricles, are highly complex, of dynamic nature, and involve interactions across multiple temporal and spatial scales, often leading to unpredictable outcomes and emergent phenomena. Electrophysiological experimental investigations in cells, tissues and the whole animal, and the human patient (Packer, 2004; Nattel et al., 2008; Iwasaki et al., 2011; Jalife, 2011; Schotten et al., 2011; Atienza et al., 2012) have led to a rapid increase in the body of knowledge regarding the mechanisms underlying arrhythmias. However, because of this inherent complexity, it is often difficult to dissect the contributions of individual players, and to elucidate interactions at a particular spatial scale. Computer simulations of cardiac electrophysiology have provided this ability, and this review article focuses, although not exhaustively and via examples from only a few simulation studies, on how remodeling in the "passive" electrical properties of the myocardium secondary to disease can render the organ susceptible to arrhythmias.

A lot remains to be uncovered, as remodeling of the electrical properties of the myocardium in disease, both passive and active, remains an intense area of research. As this review demonstrates, uncovering the integrative behavior of the heart resulting from such remodeling through simulation of atrial and ventricular function will continue to be strongly dependent on developments in experimental methodologies, which provide data to constrain, enrich, and validate the models. Of particular importance will be to fully characterize the complex remodeling that occurs in disease. Better understanding of the specific electrophysiological characteristics of remodeled tissue (i.e., GZ) surrounding the infarct in ischemic cardiomyopathy patients will enable more detailed mechanistic models of arrhythmia initiation, maintenance, and termination. Likewise, as experimental research addresses further the properties of the fibrotic myocardium, and in particular the electrophysiological aspects of the interaction between myocytes, and fibroblasts in the fibrotic lesions in the atria, atrial models are expected to provide a comprehensive view of the factors that drive arrhythmogenesis and influence arrhythmia dynamics in AF patients. Additionally, both atrial and ventricular modeling approaches could be improved by developing better capabilities to resolve the pathophysiological structure of the heart at high spatial resolution (isotropic voxel size of 1 mm or smaller); in particular, sensitive cardiac-specific tractography, and connectivity mapping techniques could provide a wealth of information valuable for constructing models of improved structural detail. Finally, present understanding of how atrial and ventricular myocardial fibers are oriented within the 3D volume of the heart is derived primarily from DT-MRI scans conducted on a handful of hearts *ex vivo*; imaging techniques capable of acquiring patient-specific maps of fiber orientation *in vivo* could be used to validate atlas-based approximations and incorporate disease-related changes in fibrous structure.

Clearly, we are poised at an exciting moment in cardiovascular medicine. The findings of molecular biology of the heart, the emergence of new technologies for measuring the properties of cells, tissues, and organ function, and the impact of Moore's law on computational modeling are coming together to drive the creation of new, quantitative, model-based approaches to understanding the function of the heart in disease, and to cardiovascular medicine of the future.

ACKNOWLEDGMENTS

Dr. Trayanova gratefully acknowledges support from the NIH Director's Pioneer Award DP1-HL123271, as well as support from NIH grants R01-HL103428 and R01-HL105216 and NSF grants CBET-0933029 and IOS-1124804.

REFERENCES

Akoum, N., Daccarett, M., McGann, C., Segerson, N., Vergara, G., Kuppahally, S., et al. (2011). Atrial fibrosis helps select the appropriate patient and strategy in catheter ablation of atrial fibrillation: a DE-MRI guided approach. *J. Cardiovasc. Electrophysiol.* 22, 16–22. doi: 10.1111/j.1540-8167.2010.01876.x

Arevalo, H., Plank, G., Helm, P., Halperin, H., and Trayanova, N. (2013). Tachycardia in post-infarction hearts: insights from 3D image-based ventricular models. *PLoS ONE* 8:e68872. doi: 10.1371/journal.pone.0068872

Arheden, H. K., Saeed, M., Higgins, C. B., Gao, D.-W., Ursell, P. C., Bremerich, J., et al. (2000). Reperfused rat myocardium subjected to various durations of ischemia: estimation of the distribution volume of contrast material with echo-planar MR imaging 1. *Radiology* 215, 520–528. doi: 10.1148/radiology.215.2.r00ma38520

Ashihara, T., Haraguchi, R., Nakazawa, K., Namba, T., Ikeda, T., Nakazawa, Y., et al. (2012). The role of fibroblasts in complex fractionated electrograms during persistent/permanent atrial fibrillation: implications for electrogram-based catheter ablation. *Circ. Res.* 110, 275–284. doi: 10.1161/CIRCRESAHA.111.255026

Ashikaga, H., Arevalo, H., Vadakkumpadan, F., Blake, R. C. 3rd., Bayer, J. D., Nazarian, S., et al. (2013). Feasibility of image-based simulation to estimate ablation target in human ventricular arrhythmia. *Heart Rhythm* 10, 1109–1116. doi: 10.1016/j.hrthm.2013.04.015

Ashikaga, H., Sasano, T., Dong, J., Zviman, M. M., Evers, R., Hopenfeld, B., et al. (2007). Magnetic resonance–based anatomical analysis of scar-related ventricular tachycardia implications for catheter ablation. *Circ. Res.* 101, 939–947. doi: 10.1161/CIRCRESAHA.107.158980

Aslanidi, O. V., Sleiman, R. N., Boyett, M. R., Hancox, J. C., and Zhang, H. (2010). Ionic mechanisms for electrical heterogeneity between rabbit Purkinje fiber and ventricular cells. *Biophys. J.* 98, 2420–2431. doi: 10.1016/j.bpj.2010.02.033

Assomull, R. G., Prasad, S. K., Lyne, J., Smith, G., Burman, E. D., Khan, M., et al. (2006). Cardiovascular magnetic resonance, fibrosis, and prognosis in dilated cardiomyopathy. *J. Am. Coll. Cardiol.* 48, 1977–1985. doi: 10.1016/j.jacc.2006.07.049

Atienza, F., Martins, R. P., and Jalife, J. (2012). Translational research in atrial fibrillation: a quest for mechanistically based diagnosis and therapy. *Circ. Arrhythm. Electrophysiol.* 5, 1207–1215. doi: 10.1161/CIRCEP.111.970335

Bayer, J., Blake, R., Plank, G., and Trayanova, N. (2012). A novel rule-based algorithm for assigning myocardial fiber orientation to computational heart models. *Ann. Biomed. Eng.* 40, 2243–2254. doi: 10.1007/s10439-012-0593-5

Bishop, M. J., Plank, G., Burton, R. A., Schneider, J. E., Gavaghan, D. J., Grau, V., et al. (2010). Development of an anatomically detailed MRI-derived rabbit ventricular model and assessment of its impact on simulations of electrophysiological function. *Am. J. Physiol. Heart Circ. Physiol.* 298, H699–H718. doi: 10.1152/ajpheart.00606.2009

Boyle, P. M., Park, C. J., Arevalo, H. J., Vigmond, E. J., and Trayanova, N. A. (2014). Sodium current reduction unmasks a structure-dependent substrate for arrhythmogenesis in the normal ventricles. *PLoS ONE* 9:e86947. doi: 10.1371/journal.pone.0086947

Boyle, P. M., Williams, J. C., Ambrosi, C. M., Entcheva, E., and Trayanova, N. A. (2013). A comprehensive multiscale framework for simulating optogenetics in the heart. *Nat. Commun.* 4, 2370. doi: 10.1038/ncomms3370

Burstein, B., Comtois, P., Michael, G., Nishida, K., Villeneuve, L., Yeh, Y. H., et al. (2009). Changes in connexin expression and the atrial fibrillation substrate in congestive heart failure. *Circ. Res.* 105, 1213–1222. doi: 10.1161/CIRCRESAHA.108.183400

Burstein, B., and Nattel, S. (2008). Atrial fibrosis: mechanisms and clinical relevance in atrial fibrillation. *J. Am. Coll. Cardiol.* 51, 802–809. doi: 10.1016/j.jacc.2007.09.064

Camelliti, P., Green, C. R., Legrice, I., and Kohl, P. (2004). Fibroblast network in rabbit sinoatrial node: structural and functional identification of homogeneous and heterogeneous cell coupling. *Circ. Res.* 94, 828–835. doi: 10.1161/01.RES.0000122382.19400.14

Chen, P.-S., Chen, L. S., Fishbein, M. C., Lin, S.-F., and Nattel, S. (2014). Role of the autonomic nervous system in atrial fibrillation pathophysiology and therapy. *Circ. Res.* 114, 1500–1515. doi: 10.1161/CIRCRESAHA.114.303772

Clayton, R., and Bishop, M. (in press). Computational models of ventricular arrhythmia mechanisms: recent developments and future prospects. *Drug Discov. Today*. doi: 10.1016/j.ddmod.2014.04.002

Comtois, P., and Nattel, S. (2011). Interactions between cardiac fibrosis spatial pattern and ionic remodeling on electrical wave propagation. *Conf. Proc. IEEE Eng. Med. Biol. Soc.* 2011, 4669–4672. doi: 10.1109/IEMBS.2011.6091156

Courtemanche, M., Ramirez, R. J., and Nattel, S. (1998). Ionic mechanisms underlying human atrial action potential properties: insights from a mathematical model. *Am. J. Physiol.* 275, H301–H321.

Dossel, O., Krueger, M. W., Weber, F. M., Wilhelms, M., and Seemann, G. (2012). Computational modeling of the human atrial anatomy and electrophysiology. *Med. Biol. Eng. Comput.* 50, 773–799. doi: 10.1007/s11517-012-0924-6

Eckstein, J., Maesen, B., Linz, D., Zeemering, S., Van Hunnik, A., Verheule, S., et al. (2011). Time course and mechanisms of endo-epicardial electrical dissociation during atrial fibrillation in the goat. *Cardiovasc. Res.* 89, 816–824. doi: 10.1093/cvr/cvq336

Estner, H. L., Zviman, M. M., Herzka, D., Miller, F., Castro, V., Nazarian, S., et al. (2011). The critical isthmus sites of ischemic ventricular tachycardia are in zones of tissue heterogeneity, visualized by magnetic resonance imaging. *Heart Rhythm* 8, 1942–1949. doi: 10.1016/j.hrthm.2011.07.027

Fink, M., Noble, D., Virag, L., Varro, A., and Giles, W. R. (2008). Contributions of HERG K+ current to repolarization of the human ventricular action potential. *Prog. Biophys. Mol. Biol.* 96, 357–376. doi: 10.1016/j.pbiomolbio.2007.07.011

Fishman, G. I., Chugh, S. S., Dimarco, J. P., Albert, C. M., Anderson, M. E., Bonow, R. O., et al. (2010). Sudden cardiac death prediction and prevention: report from a National Heart, Lung, and Blood Institute and Heart Rhythm Society Workshop. *Circulation* 122, 2335–2348. doi: 10.1161/CIRCULATIONAHA.110.976092

Grandi, E., Pandit, S. V., Voigt, N., Workman, A. J., Dobrev, D., Jalife, J., et al. (2011). Human atrial action potential and Ca2+ model: sinus rhythm and chronic atrial fibrillation. *Circ. Res.* 109, 1055–1066. doi: 10.1161/CIRCRESAHA.111.253955

Grandi, E., Pasqualini, F. S., and Bers, D. M. (2010). A novel computational model of the human ventricular action potential and Ca transient. *J. Mol. Cell. Cardiol.* 48, 112–121. doi: 10.1016/j.yjmcc.2009.09.019

Gurev, V., Lee, T., Constantino, J., Arevalo, H., and Trayanova, N. A. (2011). Models of cardiac electromechanics based on individual hearts imaging data: image-based electromechanical models of the heart. *Biomech. Model. Mechanobiol.* 10, 295–306. doi: 10.1007/s10237-010-0235-5

Heijman, J., Voigt, N., Nattel, S., and Dobrev, D. (2014). Cellular and molecular electrophysiology of atrial fibrillation initiation, maintenance, and progression. *Circ. Res.* 114, 1483–1499. doi: 10.1161/CIRCRESAHA.114.302226

Helm, P. A., Tseng, H. J., Younes, L., McVeigh, E. R., and Winslow, R. L. (2005). *Ex vivo* 3D diffusion tensor imaging and quantification of cardiac laminar structure. *Magn. Reson. Med.* 54, 850–859. doi: 10.1002/mrm.20622

Hu, Y., Gurev, V., Constantino, J., and Trayanova, N. (2014). Optimizing cardiac resynchronization therapy to minimize ATP consumption heterogeneity throughout the left ventricle: a simulation analysis using a canine heart failure model. *Heart Rhythm* 11, 1063–1069. doi: 10.1016/j.hrthm.2014.03.021

Iwasaki, Y. K., Nishida, K., Kato, T., and Nattel, S. (2011). Atrial fibrillation pathophysiology: implications for management. *Circulation* 124, 2264–2274. doi: 10.1161/CIRCULATIONAHA.111.019893

Jacquemet, V., and Henriquez, C. S. (2009). Genesis of complex fractionated atrial electrograms in zones of slow conduction: a computer model of microfibrosis. *Heart Rhythm* 6, 803–810. doi: 10.1016/j.hrthm.2009.02.026

Jacquemet, V., Kappenberger, L., and Henriquez, C. S. (2008). Modeling atrial arrhythmias: impact on clinical diagnosis and therapies. *IEEE Rev. Biomed. Eng.* 1, 94–114. doi: 10.1109/RBME.2008.2008242

Jalife, J. (2011). Deja vu in the theories of atrial fibrillation dynamics. *Cardiovasc. Res.* 89, 766–775. doi: 10.1093/cvr/cvq364

Janse, M. J. (2004). Electrophysiological changes in heart failure and their relationship to arrhythmogenesis. *Cardiovasc. Res.* 61, 208–217. doi: 10.1016/j.cardiores.2003.11.018

Jie, X., Gurev, V., and Trayanova, N. (2010). Mechanisms of mechanically induced spontaneous arrhythmias in acute regional ischemia. *Circ. Res.* 106, 185–192. doi: 10.1161/CIRCRESAHA.109.210864

Jie, X., Rodriguez, B., De Groot, J. R., Coronel, R., and Trayanova, N. (2008). Reentry in survived subepicardium coupled to depolarized and inexcitable midmyocardium: insights into arrhythmogenesis in ischemia phase 1B. *Heart Rhythm* 5, 1036–1044. doi: 10.1016/j.hrthm.2008.03.025

Jie, X., and Trayanova, N. A. (2010). Mechanisms for initiation of reentry in acute regional ischemia phase 1B. *Heart Rhythm* 7, 379–386. doi: 10.1016/j.hrthm.2009.11.014

John, R. M., Tedrow, U. B., Koplan, B. A., Albert, C. M., Epstein, L. M., Sweeney, M. O., et al. (2012). Ventricular arrhythmias and sudden cardiac death. *Lancet* 380, 1520–1529. doi: 10.1016/S0140-6736(12)61413-5

Kostin, S., Klein, G., Szalay, Z., Hein, S., Bauer, E. P., and Schaper, J. (2002). Structural correlate of atrial fibrillation in human patients. *Cardiovasc. Res.* 54, 361–379. doi: 10.1016/S0008-6363(02)00273-0

Krogh-Madsen, T., Abbott, G. W., and Christini, D. J. (2012). Effects of electrical and structural remodeling on atrial fibrillation maintenance: a simulation study. *PLoS Comput. Biol.* 8:1002390. doi: 10.1371/journal.pcbi.1002390

Krueger, M. W., Rhode, K. S., O'Neill, M. D., Rinaldi, C. A., Gill, J., Razavi, R., et al. (2014). Patient-specific modeling of atrial fibrosis increases the accuracy of sinus rhythm simulations and may explain maintenance of atrial fibrillation. *J. Electrocardiol.* 47, 324–328. doi: 10.1016/j.jelectrocard.2013.11.003

Krueger, M. W., Schmidt, V., Tobón, C., Weber, F. M., Lorenz, C., Keller, D. U., et al. (2011). "Modeling atrial fiber orientation in patient-specific geometries: a semi-automatic rule-based approach," in *Functional Imaging and Modeling of the Heart*, eds D. N. Metaxas and L. Axel (Berlin; Heidelberg: Springer), 223–232.

Li, P., and Rudy, Y. (2011). A model of canine Purkinje cell electrophysiology and Ca(2+) cycling: rate dependence, triggered activity, and comparison to ventricular myocytes. *Circ. Res.* 109, 71–79. doi: 10.1161/CIRCRESAHA.111.246512

Maleckar, M. M., Greenstein, J. L., Giles, W. R., and Trayanova, N. A. (2009a). Electrotonic coupling between human atrial myocytes and fibroblasts alters myocyte excitability and repolarization. *Biophys. J.* 97, 2179–2190. doi: 10.1016/j.bpj.2009.07.054

Maleckar, M. M., Greenstein, J. L., Giles, W. R., and Trayanova, N. A. (2009b). K+ current changes account for the rate dependence of the action potential in the human atrial myocyte. *Am. J. Physiol. Heart Circ. Physiol.* 297, H1398–H1410. doi: 10.1152/ajpheart.00411.2009

McDowell, K. S., Arevalo, H. J., Maleckar, M. M., and Trayanova, N. A. (2011). Susceptibility to arrhythmia in the infarcted heart depends on myofibroblast density. *Biophys. J.* 101, 1307–1315. doi: 10.1016/j.bpj.2011.08.009

McDowell, K. S., Vadakkumpadan, F., Blake, R., Blauer, J., Plank, G., Macleod, R. S., et al. (2012). Methodology for patient-specific modeling of atrial fibrosis as a substrate for atrial fibrillation. *J. Electrocardiol.* 45, 640–645. doi: 10.1016/j.jelectrocard.2012.08.005

McDowell, K. S., Vadakkumpadan, F., Blake, R., Blauer, J., Plank, G., Macleod, R. S., et al. (2013). Mechanistic inquiry into the role of tissue remodeling in fibrotic lesions in human atrial fibrillation. *Biophys. J.* 104, 2764–2773. doi: 10.1016/j.bpj.2013.05.025

Moreno, J. D., Zhu, Z. I., Yang, P.-C., Bankston, J. R., Jeng, M.-T., Kang, C., et al. (2011). A computational model to predict the effects of class I anti-arrhythmic drugs on ventricular rhythms. *Sci. Transl. Med.* 3, 98ra83. doi: 10.1126/scitranslmed.3002588

Nattel, S., Burstein, B., and Dobrev, D. (2008). Atrial remodeling and atrial fibrillation: mechanisms and implications. *Circ. Arrhythm. Electrophysiol.* 1, 62–73. doi: 10.1161/CIRCEP.107.754564

Nazarian, S., Bluemke, D. A., Lardo, A. C., Zviman, M. M., Watkins, S. P., Dickfeld, T. L., et al. (2005). Magnetic resonance assessment of the substrate for inducible ventricular tachycardia in nonischemic cardiomyopathy. *Circulation* 112, 2821–2825. doi: 10.1161/CIRCULATIONAHA.105.549659

Ng, J., Jacobson, J. T., Ng, J. K., Gordon, D., Lee, D. C., Carr, J. C., et al. (2012). Virtual electrophysiological study in a 3-dimensional cardiac magnetic resonance imaging model of porcine myocardial infarction. *J. Am. Coll. Cardiol.* 60, 423–430. doi: 10.1016/j.jacc.2012.03.029

Nielsen, P. M., Le Grice, I. J., Smaill, B. H., and Hunter, P. J. (1991). Mathematical model of geometry and fibrous structure of the heart. *Am. J. Physiol.* 260, H1365–H1378.

Noble, D. (2002). Modeling the heart–from genes to cells to the whole organ. *Science* 295, 1678–1682. doi: 10.1126/science.1069881

Nygren, A., Fiset, C., Firek, L., Clark, J. W., Lindblad, D. S., Clark, R. B., et al. (1998). Mathematical model of an adult human atrial cell: the role of K+ currents in repolarization. *Circ. Res.* 82, 63–81. doi: 10.1161/01.RES.82.1.63

Oakes, R. S., Badger, T. J., Kholmovski, E. G., Akoum, N., Burgon, N. S., Fish, E. N., et al. (2009). Detection and quantification of left atrial structural remodeling with delayed-enhancement magnetic resonance imaging in patients with atrial fibrillation. *Circulation* 119, 1758–1767. doi: 10.1161/CIRCULATIONAHA.108.811877

O'Hara, T., Virag, L., Varro, A., and Rudy, Y. (2011). Simulation of the undiseased human cardiac ventricular action potential: model formulation and experimental validation. *PLoS Comput. Biol.* 7:e1002061. doi: 10.1371/journal.pcbi.1002061

Packer, D. L. (2004). Evolution of mapping and anatomic imaging of cardiac arrhythmias. *J. Cardiovasc. Electrophysiol.* 15, 839–854. doi: 10.1046/j.1540-8167.2004.04275.x

Pedrotty, D. M., Klinger, R. Y., Kirkton, R. D., and Bursac, N. (2009). Cardiac fibroblast paracrine factors alter impulse conduction and ion channel expression of neonatal rat cardiomyocytes. *Cardiovasc. Res.* 83, 688–697. doi: 10.1093/cvr/cvp164

Plank, G., Prassl, A. J., Wang, J. I., Seeman, G., Scherr, D., Sanchez-Quintana, D., et al. (2008a). Atrial fibrosis promotes the transition of pulmonary vein ectopy into reentrant arrhythmias. *Heart Rhythm.* 5(Suppl. 5), S162.

Plank, G., Zhou, L., Greenstein, J. L., Cortassa, S., Winslow, R. L., O'Rourke, B., et al. (2008b). From mitochondrial ion channels to arrhythmias in the heart: computational techniques to bridge the spatio-temporal scales. *Philos. Trans. A Math. Phys. Eng. Sci.* 366, 3381–3409. doi: 10.1098/rsta.2008.0112

Pop, M., Sermesant, M., Mansi, T., Crystal, E., Ghate, S., Peyrat, J. M., et al. (2011). Correspondence between simple 3-D MRI-based computer models and *in-vivo* EP measurements in swine with chronic infarctions. *IEEE Trans. Biomed. Eng.* 58, 3483–3486. doi: 10.1109/TBME.2011.2168395

Prakosa, A., Malamas, P., Zhang, S., Pashakhanloo, F., Arevalo, H., Herzka, D. A., et al. (2014). Methodology for image-based reconstruction of ventricular geometry for patient-specific modeling of cardiac electrophysiology. *Prog. Biophys. Mol. Biol.* 115, 226–234. doi: 10.1016/j.pbiomolbio.2014.08.009

Rantner, L. J., Arevalo, H. J., Constantino, J. L., Efimov, I. R., Plank, G., and Trayanova, N. A. (2012). Three-dimensional mechanisms of increased vulnerability to electric shocks in myocardial infarction: altered virtual electrode polarizations and conduction delay in the peri-infarct zone. *J. Physiol.* 590, 4537–4551. doi: 10.1113/jphysiol.2012.229088

Rodriguez, B., and Trayanova, N. (2003). Upper limit of vulnerability in a defibrillation model of the rabbit ventricles. *J. Electrocardiol.* 36(Suppl.), 51–56. doi: 10.1016/j.jelectrocard.2003.09.066

Roes, S. D., Borleffs, C. J. W., Van Der Geest, R. J., Westenberg, J. J., Marsan, N. A., Kaandorp, T. A., et al. (2009). Infarct tissue heterogeneity assessed with contrast-enhanced MRI predicts spontaneous ventricular arrhythmia in patients with ischemic cardiomyopathy and implantable cardioverter-defibrillator. *Circulation* 2, 183–190. doi: 10.1161/CIRCIMAGING.108.826529

Rohr, S. (2009). Myofibroblasts in diseased hearts: new players in cardiac arrhythmias? *Heart Rhythm* 6, 848–856. doi: 10.1016/j.hrthm.2009.02.038

Rubart, M., and Zipes, D. P. (2005). Mechanisms of sudden cardiac death. *J. Clin. Invest.* 115, 2305–2315. doi: 10.1172/JCI26381

Rudy, Y., Ackerman, M. J., Bers, D. M., Clancy, C. E., Houser, S. R., London, B., et al. (2008). Systems approach to understanding electromechanical activity in the human heart: a national heart, lung, and blood institute workshop summary. *Circulation* 118, 1202–1211. doi: 10.1161/CIRCULATIONAHA.108.772715

Sampson, K. J., Iyer, V., Marks, A. R., and Kass, R. S. (2010). A computational model of Purkinje fibre single cell electrophysiology: implications for the long QT syndrome. *J. Physiol.* 588, 2643–2655. doi: 10.1113/jphysiol.2010.187328

Schmidt, A., Azevedo, C. F., Cheng, A., Gupta, S. N., Bluemke, D. A., Foo, T. K., et al. (2007). Infarct tissue heterogeneity by magnetic resonance imaging identifies enhanced cardiac arrhythmia susceptibility in patients with left ventricular dysfunction. *Circulation* 115, 2006–2014. doi: 10.1161/CIRCULATIONAHA.106.653568

Schotten, U., Verheule, S., Kirchhof, P., and Goette, A. (2011). Pathophysiological mechanisms of atrial fibrillation: a translational appraisal. *Physiol. Rev.* 91, 265–325. doi: 10.1152/physrev.00031.2009

Stevenson, W. G., Brugada, P., Waldecker, B., Zehender, M., and Wellens, H. J. (1985). Clinical, angiographic, and electrophysiologic findings in patients with aborted sudden death as compared with patients with sustained ventricular tachycardia after myocardial infarction. *Circulation* 71, 1146–1152. doi: 10.1161/01.CIR.71.6.1146

Stewart, P., Aslanidi, O. V., Noble, D., Noble, P. J., Boyett, M. R., and Zhang, H. (2009). Mathematical models of the electrical action potential of Purkinje fibre cells. *Philos. Trans. A Math. Phys. Eng. Sci.* 367, 2225–2255. doi: 10.1098/rsta.2008.0283

Tanaka, K., Zlochiver, S., Vikstrom, K. L., Yamazaki, M., Moreno, J., Klos, M., et al. (2007). Spatial distribution of fibrosis governs fibrillation wave dynamics in the posterior left atrium during heart failure. *Circ. Res.* 101, 839–847. doi: 10.1161/CIRCRESAHA.107.153858

Tandri, H., Weinberg, S. H., Chang, K. C., Zhu, R., Trayanova, N. A., Tung, L., et al. (2011). Reversible cardiac conduction block and defibrillation with high-frequency electric field. *Sci. Transl. Med.* 3, 102ra196-102ra196. doi: 10.1126/scitranslmed.3002445

Ten Tusscher, K. H., and Panfilov, A. V. (2006). Alternans and spiral breakup in a human ventricular tissue model. *Am. J. Physiol. Heart Circ. Physiol.* 291, H1088–H1100. doi: 10.1152/ajpheart.00109.2006

Tice, B. M., Rodríguez, B., Eason, J., and Trayanova, N. (2007). Mechanistic investigation into the arrhythmogenic role of transmural heterogeneities in regional ischaemia phase 1A. *Europace* 9, vi46-vi58. doi: 10.1093/europace/eum204

Trayanova, N. A. (2011). Whole-heart modeling: applications to cardiac electrophysiology and electromechanics. *Circ. Res.* 108, 113–128. doi: 10.1161/CIRCRESAHA.110.223610

Trayanova, N. A. (2012). Computational cardiology: the heart of the matter. *ISRN Cardiol.* 2012, 269680. doi: 10.5402/2012/269680

Trayanova, N. A. (2014). Mathematical approaches to understanding and imaging atrial fibrillation significance for mechanisms and management. *Circ. Res.* 114, 1516–1531. doi: 10.1161/CIRCRESAHA.114.302240

Trayanova, N. A., and Boyle, P. M. (2014). Advances in modeling ventricular arrhythmias: from mechanisms to the clinic. *Wiley Interdiscip. Rev. Syst. Biol. Med.* 6, 209–224. doi: 10.1002/wsbm.1256

Trayanova, N. A., O'Hara, T., Bayer, J. D., Boyle, P. M., McDowell, K. S., Constantino, J., et al. (2012). Computational cardiology: how computer simulations could be used to develop new therapies and advance existing ones. *Europace* 14(Suppl. 5), v82–v89. doi: 10.1093/europace/eus277

Vadakkumpadan, F., Arevalo, H., Ceritoglu, C., Miller, M., and Trayanova, N. (2012). Image-based estimation of ventricular fiber orientations for personalized modeling of cardiac electrophysiology. *IEEE Trans. Med. Imaging* 31, 1051–1060. doi: 10.1109/TMI.2012.2184799

Vadakkumpadan, F., Arevalo, H., Prassl, A. J., Chen, J., Kickinger, F., Kohl, P., et al. (2010). Image-based models of cardiac structure in health and disease. *Wiley Interdiscip. Rev. Syst. Biol. Med.* 2, 489–506. doi: 10.1002/wsbm.76

Vaidyanathan, R., O'Connell, R. P., Deo, M., Milstein, M. L., Furspan, P., Herron, T. J., et al. (2013). The ionic bases of the action potential in isolated mouse cardiac Purkinje cell. *Heart Rhythm* 10, 80–87. doi: 10.1016/j.hrthm.2012.10.002

Vetter, F. J., and McCulloch, A. D. (1998). Three-dimensional analysis of regional cardiac function: a model of rabbit ventricular anatomy. *Prog. Biophys. Mol. Biol.* 69, 157–183. doi: 10.1016/S0079-6107(98)00006-6

Vigmond, E. J., Aguel, F., and Trayanova, N. A. (2002). Computational techniques for solving the bidomain equations in three dimensions. *IEEE Trans. Biomed. Eng.* 49, 1260–1269. doi: 10.1109/TBME.2002.804597

Vigmond, E. J., Hughes, M., Plank, G., and Leon, L. J. (2003). Computational tools for modeling electrical activity in cardiac tissue. *J. Electrocardiol.* 36, 69–74. doi: 10.1016/j.jelectrocard.2003.09.017

Vigmond, E., Vadakkumpadan, F., Gurev, V., Arevalo, H., Deo, M., Plank, G., et al. (2009). Towards predictive modelling of the electrophysiology of the heart. *Exp. Physiol.* 94, 563–577. doi: 10.1113/expphysiol.2008.044073

Winslow, R. L., Trayanova, N., Geman, D., and Miller, M. I. (2012). Computational medicine: translating models to clinical care. *Sci. Transl. Med.* 4, 158rv111. doi: 10.1126/scitranslmed.3003528

Xu, J., Cui, G., Esmailian, F., Plunkett, M., Marelli, D., Ardehali, A., et al. (2004). Atrial extracellular matrix remodeling and the maintenance of atrial fibrillation. *Circulation* 109, 363–368. doi: 10.1161/01.CIR.0000109495.02213.52

Yan, A. T., Shayne, A. J., Brown, K. A., Gupta, S. N., Chan, C. W., Luu, T. M., et al. (2006). Characterization of the peri-infarct zone by contrast-enhanced cardiac magnetic resonance imaging is a powerful predictor of post–myocardial infarction mortality. *Circulation* 114, 32–39. doi: 10.1161/CIRCULATIONAHA.106.613414

Yue, L., Xie, J., and Nattel, S. (2011). Molecular determinants of cardiac fibroblast electrical function and therapeutic implications for atrial fibrillation. *Cardiovasc. Res.* 89, 744–753. doi: 10.1093/cvr/cvq329

3

Myocardial electrotonic response to submaximal exercise in dogs with healed myocardial infarctions: Evidence for β-adrenoceptor mediated enhanced coupling during exercise testing

Carlos L. del Rio[1,2,3], Bradley D. Clymer[2,4] and George E. Billman[1,5]*

[1] Department of Physiology and Cell Biology, The Ohio State University, Columbus, OH, USA
[2] Department of Electrical and Computer Engineering, The Ohio State University, Columbus, OH, USA
[3] Safety Pharmacology, QTest Labs, Columbus, OH, USA
[4] Biomedical Engineering, The Ohio State University, Columbus, OH, USA
[5] Davis Heart and Lung Research Institute, The Ohio State University, Columbus, OH, USA

***Correspondence:**
George E. Billman, Department of Physiology and Cell Biology, The Ohio State University, 1645 Neil Avenue, 305 Hamilton Hall, Columbus, OH, USA
e-mail: billman.1@osu.edu

Introduction: Autonomic neural activation during cardiac stress testing is an established risk-stratification tool in post-myocardial infarction (MI) patients. However, autonomic activation can also modulate myocardial electrotonic coupling, a known factor to contribute to the genesis of arrhythmias. The present study tested the hypothesis that exercise-induced autonomic neural activation modulates electrotonic coupling (as measured by myocardial electrical impedance, MEI) in post-MI animals shown to be susceptible or resistant to ventricular fibrillation (VF).

Methods: Dogs ($n = 25$) with healed MI instrumented for MEI measurements were trained to run on a treadmill and classified based on their susceptibility to VF (12 susceptible, 9 resistant). MEI and ECGs were recorded during 6-stage exercise tests (18 min/test; peak: 6.4 km/h @ 16%) performed under control conditions, and following complete β-adrenoceptor (β-AR) blockade (propranolol); MEI was also measured at rest during escalating β-AR stimulation (isoproterenol) or overdrive-pacing.

Results: Exercise progressively increased heart rate (HR) and reduced heart rate variability (HRV). In parallel, MEI decreased gradually (enhanced electrotonic coupling) with exercise; at peak exercise, MEI was reduced by 5.3 ± 0.4% (or -23 ± 1.8Ω, $P < 0.001$). Notably, exercise-mediated electrotonic changes were linearly predicted by the degree of autonomic activation, as indicated by changes in either HR or in HRV ($P < 0.001$). Indeed, β-AR blockade attenuated the MEI response to exercise while direct β-AR stimulation (at rest) triggered MEI decreases comparable to those observed during exercise; ventricular pacing had no significant effects on MEI. Finally, animals prone to VF had a significantly larger MEI response to exercise.

Conclusions: These data suggest that β-AR activation during exercise can acutely enhance electrotonic coupling in the myocardium, particularly in dogs susceptible to ischemia-induced VF.

Keywords: electrotonic coupling, β-adrenoceptor stimulation, exercise, arrhythmic risk, myocardial infarction

INTRODUCTION

Myocardial infarction is a well-established risk factor for sudden cardiac death (SCD) due to malignant arrhythmias (Adabag et al., 2010; Zaman and Kovoor, 2014). However, despite significant advances in the understanding of the physiological substrate(s) mediating/facilitating the onset of arrhythmias, risk stratification for SCD in post-MI patients remains difficult and insufficient (Goldberger et al., 2014; Wellens et al., 2014; Zaman and Kovoor, 2014). Indeed, the majority of SCD episodes occur in patients with either low-/intermediate- or without known risk factors (e.g., Wellens et al., 2014).

In these patients, underlying ionic current abnormalities, particularly those mediating repolarization, either co-exist with and/or are exacerbated by autonomic imbalances favoring enhanced sympathetic drive (e.g., Chen et al., 2007; Pokornı et al., 2011; Wellens et al., 2014). As such, multi-modality stratifications techniques, encompassing electrocardiographic evaluation of repolarization abnormalities during states of autonomic activation, such as exercise, are favored (Goldberger et al., 2014; Wellens et al., 2014). For instance, the assessment of microvolt T-wave alternans (TWA or MTWA) during low-intensity exercise has been shown to predict not only arrhythmic events in post-MI patients but also arrhythmia-free survival in patients with LV dysfunction (Cantillon et al., 2007; Amit et al., 2010; Verrier et al., 2011; Merchant et al., 2012; Shizuta et al., 2012).

Interestingly, activation of the autonomic nervous system (e.g., during exercise), and its concomitant catecholamine release, may in turn also modulate the passive electrical properties that govern electrotonic interactions in the myocardium. For example, several studies have shown that catecholamines (and increased cAMP levels) enhance junctional coupling in myocytes (e.g., see De Mello, 1996a; Dhein, 2004; Salameh and Dhein, 2011). Notably, electrotonic coupling is a well-established factor modulating both repolarization disturbances and arrhythmic risk, as poorly coupled cells are more likely to exhibit pro-arrhythmic behaviors (e.g., Pastore and Rosenbaum, 2000; De Groot and Coronel, 2004; Saffitz and Kléber, 2012; Wit and Peters, 2012). For instance, enhanced electrotonic coupling has been shown to suppress early after-depolarizations (EADs) (Huelsing et al., 2000; Himel et al., 2013), and reduce transmural dispersion of repolarization (Quan et al., 2007). Similarly, preserved electrotonic interaction has been shown to modulate TWA *in silico,* and more recently, also *in vivo* (Pastore and Rosenbaum, 2000; Watanabe et al., 2001; Cherry and Fenton, 2004; Sato et al., 2006; Kjølbye et al., 2008; Jia et al., 2012). Remarkably, no study to date has investigated concomitant passive electrical (electrotonic) changes during autonomic neural activation *in vivo*.

It was, therefore, the purpose of this study to investigate myocardial electrotonic coupling changes induced by submaximal exercise in the left-ventricle of post-MI animals, as measured by myocardial electrical impedance (MEI). Specifically, the hypothesis that exercise-induced autonomic activation can modulate myocardial electrotonic coupling (i.e., MEI) was tested in animals with healed myocardial infarctions later demonstrated to be either susceptible or resistant to ischemia-induced VF. Briefly, β-adrenoceptor (β-AR) activation during submaximal exercise acutely decreased the electrical impedance of the surviving myocardium, particularly in animals susceptible to VF, consistent with an increased electrotonic coupling.

MATERIALS AND METHODS

The principles governing the care and treatment of animals, as expressed by the American Physiological Society, were followed at all times during this study. In addition, the animal protocols and experimental procedures were approved by The Ohio State University's Institutional Lab Animal Care and Use Committee (ILACUC) at this institution, and adhered to the statutes of the Animal Welfare Act and the guidelines of the Public Health Service.

SURGICAL PREPARATION

The studies were performed using a well-characterized canine model of sudden cardiac death, known to mimic/combine the most prevalent features associated with this disease in the clinic: healed myocardial ischemic injury, acute myocardial ischemia, and cardiac autonomic activation (see Billman, 2006).

Briefly, thirty-five ($n = 35$) heartworm-free purpose bred mixed-breed dogs (weight: 16.1–24.1 kg, 19.0 ± 0.4 kg) were sedated (morphine sulfate 15 mg IM, and thiopental sodium 20 mg/kg IV), and connected to a respirator via an endotracheal cuffed tube. Anesthesia was maintained with inhaled isoflurane (1–1.5%) mixed with oxygen (100%). Under sterile conditions, the chest was opened via a left thoracotomy (fifth intercostal space); the heart was exposed, and suspended with a pericardial cradle. Subsequently, an antero-lateral myocardial infarction (MI) was created by a two-stage ligature of the left anterior descending (LAD) coronary artery. The left circumflex (LCX) coronary artery was dissected free of the surrounding tissue near its origin (under the edge of the left atrial appendage) and was instrumented with a 20 MHz Doppler-flow transducer, and a hydraulic coronary artery occluder; inflation of this balloon would later render a portion of the LCX distribution acutely ischemic (see *Arrhythmia Susceptibility*).

As required for MEI measurements (see below), a bipolar pacing electrode (Medtronic Inc., model Streamline™ 6495) was placed remote to the infarct, in the distal (non-ischemic) distribution of the LCX coronary artery. In a subset of animals ($n = 10$), a second MEI electrode was placed in the healthy (*non-infarcted*) anterior myocardium for pacing purposes (see *Experimental Protocol*). The leads were inserted into the mid-myocardial wall (parallel to the local fiber alignment), and were firmly secured in place with non-absorbable sutures (prolene 2-0). The pericardial cradle was released, the chest closed in layers and evacuated of air restoring the negative intra-thoracic pressure. All leads were tunneled under the skin, exited at the neck, and were carefully bandaged.

EXERCISE TEST PROTOCOL

The animals were allowed to recover for 3–4 weeks, and subsequently, were trained to run on a motor-driven treadmill. A 6-stage submaximal exercise stress-test (SMT), as initially described by Stone (1977), was used to activate the autonomic nervous system. This protocol is summarized in **Figure 1**, and consisted of a 3 min warm-up walking period (4.8 km/h, 0% grade; level L1), followed by running (6.4 km/h) for 15 min with the grade

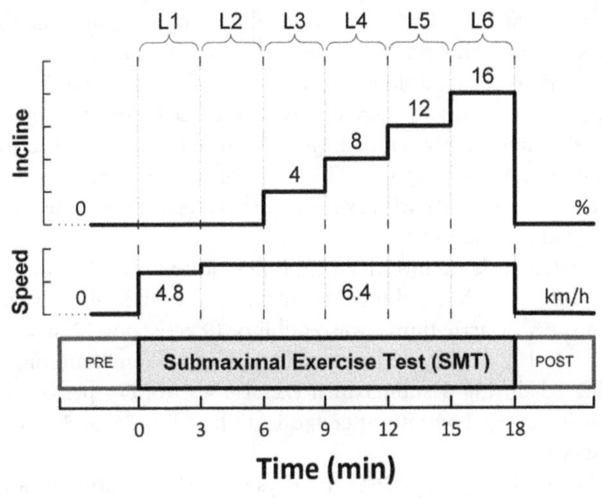

FIGURE 1 | Schematic representation of the six-level submaximal exercise test (SMT).

(incline) increased every 3 min (i.e., 0, 4, 8, 12, and 16%; levels L2-L6).

ARRHYTHMIA SUSCEPTIBILITY

The susceptibility to ischemia-induced ventricular fibrillation was assessed at the end of the study using a standardized protocol, generally referred as the "exercise-plus-ischemia" test (see Billman, 2006). In short, a submaximal exercise bout was performed (as described above) and during the last minute of exercise, the animals were subjected to a brief (2 min) LCX occlusion (i.e., while running at 6.4 km/h, 16%). This combination of exercise plus ischemia, when applied post-MI, yields two stable and well-differentiated populations of animals: one susceptible and the other resistant to ischemia-induced malignant arrhythmias, such as ventricular fibrillation [see Billman (2006) for review]. In this study, 12 animals developed VF (susceptible, S) and 9 did not (resistant, R) during the exercise-plus-ischemia test. Four animals ($n = 4$) could not be classified due to equipment failure (e.g., occluder rupture).

MYOCARDIAL ELECTRICAL IMPEDANCE (MEI)

As has previously been described, a computer controlled circuit developed in this laboratory was used to measure the complex electrical impedance of the myocardium (Howie et al., 2001; Dzwonczyk et al., 2004; Del Rio et al., 2005, 2008a,b). In short, using a bipolar pacing lead (see above) the myocardium was probed with a sub-threshold zero-mean bipolar current, consisting of two rectangular pulse of alternating polarity ($\pm$ 5 µA, 100 µs wide) generated 200 ms apart. The complex MEI spectrum was calculated in the frequency domain, as the ratio (at each frequency) of the current and voltage spectra resulting from the ensemble averages of 10 stimulus pulses and their respective (voltage) responses. The mean modulus of the complex MEI spectrum in the 0.27–5.90 kHz frequency range was examined (Del Rio et al., 2008a).

EXPERIMENTAL PROTOCOL

As described above, thirty-five animals ($n = 35$) were instrumented with MEI electrodes in the remote, non-infarcted myocardium. However, five animals ($n = 5$) experienced lead malfunctions (e.g., dislodgement) either before or at the time of experimentation, and therefore, were excluded from the analysis, while another five animals ($n = 5$) failed to acclimatize to the treadmill exercise protocol. Thus, the studies were performed in 30 animals ($n = 30$), with exercise-data successfully collected and analyzed in 25 dogs ($n = 25$).

First, in order to investigate the time-course of the electrotonic coupling (i.e., MEI) during submaximal exercise, all animals, regardless of arrhythmias susceptibility (9 resistant, 12 susceptible, and 4 unable to be classified), had MEI measurements collected during a submaximal exercise test (SMT) performed approximately 1-month after the LAD ligature (28 $\pm$ 1.7 days post-MI).

On a different day (26 $\pm$ 1.7 days post-MI), a subset of animals (5 resistant, 7 susceptible, and 4 unable to be classified; $n = 16$) performed the submaximal exercise test, but after pretreatment with the β-adrenoceptor antagonist propranolol HCl (1.0 mg/kg IV, Sigma Chemical, St. Louis, MO). Previous studies demonstrated that this dose of propranolol (1) completely abolished the cardiac response to the β-adrenoceptor agonist isoproterenol HCl (1 µg/kg IV) (Collins and Billman, 1989), and (2) did not compromise the exercise capacity during the submaximal exercise test in the presence of a 1-month-old anterior wall myocardial infarction (Brice and Stone, 1986). Propranolol was given intravenously (cephalic vein) as a bolus injection 3 min before the onset of exercise. A partially counter-balanced design was used: some dogs (6/16) were first exercise-tested under the influence of this β-adrenoceptor antagonist, and on a later day, had a control test (i.e., with no drug) performed; whereas in the remaining animals (10/16) the response to the submaximal exercise test (SMT) was first studied under control conditions, and on a subsequent day, following β-adrenoceptor blockade. In all cases, MEI measurements during the exercise tests were taken (continuously) from the distal LCX distribution (remote non-ischemic region) in awake, unsedated, and otherwise unstressed, post-MI animals (in a quiet and dimly lit room).

In order to investigate further the role of exercise-induced autonomic neural activation on myocardial electrotonic coupling (MEI), the total β-adrenoceptor response was quantified at rest in some animals ($n = 10$). Briefly, the dogs were lightly sedated with acepromazine (0.5 mg/kg IM; Ft. Dodge Animal Health, Ft. Dodge, IA), and a (cephalic vein) catheter was percutaneously placed for the administration of isoproterenol HCl (Sigma Chemical, St. Louis, MO); five increasing doses of this β-adrenoceptor agonist were given: 0.005, 0.015, 0.05, 0.15, and 0.5 µg/min/kg. MEI measurements were obtained continuously during isoproterenol infusion and washout. Data are reported (averaged over 30s) when a steady-state response was achieved at each dose, and 2 min after dosing discontinuation.

Finally, the possible confounding effects of exercise-mediated heart rate changes were evaluated in another subset of dogs ($n = 10$) via overdrive left-ventricular pacing at rest. Briefly, with the animal standing on the treadmill (awake and unsedated), an impulse generator (Grass Medical Instruments, model Grass S44, via impulse-isolation unit model SIU105-B) was used to maintain ventricular rates of 180 and 210 beats/min, mimicking those observed during moderate (L2; 6.4 km/h, 0%) and peak exercise (L6; 6.4 km/h, 16%). In these animals, a second bipolar MEI/pacing electrode was placed at the time of instrumentation (see *Surgical Preparation* above); the pacing protocol was repeated from each lead (while MEI was simultaneously recorded from the other, i.e., the non-stimulating electrode), and, as similar impedance responses were obtained, the results for the two sites (leads) were combined. MEI data collected before pacing onset, and after stabilization at each pacing rate, are reported (averaged over at least a 30s interval).

Data analysis

A single-lead bipolar electrocardiogram (ECG) was recorded during each presentation of the submaximal exercise test. The ECG signals were band-pass filtered and digitally sampled (1 kHz)/analyzed (on-line) using a heart rate variability (HRV) monitor (Delta-Biometrics, Inc.; Urbana-Champaign, IL). Briefly, using a previously well-described (Billman and

Hoskins, 1989; Billman and Dujardin, 1990) R-R interval time-series analysis technique, the heart rate (HR) mean and its variability (i.e., HRV) were determined continuously from non-overlapping 30s-segments of the ECG. Two kinds of HRV indices were studied simultaneously: (1) two measures of statistical dispersion, namely the standard deviation (RR_{SD}) and the range (RR_{RNG}; longest—shortest R-R interval) of the R-R intervals within each 30 s analysis-window; and (2) an index estimating the amplitude of the respiratory sinus arrhythmia (R-R interval variability in the 0.24—1.04 Hz frequency range), or vagal tone index (VT). MEI, HR and HRV data are reported (averaged over 30 s) at eight time-points sampled before (one), during (six), and after (one) the bouts of submaximal exercise. Pre- (baseline) and post-exercise (recovery) values were taken 2 min before/after exercise onset/offset (i.e., at $t = -2$ min, and $t = 20$ min, see **Figure 1A**) with the animals standing on the treadmill. Meanwhile, the six exercise data-points were recorded during the last 30s of each stage in the submaximal stress protocol (i.e., L1—L6).

In addition, exercise-induced changes in the ECG morphology as well as on ECG-derived indices of the duration and heterogeneity of ventricular repolarization were evaluated in a subset of animals ($n = 19$). In short, with the aid of pattern-recognition software (ECG Auto; EMKA Technologies, France), fiducial points/intervals were determined and measured offline from two sets of thirty consecutive ECG complexes (beats), one recorded before (i.e., at rest) and the other immediately following a control submaximal exercise test (i.e., within 5 beats of stopping the treadmill). The effects of exercise on the duration of the T-wave's terminal portion (i.e., peak-to-end interval, TPE (Yan and Antzelevitch, 1998; Opthof et al., 2007) and on the QT-interval's length, as well as on the relationship between cardiac electrical systole and diastole (i.e., ratio of QT- and TQ-intervals, QT/TQ) (Fossa et al., 2007; Kijtawornrat et al., 2010) were evaluated; both absolute (QT) and rate-corrected (QTc, via van de Water's formula; Van de Water et al., 1989) QT-intervals are reported. In addition, the standard deviation of the T-wave amplitude within each 30-beat epoch (T_{SD}) was calculated and used as a surrogate-marker of temporal repolarization variability (e.g., T-wave alternans; Nearing and Verrier, 2002).

All data are presented as mean ± standard error of the mean (SEM). Statistical analyses were performed with SigmaStat (Systat Software, Inc., San Jose, CA) and NCSS (NCSS, Inc., Kaysville, UT). The mean time-course of electrotonic coupling (i.e., MEI), and ECG-derived variables during the submaximal exercise tests (SMT) was evaluated using a One-Way (exercise level: baseline, L1–L6, and recovery) analysis of variance (ANOVA) with repeated measures. Intergroup comparisons (i.e., resistant vs. susceptible) were made using a Two-Way (exercise level, and group: susceptible/resistant) ANOVA with repeated measures on one factor (exercise level). Similarly, the responses to exercise, recorded under control conditions (control) and after β-adrenoceptor blockade (beta), were compared using a Two-Way (exercise level, and control/beta tests) ANOVA with repeated measures on both factors. Finally, the statistical significance of any impedance changes induced by either pacing (3 levels: baseline/two rates) and/or by isoproterenol infusion/washout (7 levels: baseline/five doses/recovery) was evaluated using One-Way ANOVA with repeated measures. The sphericity assumption (i.e., homogeneity of the covariance matrix) was verified using the Mauchley's test (NCSS, Inc.). If this assumption was not met, then a non-parametric repeated measurements ANOVA on Ranks (Friedman) test was used. In all cases, if significant F-values (or Q-values in the non-parametric case) were observed, *post-hoc* pair-wise comparisons were made using the Tukey test.

Linear regression analyses were performed as well in order to study the relationship (interaction) between exercise-induced changes in electrotonic coupling (i.e., ΔMEI) and in two indices of autonomic activation, the heart rate (ΔHR) and the vagal-tone index (ΔVT); the regression data were "centered," i.e., deviations from each animal's mean values (over the whole exercise bout) were studied. The equality of the ΔMEI/ΔHR (and ΔMEI/ΔVT) linear models fitted to the different groups and conditions studied (susceptible vs. resistant, and control vs. β-AR blockade) was tested by multiple linear regression analysis, considering both qualitative (group) and interaction terms (i.e., simultaneously testing the differences in slope and intersect of the regression functions). For all analyses, $P < 0.05$ was considered, a priori, to be statistically significant.

RESULTS

EFFECTS OF EXERCISE

As expected and consistent with previous studies (Billman and Hoskins, 1989; Billman and Dujardin, 1990; Billman, 2006), submaximal treadmill exercise resulted in a progressive acceleration of heart rate and a concomitant decrease in heart rate variability (see **Figure 2** and **Table 1**). At peak exercise (L6; 6.4 km/h, 16%) heart rate increased on average 78 ± 4.3% (HR: from 119 ± 4 at rest to 208 ± 4 bpm at L6, $P < 0.05$), while the cardiac vagal-tone index, for instance, decreased 86 ± 2.3% (VT: from 7.9 ± 0.3 at rest to 1.2 ± 0.2 ln ms^2 at L6, $P < 0.05$). In parallel with these changes indicative of strong cardiac autonomic neural activation, MEI decreased progressively during exercise in all animals studied (see **Figure 2** and **Table 1**), suggesting enhanced electrotonic coupling. For example, at the highest exercise level (i.e., L6) MEI decreased −23 ± 1.8Ω (or 5.3 ± 0.4%) from the pre-exercise (at rest) values (MEI: from 446 ± 16 to 423 ± 16Ω at L6, $P < 0.05$). Moreover, following discontinuation of exercise offset (i.e., recovery), all parameters returned toward the pre-exercise (baseline) values.

Notably, exercise-mediated impedance changes (ΔMEI) were linearly predicted by (i.e., correlated with) the degree of autonomic neural activation, as indicated by either changes in heart rate (ΔHR; slope ΔMEI vs. ΔHR = −0.249Ω/bpm; $R^2 = 0.83$, $P < 0.05$), or in vagal tone index (ΔVT; slope ΔMEI vs. ΔVT = 3.134 Ω/ln(ms^2); $R^2 = 0.77$, $P < 0.05$) (see **Figure 3** and **Table 1**).

Indeed, pretreatment with the (non-selective) β-AR antagonist propranolol significantly attenuated the MEI response to exercise (e.g., at L6, CTRL: −23 ± 2.5 Ω vs. BB: −11 ± 2.0Ω; $P < 0.05$, $n = 15$) (see **Figure 4**, **Table 2**), markedly reducing the slope of the ΔMEI vs. ΔHR (−0.250 vs. −0.139 Ω/bpm; $R^2 = 0.78$, $P < 0.05$) and the ΔMEI vs. ΔVT relationships (Ω/ln(ms^2); $R^2 = 0.77$, $P < 0.05$). Similarly, as expected, β-AR blockade blunted the exercise-induced heart rate increase (e.g., at L6, CTRL: +47 ± 6

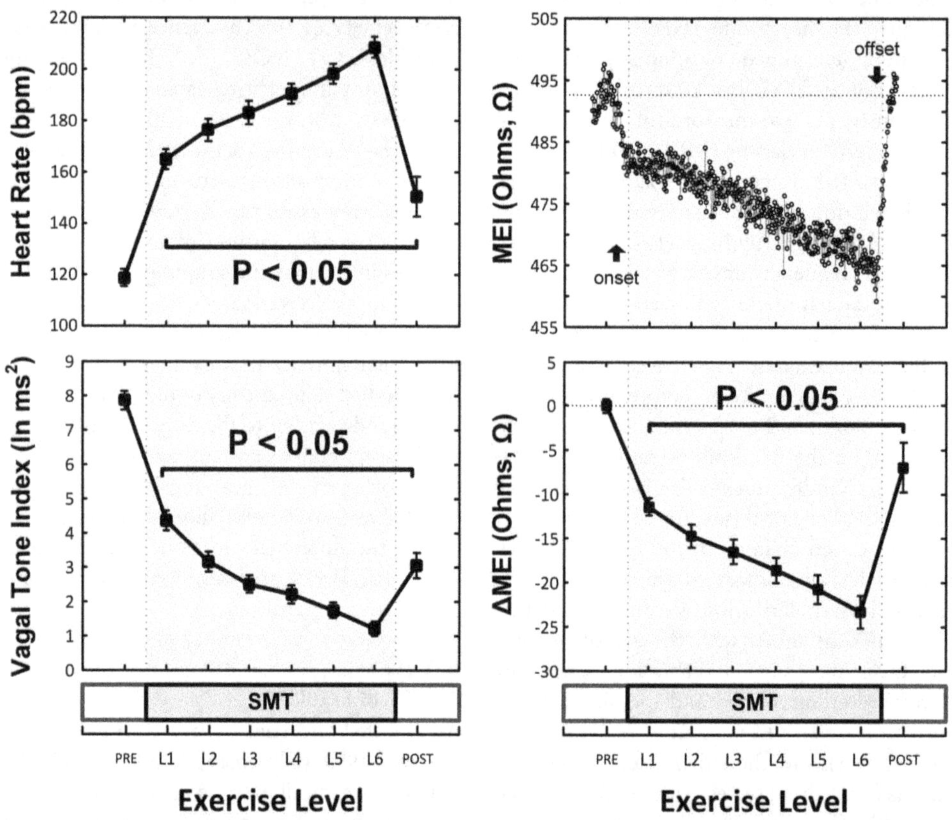

FIGURE 2 | Exercise-Induced changes in the heart-rate (HR, top-left) and ECG-derived vagal-tone index (bottom-left) and well as in the myocardial electrical impedance (MEI, bottom-right with representative response in top-right) of awake-unsedated dogs with healed left-anterior descending (LAD) myocardial infarcts ($n = 25$, except at recovery where $n = 14$).

Table 1 | Myocardial electrical impedance (MEI), heart-rate (HR) and ECG-derived indices of heart rate variability in awake-unsedated dogs with healed left-anterior descending (LAD) myocardial infarcts, both before (baseline) as well as during a submaximal exercise test.

	Baseline	Submaximal exercise test (SMT)			Correlation
Parameter	0 km/h, 0%	6.4 km/h, 0%	6.4 km/h, 8%	6.4 km/h, 16%	vs. ΔMEI
MEI (Ohms)	446 ± 16	431 ± 16*	427 ± 16*	423 ± 16*	–
Heart rate (bpm)	119 ± 3	176 ± 4*	190 ± 4*	208 ± 4*	(–) $R^2 = 0.83$
Vagal Tone (ln ms^2)	7.9 ± 0.3	3.1 ± 0.3*	2.2 ± 0.3*	1.2 ± 0.2*	(+) $R^2 = 0.77$
RR_{SD} (ms)	71 ± 6	22 ± 2*	14 ± 1*	8 ± 1*	n/s
RR_{RNG} (ms)	329 ± 30	101 ± 8*	63 ± 7*	38 ± 4*	n/s

*$P < 0.05$ vs. Baseline.
n/s, not studied.

vs. BB: +30 ± 5 bpm; see **Figure 4**), but accentuated cardiac parasympathetic withdrawal (e.g., lower vagal tone index values were recorded). Moreover, direct β-adrenoceptor stimulation at rest (with isoproterenol infusions) triggered a dose-dependent MEI response (decrease) comparable to that observed during submaximal exercise (see **Figure 5**). On average, at the highest dose-level assayed (i.e., at 0.5 μg/min·kg), isoproterenol decreased MEI by $-14 \pm 1.7\Omega$ (from 453 ± 40 to 440 ± 45Ω, $P < 0.05$). Thus, when considered together, these data suggest that the acute electrotonic (impedance) changes induced by exercise are predominantly mediated by sympathetic β-adrenoceptor activation.

On the other hand, while both submaximal exercise and direct β-adrenoceptor stimulation (at rest) led to acute MEI reductions, suggestive of favored increased electrotonic coupling, elevations in heart-rate via overdrive left-ventricular pacing had no significant effects on the passive electrical properties of the myocardium (see **Figure 6**). For instance, when resting animals were paced at

210 beats/min (from a basal rate of 123 ± 7 bpm) MEI changed only +2 ± 0.8Ω (from 426 ± 28Ω at baseline to 428 ± 29Ω, $n = 10$; N.S.); meanwhile, when the same subset of animals performed a submaximal exercise test, MEI decreased −20 ± 3.3Ω (from 435 ± 38Ω at rest to 414 ± 38.3Ω at L6, $n = 8$; $P < 0.05$) although heart rate increased similarly (from 124 ± 7 at rest to 213 ± 9 bpm at L6, $P < 0.05$). These data support the conclusion that the effects of exercise on electrotonic coupling (enhancement) are not mediated by its concomitant chronotropic effects (i.e., rate acceleration).

ARRHYTHMIA SUSCEPTIBILITY

Although (as mentioned above), MEI decreased with exercise onset in all animals studied, the degree of reduction was modulated by the underlying arrhythmic susceptibility of each animal: Animals prone to ischemia-induced VF had a significantly larger MEI response to submaximal exercise (see **Figure 7**, **Table 2**). At the peak exercise level (i.e., at L6), for instance, MEI decreased −30 ± 1.6Ω in dogs susceptible to VF (S, $n = 12$) and only −17 ± 2.1Ω in those resistant (R, $n = 9$) ($P < 0.05$), albeit comparable heart rates (e.g., S: 211 ± 5 vs. R: 210 ± 6 bpm at L6, N.S.) and heart rate variability indices (e.g., VT; S: 1.3 ± 0.3 vs. R: 0.7 ± 0.2 ln ms^2 at L6, N.S.) were reached by both groups; these observations suggest an increased impedance responsiveness to exercise-induced autonomic neural activation in dogs prone to arrhythmias.

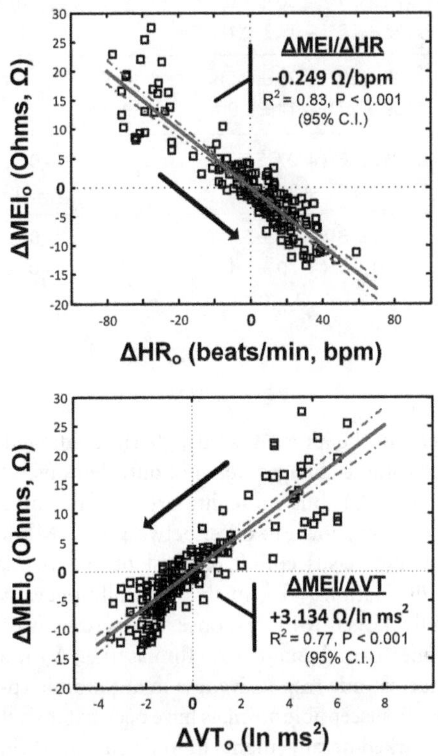

FIGURE 3 | Relationship(s) between the exercise-induced changes in the heart-rate (top) and ECG-derived vagal-tone index (bottom) with the concomitant reductions in myocardial electrical impedance (MEI); relationships were "centered," i.e., deviations from each animal's mean values (over the whole exercise bout) were studied.

In fact, susceptible animals had significantly ($P < 0.001$, see **Table 2**) steeper relationships between the exercise-mediated changes in impedance (ΔMEI) and those recorded for the heart rate (slope of ΔMEI vs. ΔHR; S: −0.295 vs. R: −0.180 Ω/bpm, $R^2 = 0.87$) and/or the vagal tone index (slope of ΔMEI vs. ΔVT; S: 4.11 vs. R: 2.09 Ω/ln ms^2, $R^2 = 0.85$). Notably, such marked intergroup differences were evident even when the slopes of the ΔMEI vs. ΔHR (S: −0.31 ± 0.2 vs. R: −0.18 ± 0.2 Ω/bpm, $P = 0.001$) and/or the ΔMEI vs. ΔVT (S: 4.3 ± 0.27 vs. R: 2.4 ± 0.46 Ω/ln ms^2, $P = 0.002$) relationships were calculated individually for each animal, rather than from the study groups. Moreover, complete β-AR blockade (with propranolol) blunted the exercise-induced impedance differences between animals susceptible (S, $n = 7$) and resistant (R, $n = 5$) to ischemia-induced arrhythmias (during control test; S: −30 ± 2.4 vs. R: −17 ± 2.7 Ω, $P < 0.05$, but after β-AR blockade; S: −16 ± 1.5 vs. R: −10 ± 4.1Ω, N.S.).

ELECTROCARDIOGRAPHIC DATA (RESPONSE TO EXERCISE)

Concomitantly with the above mentioned changes on indices of autonomic neural activation (cardio-acceleration, decreased heart-rate variability), exercise shortened the PR-interval and flattened the T-wave (data not shown) while decreasing indices of ventricular repolarization temporal duration (QTc, TPE) (see **Table 3**). For instance, on average, exercise shortened the rate-corrected QT-interval from 251 ± 4 msc at rest to 229 ± 4 msc ($P < 0.05$), suggesting a faster and/or more homogeneous repolarization. On the other hand, exercise increased the QT/TQ ratio (an index of the steepness of ventricular restitution, Fossa et al., 2007; Kijtawornrat et al., 2010) as well as the standard deviation of the T-wave amplitude (a marker of repolarization variability and/or T-wave "alternans"). Notably, exercise-induced changes on the T-wave amplitude variability were larger in animals susceptible to ischemia-induced VF (from 20.5 ± 3.1 μV at rest to 50.5 ± 9.0 μV post-exercise, $P < 0.05$) than in those resistant such arrhythmias (from 25.8 ± 4.7 μV at rest to 39.2 ± 5.6 μV post-exercise, N.S.); no other significant electrocardiographic differences, either at rest or following exercise, were noted between animals susceptible and resistant to VF.

DISCUSSION

The present study investigated the acute effects of submaximal exercise and its resulting autonomic neural activation on the myocardial electrotonic coupling of dogs with healed myocardial infarctions, as described by changes in the electrical impedance of surviving remote (i.e., non-infarcted) myocardium. This study demonstrated that acute β-adrenoceptor activation (either during bouts of exercise or via a direct pharmacological challenge) acutely increased passive (electrotonic) coupling in the myocardium, with the largest changes noted in those animals that were subsequently shown to be susceptible to malignant ventricular arrhythmias. In short, myocardial impedance was shown to decrease gradually as the level of exercise and autonomic neural activation increased. In contrast, ventricular overdrive pacing (at heart rates matched to those seen with exercise) had no significant effects on MEI.

As noted by Kléber et al. (1987), the gross myocardial electrical impedance measurements used in this study as a surrogate

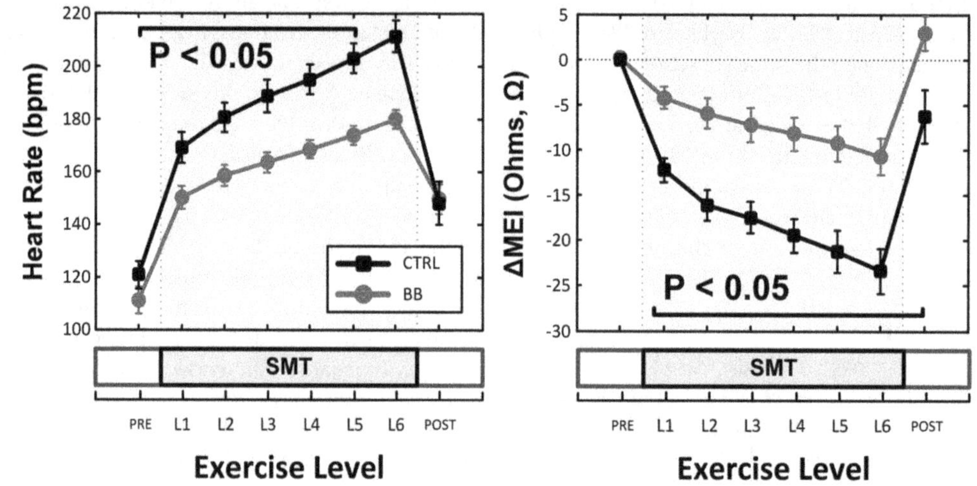

FIGURE 4 | Effects of (non-selective) β-adrenoceptor blockade (+BB, propranolol) in the myocardial electrical impedance (MEI, right), and heart-rate (HR, left) response(s) to exercise; β-adrenoceptor blockade blunted the MEI response to exercise. SMT, submaximal exercise test.

Table 2 | Exercise-induced changes in both the myocardial electrical impedance (MEI) and the heart-rate (HR) of awake-unsedated dogs with healed left-anterior descending (LAD) myocardial infarct; comparative effects of the underlying susceptibility to malignant arrhythmias (S vs. R), and of β-adrenoceptor blockade (+BB).

	Parameter/Sub-Group	Baseline 0 km/h, 0%	SMT (Peak) 6.4 km/h, 16%	Slope (Correlation) vs. ΔMEI
MEI (Ohms)	Susceptible (S, $n = 12$)	454 ± 24	424 ± 24*(− 30 ± 1.6)	*n/a*
	Resistant (R, $n = 9$)	439 ± 28	422 ± 26*(− 17 ± 2.1)†	
	Control ($n = 16$)	433 ± 22	409 ± 22*(− 23 ± 2.5)	*n/a*
	+BB ($n = 16$)	470 ± 26	459 ± 27*(− 11 ± 2.0)‡	
Heart Rate (bpm)	Susceptible ($n = 12$)	114 ± 4	211 ± 6*(+ 97 ± 5)	−0.30 ± 0.02
	Resistant ($n = 9$)	124 ± 8	210 ± 6*(+ 86 ± 4)	−0.19 ± 0.03
	Control (n =16)	121 ± 5	211 ± 6*(+ 91 ± 5)	−0.25 ± 0.03
	+BB ($n = 16$)	111 ± 5‡	180 ± 4*(+ 70 ± 5)‡	−0.16 ± 0.03

**P < 0.05 vs. Baseline.*
†P < 0.05 vs. Susceptible.
‡P < 0.05 vs. Control.

of electrotonic coupling represent the combined passive electrical properties of the intra-, extra- and inter- (i.e., junctional) cellular pathways. Thus, the observed changes (i.e., decreases) in impedance can be a reflection of both direct changes (increases) in cell-to-cell coupling at the gap-junctions, and/or geometrical effects affecting the myocyte/interstitial space ratios during exercise (Fleischhauer et al., 1995; De Mello, 2010) (see below). Notably, pharmacological interventions that result in stimulation of the β-AR/adenylyl-cyclase/PKA pathway and increase cAMP concentration have been shown to enhance gap junctional coupling in many preparations (e.g., see Manoach et al., 1995; De Mello, 1996a; Dhein, 2004). In agreement with these *in vitro* reports, complete β-AR blockade attenuated the MEI response to exercise while direct β-AR stimulation (at rest with isoproterenol) triggered MEI decreases comparable to those observed during exercise.

Moreover, in the present study, β-AR meditated exercise-induced electrotonic changes were not only demonstrated *in vivo* (conscious animals), but more importantly, the magnitude of these changes were shown to differ between post-MI dogs subsequently shown to be susceptible or resistant to ischemia-induced ventricular fibrillation (VF). In this clinically-relevant scenario, a significantly larger MEI response to exercise was noted in animals prone to malignant arrhythmias (i.e., VF), suggesting increased electrotonic responsiveness to autonomic (β-AR) activation. The VF-susceptible animals have been extensively studied, presenting marked derangements in ionic current (Sridhar et al., 2008; Bonilla et al., 2012), electrotonic coupling (Del Rio et al., 2008b), intracellular calcium homeostasis (Belevych et al., 2009, 2012), and autonomic control (see Billman, 2006). For instance, susceptible dogs have been shown to have a larger degree of electrotonic remodeling post-MI (Del Rio et al., 2008b), presenting

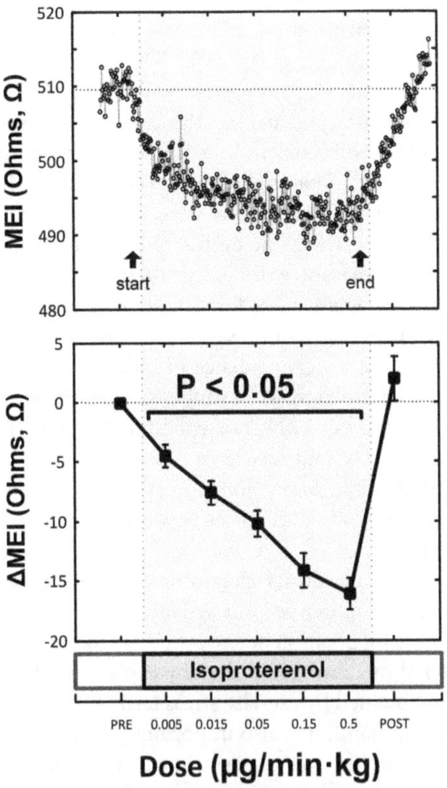

FIGURE 5 | Representative (top) and overall/mean (bottom) myocardial electrical impedance (MEI) response to direct β-adrenoceptor stimulation at rest (via escalating-dose infusion of isoproterenol), showing dose-dependent MEI decrease.

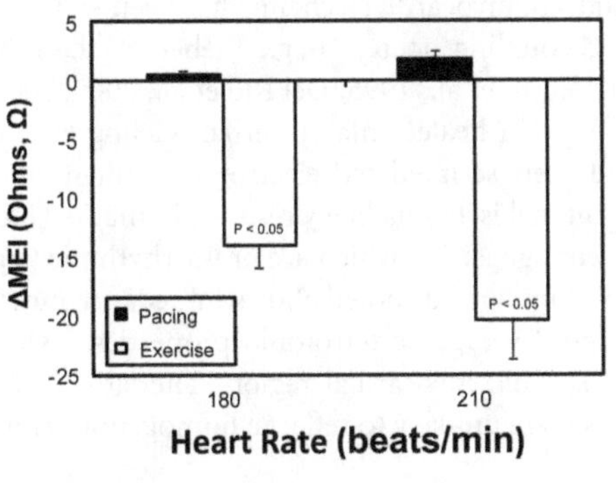

FIGURE 6 | Comparative myocardial electrical impedance (MEI) response to either submaximal exercise (white) or acute rate-matched ventricular pacing (black); only exercise decreased MEI.

moderately (albeit not statistically significant) higher remote MEI values at rest which could favor the observed increased electrotonic responsiveness. Indeed, in this study, animals prone to arrhythmias tended to have slightly higher baseline (i.e., pre-exercise) impedances but reached similar (absolute) values during exercise, suggesting, perhaps, a role of basal electrotonic derangements to their increased passive electrical responses to β-AR activation. Interestingly, the post-MI remodeling (e.g., down-regulation) of junctional proteins mediating electrotonic coupling is a well-established risk factor for malignant arrhythmias (e.g., see Saffitz and Kléber, 2012). On the other hand, susceptible animals also exhibit enhanced cardiac β-AR responsiveness, presenting a dominant functional contribution of the β_2-adrenergic receptors following MI, both *in vivo* and *in vitro* (Billman et al., 1997; Houle et al., 2001). Notably, acute β_2-AR stimulation can increase junctional conductance and protein expression in cardiac myocytes (Xia et al., 2009), likely via the exchange protein directly activated by cAMP (Epac)/Rap1 signaling pathway (Somekawa et al., 2005; Duquesnes et al., 2010; Mostafavi et al., 2014).

It also should be noted that much like patients prone to SCD (Rubart and Zipes, 2005), post-MI VF-susceptible dogs have well-documented abnormalities in myocardial calcium handling, being characterized by leaky and oxydized ryanodine receptors (Belevych et al., 2009) as well as increased calcium (Ca^{2+}) entry and Ca^{2+} transients, particularly during β-AR stimulation (Billman et al., 1997; Altschuld and Billman, 2000; Belevych et al., 2012). Moreover, in these animals, β_2-AR mediated increases in Ca^{2+}-transient amplitudes and Ca^{2+}-entry have been reported (Billman et al., 1997), rendering them exceptionally responsive (i.e., anti-arrhythmic protection) to the pharmacological blockade of L-type current (Billman, 1989). Interestingly, intracellular Ca^{2+} and junctional/electrotonic conductance are tightly coupled. For instance, inhibition of junctional communication can attenuate Ca^{2+} transients and sparks (Li et al., 2012). Meanwhile, pathologically-elevated intracellular Ca^{2+} levels (e.g., during a sustained ischemic insult) have been shown to decrease junctional conductance leading to electrotonic uncoupling (Cascio et al., 1990, 2005; Kléber, 1992; Smith et al., 1995; Owens et al., 1996; García-Dorado et al., 2004; De Groot and Coronel, 2004), likely as a protective mechanism against the spread of calcium overload (i.e., myocytes live and work together but die alone; quote from Engelmann (1875) in Janse et al., 2002). In contrast, moderate (i.e., within physiological levels) intracellular Ca^{2+} changes can enhance junctional coupling (perhaps via Ca^{2+}-activated kinases) (e.g., see Delage and Délèze, 1999). Indeed, Joyner et al. (1996) using a hybrid (both *in vitro and in silico*) paired-myocyte model showed that both β-AR stimulation (with isoproterenol) and direct opening of the L-type Ca^{2+} channels (with Bay K8644), facilitated cell-to-cell coupling and impulse propagation (an effect prevented by the L-type Ca^{2+} channel antagonist nifedipine). Thus, β-AR mediated electrotonic changes can provide mechanistic explanation(s) for the enhanced electrotonic responsiveness observed in the present study, particularly when the fact that complete β-AR blockade abolished the exercise-induced (electrotonic) differences with their VF-resistant counterparts is considered.

CLINICAL IMPLICATIONS

Regardless of the potential mechanism(s), the observed increase in electrotonic coupling during exercise and/or β-adrenergic autonomic activation may have important clinical implications. Notably, enhancements in electrotonic coupling can reduce repolarization heterogeneities thereby blunting or masking intrinsic pro-arrhythmic ionic substrates. Indeed, increased electrotonic coupling has been shown to suppress early after-depolarizations (EADs) and reduce pro-arrhythmic dispersion of repolarization (e.g., Huelsing et al., 2000; Quan et al., 2007; Himel et al., 2013). Interestingly, Vanoli et al. (1995) showed that adrenergic activation via either left stellate ganglion stimulation (*in vivo*) or isoproterenol administration (*in vitro*) blunted the d-sotalol-mediated prolongation of the action potential duration. Similarly, Järvenpää et al. (2007) reported that post-MI patients susceptible to VF have an impaired capacity of the autonomic nervous system to alter (i.e., prolong) electrocardiographic indices of repolarization. These observations are in agreement with the results of the present study; namely, the observed shortening of both the rate-corrected QT interval and the terminal portion of the T-wave (reflecting spatial repolarization heterogeneities); changes that are consistent with the exercise-mediated increases in myocardial electrotonic coupling.

Finally, substantial evidence supports the role of abnormal repolarization and calcium mishandling during neural autonomic activation in the onset and maintenance of lethal arrhythmias, particularly in the setting of both congenital and acquired (e.g., post-MI) electro-mechanical remodeling. For instance, exercise testing has been shown to amplify the arrhythmic genotype-phenotype relationship in patients with both long-QT syndrome (Takenaka et al., 2003) and catecholaminergic polymorphic ventricular tachycardia (Obeyesekere et al., 2011). However, in a stark contrast, exercise-driven risk stratification of post-MI patients (particularly those with preserved ejection fraction) remains difficult and, at times, counter-intuitive. For instance, in a recent meta-analysis, Chan et al. (2010) showed that abnormal microvolt TWA results were more likely to reflect an increased risk for arrhythmic events only when β-adrenoceptor blocker therapy was not withheld prior to testing. In a similar manner, cardiac pacing elicited not only positive TWA responses in susceptible patients (Hohnloser et al., 1997; Raatikainen et al., 2005), but led to a lower incidence of indeterminate test results when compared to exercise testing (Kraaier et al., 2009). In this study, exercise not only shortened the Tpeak to Tend interval (TPE), an index that has been reported to prolong during pro-arrhythmic stimulation (Johnson et al., 2013), but failed to induce significant TWA differences between susceptible and resistant animals (i.e., S: 50.5 ± 9.0 vs. R: 39.2 ± 5.6 μV, N.S.). Thus, enhanced myocardial electrotonic coupling mediated by exercise-induced β-adrenoceptor activation could mask (e.g., via reductions in repolarization heterogeneities) changes in indices of risk for arrhythmia and could thereby explain the false negative results often obtained by exercise stress testing.

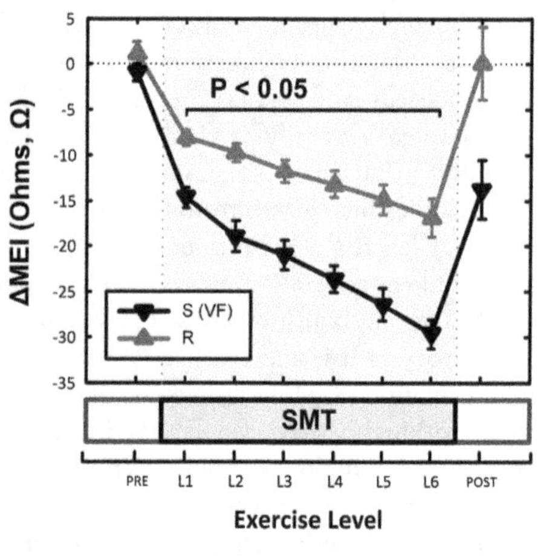

FIGURE 7 | Effects of underlying arrhythmic susceptibility of each animal in the myocardial electrical impedance (MEI) response to exercise; animals prone to ischemia-induced VF (i.e., S; $n = 12$) had a significantly larger MEI response to submaximal exercise, when compared those that were resistant (i.e., R; $n = 9$).

On the other hand, it is also important to note that improved electrotonic coupling has been shown to blunt myocardial ionic heterogeneities (e.g., Huelsing et al., 2000; Quan et al., 2007; Himel et al., 2013), masking and even reducing pro-arrhythmic risk (e.g., via pharmacological gap-junction modulation,; Hennan et al., 2006; Kjølbye et al., 2008). However any improvement in electrotonic coupling that was induced by acute exercise was of insufficient magnitude to prevent the onset of ischemic (coronary artery occlusion) arrhythmias in susceptible animals. Indeed, myocardial ischemia has been shown to depress electrotonic coupling acutely (e.g., Kléber et al., 1987; Cascio et al., 1990; Smith et al., 1995; Del Rio et al., 2005, 2008a). Thus, in the setting of a healed infarction/remodeling (Del Rio et al., 2008b) and exercise-mediated electrotonic enhancements, concomitant regional ischemia likely resulted in marked local passive electrical heterogeneities, which are pro-arrhythmic (e.g., Bishop et al., 2014). Similarly, as noted above, impedance measurements represent the "average" electrotonic properties, (Kléber et al., 1987) of a specific myocardial region. Therefore, the observed MEI decreases are unlikely to reflect a homogenous enhancement

Table 3 | Electrocardiographic response(s) to submaximal exercise.

Time	RR(ms)	PR (ms)	QRS (ms)	QT (ms)	QT_c(msc)	TPE (ms)	QT/TQ (n/u)	T_{SD}(μV)
Baseline	479 ± 19	92 ± 3	66 ± 2	206 ± 5	251 ± 4	51 ± 4	0.79 ± 0.04	25 ± 3
Exercise	329 ± 8	79 ± 3	65 ± 3	170 ± 4	229 ± 4	39 ± 2	1.11 ± 0.06	45 ± 5
***P < 0.05*†**	↓	↓	–	↓	↓	↓	↑	↑

Data collected immediately after the discontinuation of exercise.

†Arrows (↓,↑): P < 0.05 Exercise vs. Baseline (rest).

QTc, van der Water's rate-corrected QT interval; TPE, Tpeak-Tend; QT/TQ, index reflecting the steepness of restitution; TSD, Standard deviation of the T-Wave amplitude.

of electrotonic coupling. Indeed, the heterogeneous distribution of the myocardial autonomic innervation, would favor the onset of "focal" arrhythmias during β-AR stimulation (Myles et al., 2012).

STUDY LIMITATIONS

This study demonstrated that β-adrenoceptor activation mediates exercise-driven changes (increased) in myocardial electrotonic coupling. However, it also should be noted that despite complete β-adrenoceptor blockade, a moderate decrease in MEI was observed during exercise. Several factors, that were not assessed in the present study, may have contributed to the residual (non-β-AR mediated) increases in myocardial electrotonic coupling during exercise.

For instance, during exercise, circulating cathecholamines activate both β- and α-adrenoceptors. Interestingly, sub-chronic α-adrenergic stimulation has been reported to exert PKC-mediated enhancements in connexin43 expression (Salameh et al., 2006). Furthermore, Rojas-Gomez et al. (2008) found that phenylephrine (an α-adrenergic receptor agonist) enhanced Cx43 expression in neonatal rat cardiac myocytes, resulting in enhanced gap-junction conductance. However, it also should be noted that opposite electrotonic (i.e., reductions in junctional conductance) have been reported during acute α-adrenoceptor stimulation (De Mello, 1997; de Boer et al., 2007), albeit these effects may vary in the setting of concomitant β-adrenoceptor stimulation (Salameh et al., 2010). Similarly, the renin-angiotensin system is also acutely activated during exercise, increasing the circulating levels of angiotensin-II, which can modulate the passive electrical properties of the myocardium (De Mello, 1996b, 2014; Sovari et al., 2013).

Also, as noted above, changes in both spatial/geometrical and/or ionic composition of the myocardium can alter its electrotonic properties. For example, Veeraraghavan et al. (2012) recently reported that changes in interstitial volume can modulate both conduction velocity and its dependence on gap-junction conductance. Changes in interstitial and/or myocyte volumes during exercise are likely, particularly given the reported ionic, metabolic, and plasma-volume changes during exercise (Paterson, 1996); interestingly, β-AR activation has been implicated in the volume-regulation (i.e., decrease) of cardiac myocytes (Wang et al., 1997). Thus, β-adrenoceptor mediated changes in myocyte volume could also contribute to the exercise-induced changes MEI reported in the present study.

Similarly, changes in both cell-to-cell coupling (e.g., Burt and Spray, 1988; Saffitz and Yamada, 1998; Salameh and Dhein, 2013) and global indices of myocardial passive electrical properties (e.g., Sasaki et al., 1994; Dekker et al., 1996; Howie et al., 2001) have been linked/associated with alterations in the mechanical properties of the myocardium. Indeed, in isolated myocytes, positive/negative inotropic agents have been shown to enhance/depress (respectively) junctional coupling in parallel with their functional effects (Burt and Spray, 1988; Dhein, 2004). In the present study, both exercise and direct pharmacological β-AR stimulation (with isoproterenol), two well-defined inotropic interventions, decreased MEI, consistent with an enhanced electrotonic coupling. Although neither systemic/cardiac hemodynamics nor mechanics were assessed directly in the present study, previous studies have extensively documented the hemodynamic/functional responses of susceptible/resistant post-MI dogs, both at rest and during exercise (e.g., Billman et al., 1985, 1997; De Ferrari et al., 1993; Avendano and Billman, 1994). For instance, Billman et al. (1985) reported comparable increases in the peak rate of left-ventricular pressure change (i.e., dP/dtmax—an inotropic index) during exercise in both groups of post-MI dogs, with animals prone to arrhythmias showing larger elevations in ventricular filling (end-diastolic) pressures (consistent with the exercise-driven preload changes, Miyazaki et al., 1990) and blunted increases in systolic pressures. Meanwhile, Avendano and Billman (1994) described similar inotropic/hemodynamic changes (i.e., dP/dtmax and systolic pressure increases) following isoproterenol administration (and other interventions that increased cAMP levels) in post-MI dogs and, in contrast to exercise, moderate isoproterenol-mediated end-diastolic pressure reductions were also noted (consistent with pre-load reductions Barnes et al., 1979). Hence, as mechanical stretch can alter intercellular coupling (Salameh and Dhein, 2013), it is possible that exercise-mediated changes in myocardial wall-tension could also play a role in the passive electrical changes that were observed in the present study. Finally, neither myocardial nor core body temperature were measured during exercise in this study. Notably, the resistivity of a medium can decrease as temperature increases (e.g., 2%/°C; Tsai et al., 2002). However, previously unpublished data from our laboratory (Billman GE, and del Rio CL) found that core body temperature not only increased moderately (~1°C) during exercise, but also, recovered slowly post-exercise (consistent with the limited heat-dissipation of dogs); an observation that contrasts with the rapid restoration of electrotonic coupling following the termination of exercise. Thus, changes in myocardial temperature induced by exercise probably did not contribute to the MEI changes noted in the present study.

In conclusion, the results of the present study demonstrate that β-AR activation during exercise can acutely enhance passive electrical properties (i.e., electrotonic coupling) of the myocardium, particularly in post-MI dogs susceptible to ischemia-induced VF. Increased coupling during β-AR stimulation may have important clinical implications, as it could mask intrinsic (and/or acquired) pro-arrhythmic repolarization abnormalities during states of autonomic activation (e.g., exercise) *in vivo*.

ACKNOWLEDGMENTS

This study was supported in part by a National Heart, Lung, and Blood Institute Grant, HL-68609 (GEB).

REFERENCES

Adabag, A. S., Luepker, R. V., Roger, V. L., and Gersh, B. J. (2010). Sudden cardiac death: epidemiology and risk factors. *Nat. Rev. Cardiol.* 7, 216–225. doi: 10.1038/nrcardio.2010.3

Altschuld, R. A., and Billman, G. E. (2000). Beta(2)-Adrenoceptors and ventricular fibrillation. *Pharmacol. Ther.* 88, 1–14. doi: 10.1016/S0163-7258(00)00075-9

Amit, G., Rosenbaum, D. S., Super, D. M., and Costantini, O. (2010). Microvolt T-wave alternans and electrophysiologic testing predict distinct arrhythmia substrates: implications for identifying patients at risk for sudden cardiac death. *Heart Rhythm* 7, 763–768. doi: 10.1016/j.hrthm.2010.02.012

Avendano, C. E., and Billman, G. E. (1994). Effect of interventions that increase cyclic AMP levels on susceptibility to ventricular fibrillation in unanesthetized dogs. *Eur. J. Pharmacol.* 255, 99–109.

Barnes, G. E., Horwitz, L. D., and Bishop, V. S. (1979). Reliability of the maximum derivatives of left ventricular pressure and internal diameter as indices of the inotropic state of the depressed myocardium. *Cardiovasc. Res.* 13, 652–662.

Belevych, A. E., Terentyev, D., Terentyeva, R., Ho, H. T., Gyorke, I., Bonilla, I. M., et al. (2012). Shortened Ca2+ signaling refractoriness underlies cellular arrhythmogenesis in a postinfarction model of sudden cardiac death. *Circ. Res.* 110, 569–577. doi: 10.1161/CIRCRESAHA.111.260455

Belevych, A. E., Terentyev, D., Viatchenko-Karpinski, S., Terentyeva, R., Sridhar, A., Nishijima, Y., et al. (2009). Redox modification of ryanodine receptors underlies calcium alternans in a canine model of sudden cardiac death. *Cardiovasc. Res.* 84, 387–395. doi: 10.1093/cvr/cvp246

Billman, G. E. (1989). Effect of calcium channel antagonists on susceptibility to sudden cardiac death: protection from ventricular fibrillation. *J. Pharmacol. Exp. Ther.* 248, 1334–1342.

Billman, G. E. (2006). A comprehensive review and analysis of 25 years of data from an *in vivo* canine model of sudden cardiac death: implications for future anti-arrhythmic drug development. *Pharmacol. Ther.* 111, 808–835. doi: 10.1016/j.pharmthera.2006.01.002

Billman, G. E., Castillo, L. C., Hensley, J., Hohl, C. M., and Altschuld, R. A. (1997). Beta2-adrenergic receptor antagonists protect against ventricular fibrillation: *in vivo* and *in vitro* evidence for enhanced sensitivity to beta2-adrenergic stimulation in animals susceptible to sudden death. *Circulation* 96, 1914–1922.

Billman, G. E., and Dujardin, J. P. (1990). Dynamic changes in cardiac vagal tone as measured by time-series analysis. *Am. J. Physiol.* 258(Pt 2), H896–H902.

Billman, G. E., and Hoskins, R. S. (1989). Time-series analysis of heart rate variability during submaximal exercise. Evidence for reduced cardiac vagal tone in animals susceptible to ventricular fibrillation. *Circulation* 80, 146–157.

Billman, G. E., Schwartz, P. J., Gagnol, J. P., and Stone, H. L. (1985). Cardiac response to submaximal exercise in dogs susceptible to sudden cardiac death. *J. Appl. Physiol.* 59, 890–897.

Bishop, M. J., Connolly, A., and Plank, G. (2014). Structural heterogeneity modulates effective refractory period: a mechanism of focal arrhythmia initiation. *PLoS ONE* 9:e109754. doi: 10.1371/journal.pone.0109754

Bonilla, I. M., Belevych, A. E., Sridhar, A., Nishijima, Y., Ho, H. T., He, Q., et al. (2012). Endurance exercise training normalizes repolarization and calcium-handling abnormalities, preventing ventricular fibrillation in a model of sudden cardiac death. *J. Appl. Physiol.* 113, 1772–1783. doi: 10.1152/japplphysiol.00175.2012

Brice, G., and Stone, H. L. (1986). Exercise tolerance and compensatory sympathetic tone during beta-blockade after myocardial infarction. *Med. Sci. Sports Exerc.* 18, 396–401.

Burt, J. M., and Spray, D. C. (1988). Inotropic agents modulate gap junctional conductance between cardiac myocytes. *Am. J. Physiol.* 254(Pt 2), H1206–H1210.

Cantillon, D. J., Stein, K. M., Markowitz, S. M., Mittal, S., Shah, B. K., Morin, D. P., et al. (2007). Predictive value of microvolt T-wave alternans in patients with left ventricular dysfunction. *J. Am. Coll. Cardiol.* 50, 166–173. doi: 10.1016/j.jacc.2007.02.069

Cascio, W. E., Yang, H., Muller-Borer, B. J., and Johnson, T. A. (2005). Ischemia-induced arrhythmia: the role of connexins, gap junctions, and attendant changes in impulse propagation. *J. Electrocardiol.*38, 55–59. doi: 10.1016/j.jelectrocard.2005.06.019

Cascio, W. E., Yan, G. X., and Kléber, A. G. (1990). Passive electrical properties, mechanical activity, and extracellular potassium in arterially perfused and ischemic rabbit ventricular muscle. Effects of calcium entry blockade or hypocalcemia. *Circ. Res.* 66, 1461–1473.

Chan, P. S., Gold, M. R., and Nallamothu, B. K. (2010). Do Beta-blockers impact microvolt T-wave alternans testing in patients at risk for ventricular arrhythmias? a meta-analysis. *J. Cardiovasc. Electrophysiol.* 21, 1009–1014. doi: 10.1111/j.1540-8167.2010.01757.x

Chen, L. S., Zhou, S., Fishbein, M. C., and Chen, P. S. (2007). New perspectives on the role of autonomic nervous system in the genesis of arrhythmias. *J. Cardiovasc. Electrophysiol.* 18, 123–127. doi: 10.1111/j.1540-8167.2006.00590.x

Cherry, E. M., and Fenton, F. H. (2004). Suppression of alternans and conduction blocks despite steep APD restitution: electrotonic, memory, and conduction velocity restitution effects. *Am. J. Physiol. Heart Circ. Physiol.* 286, H2332–H2341. doi: 10.1152/ajpheart.00747.2003

Collins, M. N., and Billman, G. E. (1989). Autonomic response to coronary occlusion in animals susceptible to ventricular fibrillation. *Am. J. Physiol.* 257(Pt 2), H1886–H1894.

de Boer, T. P., van Rijen, H. V., Van der Heyden, M. A., Kok, B., Opthof, T., Vos, M. A., et al. (2007). Beta-, not alpha-adrenergic stimulation enhances conduction velocity in cultures of neonatal cardiomyocytes. *Circ. J.* 71, 973–981. doi: 10.1253/circj.71.973

De Ferrari, G. M., Salvati, P., Grossoni, M., Ukmar, G., Vaga, L., Patrono, C., et al. (1993). Pharmacologic modulation of the autonomic nervous system in the prevention of sudden cardiac death. A study with propranolol, methacholine and oxotremorine in conscious dogs with a healed myocardial infarction. *J. Am. Coll. Cardiol.* 22, 283–290.

De Groot, J. R., and Coronel, R. (2004). Acute ischemia-induced gap junctional uncoupling and arrhythmogenesis. *Cardiovasc. Res.* 62, 323–334. doi: 10.1016/j.cardiores.2004.01.033

Dekker, L. R., Fiolet, J. W., VanBavel, E., Coronel, R., Opthof, T., Spaan, J. A., et al. (1996). Intracellular Ca2+, intercellular electrical coupling, and mechanical activity in ischemic rabbit papillary muscle. Effects of preconditioning and metabolic blockade. *Circ. Res.* 79, 237–246.

Delage, B., and Délèze, J. (1999). Chapter 9: a reexamination of calcium effects on gap junctions in heart myocytes. *Curr. Top Membr.* 49, 189–206.

Del Rio, C. L., Dawson, T. A., Clymer, B. D., Paterson, D. J., and Billman, G. E. (2008a). Effects of acute vagal nerve stimulation on the early passive electrical changes induced by myocardial ischaemia in dogs: heart rate-mediated attenuation. *Exp. Physiol.* 93, 931–944. doi: 10.1113/expphysiol.2007.041558

Del Rio, C. L., McConnell, P. I., Clymer, B. D., Dzwonczyk, R., Michler, R. E., Billman, G. E., et al. (2005). Early time course of myocardial electrical impedance during acute coronary artery occlusion in pigs, dogs, and humans. *J. Appl. Physiol.* 99, 1576–1581. doi: 10.1152/japplphysiol.00830.2004

Del Rio, C. L., McConnell, P. I., Kukielka, M., Dzwonczyk, R., Clymer, B. D., Howie, M. B., et al. (2008b). Electrotonic remodeling following myocardial infarction in dogs susceptible and resistant to sudden cardiac death. *J. Appl. Physiol.* 104, 386–393. doi: 10.1152/japplphysiol.01106.2007

De Mello, W. C. (1996a). Impaired regulation of cell communication by beta-adrenergic receptor activation in the failing heart. *Hypertension* 27, 265–268.

De Mello, W. C. (1996b). Renin-angiotensin system and cell communication in the failing heart. *Hypertension* 27, 1267–1272.

De Mello, W. C. (1997). Influence of alpha-adrenergic-receptor activation on junctional conductance in heart cells: interaction with beta-adrenergic adrenergic agonists. *J. Cardiovasc. Pharmacol.* 29, 273–277.

De Mello, W. C. (2010). Cell swelling impairs dye coupling in adult rat ventricular myocytes. Cell volume as a regulator of cell communication. *Mol. Cell. Biochem.* 343, 107–113. doi: 10.1007/s11010-010-0504-8

De Mello, W. C. (2014). Angiotensin (1-7) re-establishes heart cell communication previously impaired by cell swelling: implications for myocardial ischemia. *Exp. Cell. Res.* 323, 359–365. doi: 10.1016/j.yexcr.2014.03.006

Dhein, S. (2004). Pharmacology of gap junctions in the cardiovascular system. *Cardiovasc. Res.* 62, 287–298. doi: 10.1016/j.cardiores.2004.01.019

Duquesnes, N., Derangeon, M., Métrich, M., Lucas, A., Mateo, P., Li, L., et al. (2010). Epac stimulation induces rapid increases in connexin43 phosphorylation and function without preconditioning effect. *Pflugers Arch.* 460, 731–741. doi: 10.1007/s00424-010-0854-9

Dzwonczyk, R., del Rio, C., Brown, D. A., Michler, R. E., Wolf, R. K., and Howie, M. B. (2004). Myocardial electrical impedance responds to ischemia and reperfusion in humans. *IEEE Trans. Biomed. Eng.* 51, 2206–2209. doi: 10.1109/TBME.2004.834297

Fleischhauer, J., Lehmann, L., and Kléber, A. G. (1995). Electrical resistances of interstitial and microvascular space as determinants of the extracellular electrical field and velocity of propagation in ventricular myocardium. *Circulation* 92, 587–594.

Fossa, A. A., Wisialowski, T., Crimin, K., Wolfgang, E., Couderc, J. P., Hinterseer, M., et al. (2007). Analyses of dynamic beat-to-beat QT-TQ interval (ECG restitution) changes in humans under normal sinus rhythm and prior to an event of torsades de pointes during QT prolongation caused by sotalol. *Ann. Noninvasive. Electrocardiol.* 12, 338–348. doi: 10.1111/j.1542-474X.2007.00183.x

García-Dorado, D., Rodríguez-Sinovas, A., and Ruiz-Meana, M. (2004). Gap junction-mediated spread of cell injury and death during myocardial ischemia-reperfusion. *Cardiovasc. Res.* 61, 386–401. doi: 10.1016/j.cardiores.2003.11.039

Goldberger, J. J., Basu, A., Boineau, R., Buxton, A. E., Cain, M. E., Canty, J. M. Jr., et al. (2014). Risk stratification for sudden cardiac death: a plan for the future. *Circulation* 129, 516–526. doi: 10.1161/CIRCULATIONAHA.113.007149

Hennan, J. K., Swillo, R. E., Morgan, G. A., Keith, J. C. Jr., Schaub, R. G., Smith, R. P., et al. (2006). Rotigaptide (ZP123) prevents spontaneous ventricular arrhythmias and reduces infarct size during myocardial ischemia/reperfusion injury in open-chest dogs. *J. Pharmacol. Exp. Ther.* 317, 236–243. doi: 10.1124/jpet.105.096933

Himel, H. D. 4th., Garny, A., Noble, P. J., Wadgaonkar, R., Savarese, J., Liu, N., et al. (2013). Electrotonic suppression of early afterdepolarizations in the neonatal rat ventricular myocyte monolayer. *J. Physiol.* 591(Pt 21), 5357–5364. doi: 10.1113/jphysiol.2013.262923

Hohnloser, S. H., Klingenheben, T., Zabel, M., Li, Y. G., Albrecht, P., and Cohen, R. J. (1997). T wave alternans during exercise and atrial pacing in humans. *J. Cardiovasc. Electrophysiol.* 8, 987–993.

Houle, M. S., Altschuld, R. A., and Billman, G. E. (2001). Enhanced *in vivo* and *in vitro* contractile responses to beta(2)-adrenergic receptor stimulation in dogs susceptible to lethal arrhythmias. *J. Appl. Physiol.* 91, 1627–1637.

Howie, M. B., Dzwonczyk, R., and McSweeney, T. D. (2001). An evaluation of a new two-electrode myocardial electrical impedance monitor for detecting myocardial ischemia. *Anesth Analg.* 92, 12–18.

Huelsing, D. J., Spitzer, K. W., and Pollard, A. E. (2000). Electrotonic suppression of early afterdepolarizations in isolated rabbit Purkinje myocytes. *Am. J. Physiol. Heart Circ. Physiol.* 279, H250–H259.

Janse, M. J., Tan, H. L., Dekker, L. R. C., and Kléber, A. G. (2002). "Cellular electrical uncoupling during ischemia," in *Heart Cell Coupling and Impulse Propagation in Health and Disease*, eds W. C. de Mello, M. J. Janse (Boston; Dordrecht; London: Kluwer Academic Publishers), 257–282.

Järvenpää, J., Oikarinen, L., Korhonen, P., Väänänen, H., Toivonen, L., and Viitasalo, M. (2007). Changing capacity of electrocardiographic ventricular repolarization in post-myocardial infarction patients with and without nonfatal cardiac arrest. *Am. J. Cardiol.* 99, 295–299. doi: 10.1016/j.amjcard.2006.08.027

Jia, Z., Bien, H., Shiferaw, Y., and Entcheva, E. (2012). Cardiac cellular coupling and the spread of early instabilities in intracellular Ca2+. *Biophys. J.* 102, 1294–1302. doi: 10.1016/j.bpj.2012.02.034

Johnson, D. M., Heijman, J., Bode, E. F., Greensmith, D. J., van der Linde, H., Abi-Gerges, N., et al. (2013). Diastolic spontaneous calcium release from the sarcoplasmic reticulum increases beat-to-beat variability of repolarization in canine ventricular myocytes after β-adrenergic stimulation. *Circ. Res.* 112, 246–256. doi: 10.1161/CIRCRESAHA.112.275735

Joyner, R. W., Kumar, R., Wilders, R., Jongsma, H. J., Verheijck, E. E., Golod, D. A., et al. (1996). Modulating L-type calcium current affects discontinuous cardiac action potential conduction. *Biophys. J.* 71, 237–245.

Kijtawornrat, A., Panyasing, Y., Del Rio, C., and Hamlin, R. L. (2010). Assessment of ECG interval and restitution parameters in the canine model of short QT syndrome. *J. Pharmacol. Toxicol. Methods* 61, 231–237. doi: 10.1016/j.vascn.2010.02.001

Kjølbye, A. L., Dikshteyn, M., Eloff, B. C., Deschênes, I., and Rosenbaum, D. S. (2008). Maintenance of intercellular coupling by the antiarrhythmic peptide rotigaptide suppresses arrhythmogenic discordant alternans. *Am. J. Physiol. Heart Circ. Physiol.* 294, H41–H49. doi: 10.1152/ajpheart.01089.2006

Kléber, A. G., Riegger, C. B., and Janse, M. J. (1987). Electrical uncoupling and increase of extracellular resistance after induction of ischemia in isolated, arterially perfused rabbit papillary muscle. *Circ. Res.* 61, 271–279.

Kléber, G. (1992). The potential role of Ca2+ for electrical cell-to-cell uncoupling and conduction block in myocardial tissue. *Basic Res. Cardiol.* 87, 131–143.

Kraaier, K., Verhorst, P. M., van der Palen, J., van Dessel, P. F., Wilde, A. A., and Scholten, M. F. (2009). Microvolt T-wave alternans during exercise and pacing are not comparable. *Europace* 11, 1375–1380. doi: 10.1093/europace/eup253

Li, C., Meng, Q., Yu, X., Jing, X., Xu, P., and Luo, D. (2012). Regulatory effect of connexin 43 on basal Ca2+ signaling in rat ventricular myocytes. *PLoS ONE* 7:e36165. doi: 10.1371/journal.pone.0036165

Manoach, M., Varon, D., and Erez, M. (1995). The role of catecholamines on intercellular coupling, myocardial cell synchronization and self-ventricular defibrillation. *Mol. Cell Biochem.* 147, 181–185.

Merchant, F. M., Ikeda, T., Pedretti, R. F., Salerno-Uriarte, J. A., Chow, T., Chan, P. S., et al. (2012). Clinical utility of microvolt T-wave alternans testing in identifying patients at high or low risk of sudden cardiac death. *Heart Rhythm.* 9, 1256.e2–1264.e2. doi: 10.1016/j.hrthm.2012.03.014

Miyazaki, S., Guth, B. D., Miura, T., Indolfi, C., Schulz, R., Ross, J., et al. (1990). Changes of left ventricular diastolic function in exercising dogs without and with ischemia. *Circulation* 81, 1058–1070.

Mostafavi, H., Khaksarian, M., Joghataei, M. T., Soleimani, M., Hassanzadeh, G., Eftekhari, S., et al. (2014). Selective β2 adrenergic agonist increases Cx43 and miR-451 expression via cAMP-Epac. *Mol. Med. Rep.* 9, 2405–2410. doi: 10.3892/mmr.2014.2120

Myles, R. C., Wang, L., Kang, C., Bers, D. M., and Ripplinger, C. M. (2012). Local β-adrenergic stimulation overcomes source-sink mismatch to generate focal arrhythmia. *Circ. Res.* 110, 1454–1464. doi: 10.1161/CIRCRESAHA.111.262345

Nearing, B. D., and Verrier, R. L. (2002). Modified moving average analysis of T-wave alternans to predict ventricular fibrillation with high accuracy. *J. Appl. Physiol.* 92, 541–549. doi: 10.1152/japplphysiol.00592.2001

Obeyesekere, M. N., Klein, G. J., Modi, S., Leong-Sit, P., Gula, L. J., Yee, R., et al. (2011). How to perform and interpret provocative testing for the diagnosis of Brugada syndrome, long-QT syndrome, and catecholaminergic polymorphic ventricular tachycardia. *Circ. Arrhythm. Electrophysiol.* 4, 958–964. doi: 10.1161/CIRCEP.111.965947

Opthof, T., Coronel, R., Wilms-Schopman, F. J., Plotnikov, A. N., Shlapakova, I. N., Danilo, P. Jr., et al. (2007). Dispersion of repolarization in canine ventricle and the electrocardiographic T wave: Tp-e interval does not reflect transmural dispersion. *Heart Rhythm.* 4, 341–348. doi: 10.1016/j.hrthm.2006.11.022

Owens, L. M., Fralix, T. A., Murphy, E., Cascio, W. E., and Gettes, L. S. (1996). Correlation of ischemia-induced extracellular and intracellular ion changes to cell-to-cell electrical uncoupling in isolated blood-perfused rabbit hearts. *Circulation* 94, 10–13.

Pastore, J. M., and Rosenbaum, D. S. (2000). Role of structural barriers in the mechanism of alternans-induced reentry. *Circ. Res.* 87, 1157–1163. doi: 10.1161/01.RES.87.12.1157

Paterson, D. J. (1996). Antiarrhythmic mechanisms during exercise. *J. Appl. Physiol.* 80, 1853–1862.

Pokornı J., Stanìk, V., and Vrána, M. (2011). Sudden cardiac death thirty years ago and at present. The role of autonomic disturbances in acute myocardial infarction revisited. *Physiol. Res.* 60, 715–728.

Quan, X. Q., Bai, R., Liu, N., Chen, B. D., and Zhang, C. T. (2007). Increasing gap junction coupling reduces transmural dispersion of repolarization and prevents torsade de pointes in rabbit LQT3 model. *J. Cardiovasc. Electrophysiol.* 18, 1184–1189. doi: 10.1111/j.1540-8167.2007.00923.x

Raatikainen, M. J., Jokinen, V., Virtanen, V., Hartikainen, J., Hedman, A., and Huikuri, H. V. (2005). (CARISMA Investigators). Microvolt T-wave alternans during exercise and pacing in patients with acute myocardial infarction. *Pacing Clin. Electrophysiol.* 28. S193–S197. doi: 10.1111/j.1540-8159.2005.00110.x

Rojas-Gomez, D. M., Schulte, J. S., Mohr, F. W., and Dhein, S. (2008). Alpha-1-adrenoceptor subtype selective regulation of connexin 43 expression in rat cardiomyocytes. *Naunyn. Schmiedebergs Arch. Pharmacol.* 377, 77–85. doi: 10.1007/s00210-007-0244-9

Rubart, M., and Zipes, D. P. (2005). Mechanisms of sudden cardiac death. *J. Clin. Invest.* 115, 2305–2315. doi: 10.1172/JCI26381

Saffitz, J. E., and Kléber, A. G. (2012). Gap junctions, slow conduction, and ventricular tachycardia after myocardial infarction. *J. Am. Coll. Cardiol.* 60, 1111–1113. doi: 10.1016/j.jacc.2012.05.020

Saffitz, J. E., and Yamada, K. A. (1998). Do alterations in intercellular coupling play a role in cardiac contractile dysfunction? *Circulation* 97, 630–632.

Salameh, A., and Dhein, S. (2011). Adrenergic control of cardiac gap junction function and expression. *Naunyn. Schmiedebergs Arch. Pharmacol.* 383, 331–346. doi: 10.1007/s00210-011-0603-4

Salameh, A., and Dhein, S. (2013). Effects of mechanical forces and stretch on intercellular gap junction coupling. *Biochim. Biophys. Acta* 1828, 147–156. doi: 10.1016/j.bbamem.2011.12.030

Salameh, A., Frenzel, C., Boldt, A., Rassler, B., Glawe, I., Schulte, J., et al. (2006). Subchronic alpha- and beta-adrenergic regulation of cardiac gap junction protein expression. *FASEB J.* 20, 365–367. doi: 10.1096/fj.05-4871fje

Salameh, A., Karl, S., Djilali, H., Dhein, S., Janousek, J., and Daehnert, I. (2010). Opposing and synergistic effects of cyclic mechanical stretch and α- or β-adrenergic stimulation on the cardiac gap junction protein Cx43. *Pharmacol. Res.* 62, 506–513. doi: 10.1016/j.phrs.2010.08.002

Sasaki, E., Conger, J. L., Kadipasaoglu, K. A., Pehlivanoglu, S., and Frazier, O. H. (1994). Simultaneous evaluation of cardiac wall motion and myocardial ischemic injury by measurement of electrical impedance. *ASAIO J.* 40, M826–M829.

Sato, D., Shiferaw, Y., Garfinkel, A., Weiss, J. N., Qu, Z., and Karma, A. (2006). Spatially discordant alternans in cardiac tissue: role of calcium cycling. *Circ. Res.* 99, 520–527. doi: 10.1161/01.RES.0000240542.03986.e7

Shizuta, S., Ando, K., Nobuyoshi, M., Ikeda, T., Yoshino, H., Hiramatsu, S., et al. (2012). (PREVENT-SCD Investigators). Prognostic utility of T-wave alternans in a real-world population of patients with left ventricular dysfunction: the PREVENT-SCD study. *Clin. Res. Cardiol.* 101, 89–99. doi: 10.1007/s00392-011-0368-2

Smith, W. T. IV, Fleet, W. F., Johnson, T. A., Engle, C. L., and Cascio, W. E. (1995). The Ib phase of ventricular arrhythmias in ischemic *in situ* porcine heart is related to changes in cell-to-cell electrical coupling. *Circulation* 92, 3051–3060.

Somekawa, S., Fukuhara, S., Nakaoka, Y., Fujita, H., Saito, Y., and Mochizuki, N. (2005). Enhanced functional gap junction neoformation by protein kinase A-dependent and Epac-dependent signals downstream of cAMP in cardiac myocytes. *Circ. Res.* 97, 655–662. doi: 10.1161/01.RES.0000183880.49270.f9

Sovari, A. A., Rutledge, C. A., Jeong, E. M., Dolmatova, E., Arasu, D., Liu, H., et al. (2013). Mitochondria oxidative stress, connexin43 remodeling, and sudden arrhythmic death. *Circ. Arrhythm. Electrophysiol.* 6, 623–631. doi: 10.1161/CIRCEP.112.976787

Sridhar, A., Nishijima, Y., Terentyev, D., Terentyeva, R., Uelmen, R., Kukielka, M., et al. (2008). Repolarization abnormalities and afterdepolarizations in a canine model of sudden cardiac death. *Am. J. Physiol. Regul. Integr. Comp. Physiol.* 295, R1463–R1472. doi: 10.1152/ajpregu.90583.2008

Stone, H. L. (1977). Cardiac function and exercise training in conscious dogs. *J. Appl. Physiol.* 42, 824–832.

Takenaka, K., Ai, T., Shimizu, W., Kobori, A., Ninomiya, T., Otani, H., et al. (2003). Exercise stress test amplifies genotype-phenotype correlation in the LQT1 and LQT2 forms of the long-QT syndrome. *Circulation* 107, 838–844. doi: 10.1161/01.CIR.0000048142.85076.A2

Tsai, J. Z., Will, J. A., Hubbard-Van Stelle, S., Cao, H., Tungjitkusolmun, S., Choy, Y. B., et al. (2002). Error analysis of tissue resistivity measurement. *IEEE Trans. Biomed. Eng.* 49, 484–494. doi: 10.1109/10.995687

Van de Water, A., Verheyen, J., Xhonneux, R., and Reneman, R. S. (1989). An improved method to correct the QT interval of the electrocardiogram for changes in heart rate. *J. Pharmacol. Methods* 22, 207–117.

Vanoli, E., Priori, S. G., Nakagawa, H., Hirao, K., Napolitano, C., Diehl, L., et al. (1995). Sympathetic activation, ventricular repolarization and Ikr blockade: implications for the antifibrillatory efficacy of potassium channel blocking agents. *J. Am. Coll. Cardiol.* 25, 1609–1614.

Veeraraghavan, R., Salama, M. E., and Poelzing, S. (2012). Interstitial volume modulates the conduction velocity-gap junction relationship. *Am. J. Physiol. Heart Circ. Physiol.* 302, H278–H286. doi: 10.1152/ajpheart.00868.2011

Verrier, R. L., Klingenheben, T., Malik, M., El-Sherif, N., Exner, D. V., Hohnloser, S. H., et al. (2011). Microvolt T-wave alternans physiological basis, methods of measurement, and clinical utility–consensus guideline by international society for holter and noninvasive electrocardiology. *J. Am. Coll. Cardiol.* 58, 1309–1324. doi: 10.1016/j.jacc.2011.06.029

Wang, Z., Mitsuiye, T., Rees, S. A., and Noma, A. (1997). Regulatory volume decrease of cardiac myocytes induced by beta-adrenergic activation of the Cl-channel in guinea pig. *J. Gen. Physiol.* 110, 73–82.

Watanabe, M. A., Fenton, F. H., Evans, S. J., Hastings, H. M., and Karma, A. (2001). Mechanisms for discordant alternans. *J. Cardiovasc. Electrophysiol.* 12, 196–206. doi: 10.1046/j.1540-8167.2001.00196.x

Wellens, H. J., Schwartz, P. J., Lindemans, F. W., Buxton, A. E., Goldberger, J. J., Hohnloser, S. H., et al. (2014). Risk stratification for sudden cardiac death: current status and challenges for the future. *Eur. Heart J.* 35, 1642–1651. doi: 10.1093/eurheartj/ehu176

Wit, A. L., and Peters, N. S. (2012). The role of gap junctions in the arrhythmias of ischemia and infarction. *Heart Rhythm.* 9, 308–311. doi: 10.1016/j.hrthm.2011.09.056

Xia, Y., Gong, K. Z., Xu, M., Zhang, Y. Y., Guo, J. H., Song, Y., et al. (2009). Regulation of gap-junction protein connexin 43 by beta-adrenergic receptor stimulation in rat cardiomyocytes. *Acta Pharmacol. Sin.* 30, 928–934. doi: 10.1038/aps.2009.92

Yan, G. X., and Antzelevitch, C. (1998). Cellular basis for the normal T wave and the electrocardiographic manifestations of the long-QT syndrome. *Circulation* 98, 1928–1936.

Zaman, S., and Kovoor, P. (2014). Sudden cardiac death early after myocardial infarction: pathogenesis, risk stratification, and primary prevention. *Circulation* 129, 2426–2435. doi: 10.1161/CIRCULATIONAHA.113.007497

4

Passive ventricular remodeling in cardiac disease: Focus on heterogeneity

Elise L. Kessler[1], Mohamed Boulaksil[1,2], Harold V. M. van Rijen[1], Marc A. Vos[1] and Toon A. B. van Veen[1]*

[1] *Division of Heart and Lungs, Department of Medical Physiology, University Medical Center Utrecht, Utrecht, Netherlands*
[2] *Department of Cardiology, Radboud University Medical Center, Nijmegen, Netherlands*

***Correspondence:**
Toon A. B. van Veen, University Medical Center Utrecht, Department of Medical Physiology, Division of Heart and Lungs, Yalelaan 50, Utrecht 3584 CM, Netherlands
e-mail: a.a.b.vanveen@umcutrecht.nl

Passive ventricular remodeling is defined by the process of molecular ventricular adaptation to different forms of cardiac pathophysiology. It includes changes in tissue architecture, such as hypertrophy, fiber disarray, alterations in cell size and fibrosis. Besides that, it also includes molecular remodeling of gap junctions, especially those composed by Connexin43 proteins (Cx43) in the ventricles that affect cell-to-cell propagation of the electrical impulse, and changes in the sodium channels that modify excitability. All those alterations appear mainly in a heterogeneous manner, creating irregular and inhomogeneous electrical and mechanical coupling throughout the heart. This can predispose to reentry arrhythmias and adds to a further deterioration into heart failure. In this review, passive ventricular remodeling is described in Hypertrophic Cardiomyopathy (HCM), Dilated Cardiomyopathy (DCM), Ischemic Cardiomyopathy (ICM), and Arrhythmogenic Cardiomyopathy (ACM), with a main focus on the heterogeneity of those alterations mentioned above.

Keywords: gap junction, sodium channel, fibrosis, arrhythmias, heterogeneity

INTRODUCTION

The lifelong purpose of the heart is maintenance of cardiac output and supply of all organs with an appropriate amount of oxygen and nutrients. At the same time it steers the controlled homeostasis of the blood via clearance of waste products, drugs and imbalanced levels of ions and proteins in the lungs, liver, and kidneys. To be able to fulfill this task, the heart has to adapt its workload to the needs of the body (Kemp and Conte, 2012). Many different diseases like coronary artery disease, myocardial infarction, hypertension, dysfunction of valves, congenital heart disease, lung diseases, diabetes, anemia, hyperthyroidism, and or arrhythmia/dysrhythmia can alter the performance of the heart (Lloyd-Jones et al., 2002; van Rijen et al., 2006; Roger et al., 2011). In order to preserve cardiac output under these conditions, the heart will start several compensatory mechanisms, like the Frank Starling mechanism, neurohumoral activation, and inflammational responses (Westerhof and O'Rourke, 1995; Lee and Tkacs, 2008). Moreover, the heart starts to modify the gene program that shapes the individual cells that compose the organ. This in an attempt to adapt chronically to the new requirements of its environment. These adaptations together will result in myocardial remodeling that most often has heterogeneous characteristics (Swynghedauw, 1999).

By nature, the heart itself is a rather heterogeneous organ: morphologically, the right and left side as well as atria and ventricles show various differences in cell constellations, hemodynamics and their respective electrical characteristics (Zimmer, 1994). The different resistances in peripheral and pulmonary circulation for instance are causative for the differences between left and right ventricle anatomy (right ventricular wall is much thinner than the left wall). Also with respect to molecular make-up and microarchitecture of the cardiac muscle significant differences exist. The way the fibers are orientated within the left and right ventricle is not comparable. Electrical impulse propagation faces differences in conduction velocity between left and right ventricles but also with the specialized conduction system. Part of that relies on differences in expression level and pattern of gap junction channels and the ion channels that underlie action potential generation.

The sodium channel protein Nav1.5, for instance, is heterogeneously distributed throughout the ventricles and the cardiac conduction system in healthy hearts (Remme et al., 2009). Besides that, two pools of Nav1.5 channels can be found in cardiomyocytes: a lateral pool and a pool in the intercalated disc that coexist and interact with different proteins (Petitprez et al., 2011). Also Cx43 is found in different densities within the healthy heart e.g., regarding the posterior and anterior wall of the ventricles (Strom et al., 2010).

Beyond the natural heterogeneity that is found under the normal physiological functioning of the heart, this review will focus on the heterogenic aspect that is involved in passive remodeling of the ventricles under pathophysiological conditions. Passive remodeling is defined as the chronic molecular and structural adaptations in ventricular cardiomyocytes and alterations in gene expression as induced by different forms of heart disease. Active remodeling, in contrast, is defined as phosphorylation processes that e.g., result from sympathic and parasympathic imbalance. This is exampled by the increase in heart rate that is facilitated through alterations in phosphorylation of ion channels (e.g., L–type calcium channels) in the sinus node.

One of the most crucial and maladaptive factors of passive remodeling in the ventricles is heterogeneity in electrical and structural remodeling. In that perspective we will discuss factors associated with conduction and propagation of excitation, but not with respect to repolarization (e.g., potassium currents, heterogeneity in action potential duration), and contraction (e.g., calcium-handling and sarcomeric proteins). During remodeling, heterogeneous alterations in three factors contribute to increase the propensity to arrhythmias and to develop heart failure: (1) tissue architecture such as hypertrophy, fibrosis, fiber disarray, and cell size, (2) electrical coupling by means of gap junctions and especially those composed of Cx43, and (3) electrical excitability due to changes in sodium channels that are mainly composed of Nav1.5 (Kleber and Rudy, 2004; van Rijen et al., 2006; Bowers et al., 2010).

We will address remodeling of these factors during Dilated Cardiomyopathy (DCM), Hypertrophic Cardiomyopathy (HCM), Ischemic Cardiomyopathy (ICM) and Arrhythmogenic Cardiomyopathy (ACM), previously known as Arrhythmogenic Right Ventricular Cardiomyopathy/Dysplasia (ARVC/D). In general, DCM can be identified by cardiac chamber dilatation and reduced systolic function often leading to congestive heart failure. It is the most commonly occurring cardiomyopathy in adults and children and is associated with muscle dysfunction and/or volume overload. On the other hand, in children DCM is mostly caused by myocarditis and neurohumoral diseases (Towbin et al., 2006). DCM is defined as the presence of left ventricular fractional shortening (<25%) and/or LVEF < 45% and left ventricular end-diastolic dimensions (LVEDD) of >117% of the predicted value by the Henry formula (Mestroni et al., 1999). It can also be caused by a variety of genetic mutations that are uncovered upon analysis of family history and molecular genetic testing. These forms, however, are referred to as familial dilated cardiomyopathy (FDC) (Hershberger and Morales, 2013). HCM has been defined by the World Health Organization as the presence of left or biventricular hypertrophy, in absence of any cardiac or systemic cause (Richardson et al., 1996). When this definition is used, the general prevalence is about 1:500 (Maron, 2002). However, HCM can also be caused by mutations in genes encoding for cardiac sarcomeric and myofilament proteins; for the latter already more than 1400 mutations have been identified increasing the prevalence even more (Maron et al., 2012; Efthimiadis et al., 2014).

ICM results from myocardial ischemia and is characterized by remodeling due to myocardial infarction which eventually triggers loss of contractility, still being the leading cause of ventricular dysfunction worldwide (reviewed in Wu, 2007).

Finally, ACM is a non-ischemic progressive and predominantly heritable heart disease associated with cardiac arrhythmias and sudden cardiac death (Corrado et al., 2000). ACM is characterized through replacement of cardiomyocytes by fibro-fatty tissue (Thiene et al., 1988; Saffitz et al., 2009). About 60% of the cases have a hereditary basis and mutations causing ACM have been found in several desmosomal genes like desmoplakin (Rampazzo et al., 2002), plakoglobin (Asimaki et al., 2007), plakophilin2 (Gerull et al., 2004; van Tintelen et al., 2006), desmocollin2 (Heuser et al., 2006; Syrris et al., 2006), and desmoglein (Pilichou et al., 2006). Moreover, genes not related to the desmosome can be affected such as the transmembrane protein 43 (TMEM43), phospholamban (PLN), desmin and transforming growth factor beta3 (TGFβ3) (Beffagna et al., 2005; Merner et al., 2008; Otten et al., 2010; van der Zwaag et al., 2012).

In addition, a variety of mutations in several ion channels that add to action potential generation have been described to trigger pro-arrhythmic remodeling of the heart. This subset of arrhythmogenic cardiac diseases is, however, beyond the scope of this review.

TISSUE ARCHITECTURE

Several extrinsic and intrinsic factors can lead to alterations in cardiac workload. Those changes can trigger growth of individual myocytes leading to cardiac hypertrophy. An increased amount of hypertrophy is associated with a decreased conduction velocity of the electrical impulse (Winterton et al., 1994; Cooklin et al., 1997; McIntyre and Fry, 1997). Moreover, metaplasia of fibroblasts into myofibroblasts, a more contractile and collagen producing cell type can increase the deposition of the extracellular matrix (ECM) leading to fibrosis (Davis and Molketin, 2013). This is further supported by an increased rate of cell death—necrosis and apoptosis—and inflammatory processes such as the secretion of TNF-alpha or IL-6 (Gill et al., 2002; Nian et al., 2004). Besides that, also alterations in myocardial fiber orientation can importantly affect characteristics of cardiac impulse propagation (Vetter et al., 2005).

HYPERTROPHY AND CELL SIZE

The key feature of hypertrophy in general is an increased cell size that electrically can be measured as an increase in cell-capacitance. Hypertrophy and increased cell size counteract the increased wall tension as caused by changes in cardiac workload (Laplace's law). Therefore, hypertrophy is seen as a compensatory mechanism. However, cardiac impulse propagation as well as conduction velocity gradually decrease with increasing severity of hypertrophy (Winterton et al., 1994; Cooklin et al., 1997; McIntyre and Fry, 1997) leading to an elevated risk for heart failure and sudden cardiac death (Meyerburg et al., 1992).

In DCM mainly the cell length is increased and this is associated by dilation and systolic disturbances of predominantly the left ventricle. Also both ventricles can be impaired, but generally with normal left ventricular wall thickness (Richardson et al., 1996; DuPont et al., 2001). The effect of eccentric hypertrophy on electrical signaling has been addressed in several animal models. An increase in conduction velocity was shown in a rabbit model, where a combined pressure- and volume overload increased heart weight by about 100%, and both cell length and width were increased by about 30%. Delayed activation was indicated by an increase in QRS duration from 50 ms in control to 58 ms in rabbits with DCM. Parallel and transverse to fiber orientation, however, epicardial conduction velocity appeared increased by 18 and 16%, respectively while transmural conduction velocity was unchanged. The authors of this study concluded that the increased cell size was responsible for the increase in longitudinal and transverse conduction velocity. Moreover, they concluded that the increased conduction velocity could not sufficiently compensate for the increased heart size, which was causative for the prolonged QRS durations (Wiegerinck et al., 2006). In a dog model of rapid pacing, it has been shown that QRS duration and cell length were increased, while cell width was reduced. Besides, transmural conduction velocity was reduced in both RV and LV, while Cx43 expression was reduced only in LV. As such, reduced cell width seems to play a dominant role in the reduced conduction velocity (Akar et al., 2004). In mice models, where DCM was induced by transverse aortic constriction (TAC), cell size, and the amount of hypertrophy was significantly increased after 6 weeks of TAC. This was leading to prolongations of PQ, QT, and QRS intervals, and slowing of right ventricular conduction velocity parallel to the fiber orientation (Boulaksil et al., 2010b). Data of a recent study with DCM patients showed elevated levels of myosin light-chain kinase and CRP that could possibly serve as diagnostic biomarkers for hypertrophy (Branishte et al., 2013).

In HCM, primarily cell width is increased (Formigli et al., 2003) leading to hypertrophy without dilation of the ventricles (Maron, 2002). This affects conduction of the electrical impulse as has been shown using computer modeling, where conduction velocity increased with cell size, and cell size was determined to be the dominant factor affecting conduction velocity (Spach et al., 2000). Also for HCM, several animal models have been described. In a rat model, where RV-HCM was induced by injections with monocrotaline (leading to pulmonary hypertension), increased cell width and lateralized Cx43 expression were found, while cell length was unaffected. Conduction velocity parallel to the fiber orientation was decreased, although perpendicular to the fiber orientation the conduction velocity was unchanged (Uzzaman et al., 2000). Similar results were obtained in another study that used the same rat model with monocrotaline induced pressure overload. In this study, RV cell width was increased, but again cell length remained unaffected. In the left ventricle, cell width and length were both decreased. Moreover, longer action potentials (at 90% repolarization), prolongation of the effective refractory period, and slowing of the longitudinal conduction velocity occurred (Hardziyenka et al., 2012). Besides the rat model, LV epicardial mapping was also performed in patients after chronic thromboembolic pulmonary hypertension. Comparable to the experimental model, these patients also showed prolongation of the effective refractory period and conduction slowing (Hardziyenka et al., 2012).

In ICM, cardiac hypertrophy can be found in the majority of patients (Kannel et al., 1961; Zaino and Tabor, 1963). In MRL (Murphy Roths Large) mice exhibiting an ICM phenotype, increased cell size and hypertrophy lead to a faster progression toward heart failure than in controls (Smiley et al., 2014). Moreover, electrocardiographic left ventricular hypertrophy embedded a predictive value for arrhythmias and mortality in ICM patients, making it an important factor to consider during diagnosis (Bender et al., 2012). In ACM no gross cardiac hypertrophy has been reported and the individual cell size is not increased either. Therefore, hypertrophy is not included as a parameter into the revised Task Force Criteria that are used to diagnose ACM (Marcus et al., 2010).

FIBROSIS AND MYOCARDIAL FIBER DISARRAY

In the healthy heart, cardiac myocytes are embedded in the ECM, a network of multiple molecules, proteins and thin intertwining strands of collagen fibers, synthesized by cardiac fibroblasts (Manabe et al., 2002). This network ensures tissue strength and allows cell-cell contact between neighboring cells (Weber et al., 1994). Cardiac fibrosis is the inappropriately high amount of collagen deposition in the heart during pathophysiological remodeling which hampers electrical conduction and enables the development of arrhythmias (Krenning et al., 2010). In addition, also cardiomyocyte fiber orientation plays an important role in the propagation of the electrical signal and fiber disarray can further facilitate the generation of ventricular arrhythmias (Brugada et al., 1991; Punske et al., 2005) This was recently shown in a study that combined data from neonatal rat cardiomyocytes and computer models (Kudryashova et al., 2014).

Fibrosis can be divided into replacement fibrosis (compact and patchy) and reactive fibrosis (interstitial and diffuse) (Swynghedauw, 1999). Typical examples of these four different forms we published before and are expressed in **Figure 1** of a review article by the de Jong et al. (2011). Replacement fibrosis occurs after clearance of dead myocytes, where cardiac cells will be replaced by collagen fibers facilitating the preservation of the structure of the myocardium as well as the clearance of debris (de Jong et al., 2011). This normally includes compact or patchy fibrosis that is generated after an infarct or in due to chronic pressure overload. These processes have been described both in patients and in experimental animal models (Xia et al., 2009). Compact fibrosis is created, when a whole area is replaced by fibrosis and no viable myocytes are left. Although this seems to be dramatic for the cardiac contractile performance, this form is the least arrhythmogenic (de Bakker et al., 1988). Patchy fibrosis describes areas, where fibrosis and myocardial cells are confounded. In this case, collagen fibers are long strands disturbing the electrical signal propagation (de Bakker et al., 1993). Reactive fibrosis describes the process when more collagen is produced than degraded without a loss of viable cardiomyocytes. This includes interstitial and diffuse fibrosis and can be caused by mutations and changes in gene expression, a phenotypical switch from fibroblasts into myofibroblasts, as well as due to aging (Biernacka and Frangogiannis, 2011). Interstitial fibrosis is localized in between the individual cells. High interstitial collagen content causes reduced compliance and electrical impairment (Rohr, 2009) possibly leading to arrhythmias and heart failure (Janicki and Brower, 2002). Diffuse fibrosis is comparable to patchy fibrosis, however, the collagen strands are short and this form is less arrhythmogenic (Kawara et al., 2001).

In murine animal models that can be followed and analyzed at different time points after the experimental intervention has been made, chronic pressure overload initially leads to reactive fibrosis and in later stages this may change into a heterogeneous deposition of replacement fibrosis. The switch is likely caused by the fact that at a certain time point proper nutrient supply to the cells fails

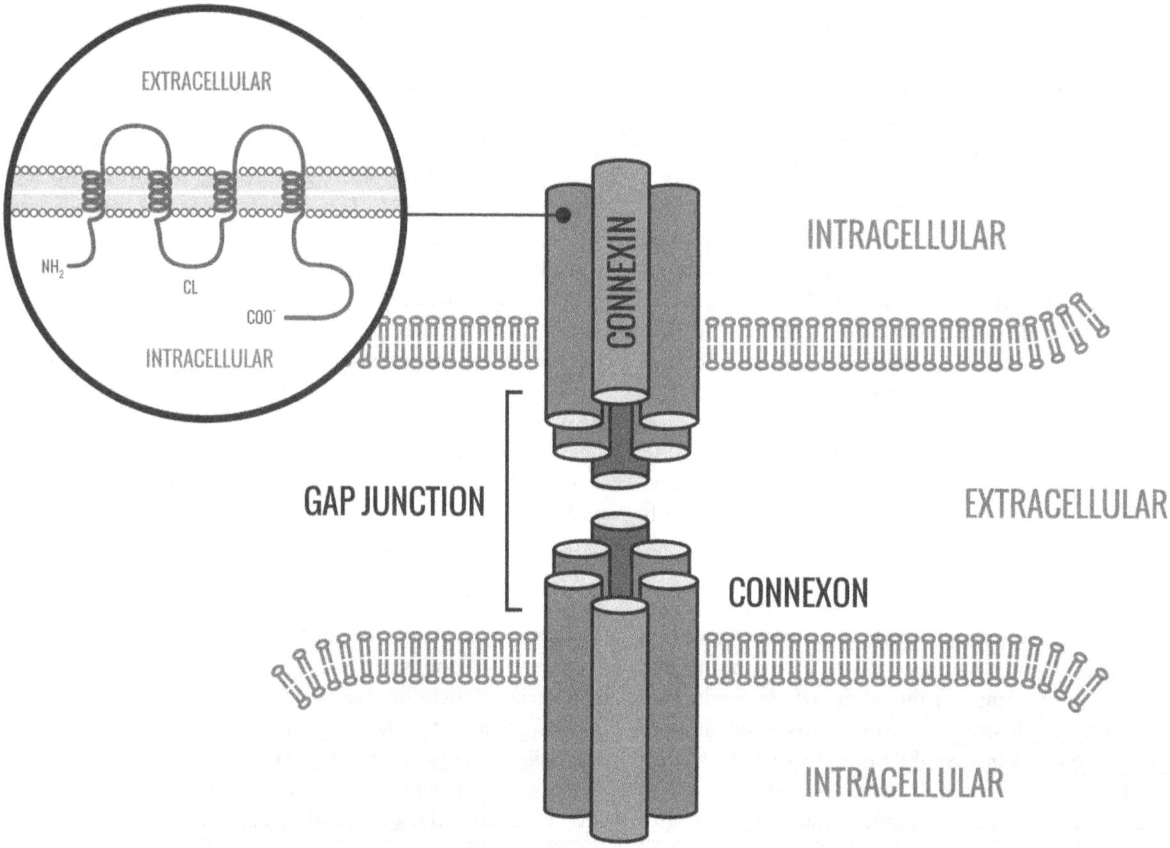

FIGURE 1 | The cardiac gap junction. Gap junctions are located in the intercalated disc. They consist of two hemichannels (connexons) connecting across the intercellular space. Each hemichannel is provided by one cell and connexons are composed of six hexagonally arranged connexin proteins.

to maintain a minimal level (Isoyama and Nitta-Komatsubara, 2002).

Myocardial fiber disarray is the result of altered fiber orientation after e.g., an infarct. Adjacent cardiomyocytes are then mostly aligned in a perpendicular way or obliquely to each other in or around the collagen (Hughes, 2004). Nowadays, predominantly computer models are used to simulate possible alterations and effects on electrical propagation caused by fiber disarray. Computer models are by definition artificial and similarly to genetic engineered animal models, care should be taken by extrapolating these results to the human heart. However, these mathematical models may provide valuable additive insight, since they allow studying the effects induced by individual alterations but also the summation of more than one altered factor can be studied systemically. With such models models, risk of cardiac death can be predicted in e.g., long QT patients and various factors can be implemented at the same time like cell size, wall thickness, action potential duration and fibrosis (Hoefen et al., 2012; Zhao et al., 2013).

In DCM predominantly patchy areas of interstitial and replacement fibrosis can be found, but also perivascular patterns have been described (Nakayama et al., 1987; Swynghedauw, 1999). In HCM patients, interstitial fibrosis predominates (Swynghedauw, 1999). In mice with chronic pressure overload, next to hypertrophy, increased levels of interstitial fibrosis have been reported in many cases (Xia et al., 2009; Boulaksil et al., 2010a,b). Moreover, myocardial disarray is one of the hallmarks of HCM (Hughes, 2004). Although it is also present in other cardiac diseases and even in physiologically aged hearts, through the presence in high quantities it is specific for HCM making it a highly sensitive and useful marker (Hughes and McKenna, 2005).

In ICM, infarcted myocytes are replaced predominantly by heterogeneously distributed replacement- and interstitial fibrosis creating islands of cardiomyocytes surrounded by scar tissue. This so-called "labyrinth" of viable strands of cardiomyocytes surrounded by insulating areas of fibrosis creates disconnection of myocytes that leads to excitation blocks and arrhythmias (Fenoglio et al., 1983; Weber et al., 2008). In murine infarct models, fiber disarray has been reported in the infarct border zone, although to a much lesser extent than in HCM (Smith et al., 1991).

ACM is characterized by degeneration of cardiomyocytes and fibro-fatty replacement (Thiene et al., 1988). One theory is that altered cell-cell adhesion due to mutations in genes encoding for structures of the intercalated disc, e.g., the desmosomes, causes injuries to myocytes. This promotes cell death and leads to replacement by fibro-fatty tissue (Saffitz et al., 2009). Histologically, analysis of fibrosis and fiber orientation can help to diagnose any of the above described diseases. Moreover, in all diseases, fibrosis leads to conduction blocks, which increases the propensity to develop reentry arrhythmias, or promotes the manifestation of ectopic impulse generation in relatively uncoupled clusters of cardiomyocytes due to disease-induced remodeling of the expressed ion channels.

ELECTRICAL COUPLING—GAP JUNCTIONS

Gap junctions in the heart are agglomerates of channels that connect the cytoplasm of two adjoining cells allowing electrical coupling between the cardiomyocytes as well as the exchange of certain small molecules, metabolites and ions up to a size of approximately 1 kDa (Elfgang et al., 1995; Noorman et al., 2009). One gap junction channel consists of two hemi-channels (connexons), each delivered by one of the two adjoining cells (**Figure 1**). The two connexons dock in the intercellular space to form a functional channel.

The connexons are composed of connexin proteins. In cardiomyocytes the three main isoforms that are expressed are Connexin 40 (Cx40), Connexin 45 (Cx45), and Connexin 43 (Cx43) with Cx43 being predominant in ventricular cardiomyocytes. Together with adherens junctions and desmosomes, gap junctions are localized in the intercalated disc (ICD), a step-like specialized membrane structure at the longitudinal cell edges between two cells (**Figure 2**). In those ICD's, gap junctions are normally present in the regions parallel (interplicate) to the longitudinal axis of the cardiomyocytes (Smith et al., 1991).

In patients of all four types of cardiac disease, a reduction in ventricular Cx43 localized at the ICD has been found (Peters et al., 1993; DuPont et al., 2001; Kaplan et al., 2004a). Using genetically engineered animal models, a plethora of data have been collected regarding to role of Cx43, using Cx43 knock out animal models. In 1995, the first Cx43 KO model revealed that these mice died perinatally due to major heart problems (malformation of the outflow tract) and cardiac failure (Reaume et al., 1995). Since then, conditional Cx43 KO mice and haploinsufficient animals have been generated. Nevertheless, results obtained from studies with heterozygous KO animals are contradicting. Mice showed reduced expression of Cx43 up to 50%, and in some studies this reduction resulted in reduced conduction velocity (Guerrero et al., 1997; Thomas et al., 1998; Eloff et al., 2001) while other

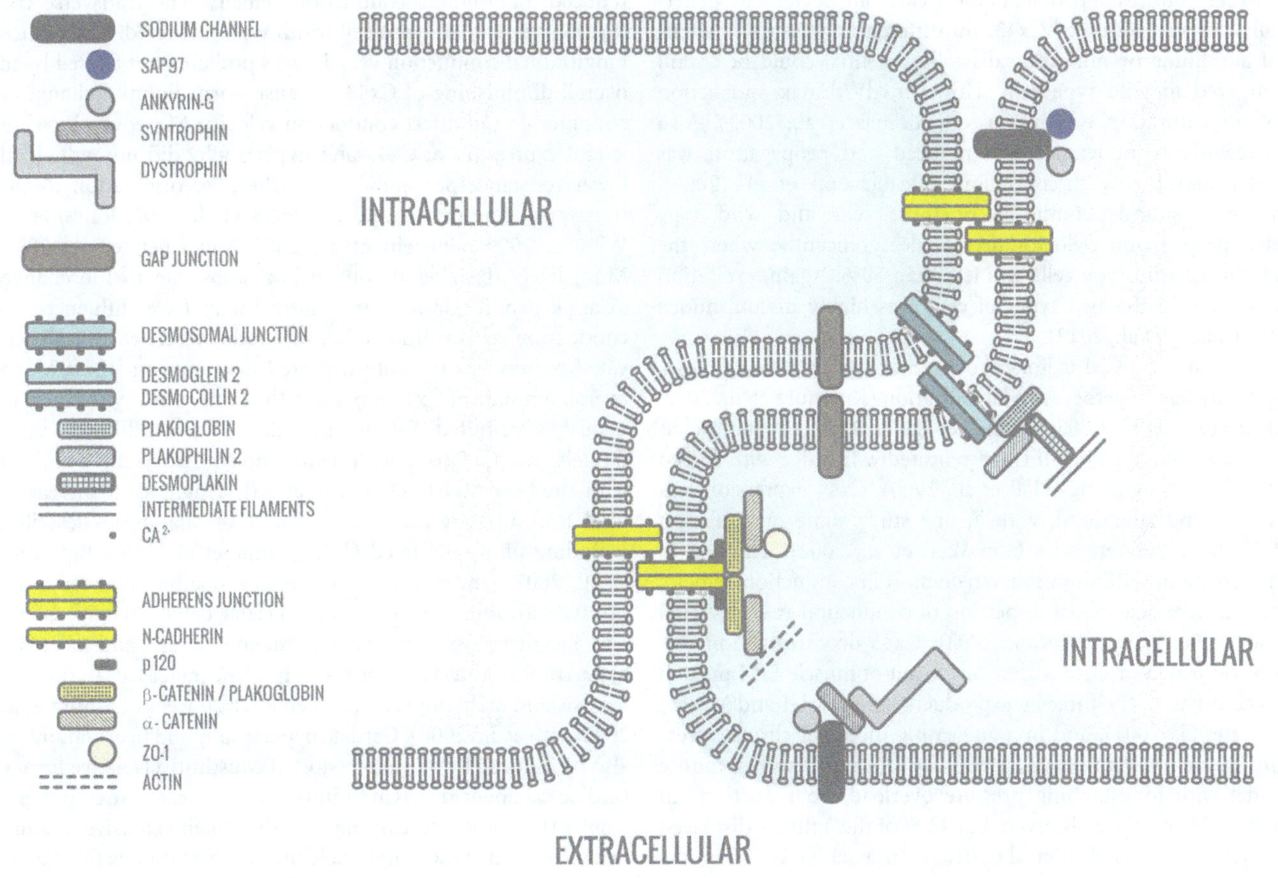

FIGURE 2 | The intercalated disc (ICD). The intercalated disc is the region between two cardiomyocytes, where different junctions are located: Gap junctions, adherens junctions, and desmosomal junctions as well as ion channels. They all form macromolecular protein complexes with different functions.

studies in which a similar reduction in Cx43 was achieved no alterations in conduction velocity were reported (Morley et al., 1999; van Rijen et al., 2004; Stein et al., 2009, 2011). These contradicting results triggered to invent a different approach to reduce Cx43 expression, and also to circumvent the problem of perinatal death in homozygous KO mice. This was achieved through generation of two conditional KO mice models (Orban et al., 1992).

In the first model, one coding region of the Cx43 gene was replaced by the fusion construct Cre-ER(t) and the other Cx43 allele was flanked by loxP (Feil et al., 1996) resulting in a 50% reduced expression of Cx43 under basic conditions ($Cx43^{CreER(t)/fl}$). Exposure to an agent activating the Cre recombinase (e.g., Tamoxifen) resulted in a further reduction of Cx43 expression up to maximally 95% (van Rijen et al., 2004). In the second model, the Cre gene was placed behind an alpha-myosin-heavy-chain (αMHC) promoter resulting in the deletion of the floxed Cx43 gene ($\alpha MHC\text{-}Cre/Cx43^{fl/fl}$) once the promoter got activated (Gutstein et al., 2001). In this way, the Cx43 gene was knocked out around birth allowing those animals to develop normally during gestational stages. In both models, mice died due to arrhythmias. In the case of the $\alpha MHC\text{-}Cre/Cx43^{fl/fl}$ mice death occurs around 1 or 2 months after birth (Gutstein et al., 2001) and in the case of the $Cx43^{CreER(t)/fl}$ mice within 1 month after induction of the deletion (Eckardt et al., 2004).

In cell cultures of neonatal mouse cardiomyocytes with genetically reduced levels of Cx43, no differences in action potential amplitude or minimum diastolic potential could be found compared to wild type cells. However, dV/dtmax and action potential duration was increased (Thomas et al., 2003). Also intercellular conductance was reduced and propagation was slower and highly discontinuous (Beauchamp et al., 2004). In tissue strands composed of these cells and wild type cells, propagation velocity decreased significantly, when the amount of wild type cells was less than 50%. Again, excitation between wild the two types of cells was highly discontinuous (Beauchamp et al., 2012).

In humans, DCM is linked to a reduced expression of Cx43, especially seen together with lateralization (Kitamura et al., 2002, 2003; Kostin et al., 2003; Salameh et al., 2009). In animal models this observation was confirmed repeatedly. In mice with forced retinoic acid signaling (Hall et al., 2000), Cx43 expression was reduced and lateralized, with in one study some upregulation of Cx40 in the ventricles (van Veen et al., 2002). This led to an increase in QRS duration, a reduction in conduction velocity and an increased spatial dispersion of conduction velocity (Hall et al., 2000; van Veen et al., 2002). Cx43 downregulation was also confirmed in mice with a knock-out of muscle LIM protein (an acronym of the three gene products Lin-11, Isl-1 and Mec-3) (Ehler et al., 2001), and in a guinea pig model of chronic pressure overload (Wang et al., 1999). However, in another mouse model with longstanding pressure overload, no reductions in total Cx43 could be observed, but 44% of the animals displayed arrhythmias (Boulaksil et al., 2010a). In a rabbit DCM model of a combined volume and pressure overload, reduced mid-myocardial Cx43 was reported, QRS duration was prolonged and arrhythmias were inducible (Wiegerinck et al., 2006). Besides this animal model, another DCM rabbit model induced by volume overload showed a reduction in Cx43 expression in different groups (Goldfine et al., 1999; Haugan et al., 2006). In a dog model of DCM (induced by RV pacing), lateralized Cx43 expression was described and immunofluorescent signals were decreased in the left ventricle, but not in the right. Moreover, arrhythmias could be induced and QRS duration was prolonged. This was associated with a reduced longitudinal and transversal conduction velocity in both LV and RV (Akar et al., 2007). It was also reported that downregulation of Cx43 triggered fibrosis formation after pressure overload thereby connecting the different passive changes in the heart (Jansen et al., 2012a). The latter study showed that the severity of fibrosis could directly be related to the amount of Cx43 downregulation.

In HCM patients, in an early stage of the disease, an initial increase in Cx43 expression was described together with extensive lateral staining. In later stages, Cx43 was reduced and heterogeneously distributed (Kostin et al., 2004). Other groups showed a reduction in Cx43 without lateralization, or even lateralization without changes in Cx43 expression levels (Peters et al., 1993; Sepp et al., 1996). Animal models confirm some of the observed changes in humans. As already described in the hypertrophy section, in a rat model where HCM was induced using monocrotaline, a decrease in Cx43 expression at the ICD with lateralization was shown (Uzzaman et al., 2000) resulting in a, reduced longitudinal conduction velocity. The transverse conduction velocity and also cell width were unaltered. The reduced longitudinal conduction velocity was probably not caused by the overall diminishing of Cx43, because normally mild changes in coupling do not affect conduction velocity. Moreover, increased lateral expression of Cx43 and hypertrophy did not sufficiently lower resistance perpendicular to the fiber orientation to alter transversal conduction velocity (Palka et al., 1997; Jongsma and Wilders, 2000; Gutstein et al., 2001; van Rijen et al., 2004). More likely the altered source/sink ratios due to the changed axial/perpendicular resistance ratio might have influenced the conduction velocity. In another rat model, where chronically elevated pulmonary pressure triggered development of HCM, the overall amount of Cx43 remained the same, but it was heterogeneously distributed (Sasano et al., 2007). In two different rabbit models of HCM (one with a mutation in troponin 1 and one with the beta-MyHC-Q403 mutation), a significant increase in total mid-myocardial expression of Cx43 has been described, including phosphorylated Cx43 (Sanbe et al., 2005; Ripplinger et al., 2007). In an UM-X7.1 cardiomyopathic hamster model of HCM (leading to loss of cytoskeletal delta-sarcoglycan protein and therefore to cardiac remodeling, failure, and mortality) hypertrophy, a decrease in Cx43 mRNA, increased amounts of fibrosis and arrhythmias were seen after 20 weeks (Ambra et al., 2002; Sato et al., 2008). Cardiac hypertrophy and heart failure can also be induced by overexpression of constitutively active form of cardiac calcineurin-A (CnA) in the mouse heart. Next to hypertrophy these mice develop rapidly after birth extensive amounts of fibrosis and show a high incidence of arrhythmias (Molkentin et al., 1998). In this model reduced Cx43 signals in the ICD's and decreased conduction velocity can be observed (Bierhuizen et al., 2008). In mice undergoing TAC, heterogeneous and partly reduced signals of Cx43 have been reported leading to dispersed impulse conduction (Boulaksil et al., 2010a,b).

In ICM, ischemia reduces gap junction permeability (Dhein, 2006) and induces lateralization of Cx43 (Peters et al., 1993; Beardslee et al., 2000). The infarct border zone (the region bordering healthy and infarcted tissue) will, in that respect, be most at risk of remodeling. Already in 1991, Smith et al. reported gap junction remodeling in this zone, including reduced and lateralized Cx43 signals (Smith et al., 1991). This was also confirmed in dogs (Peters et al., 1997; Huang et al., 1999; Cabo et al., 2006), and patients (DuPont et al., 2001). In patients, alterations were even detected at areas distant from the border zone (Kostin et al., 2003). Moreover, an upregulation in Cx45 could be observed in the border zone, resulting in reduced gap junctional communication due to the intrinsic different properties of the Cx45 gap junction channels (Yamada et al., 2003). The observation of reduced and heterogeneously distributed Cx43 could also be confirmed in rabbit models (Tansey et al., 2006). However, in transgenic mice with 50% of the normal Cx43 expression level, the post-infarction area was smaller than in controls (Kanno et al., 2003). This would suggest that preservation of Cx43 is not *per se* beneficial for maintenance of function of the infarcted heart. Zhang et al. (2010) even proposed to be careful with increasing Cx43 expression in heart diseases until the meaning of alterations in expression of Cx43 upon myocardial infarction is fully understood. We have to keep in mind, however, that Cx43 gap junction channels not only are responsible for propagation of the electrical impulse in the heart, but also for metabolic coupling of the cardiomyocytes. In that respect, a smaller infarct size might rely on a reduced spreading of pro-apoptotic death signals due to a reduced level of intercellular coupling.

In ACM, reduced Cx43 expression has been reported in several studies. Theories are that Cx43 remodeling is triggered by abnormal mechanical coupling (Kaplan et al., 2004a) due to mutations in proteins composing junctions that support the structure of the cardiomyocytes. The different junctions in the intercalated disc assemble and form clusters. Therefore, dysfunction of one junction/protein influences the functioning of others (Agullo-Pascual et al., 2014). In human studies, heterogeneous disturbances in Cx43 signals, decreased presence in the intercalated disc, and lateralization of the signal has been reported in all different forms of ACM (Kaplan et al., 2004a; Noorman et al., 2013a). Although previously thought that this would predominantly be in the right ventricle, these changes are not exclusive and can also be found in the left ventricle and the septum (Noorman et al., 2013b). In general, this leads to scattered impulse conduction, which increases the susceptibility to arrhythmias (Boulaksil et al., 2010a). In the first attempts to investigate ACM in animal models, PKP2 mutations (the most abundant mutated desmosomal protein in humans) were used. In mice, homozygous null mutations in PKP2 are lethal whereas heterozygous mutations do not show any or only little phenotype (Ruiz et al., 1996; Grossman et al., 2004). Therefore, it is suggested that the abundant phenotypical presentation of ACM in patients is, on top of the genetic mutation, dependent on additional factors (e.g., inflammation, exercise). To study the familial cases, initially, two different familial forms of ACM have been studied with mutations in desmosomal genes different from PKP2: Naxos disease [mutation in plakoglobin (PKG)] (Protonotarios et al., 1986; McKoy et al., 2000; Protonotarios and Tsatsopoulou, 2004); and Carvajal-syndrome [desmoplakin (DPK)] (Carvajal-Huerta, 1998; Norgett et al., 2000). In patients, in both diseases, Cx43 is reduced in both ventricles in the early phase of the disease and an increase in non-phosphorylated Cx43 was detected that might be associated with accelerated down-regulation of the protein (Kaplan et al., 2004a,b). An *in vitro* model for Naxos disease using neonatal rat cardiomyocytes transfected with an adenovirus encoding the PKG 2057del2 mutation recapitulated all abnormalities seen in patients: reduced plakoglobin and Cx43 signal at the ICD's, increased apoptosis and secretion of inflammatory mediators (Asimaki et al., 2014). Moreover, a zebrafish model with the same mutation was used to screen for potential drugs to intervene with the development and progression of ACM (Asimaki et al., 2014). This latter study revealed promising results for future therapy since disease-causing targets could be identified and *in vitro* studies showed prevention and even regression of the disease when the intervention was applied in the early phases of cardiac remodeling.

EXCITABILITY

Proper contraction of the heart also results from a finely tuned impulse generation, which feeds propagation. In ventricular cardiomyocytes, action potential generation is initiated by the fast and robust depolarization as caused by the opening of the voltage-dependent Na^+ channels (Clancy and Kass, 2002). Already in 1921, Daly and Clark (1921) showed in frogs that rate, propagation velocity and force of the cardiac contraction were reduced in solutions containing a reduced (extra-cellular) sodium concentration.

The human sodium channel consists of one alpha and four beta subunits. The alpha subunit consists of four homologous domains connected by cytoplasmic linkers (**Figure 3**). Each of those domains consists in turn of six transmembrane sequences (Balser, 1999). In cardiomyocytes two different pools of Nav1.5 channels co-exist, namely at the lateral membranes where the channel interacts with the dystrophin-syntrophin complex and in the intercalated disc where it binds SAP97 (**Figure 2**) (Petitprez et al., 2011). Both pools are thought to interact with different proteins. At the ICD, it is envisioned that Nav1.5 can influence e.g., Cx43 in the gap junctions and *vice versa* (Delmar, 2012).

Initially, much work on excitability has been performed *in vitro* using neonatal rat cardiomyocytes. Lateron, *in vivo* experiments on reduced excitability have been performed in genetically engineered mice models. SCN5a haploinsufficient mice showed about a 50% reduction of sodium current, while having a normal survival rate (Papadatos et al., 2002). ECG analysis showed a prolonged RR interval, P-wave duration, PR interval, QRS duration, and QT interval together with an age related aggravation of the phenotype (Royer et al., 2005). In those SCN5a haploinsuffient mice, QRS prolongation and conduction slowing was observed. However, in young mice, epicardial conduction velocity was not reduced in the left ventricle and only mildly reduced in the right. The reduction in conduction velocity became more dominant in both ventricles in older mice (12–17 months) where it was

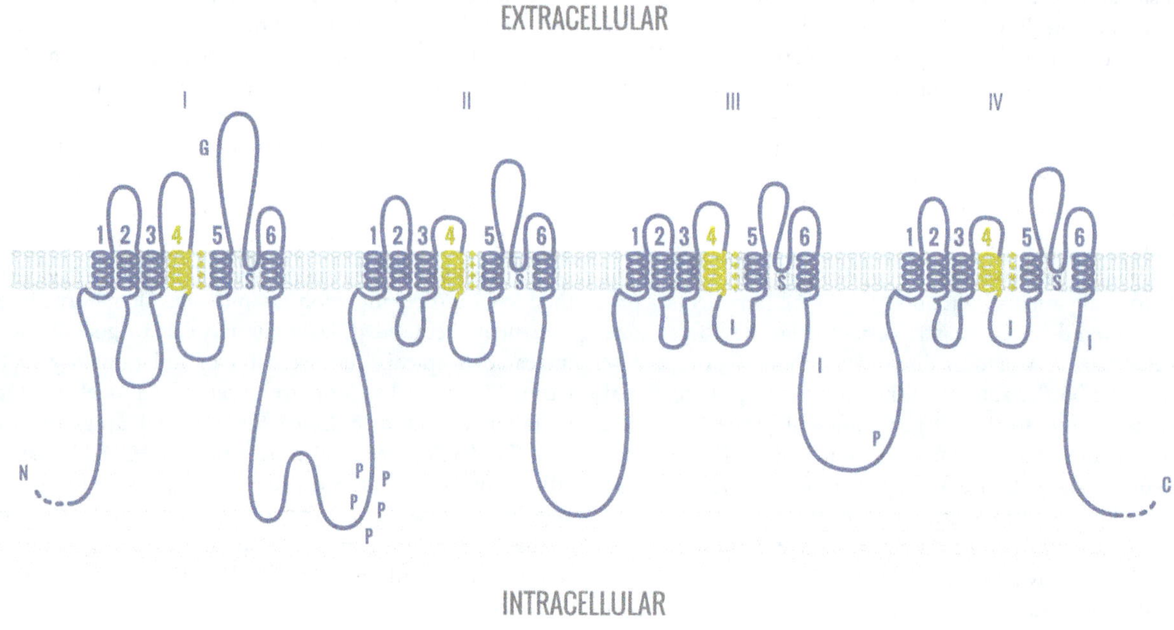

FIGURE 3 | The alpha subunit of the human sodium channel. The alpha subunit of the human sodium channel consists of four homologous domains connected by cytoplasmic linkers. Each domain is composed of six trans-membrane sequences. G, glycosylation; P, phosphorylation; S, ion selectivity; I, inactivation sites. Positive (+) charges in S4 are crucial for transmembrane voltage sensing.

associated with increased fibrosis and altered Cx43 expression (van Veen et al., 2005).

In patients with the 1795InsD mutation in the SCN5a gene, bradycardia, conduction delay, QT prolongation, and right precordial ST-elevation can be detected. To investigate the cause of sodium channel related diseases, and in particular the above mentioned one, Remme et al. created a 1798InsD mouse model (1798InsD is the mouse analog of 1795InsD in human), where indeed a single mutation leads to a phenotype of bradycardia, right ventricular conduction slowing, and QT prolongation (Remme et al., 2006). Given the enormous amount of sodium channel mutations leading to a pro-arrhythmic phenotype in patients, generation of such mouse models significantly has contributed to a better understanding of the underlying etiology. In a DCM dog model, in which disease was induced through RV pacing, neither sodium current density, nor upstroke velocity of the action potential in left ventricular endo- or epicardial myocytes differed from control individuals (Kaab et al., 1996; Akar et al., 2004). Similarly, in a DCM rabbit model, sodium current density did not differ from controls in left ventricular myocytes (Wiegerinck et al., 2006). Recent data from a Torsade de Pointes sensitive canine heart model after chronic AV block (CAVB) confirm that no changes in I_{Na} appear, although increased cell size was reported (Boulaksil et al., 2011).

HCM patients showed increased CaMKII phosphorylation of Nav1.5 channels, which is in general associated with a delayed inactivation of the current (Wagner et al., 2006; Coppini et al., 2013). Increased late sodium current leads to prolonged repolarization (and therefore an increased action potential duration) and arrhythmias as has been shown in patients and several animal models (Jelicks and Siri, 1995; Undrovinas et al., 1999; Gray et al., 2001; Mészáros et al., 2001; Coppini et al., 2013). Increased late sodium current also causes changes in calcium metabolism and homeostasis, influencing cell metabolism and contractile functioning of the cells. This in turn may lead to hypertrophy (Coppini et al., 2013). In mice with calcineurin-induced cardiac hypertrophy, reduced Nav1.5 protein and RNA amounts could be found in the ICD's (Bierhuizen et al., 2008).

ICM is also associated with increased late I_{Na} (Ju et al., 1996; Huang et al., 2001). Various causes can lead to an increase of intracellular sodium concentration in ischemic cardiomyocytes. First, ischemia seems to increase the amplitude of the late I_{Na} significantly (Hammarstrom and Gage, 2002). Anaerobic glycolysis, due to lack of sufficient oxygen supply to the cells, leads to a decrease of ATP and leaking of protons via the cardiac Na/H exchanger (NHE1). Because of that, more sodium enters the cell (Tani and Neely, 1989). Moreover, a reduction of Na^+/K^+ ATPase pump activity will cause an additional decrease of sodium extrusion (Xiao and Allen, 1999). Increased sodium levels will activate the Na/Ca exchanger. This, in turn, leads to an increased concentration of calcium in the cell and a reduction in intracellular pH. The altered ion concentrations will lead to drastic changes in cellular metabolism, signal transduction, electrophysiological characteristics and contractile properties, probably leading to cell damage and cell death (Silverman and Stern, 1994; Imahashi et al., 1999; Allen and Xiao, 2002).

In the early stages of hypoxia, an increase in intracellular sodium concentration was observed in rat hearts that returned back to pre-infarction levels, when ischemia was of short duration (Tani and Neely, 1989). When sodium is persistently elevated, the subsequent increased calcium levels may be prevented by late sodium current inhibition through ranolazine (Soliman et al., 2012). Moreover, a NHE1 inhibitor has been reported to show cardio-protective effects after infarction in a rat model (Huber et al., 2012). Although controversial results have been published lateron about NHE1, it is still under investigation and thought to be one of the most effective post-infarct treatments (Karmazyn, 2013). Next to adherens-, gap- and desmosomal junctions, also ion channels are located in the ICD (Balse et al., 2012), and it becomes more and more clear that in ACM alterations in sub-cellular localization of sodium channels is importantly involved in the consequences of cardiac remodeling. In patients, a reduced localization of Nav1.5 in the ICD has been reported (Noorman et al., 2013a). In cultured cardiomyocytes, the reduced expression of PKP2, caused a subsequent reduction in the sodium current and a slower conduction velocity (Sato et al., 2009). Besides that, loss of expression of Ankyrin-G, an important protein that anchors the voltage-gated sodium channel, leads to disturbances in PKP2 and Cx43 expression. The other way around, loss of PKP2 causes a reduction in expression of Ankyrin-G as well as of Nav1.5 (Sato et al., 2011), thereby confirming the role of sodium channels in this disease. Besides that, in zebrafish and neonatal rat cardiomyocytes containing the mentioned 2057del2 plakoglobin (related to Naxos disease), a marked reduction in I_{Na} current density was observed (Asimaki et al., 2014). In these neonatal rat cardiomyocytes, the immunofluorescent Nav1.5 signal at the membrane was reduced, but total cell content appeared unchanged (Asimaki et al., 2014). This reduction in I_{Na} and consequently a reduced conduction velocity has also previously been shown in transgenic mice with a desmoglein-2 mutation (Rizzo et al., 2012). Moreover, reduced heterogeneous expression of Cx43 in conditional knockout mice caused decreased expression of Nav1.5, reduced sodium current and an increased vulnerability of those mice for arrhythmias (Jansen et al., 2012a). Similarly, PKP2 haploinsufficiency in mice resulted in a sodium current deficit and arrhythmogenesis when triggered with flecainide (Cerrone et al., 2012). The importance of these finding was reflected in a study of Cerrone et al. which showed that in patients with a mutation in PKP-2, provocation with flecainide triggered arrhythmias suggesting that also in these patients a concomitant sodium current deficit existed (Cerrone et al., 2014).

HETEROGENEITY

The natural mode of functional heterogeneity within the normal cardiac performance is also of importance during heart disease. Due to, e.g., pulmonary disease or aortic stenosis, different parts of the heart are affected prior to the other, leading to heterogenic alterations that conflict with the natural organization. In ACM, where disease-dependent changes often start in the right ventricle, the left ventricle can remain relatively unaffected in the early stages of disease. In an opposite fashion aortic stenosis will first remodel the left ventricle before right ventricular involvement manifests. Differently, right ventricular remodeling due to pulmonary hypertension might simultaneously trigger LV remodeling (atrophy) due to a reduced filling (Hardziyenka et al., 2012).

These different types of remodeling are part of various diseases and are by definition heterogeneous, since all of those diseases have different causes and therefore treatment options (Coronel et al., 2013).

Cardiac remodeling deteriorating into heart failure most likely depends on a combination of the mechanisms as described in this article, and it is characterized by heterogeneous remodeling of excitation-contraction coupling (Coronel et al., 2001; Lou et al., 2011). Pathophysiological heterogeneity in cardiac tissue sustains ventricular tachycardia, stabilizes reentry arrhythmias and provides substrate for sustained tachycardia (Pazo et al., 2004; Ripplinger et al., 2006).

Passive heterogeneous ventricular remodeling in the heart is one of the most destructive features of cardiac remodeling and every remodeling mechanism itself shows the worst outcome, when occurring heterogeneously. In this article, several mechanisms of passive remodeling have been described during DCM, HCM, ICM and ACM. Passive remodeling of tissue architecture was investigated focusing on fibrosis, alterations in cell size, hypertrophy and fiber disarray. Disturbances in electrical coupling were discussed by describing changes in the distribution of the gap junction protein Cx43. Remodeling of electrical excitability was studied using the sodium channel protein Nav1.5.

To summarize, different types of fibrosis occur in all of the four discussed heart diseases and act as modulators of impulse propagation ranging from conduction slowing, increased dispersion of conduction and even conduction block. Moreover, it can alter the structure of the heart, e.g., alterations in cellular dimensions, which is caused by modifications in molecular pathways that control normal cellular physiology. As a consequence this may lead to reductions in excitability and cell-to-cell conduction (Fenoglio et al., 1983; Kawara et al., 2001). Heterogeneously distributed fibrosis can even create a "labyrinth" in the heart facilitating reentry arrhythmias (Engelman et al., 2010). Therefore, this is considered to be worse than only local interstitial fibrosis since it would be more difficult for electrical signals to propagate though a labyrinth of fibrotic patches than only being obstructed by single fibers (Kawara et al., 2001; Tanaka et al., 2007). This idea was strengthened by a study where reduction of heterogeneous patchy fibrosis was one-on-one correlated to a reduction of arrhythmias (Stein et al., 2010).

Hypertrophy can be detected in HCM and ICM. Changes in cell size are the key features of HCM and DCM, whereby HCM is characterized by an increase in cell width and DCM by an increase in cell length. Myocardial fiber disarray mainly occurs in HCM, where it is even used as a biomarker. It can also be observed in ICM, but to a much lesser extend. Heterogeneously distributed hypertrophy, myocardial fiber disarray and changes in cell size can lead to alterations in impulse propagation and conduction velocity causing disturbed signaling, deregulated contractions, and eventually heart failure (Meyerburg et al., 1992; Winterton et al., 1994; Cooklin et al., 1997; McIntyre and Fry, 1997). Pathophysiological heterogeneity in the sense of right vs. left ventricles or atria can also worsen disease phenotype as is classically illustrated by the fact that progressive LV dysfunction eventually results in RV failure too with consequently, pulmonary remodeling and edema (Chen et al., 2012).

Heterogeneous distribution, de-phosphorylation and a reduction of Cx43 signals in the ICD are characteristics found in all four different heart diseases. They are one of the key features of ACM (Noorman et al., 2013a), but also occur in DCM, ICM, and late stages of HCM. This can lead to a reduction in longitudinal and an increase in transverse conduction (reducing the normal anisotropic mode of conduction) causing heterogeneous propagation (increased dispersion of conduction) and arrhythmogenesis. At these places signaling (mechanical or electrical) will be more difficult leading to de-regulated intercellular coupling (Boulaksil et al., 2010a). The heterogeneous distribution of the different proteins and structures can be sub-divided into macro and micro heterogeneity. Macro heterogeneity compares the different regions in the heart, whereas micro heterogeneity is a measure for local heterogeneity (Jansen et al., 2012a).

Changes in expression and distribution of the sodium channel protein Nav1.5 can also be seen in HCM, DCM, and ACM. Homogeneous distribution of Nav1.5 throughout different parts of the heart is crucial for normal conduction (Clancy and Kass, 2002) although functional expression levels differ between epicard, endocard, and conduction system (Remme et al., 2009). Heterogeneous distribution, caused by a local increase or decrease of sodium channels possibly facilitates arrhythmogenesis and therefore heart failure, since the sodium current will be hampered or fastened locally (Wagner et al., 2011; Shryock et al., 2013). Although these heterogeneous maladaptations can have effects when occurring alone, they are often found to trigger arrhythmias and eventually heart failure due to a combination of simultaneous alterations in different factors. Therefore, great care should be taken when investigating one single mechanism of remodeling, since a heterogeneous adaptation of one mechanism can also cause others to develop or are even linked to each other. This concept is illustrated by several studies, which report a simultaneous downregulation and de-phosphorylation of Cx43, and Nav1.5, (Stein et al., 2009; Jansen et al., 2012b; Noorman et al., 2013a) and even link this combination to an increased deposition of fibrotic materials (van Veen et al., 2005; Jansen et al., 2012a). These studies example the complexity of cardiac remodeling during pathophysiology in relation to the increase in propensity to develop arrhythmias.

Regarding the future perspective of cardiac research, one should focus on these connections between heterogeneous changes in single factors within the heart that lead to the total picture of heterogeneous remodeling. This might unravel currently unknown relationships between the various forms of maladaptation and help to improve the search for treatment options. In a study that was mentioned before, long term administration of the antihypertensive drugs eplerenone or losartan in a mouse model of extreme aging not only reduced the amount of interstitial- and patchy fibrosis, but also preserved a homogeneous pattern of gap junctional coupling. This preservation of the normal substrate for conduction resulted in a significantly reduced amount of arrhythmias (Stein et al., 2010). Beyond pharmacological interventions, pacing strategies (like cardiac resynchronization therapy) that aim to correct the abnormal sequence of activation, e.g., due to bundle branch block or electrical remodeling, will provide further future perspectives to improve performance of the remodeled heart.

ACKNOWLEDGMENTS

We acknowledge support from the Netherlands CardioVascular Research Initiative: the Dutch Heart Foundation, Dutch Federation of University Medical Centers, the Netherlands Organization for Health Research and Development, and the Royal Netherlands Academy of Sciences (CVON-PREDICT, Elise L. Kessler, Marc A. Vos, Toon A. B. van Veen).

REFERENCES

Agullo-Pascual, E., Cerrone, M., and Delmar, M. (2014). Arrhythmogenic cardiomyopathy and Brugada syndrome: diseases of the connexome. *FEBS Lett.* 588, 1322–1330. doi: 10.1016/j.febslet.2014.02.008

Akar, F. G., Nass, R. D., Hahn, S., Cingolani, E., Shah, M., Hesketh, G. G., et al. (2007). Dynamic changes in conduction velocity and gap junction properties during development of pacing-induced heart failure. *Am. J. Physiol. Heart Circ. Physiol.* 293, H1223–H1230. doi: 10.1152/ajpheart.00079.2007

Akar, F. G., Spragg, D. D., Tunin, R. S., Kass, D. A., and Tomaselli, G. F. (2004). Mechanisms underlying conduction slowing and arrhythmogenesis in nonischemic dilated cardiomyopathy. *Circ. Res.* 95, 717–725. doi: 10.1161/01.RES.0000144125.61927.1c

Allen, D. G., and Xiao, X. H. (2002). Role of the cardiac Na/H exchanger during ischemia and reperfusion. *Cardiovasc. Res.* 57, 934–941. doi: 10.1016/S0008-6363(02)00836-2

Ambra, R., Di Nardo, P., Fantini, C., Minieri, M., Canali, R., Natella, F., et al. (2002). Selective changes in DNA binding activity of transcription factors in UM-X7.1 cardiomyopathic hamsters. *Life Sci.* 71, 2369–2381. doi: 10.1016/S0024-3205(02)02020-9

Asimaki, A., et al. (2007). A novel dominant mutation in plakoglobin causes arrhythmogenic right ventricular cardiomyopathy. *Am. J. Hum. Genet.* 81, 964–973. doi: 10.1086/521633

Asimaki, A., Syrris, P., Wichter, T., Matthias, P., Saffitz, J. E., and McKenna, W. J. (2014). Identification of a new modulator of the intercalated disc in a zebrafish model of arrhythmogenic cardiomyopathy. *Sci. Transl. Med.* 6, 240ra74. doi: 10.1126/scitranslmed.3008008

Balse, E., Steele, D. F., Abriel, H., Coulombe, A., Fedida, D., and Hatem, S. N. (2012). Dynamic of ion channel expression at the plasma membrane of cardiomyocytes. *Physiol. Rev.* 92, 1317–1358. doi: 10.1152/physrev.00041.2011

Balser, J. R. (1999). Structure and function of the cardiac sodium channels. *Cardiovasc. Res.* 42, 327–338. doi: 10.1016/S0008-6363(99)00031-0

Beardslee, M. A., Lerner, D. L., Tadros, P. N., Laing, J. G., Beyer, E. C., Yamada, K. A., et al. (2000). Dephosphorylation and intracellular redistribution of ventricular connexin43 during electrical uncoupling induced by ischemia. *Circ. Res.* 87, 656–662. doi: 10.1161/01.RES.87.8.656

Beauchamp, P., Choby, C., Desplantez, T., de Peyer, K., Green, K., Yamada, K. A., et al. (2004). Electrical propagation in synthetic ventricular myocyte strands from germline connexin43 knockout mice. *Circ. Res.* 95, 170–178. doi: 10.1161/01.RES.0000134923.05174.2f

Beauchamp, P., Desplantez, T., McCain, M. L., Li, W., Asimaki, A., Rigoli, G., et al. (2012). Electrical coupling and propagation in engineered ventricular myocardium with heterogeneous expression of connexin43. *Circ. Res.* 110, 1445–1453. doi: 10.1161/CIRCRESAHA.111.259705

Beffagna, G., Occhi, G., Nava, A., Vitiello, L., Ditadi, A., Basso, C., et al. (2005). Regulatory mutations in transforming growth factor-beta3 gene cause arrhythmogenic right ventricular cardiomyopathy type 1. *Cardiovasc. Res.* 65, 366–373. doi: 10.1016/j.cardiores.2004.10.005

Bender, S. R., Friedman, D. J., Markowitz, S. M., Lerman, B. B., and Okin, P. M. (2012). Electrocardiographic left ventricular hypertrophy predicts arrhythmia and mortality in patients with ischemic cardiomyopathy. *J. Interv. Card. Electrophysiol.* 34, 237–245. doi: 10.1007/s10840-011-9661-2

Bierhuizen, M. F., Boulaksil, M., van Stuijvenberg, L., van der Nagel, R., Jansen, A. T., Mutsaers, N. A., et al. (2008). In calcineurin-induced cardiac hypertrophy expression of Nav1.5, Cx40 and Cx43 is reduced by different mechanisms. *J. Mol. Cell. Cardiol.* 45, 373–384. doi: 10.1016/j.yjmcc.2008.06.011

Biernacka, A., and Frangogiannis, N. G. (2011). Aging and cardiac fibrosis. *Aging Dis.* 2, 158–173.

Boulaksil, M., Jungschleger, J. G., Antoons, G., Houtman, M. J., de Boer, T. P., Wilders, R., et al. (2011). Drug-induced torsade de pointes arrhythmias in the chronic AV block dog are perpetuated by focal activity. *Circ. Arrhythm. Electrophysiol.* 4, 566–576. doi: 10.1161/CIRCEP.110.958991

Boulaksil, M., Noorman, M., Engelen, M. A., van Veen, T. A., Vos, M. A., de Bakker, J. M., et al. (2010b). Longitudinal arrhythmogenic remodelling in a mouse model of longstanding pressure overload. *Neth. Heart J.* 18, 509–515. doi: 10.1007/BF03091824

Boulaksil, M., Winckels, S. K., Engelen, M. A., Stein, M., van Veen, T. A., Jansen, J. A., et al. (2010a). Heterogeneous Connexin 43 distribution in heart failure is associated with dispersed conduction and enhanced susceptibility to ventricular arrhythmias. *Eur. J. Heart Fail.* 12, 913–921. doi: 10.1093/eurjhf/hfq092

Bowers, S. L., Borg, T. K., and Baudino, T. A. (2010). The dynamics of fibroblast-myocyte-capillary interactions in the heart. *Ann. N. Y. Acad. Sci.* 1188, 143–152. doi: 10.1111/j.1749-6632.2009.05094.x

Branishte, T., Jungschleger, J. G., Antoons, G., Houtman, M. J., de Boer, T. P., Wilders, R., et al. (2013). Aspects of molecular mechanisms in myocardial hypertrophy, particular morphological changes and cell bioenergetic characteristics in patients with dilated cardiomyopathy. *Rev. Med. Chir. Soc. Med. Nat. Iasi* 117, 851–856.

Brugada, J., Boersma, L., Kirchhof, C. J., Heynen, V. V., and Allessie, M. A. (1991). Reentrant excitation around a fixed obstacle in uniform anisotropic ventricular myocardium. *Circulation* 84, 1296–1306. doi: 10.1161/01.CIR.84.3.1296

Cabo, C., Yao, J., Boyden, P. A., Chen, S., Hussain, W., Duffy, H. S., et al. (2006). Heterogeneous gap junction remodeling in reentrant circuits in the epicardial border zone of the healing canine infarct. *Cardiovasc. Res.* 72, 241- 249. doi: 10.1016/j.cardiores.2006.07.005

Carvajal-Huerta, L. (1998). Epidermolytic palmoplantar keratoderma with woolly hair and dilated cardiomyopathy. *J. Am. Acad. Dermatol.* 39, 418–421. doi: 10.1016/S0190-9622(98)70317-2

Cerrone, M., Lin, X., Zhang, M., Agullo-Pascual, E., Pfenniger, A., Chkourko Gusky, H., et al. (2014). Missense mutations in plakophilin-2 cause sodium current deficit and associate with a brugada syndrome phenotype. *Circulation* 129, 1092–1103. doi: 10.1161/CIRCULATIONAHA.113.003077

Cerrone, M., Noorman, M., Lin, X., Chkourko, H., Liang, F. X., van der Nagel, R., et al. (2012). Sodium current deficit and arrhythmogenesis in a murine model of plakophilin-2 haploinsufficiency. *Cardiovasc. Res.* 95, 460–468. doi: 10.1093/cvr/cvs218

Chen, Y., Guo, H., Xu, D., Xu, X., Wang, H., Hu, X., et al. (2012). Left ventricular failure produces profound lung remodeling and pulmonary hypertension in mice: heart failure causes severe lung disease. *Hypertension* 59, 1170–1178. doi: 10.1161/HYPERTENSIONAHA.111.186072

Clancy, C. E., and Kass, R. S. (2002). Defective cardiac ion channels: from mutations to clinical syndromes. *J. Clin. Invest.* 110, 1075–1077. doi: 10.1172/JCI0216945

Cooklin, M., Wallis, W. R., Sheridan, D. J., and Fry, C. H. (1997). Changes in cell-to-cell electrical coupling associated with left ventricular hypertrophy. *Circ. Res.* 80, 765–771. doi: 10.1161/01.RES.80.6.765

Coppini, R., Ferrantini, C., Yao, L., Fan, P., Del Lungo, M., Stillitano, F., et al. (2013). Late sodium current inhibition reverses electromechanical dysfunction in human hypertrophic cardiomyopathy. *Circulation* 127, 575–584. doi: 10.1161/CIRCULATIONAHA.112.134932

Coronel, R., de Groot, J. R., and van Lieshout, J. J. (2001). Defining heart failure. *Cardiovasc. Res.* 50, 419–422. doi: 10.1016/S0008-6363(01)00284-X

Coronel, R., Wilders, R., Verkerk, A. O., Wiegerinck, R. F., Benoist, D., and Bernus, O. (2013). Electrophysiological changes in heart failure and their implications for arrhythmogenesis. *Biochim. Biophys. Acta* 1832, 2432–2441. doi: 10.1016/j.bbadis.2013.04.002

Corrado, D., Basso, C., and Thiene, G. (2000). Arrhythmogenic right ventricular cardiomyopathy: diagnosis, prognosis, and treatment. *Heart* 83, 588–595. doi: 10.1136/heart.83.5.588

Daly, I. B., and Clark, A. J. (1921). The action of ions upon the frog's heart. *J Physiol* 54, 367–383.

Davis, J., and Molketin, J. D. (2013). Myofibroblasts: trust your heart and let fate decide. *J. Mol. Cell Cardiol.* 70, 9–18. doi: 10.1016/j.yjmcc.2013.10.019

de Bakker, J. M., van Capelle, F. J., Janse, M. J., Tasseron, S., Vermeulen, J. T., de Jonge, N., et al. (1993). Slow conduction in the infarcted human heart. 'Zigzag' course of activation. *Circulation* 88, 915–926. doi: 10.1161/01.CIR.88.3.915

de Bakker, J. M., van Capelle, F. J., Janse, M. J., Wilde, A. A., Coronel, R., Becker, A. E., et al. (1988). Reentry as a cause of ventricular tachycardia in patients with chronic ischemic heart disease: electrophysiologic and anatomic correlation. *Circulation* 77, 589–606. doi: 10.1161/01.CIR.77.3.589

de Jong, S., Zwanenburg, J. J., Visser, F., der Nagel, R. V, van Rijen, H. V., Vos, M. A., et al. (2011). Direct detection of myocardial fibrosis by MRI. *J. Mol. Cell. Cardiol.* 51, 974–979. doi: 10.1016/j.yjmcc.2011.08.024

Delmar, M. (2012). Connexin43 regulates sodium current; ankyrin-G modulates gap junctions: the intercalated disc exchanger. *Cardiovasc. Res.* 93, 220–222. doi: 10.1093/cvr/cvr343

Dhein, S. (2006). Cardiac ischemia and uncoupling: gap junctions in ischemia and infarction. *Adv. Cardiol.* 42, 198–212. doi: 10.1159/000092570

DuPont, E., Matsushita, T., Kaba, R. A., Vozzi, C., Coppen, S. R., Khan, N., et al. (2001). Altered connexin expression in human congestive heart failure. *J. Mol. Cell. Cardiol.* 33, 359–371. doi: 10.1006/jmcc.2000.1308

Eckardt, D., Theis, M., Degen, J., Ott, T., van Rijen, H. V., Kirchhoff, S., et al. (2004). Functional role of connexin43 gap junction channels in adult mouse heart assessed by inducible gene deletion. *J. Mol. Cell. Cardiol.* 36, 101–110. doi: 10.1016/j.yjmcc.2003.10.006

Efthimiadis, G. K., Pagourelias, E. D., Gossios, T., and Zegkos, T. (2014). Hypertrophic cardiomyopathy in 2013, current speculations and future perspectives. *World J. Cardiol.* 6, 26–37. doi: 10.4330/wjc.v6.i2.26

Ehler, E., Horowits, R., Zuppinger, C., Price, R. L., Perriard, E., Leu, M., et al. (2001). Alterations at the intercalated disk associated with the absence of muscle LIM protein. *J. Cell Biol.* 153, 763–772. doi: 10.1083/jcb.153.4.763

Elfgang, C., Eckert, R., Lichtenberg-Fraté, H., Butterweck, A., Traub, O., Klein, R. A., et al. (1995). Specific permeability and selective formation of gap junction channels in connexin-transfected HeLa cells. *J. Cell Biol.* 129, 805–817. doi: 10.1083/jcb.129.3.805

Eloff, B. C., Lerner, D. L., Yamada, K. A., Schuessler, R. B., Saffitz, J. E., and Rosenbaum, D. S. (2001). High resolution optical mapping reveals conduction slowing in connexin43 deficient mice. *Cardiovasc. Res.* 51, 681–690. doi: 10.1016/S0008-6363(01)00341-8

Engelman, Z. J., Trew, M. L., and Smaill, B. H. (2010). Structural heterogeneity alone is a sufficient substrate for dynamic instability and altered restitution. *Circ. Arrhythm. Electrophysiol.* 3, 195–203. doi: 10.1161/CIRCEP.109.890459

Feil, R., Brocard, J., Mascrez, B., LeMeur, M., Metzger, D., and Chambon, P. (1996). Ligand-activated site-specific recombination in mice. *Proc. Natl. Acad. Sci. U.S.A.* 93, 10887–10890. doi: 10.1073/pnas.93.20.10887

Fenoglio, J. J., Ursell, P. C., Kellogg, C. F., Drusin, R. E., and Weiss, M. B. (1983). Diagnosis and classification of myocarditis by endomyocardial biopsy. *N. Engl. J. Med.* 308, 12–18. doi: 10.1056/NEJM198301063080103

Formigli, L., Ibba-Manneschi, L., Perna, A. M., Pacini, A., Polidori, L., Nediani, C., et al. (2003). Altered Cx43 expression during myocardial adaptation to acute and chronic volume overloading. *Histol. Histopathol.* 18, 359–369.

Gerull, B., Heuser, A., Wichter, T., Paul, M., Basson, C. T., McDermott, D. A., et al. (2004). Mutations in the desmosomal protein plakophilin-2 are common in arrhythmogenic right ventricular cardiomyopathy. *Nat. Genet.* 36, 1162–1164. doi: 10.1038/ng1461

Gill, C., Mestril, R., and Samali, A. (2002). Losing heart: the role of apoptosis in heart disease—a novel therapeutic target? *FASEB J.* 16, 135–146. doi: 10.1096/fj.01-0629com

Goldfine, S. M., Walcott, B., Brink, P. R., Magid, N. M., and Borer, J. S. (1999). Myocardial connexin43 expression in left ventricular hypertrophy resulting from aortic regurgitation. *Cardiovasc. Pathol.* 8, 1–6. doi: 10.1016/S1054-8807(98)00011-8

Gray, R. P., McIntyre, H., Sheridan, D. S., and Fry, C. H. (2001). Intracellular sodium and contractile function in hypertrophied human and guinea-pig myocardium. *Pflugers Arch.* 442, 117–123. doi: 10.1007/s004240000512

Grossman, K. S., Grund, C., Huelsken, J., Behrend, M., Erdmann, B., Franke, W. W., et al. (2004). Requirement of plakophilin 2 for heart morphogenesis and cardiac junction formation. *J. Cell Biol.* 167, 149–160. doi: 10.1083/jcb.200402096

Guerrero, P. A., Schuessler, R. B., Davis, L. M., Beyer, E. C., Johnson, C. M., Yamada, K. A., et al. (1997). Slow ventricular conduction in mice heterozygous for a connexin43 null mutation. *J. Clin. Invest.* 99, 1991–1998. doi: 10.1172/JCI119367

Gutstein, D. E., Liu, F. Y., Meyers, M. B., Choo, A., and Fishman, G. I. (2001). The organization of adherens junctions and desmosomes at the cardiac intercalated disc is independent of gap junctions. *J. Cell Sci.* 116, 875–885. doi: 10.1242/jcs.00258

Hall, D. G., Morley, G. E., Vaidya, D., Ard, M., Kimball, T. R., Witt, S. A., et al. (2000). Early onset heart failure in transgenic mice with dilated cardiomyopathy. *Pediatr. Res.* 48, 36–42. doi: 10.1203/00006450-200007000-00009

Hammarstrom, A. K., and Gage, P. W. (2002). Hypoxia and persistent sodium current. *Eur. Biophys.* 31, 323–333. doi: 10.1007/s00249-002-0218-2

Hardziyenka, M., Campian, M. E., Verkerk, A. O., Surie, S., van Ginneken, A. C., Hakim, S., et al. (2012). Electrophysiologic remodeling of the left ventricle in pressure overload-induced right ventricular failure. *J. Am. Coll. Cardiol.* 59, 2193–2202. doi: 10.1016/j.jacc.2012.01.063

Haugan, K., Miyamoto, T., Takeishi, Y., Kubota, I., Nakayama, J., Shimojo, H., et al. (2006). Rotigaptide (ZP123) improves atrial conduction slowing in chronic volume overload-induced dilated atria. *Basic Clin. Pharmacol. Toxicol.* 99, 71–79. doi: 10.1111/j.1742-7843.2006.pto_432.x

Hershberger, R. E., and Morales, A. (2013). "A dilated cardiomyopathy overview," in *GeneReviews®*, eds R. A. Pagon, M. P. Adam, H. H. Ardinger (Seattle, WA: University of Washington).

Heuser, A., Plovie, E. R., Ellinor, P. T., Grossmann, K. S., Shin, J. T., Wichter, T., et al. (2006). Mutant desmocollin-2 causes arrhythmogenic right ventricular cardiomyopathy. *Am. J. Hum. Genet.* 79, 1081–1018. doi: 10.1086/509044

Hoefen, R., Reumann, M., Goldenberg, I., Moss, A. J., O-Uchi, J., Gu, Y. et al. (2012). *In silico* cardiac risk assessment in patients with long QT syndrome: type 1: clinical predictability of cardiac models. *J. Am. Coll. Cardiol.* 60, 2182–2191. doi: 10.1016/j.jacc.2012.07.053

Huang, B., El-Sherif, T., Gidh-Jain, M., Qin, D., and El-Sherif, N. (2001). Alterations of sodium channel kinetics and gene expression in the postinfarction remodeled myocardium. *J. Cardiovasc. Electrophysiol.* 12, 218–225. doi: 10.1046/j.1540-8167.2001.00218.x

Huang, X. D., Sandusky, G. E., and Zipes, D. P. (1999). Heterogeneous loss of Connexin43 protein in ischemic dog hearts. *J. Cardiovasc. Electrophysiol.* 10, 79–91. doi: 10.1111/j.1540-8167.1999.tb00645.x

Huber, J. D., Bentzien, J., Boyer, S. J., Burke, J., De Lombaert, S., Eickmeier, C., et al. (2012). Identification of a potent sodium hydrogen exchanger isoform 1 (NHE1) inhibitor with a suitable profile for chronic dosing and demonstrated cardioprotective effects in a preclinical model of myocardial infarction in the rat. *J. Med. Chem.* 55, 7114–7140. doi: 10.1021/jm300601d

Hughes, S. E. (2004). The pathology of hypertrophic cardiomyopathy. *Histopathology* 44, 412–427. doi: 10.1111/j.1365-2559.2004.01835.x

Hughes, S. E., and McKenna, W. J. (2005). New insights into the pathology of inherited cardiomyopathy. *Heart* 91, 257–264. doi: 10.1136/hrt.2004.040337

Imahashi, K., Kusuoka, H., Hashimoto, K., Yoshioka, J., Yamaguchi, H., and Nishimura, T. (1999). Intracellular sodium accumulation during ischemia as the substrate for reperfusion injury. *Circ. Res.* 84, 1401–1406. doi: 10.1161/01.RES.84.12.1401

Isoyama, S., and Nitta-Komatsubara, Y. (2002). Acute and chronic adaptation to hemodynamic overload and ischemia in the aged heart. *Heart Fail. Rev.* 7, 63–69. doi: 10.1023/A:1013701923065

Janicki, J. S., and Brower, G. L. (2002). The role of myocardial fibrillar collagen in ventricular remodeling and function. *J. Card. Fail.* 8(6Suppl): 319–325. doi: 10.1054/jcaf.2002.129260

Jansen, J. A., Noorman, M., Musa, H., Stein, M., de Jong, S., van der Nagel, R., et al. (2012b). Reduced heterogeneous expression of Cx43 results in decreased Nav1.5 expression and reduced sodium current that accounts for arrhythmia vulnerability in conditional Cx43 knockout mice. *Heart Rhythm* 9, 600–607. doi: 10.1016/j.hrthm.2011.11.025

Jansen, J. A., van Veen, T. A., de Jong, S., van der Nagel, R., van Stuijvenberg, L., Driessen, H., et al. (2012a). Reduced Cx43 expression triggers increased fibrosis due to enhanced fibroblast activity. *Circ. Arrhythm. Electrophysiol.* 5, 380–390. doi: 10.1161/CIRCEP.111.966580

Jelicks, L. A., and Siri, F. M. (1995). Effects of hypertrophy and heart failure on $[Na^+]_i$ in pressure-overloaded guinea pig heart. *Am. J. Hypertens* 8, 934–943. doi: 10.1016/0895-7061(95)00219-F

Jongsma, H. J., and Wilders, R. (2000). Gap junctions in cardiovascular disease. *Circ. Res.* 86, 1193–1197. doi: 10.1161/01.RES.86.12.1193

Ju, Y. K., Saint, D. A., and Gage, P. W. (1996). Hypoxia increases persistent sodium current in rat ventricular myocytes. *J. Physiol.* 497, 337–347.

Kaab, S., Nuss, H. B., Chiamvimonvat, N., O'Rourke, B., Pak, P. H., Kass, D. A., et al. (1996). Ionic mechanism of action potential prolongation in ventricular myocytes from dogs with pacing-induced heart failure. *Circ. Res.* 78, 262–273. doi: 10.1161/01.RES.78.2.262

Kannel, W. B., Dawber, T. R., Kagan, A., Revotski, N., and Stokes, J. 3rd. (1961). Factors of risk in the development of coronary heart disease six-year follow-up experienee; the Framingham study. *Ann. Int. Med.* 55, 33–50. doi: 10.7326/0003-4819-55-1-33

Kanno, S., Kovacs, A., Yamada, K. A., and Saffitz, J. E. (2003). Connexin43 as a determinant of myocardial infarct sizefollowing coronary occlusion in mice. *J. Am. Coll. Cardiol.* 41, 681–686. doi: 10.1016/S0735-1097(02)02893-0

Kaplan, S. R., Gard, J. J., Carvajal-Huerta, L., Ruiz-Cabezas, J. C., Thiene, G., and Saffitz, J. E. (2004b). Structural and molecular pathology of the heart in Carvajal syndrome. *Cardiovasc. Pathol.* 13, 26–32. doi: 10.1016/S1054-8807(03)00107-8

Kaplan, S. R., Gard, J. J., Protonotarios, N., Tsatsopoulou, A., Spiliopoulou, C., Anastasakis, A., et al. (2004a). Remodeling of myocyte gap junctions in arrhythmogenic right ventricular cardiomyopathy due to a deletion in plakoglobin (Naxos disease). *Heart Rhythm* 1, 3–11. doi: 10.1016/j.hrthm.2004.01.001

Karmazyn, M. (2013). NHE-1: still a viable therapeutic target. *J. Mol. Cell. Cardiol.* 61, 77–82. doi: 10.1016/j.yjmcc.2013.02.006

Kawara, T., Derksen, R., de Groot, J. R., Coronel, R., Tasseron, S., Linnenbank, A. C., et al. (2001). Activation delay after premature stimulation in chronically diseased human myocardium relates to the architecture of interstitial fibrosis. *Circulation* 104, 3069–3075. doi: 10.1161/hc5001.100833

Kemp, C. D., and Conte, J. V. (2012). The pathophysiology of heart failure. *Cardiovasc. Pathol.* 21, 365–371. doi: 10.1016/j.carpath.2011.11.007

Kitamura, H., Ohnishi, Y., Yoshida, A., Okajima, K., Azumi, H., Ishida, A., et al. (2002). Heterogeneous loss of connexin43 protein in nonischemic dilated cardiomyopathy with ventricular tachycardia. *J. Cardiovasc. Electrophysiol.* 13, 865–870. doi: 10.1046/j.1540-8167.2002.00865.x

Kitamura, H., Yoshida, A., Ohnishi, Y., Okajima, K., Ishida, A., Galeano, E. J., et al. (2003). Correlation of connexin43 expression and late ventricular potentials in nonischemic dilated cardiomyopathy. *Circulation* 67, 1017–1021. doi: 10.1253/circj.67.1017

Kleber, A. G., and Rudy, Y. (2004). Basic mechanisms of cardiac impulse propagation and associated arrhythmias. *Physiol. Rev.* 84, 431–488. doi: 10.1152/physrev.00025.2003

Kostin, S., Dammer, S., Hein, S., Klovekorn, W. P., Bauer, E. P., and Schaper, J. (2004). Connexin 43 expression and distribution in compensated and decompensated cardiac hypertrophy in patients with aortic stenosis. *Cardiovasc. Res.* 62, 426–436. doi: 10.1016/j.cardiores.2003.12.010

Kostin, S., Rieger, M., Dammer, S., Hein, S., Richter, M., Klövekorn, W. P., et al. (2003). Gap junction remodeling and altered connexin43 expression in the failing human heart. *Mol. Cell. Biochem.* 242, 135–144. doi: 10.1023/A:102115 4115673

Krenning, G., Zeisberg, E. M., and Kalluri, R. (2010). The origin of fibroblasts and mechanism of cardiac fibrosis. *J. Cell. Physiol.* 255, 631–637. doi: 10.1002/jcp.22322

Kudryashova, N. N., Teplenin, A. S., Orlova, Y. V., Selina, L. V., and Agladze, K. (2014). Arrhythmogenic role of the border between two areas of cardiac cell alignment. *J. Mol. Cell. Cardiol.* 76, 227–234. doi: 10.1016/j.yjmcc.2014.09.003

Lee, C. S., and Tkacs, N. C. (2008). Current concepts of neurohormonal activation in heart failure: mediators and mechanisms. *AACN Adv. Crit. Care* 19, 364–385. doi: 10.1097/01.AACN.0000340718.93742.c4

Lloyd-Jones, D. M., Larson, M. G., Leip, E. P., Beiser, A., D'Agostino, R. B., Kannel, W. B., et al. (2002). Lifetime risk for developing congestive heart failure: the framingham heart study. *Circulation* 106, 3068–3072. doi: 10.1161/01.CIR.0000039105.49749.6F

Lou, Q., Fedorov, V. V., Glukhov, A. V., Moazami, N., Fast, V. G., and Efimov, I. R. (2011). Transmural heterogeneity and remodeling of ventricular excitation-contraction coupling in human heart failure. *Circulation* 123, 1881–1890. doi: 10.1161/CIRCULATIONAHA.110.989707

Manabe, I., Shindo, T., and Nagai, R. (2002). Gene expression in fibroblasts and fibrosis: involvement in cardiac hypertrophy. *Circ. Res.* 91, 1103–1113. doi: 10.1161/01.RES.0000046452.67724.B8

Marcus, F. I., McKenna, W. J., Sherrill, D., Basso, C., Bauce, B., Bluemke, D. A., et al. (2010). Diagnosis of arrhythmogenic right ventricular cardiomyopathy/dysplasia - proposed modification of the task force criteria. *Circulation* 121, 1533–1541. doi: 10.1161/CIRCULATIONAHA.108.840827

Maron, B. J. (2002). Hypertrophic cardiomyopathy: a systematic review. *JAMA* 287, 1308–2130. doi: 10.1001/jama.287.10.1308

Maron, B. J., Maron, M. S., and Semsarian, C. (2012). Genetics of hypertrophic cardiomyopathy after 20 years. *J. Am. Coll. Cardiol.* 60, 705–715. doi: 10.1016/j.jacc.2012.02.068

McIntyre, H., and Fry, C. H. (1997). Abnormal action potential conduction in isolated human hypertrophied left ventricular myocardium. *J. Cardiovasc. Electrophysiol.* 8, 887–894. doi: 10.1111/j.1540-8167.1997.tb00850.x

McKoy, G., Protonotarios, N., Crosby, A., Tsatsopoulou, A., Anastasakis, A., Coonar, A., et al. (2000). Identification of a deletion in plakoglobin in arrhythmogenic right ventricular cardiomyopathy with palmoplantar keratoderma and woolly hair (Naxos disease). *Lancet* 355, 2119–2124. doi: 10.1016/S0140-6736(00)02379-5

Merner, N. D., Hodgkinson, K. A., Haywood, A. F., Connors, S., French, V. M., Drenckhahn, J. D., et al. (2008). Arrhythmogenic right ventricular cardiomyopathy type 5 is a fully penetrant, lethal arrhythmic disorder caused by a missense mutation in the TMEM43 gene. *Am. J. Hum. Genet.* 82, 809–821. doi: 10.1016/j.ajhg.2008.01.010

Mestroni, L., Rocco, C., Gregori, D., Sinagra, G., Di Lenarda, A., Miocic, S., et al. (1999). Familial dilated cardiomyopathy: evidence for genetic and phenotypic heterogeneity. Heart Muscle Disease Study Group. *J. Am. Coll. Cardiol.* 34, 181–190. doi: 10.1016/S0735-1097(99)00172-2

Mészáros, J., Khananshvili, D., and Hart, G. (2001). Mechanisms underlying delayed afterdepolarizations in hypertrophied left ventricular myocytes of rats. *Am. J. Physiol. Heart Circ. Physiol.* 281, H903–H914.

Meyerburg, R. J., Kessler, K. M., and Castellanos, A. (1992). Sudden cardiac death. Structure, function, and time-dependence of risk. *Circulation* 85(1 Suppl): I2–I10.

Molkentin, J. D., Lu, J. R., Antos, C. L., Markham, B., Richardson, J., Robbins, J., et al. (1998). A calcineurin-dependent transcriptional pathway for cardiac hypertrophy. *Cell* 93, 215–228. doi: 10.1016/S0092-8674(00)81573-1

Morley, G. E., Vaidya, D., Samie, F. H., Lo, C., Delmar, M., and Jalife, J. (1999). Characterization of conduction in the ventricles of normal and heterozygous Cx43 knockout mice using optical mapping. *J. Cardiovasc. Electrophysiol.* 10, 1361–1375. doi: 10.1111/j.1540-8167.1999.tb00192.x

Nakayama, Y., Shimizu, G., Hirota, Y., Saito, T., Kino, M., Kitaura, Y., et al. (1987). Functional and histopathologic correlation in patients with dilated cardiomyopathy: an integrated evaluation by multivariate analysis. *J. Am. Coll. Cardiol.* 10, 186–192.

Nian, M., Lee, P., Khaper, N., and Liu, P. (2004). Inflammatory cytokines and postmyocardial infarction remodeling. *Circ. Res.* 94, 1543–1553. doi: 10.1161/01.RES.0000130526.20854.fa

Noorman, M., Groeneweg, J. A., Asimaki, A., Rizzo, S., Papegaaij, M., van Stuijvenberg, L., et al. (2013b). End stage of arrhythmogenic cardiomyopathy with severe involvement of the interventricular septum. *Heart Rhythm* 10, 283–289. doi: 10.1016/j.hrthm.2012.10.029

Noorman, M., Hakim, S., Kessler, E., Groeneweg, J. A., Cox, M. G., Asimaki, A., et al. (2013a). Remodeling of the cardiac sodium channel, connexin43, and plakoglobin at the intercalated disk in patients with arrhythmogenic cardiomyopathy. *Heart Rhythm* 10, 412–419. doi: 10.1016/j.hrthm.2012.11.018

Noorman, M., van der Heyden, M. A., van Veen, T. A., Cox, M. G., Hauer, R. N., de Bakker, J. M., et al. (2009). Cardiac cell-cell junctions in health and disease: electrical versus mechanical coupling. *J. Mol. Cell. Cardiol.* 47, 23–31. doi: 10.1016/j.yjmcc.2009.03.016

Norgett, E. E., Hatsell, S. J., Carvajal-Huerta, L., Cabezas, J. C., Common, J., Purkis, P. E., et al. (2000). Recessive mutation in desmoplakin disrupts desmoplakin-intermediate filament interactions and causes dilated cardiomyopathy, woolly hair and keratoderma. *Hum. Mol. Genet.* 9, 2761–2766. doi: 10.1093/hmg/9.18.2761

Orban, P. C., Chui, D., and Marth, J. D. (1992). Tissue- and site-specific DNA recombination in transgenic mice. *Proc. Natl. Acad. Sci. U.S.A.* 89, 6861–6865. doi: 10.1073/pnas.89.15.6861

Otten, E., Asimaki, A., Maass, A., van Langen, I. M., van der Wal, A., de Jonge, N., et al. (2010). Desmin mutations as a cause of right ventricular heart failure affect the intercalated disks. *Heart Rhythm* 7, 1058–1064. doi: 10.1016/j.hrthm.2010.04.023

Palka, P., Lange, A., Fleming, A. D., Donnelly, J. E., Dutka, D. P., Starkey, I. R., et al. (1997). Differences in myocardial velocity gradient measured throughout the cardiac cycle in patients with hypertrophic cardiomyopathy, athletes and patients with left ventricular hypertrophy due to hypertension. *J. Am. Coll. Cardiol.* 30, 760–768. doi: 10.1016/S0735-1097(97)00231-3

Papadatos, G. A., Wallerstein, P. M., Head, C. E., Ratcliff, R., Brady, P. A., Benndorf, K., et al. (2002). Slowed conduction and ventricular tachycardia after targeted disruption of the cardiac sodium channel gene Scn5a. *Proc. Natl. Acad. Sci. U.S.A.* 99, 6210–6215. doi: 10.1073/pnas.082121299

Pazo, D., Kramer, L., Pumir, A., Kanani, S., Efimov, I., and Krinsky, V. (2004). Pinning force in active media. *Phys. Rev. Lett.* 93, 168303-1–168303-4. doi: 10.1103/PhysRevLett.93.168303

Peters, N. S., Coromilas, J., Severs, N. J., and Wit, A. L. (1997). Disturbed connexin43 gap junction distribution correlates with the location of reentrant circuits in the epicardial border zone of healing canine infarcts that cause ventricular tachycardia. *Circulation* 95, 988–996. doi: 10.1161/01.CIR.95.4.988

Peters, N. S., Green, C. R., Poole-Wilson, P. A., and Severs, N. J. (1993). Reduced content of connexin43 gap junctions in ventricular myocardium from hypertrophied and ischemic human hearts. *Circulation* 88, 864–875. doi: 10.1161/01.CIR.88.3.864

Petitprez, S., Zmoos, A. F., Ogrodnik, J., Balse, E., Raad, N., El-Haou, S., et al. (2011). SAP97 and dystrophin macromolecular complexes determine two pools of cardiac sodium channels Nav1.5 in cardiomyocytes. *Circ. Res.* 108, 294–304. doi: 10.1161/CIRCRESAHA.110.228312

Pilichou, K., Nava, A., Basso, C., Beffagna, G., Bauce, B., Lorenzon, A., et al. (2006). Mutations in desmoglein-2 gene are associated with arrhythmogenic right ventricular cardiomyopathy. *Circulation* 113, 1171–1179. doi: 10.1161/CIRCULATIONAHA.105.583674

Protonotarios, N., and Tsatsopoulou, A. (2004). Naxos disease and carvajal syndrome: cardiocutaneous disorders that highlight the pathogenesis and broaden the spectrum of arrhythmogenic right ventricular cardiomyopathy. *Cardiovasc. Pathol.* 13, 185–194. doi: 10.1016/j.carpath.2004.03.609

Protonotarios, N., Tsatsopoulou, A., Patsourakos, P., Alexopoulos, D., Gezerlis, P., Simitsis, S., et al. (1986). Cardiac abnormalities in familial palmoplantar keratosis. *Br. Heart J.* 56, 321–326. doi: 10.1136/hrt.56.4.321

Punske, B., Taccardi, B., Steadman, B., Ershler, P. R., England, A., Valencik, M. L., et al. (2005). Effect of fiber orientation on propagation: electrical mapping of genetically altered mouse hearts. *J. Electrocardiol.* 38, 40–44. doi: 10.1016/j.jelectrocard.2005.06.097

Rampazzo, A., Nava, A., Malacrida, S., Beffagna, G., Bauce, B., Rossi, V., et al. (2002). Mutation in human desmoplakin domain binding to plakoglobin causes a dominant form of arrhythmogenic right ventricular cardiomyopathy. *Am. J. Hum. Genet.* 71, 1200–1206. doi: 10.1086/344208

Reaume, A. G., de Sousa, P. A., Kulkarni, S., Langille, B. L., Zhu, D., Davies, T. C., et al. (1995). Cardiac malformation in neonatal mice lacking connexin 43. *Science* 267, 1831–1834. doi: 10.1126/science.7892609

Remme, C. A., Verkerk, A. O., Hoogaars, W. M., Aanhaanen, W. T., Scicluna, B. P., Annink, C., et al. (2009). The cardiac sodium channel displays differential distribution in the conduction system and transmural heterogeneity in the murine ventricular myocardium. *Basic Res. Cardiol.* 104, 511–522. doi: 10.1007/s00395-009-0012-8

Remme, C. A., Verkerk, A. O., Nuyens, D., van Ginneken, A. C., van Brunschot, S., Belterman, C. N., et al. (2006). Overlap syndrome of cardiac sodium channel disease in mice carrying the equivalent mutation of human SCN5A-1795insD. *Circulation* 114, 2584–2594. doi: 10.1161/CIRCULATIONAHA.106.653949

Richardson, P., McKenna, W., Bristow, M., Maisch, B., Mautner, B., O'Connell, J., et al. (1996). Report of the 1995 World Health Organization/International Society and Federation of Cardiology Task Force on the Definition and Classification of cardiomyopathies. *Circulation* 93, 841–842. doi: 10.1161/01.CIR.93.5.841

Ripplinger, C. M., Krinsky, V. I., Nikolski, V. P., and Efimov, I. R. (2006). Mechanisms of unpinning and termination of ventricular tachycardia. *Am. J. Physiol.* 291, H184–H192. doi: 10.1152/ajpheart.01300.2005

Ripplinger, C. M., Li, W., Hadley, J., Chen, J., Rothenberg, F., Lombardi, R., et al. (2007). Enhanced transmural fiber rotation and connexin 43 heterogeneity are associated with an increased upper limit of vulnerability in a transgenic rabbit model of human hypertrophic cardiomyopathy. *Circ. Res.* 101, 1049–1057. doi: 10.1161/CIRCRESAHA.107.161240

Rizzo, S., Lodder, E. M., Verkerk, A. O., Wolswinkel, R., Beekman, L., Pilichou, K., et al. (2012). Intercalated disc abnormalities, reduced Na+ current density, and conduction slowing in desmoglein-2 mutant mice prior to cardiomyopathic changes. *Cardiovasc. Res.* 95, 409–418. doi: 10.1093/cvr/cvs219

Roger, V. L., Lloyd-Jones, D. M., Adams, R. J., Berry, J. D., Brown, T. M., Carnethon, M. R., et al. (2011). Heart disease and stroke statistics - update: a report fromthe American Heart Association. *Circulation* 123, e18–e209. doi: 10.1161/CIR.0b013e3182009701

Rohr, S. (2009). Myofibroblasts in diseased hearts: new players in cardiac arrhythmias. *Heart Rhythm* 6, 848–856. doi: 10.1016/j.hrthm.2009.02.038

Royer, A., van Veen, T. A., Le Bouter, S., Marionneau, C., Griol-Charhbili, V., Léoni, A. L., et al. (2005). Mouse model of SCN5A-linked hereditary Lenegre's disease: age-related conduction slowing and myocardial fibrosis. *Circulation* 111, 1738–1746. doi: 10.1161/01.CIR.0000160853.19867.61

Ruiz, P., Brinkmann, V., Ledermann, B., Behrend, M., Grund, C., Thalhammer, C., et al. (1996). Targeted mutation of plakoglobin in mice reveals essential functions of desmosomes in the embryonic heart. *J. Cell Biol.* 135, 215–225. doi: 10.1083/jcb.135.1.215

Saffitz, J., Asimaki, A., and Huang, H. (2009). Arrhythmogenic right ventricular cardiomyopathy: new insights into disease mechanisms and diagnosis. *J. Investig. Med.* 57, 861–864. doi: 10.231/JIM.0b013e3181c5e631

Salameh, A., Krautblatter, S., Karl, S., Blanke, K., Gomez, D. R., Dhein, S., et al. (2009). The signal transduction cascade regulating the expression of the gap junction protein connexin43 by beta-adrenoceptors. *Br. J. Pharmacol.* 158, 198–208. doi: 10.1111/j.1476-5381.2009.00344.x

Sanbe, A., James, J., Tuzcu, V., Nas, S., Martin, L., Gulick, J., et al. (2005). Transgenic rabbit model for human troponin I-based hypertrophic cardiomyopathy. *Circulation* 111, 2330–2338. doi: 10.1161/01.CIR.0000164234.24957.75

Sasano, C., Honjo, H., Takagishi, Y., Uzzaman, M., Emdad, L., Shimizu, A., et al. (2007). Internalization and dephosphorylation of connexin43 in hypertrophied right ventricles of rats with pulmonary hypertension. *Circulation* 71, 382–389. doi: 10.1253/circj.71.382

Sato, P. Y., Coombs, W., Lin, X., Nekrasova, O., Green, K. J., Isom, L. L., et al. (2011). Interactions between ankyrin-G, Plakophilin-2, and Connexin43 at the cardiac intercalated disc. *Circ. Res.* 109, 193–201. doi: 10.1161/CIRCRESAHA.111.247023

Sato, P. Y., Musa, H., Coombs, W., Guerrero-Serna, G., Patiño, G. A., Taffet, S. M., et al. (2009). Loss of plakophilin-2 expression leads to decreased sodium current and slower conduction velocity in cultured cardiac myocytes. *Circ. Res.* 105, 523–526. doi: 10.1161/CIRCRESAHA.109.201418

Sato, P. Y., Ohkusa, T., Honjo, H., Suzuki, S., Yoshida, M. A., Ishiguro, Y. S., et al. (2008). Altered expression of connexin43 contributes to the arrhythmogenic substrate during the development of heart failure in cardiomyopatic hamster. *Am. J. Physiol. Heart Circ.* 294, H1164–H1173. doi: 10.1152/ajpheart.00960.2007

Sepp, R., Severs, N. J., and Gourdie, R. G. (1996). Altered patterns of cardiac intercellular junction distribution in hypertrophic cardiomyopathy. *Heart* 76, 412–417. doi: 10.1136/hrt.76.5.412

Shryock, J. C., Song, Y., Rajamani, S., Antzelevitch, C., and Belardinelli, L. (2013). The arrhythmogenic consequences of increasing late INa in the cardiomyocyte. *Cardiovasc. Res.* 99, 600–611. doi: 10.1093/cvr/cvt145

Silverman, H. S., and Stern, M. D. (1994). Ionic basis of ischaemic cardiac injury: insights from cellular studies. *Cardiovasc. Res.* 28, 581–597. doi: 10.1093/cvr/28.5.581

Smiley, D., Smith, M. A., Carreira, V., Jiang, M., Koch, S. E., Kelley, M., et al. (2014). Increased fibrosis and progression to heart failure in MRL mice following ischemia/reperfusion injury. *Cardiovasc. Pathol.* 23, 327–334. doi: 10.1016/j.carpath.2014.06.001

Smith, J. H., Green, C. R., Peters, N. S., Rothery, S., and Severs, N. J. (1991). Altered patterns of gap junction distribution in ischemic heart disease. An immunohistochemical study of human myocardium using laser scanning confocal microscopy. *Am. J. Pathol.* 139, 801–821.

Soliman, D., Green, C. R., Peters, N. S., Rothery, S., and Severs, N. J. (2012). Late sodium current inhibition alone with ranolazine is sufficient to reduce ischemia- and cardiac glycoside-induced calcium overload and contractile dysfunction mediated by reverse-mode sodium/calcium exchange. *J. Pharmacol. Exp. Ther.* 343, 325–332. doi: 10.1124/jpet.112.196949

Spach, M. S., Heidlage, J. F., Dolber, P. C., and Barr, R. C. (2000). Electrophysiological effects of remodeling cardiac gap junctions and cell size experimental and model studies of normal cardiac growth. *Circ. Res.* 86, 302–311. doi: 10.1161/01.RES.86.3.302

Stein, M., Boulaksil, M., Jansen, J. A., Herold, E., Noorman, M., Joles, J. A., et al. (2010). Reduction of fibrosis-related arrhythmias by chronic renin-angiotensin-aldosterone system inhibitors in an aged mouse model. *Am. J. Physiol. Heart Circ. Physiol.* 299, 310–321. doi: 10.1152/ajpheart.01137.2009

Stein, M., van Veen, T. A., Hauer, R. N., de Bakker, J. M., and van Rijen, H. V. (2011). A 50% reduction of excitability but not of intercellular coupling affects conduction velocity restitution and activation delay in the mouse heart. *PLoS ONE* 6:e20310. doi: 10.1371/journal.pone.0020310

Stein, M., van Veen, T. A., Remme, C. A., Boulaksil, M., Noorman, M., van Stuijvenberg, L., et al. (2009). Combined reduction of intercellular coupling and membrane excitability differentially affects transverse and longitudinal cardiac conduction. *Cardiovasc. Res.* 83, 52–60. doi: 10.1093/cvr/cvp124

Strom, M., Wan, X., Poelzing, S., Ficker, E., and Rosenbaum, D. S. (2010). Gap junction heterogeneity as mechanism for electrophysiologically distinct properties across the ventricular wall. *Am. J. Physiol. Heart Circ. Physiol.* 298, 787–794. doi: 10.1152/ajpheart.00887.2009

Swynghedauw, B. (1999). Molecular mechanisms of myocardial remodeling. *Physiol. Rev.* 79, 215–262.

Syrris, P., Ward, D., Evans, A., Asimaki, A., Gandjbakhch, E., Sen-Chowdhry, S., et al. (2006). Arrhythmogenic right ventricular dysplasia/cardiomyopathy associated with mutations in the desmosomal gene desmocollin-2. *Am. J. Hum. Genet.* 79, 978–984. doi: 10.1086/509122

Tanaka, K., Zlochiver, S., Vikstrom, K. L., Yamazaki, M., Moreno, J., Klos, M., et al. (2007). Spatial distribution of fibrosis governs fibrillation wave dynamics in the posterior left atrium during heart failure. *Circ. Res.* 101, 839–847. doi: 10.1161/CIRCRESAHA.107.153858

Tani, M., and Neely, J. R. (1989). Role of intracellular Na^+ and Ca^{2+} overload and depressed recovery of ventricular function of reperfused ischemic rat hearts. Possible involvement of H^+-Na^+ and Na^+-Ca^{2+} exchange. *Circ. Res.* 65, 1045–1056. doi: 10.1161/01.RES.65.4.1045

Tansey, E. E., Kwaku, K. F., Hammer, P. E., Cowan, D. B., Federman, M., Levitsky, S., et al. (2006). Reduction and redistribution of gap and adherens junction proteins after ischemia and reperfusion. *Ann. Thorac. Surg.* 82, 1472–1479. doi: 10.1016/j.athoracsur.2006.04.061

Thiene, G., Nava, A., Corrado, D., Rossi, L., and Pennelli, N. (1988). Right ventricular cardiomyopathy and sudden death in young people. *N. Engl. J. Med.* 318, 129–133. doi: 10.1056/NEJM198801213180301

Thomas, S. A., Schuessler, R. B., Berul, C. I., Beardslee, M. A., Beyer, E. C., Mendelsohn, M. E., et al. (1998). Disparate effects of deficient expression of Connexin43 on atrial and ventricular conduction: evidence for chamber-specific molecular determinants of conduction. *Circulation* 97, 686–691. doi: 10.1161/01.CIR.97.7.686

Thomas, S. P., Kucera, J. P., Bircher-Lehmann, L., Rudy, Y., Saffitz, J. E., and Kléber, A. G. (2003). Impulse propagation in synthetic strands of neonatal cardiac myocytes with genetically reduced levels of connexin43. *Circ. Res.* 92, 1209–1216. doi: 10.1161/01.RES.0000074916.41221.EA

Towbin, J. A., Lowe, A. M., Colan, S. D., Sleeper, L. A., Orav, E. J., Clunie, S., et al. (2006). Incidence, causes, and outcomes of dilated cardiomyopathy in children. *JAMA* 296, 1867–1876. doi: 10.1001/jama.296.15.1867

Undrovinas, A. I., Maltsev, V. A., and Sabbah, H. N. (1999). Repolarization abnormalities in cardiomyocytes of dogs with chronic heart failure: role of sustained inward current. *Cell Mol. Life Sci.* 55, 494–505. doi: 10.1007/s000180050306

Uzzaman, M., Honjo, H., Takagishi, Y., Emdad, L., Magee, A. I., Severs, N. J., et al. (2000). Remodeling of gap junctional coupling in hypertrophied right ventricles of rats with monocrotaline-induced pulmonary hypertension. *Circ. Res.* 86, 871–878. doi: 10.1161/01.RES.86.8.871

van der Zwaag, P. A., van Rijsingen, I. A., Asimaki, A., Jongbloed, J. D., van Veldhuisen, D. J., Wiesfeld, A. C., et al. (2012). Phospholamban R14del mutation in patients diagnosed with dilated cardiomyopathy or arrhythmogenic right ventricular cardiomyopathy: evidence supporting the concept of arrhythmogenic cardiomyopathy. *Eur. J. Heart Fail.* 14, 1199–1207. doi: 10.1093/eurjhf/hfs119 van Rijen, H. V., Eckardt, D., Degen, J., Theis, M., Ott, T., Willecke, K., et al. (2004). Slow conduction and enhanced anisotropy increase the propensity for ventricular tachyarrhythmias in adult mice with induced deletion of connexin43. *Circulation* 109, 1048–1055. doi: 10.1161/01.CIR.0000117402.70689.75

van Rijen, H. V., van Veen, T. A., Gros, D., Wilders, R., and de Bakker, J. M. (2006). Connexins and cardiac arrhythmias. *Adv. Cardiol.* 42, 150–160. doi: 10.1159/000092567

van Tintelen, J. P., Entius, M. M., Bhuiyan, Z. A., Jongbloed, R., Wiesfeld, A. C., Wilde, A. A., et al. (2006). Plakophilin-2 mutations are the major determinant of familial arrhythmogenic right ventricular dysplasia/cardiomyopathy. *Circulation* 113, 1650–1658. doi: 10.1161/CIRCULATIONAHA.105.609719

van Veen, T. A., Stein, M., Royer, A., Le Quang, K., Charpentier, F., Colledge, W. H., et al. (2005). Impaired impulse propagation in Scn5a-knockout mice combined contribution of excitability, connexin expression, and tissue architecture in relation to aging. *Circ* 112, 1927–1935. doi: 10.1161/CIRCULATIONAHA.105.539072

van Veen, T. A., van Rijen, H. V., Wiegerinck, R. F., Opthof, T., Colbert, M. C., Clement, S., et al. (2002). Remodeling of gap junctions in mouse hearts hypertrophied by forced retinoic acid signaling. *J. Mol. Cell. Cardiol.* 34, 1411–1423. doi: 10.1006/jmcc.2002.2102

Vetter, F. J., Simons, S. B., Mironov, S., Hyatt, C. J., and Pertsov, A. M. (2005). Epicardial fiber organization in swine right ventricle and its impact on propagation. *Circ. Res.* 96, 244–251. doi: 10.1161/01.RES.0000153979.71859.e7

Wagner, S., Dybkova, N., Rasenack, E. C., Jacobshagen, C., Fabritz, L., Kirchhof, P., et al. (2006). Ca2+/calmodulin-dependent protein kinase II regulates cardiac Na+ channels. *J. Clin. Invest.* 116, 3127–3138. doi: 10.1172/JCI26620

Wagner, S., Ruff, H. M., Weber, S. L., Bellmann, S., Sowa, T., Schulte, T., et al. (2011). Reactive oxygen species-activated Ca/calmodulin kinase IIδ is required for late I(Na) augmentation leading to cellular Na and Ca overload. *Circ. Res.* 108, 555–565. doi: 10.1161/CIRCRESAHA.110.221911

Wang, X., Li, F., Campbell, S. E., and Gerdes, A. M. (1999). Chronic pressure overload cardiac hypertrophy and failure in guinea pigs: II. Cytoskeletal remodeling. *J. Mol. Cell. Cardiol.* 31, 319–331. doi: 10.1006/jmcc.1998.0885

Weber, K. T., Sun, Y., and Díez, J. (2008). Fibrosis: a living tissue and the infarcted heart. *J. Am. Coll. Cardiol.* 52, 2029–2031. doi: 10.1016/j.jacc.2008.09.012

Weber, K. T., Sun, Y., Tyagi, S. C., and Cleutjens, J. P. (1994). Collagen network of the myocardium: function, structural remodeling and regulatory mechanisms. *J. Mol. Cell. Cardiol.* 26, 279–292. doi: 10.1006/jmcc.1994.1036

Westerhof, N., and O'Rourke, M. F. (1995). Haemodynamic basis for the development of left ventricular failure. *J. Hypertens.* 13, 943–952.

Wiegerinck, R. F., Verkerk, A. O., Belterman, C. N., van Veen, T. A., Baartscheer, A., Opthof, T., et al. (2006). Larger cell size in rabbits with heart failure increases myocardial conduction velocity and QRS duration. *Circulation* 113, 806–813. doi: 10.1161/CIRCULATIONAHA.105.565804

Winterton, S. J., Turner, M. A., O'Gorman, D. J., Flores, N. A., and Sheridan, D. J. (1994). Hypertrophy causes delayed conduction in human and guinea pig myocardium: accentuation during ischaemic perfusion. *Cardiovasc. Res* 28, 47–54. doi: 10.1093/cvr/28.1.47

Wu, A. H. (2007). Management of patients with non–ischaemic cardiomyopathy. *Heart* 93, 403–408. doi: 10.1136/hrt.2005.085761

Xia, Y., Lee, K., Li, N., Corbett, D., Mendoza, L., and Frangogiannis, N. G. (2009). Characterization of the inflammatory and fibrotic response in a mouse model of cardiac pressure overload. *Histochem. Cell Biol.* 131, 471–481. doi: 10.1007/s00418-008-0541-5

Xiao, X. H., and Allen, D. G. (1999). Role of Na^+/H^+ exchanger during ischemia and preconditioning in the isolated rat heart. *Circ. Res.* 85, 723–730. doi: 10.1161/01.RES.85.8.723

Yamada, K. A., Rogers, J. G., Sundset, R., Steinberg, T. H., and Saffitz, J. (2003). Up-regulation of connexin45 in heart failure. *J. Cardiovasc. Electrophysiol.* 14, 1205–1212. doi: 10.1046/j.1540-8167.2003.03276.x

Zaino, E. C., and Tabor, S. H. (1963). Cardiac hypertrophy in acute myocardial infarction a study based on 100 autopsied cases. *Circulation* 28, 1081–1083. doi: 10.1161/01.CIR.28.6.1081

Zhang, Y., Wang, H., Kovacs, A., Kanter, E. M., and Yamada, K. A. (2010). Reduced expression of Cx43 attenuates ventricular remodeling after myocardial infarction via impaired TGF-beta signaling. *Am. J. Physiol. Heart Circ. Physiol.* 298, H477–H487. doi: 10.1152/ajpheart.00806.2009

Zhao, J., Stephenson, R. S., Sands, G. B., LeGrice, I. J., Zhang, H., Jarvis, J. C., et al. (2013). Atrial fibrosis and atrial fibrillation: a computer simulation in the posterior left atrium. *FIMH LNCS* 7945, 400–408. doi: 10.1007/978-3-642-38899-6_47

Zimmer, H. G. (1994). Some aspects of cardiac heterogeneity. *Basic Res. Cardiol.* 89, 101–117.

5

Potential effects of intrinsic heart pacemaker cell mechanisms on dysrhythmic cardiac action potential firing

Yael Yaniv[1]*, Kenta Tsutsui[2] and Edward G. Lakatta[2]*

[1] Biomedical Engineering Faculty, Technion-Israel Institute of Technology, Haifa, Israel
[2] Laboratory of Cardiovascular Science, Biomedical Research Center, Intramural Research Program, National Institute on Aging, National Institutes of Health, Baltimore, MD, USA

***Correspondence:**
Yael Yaniv, Biomedical Engineering Faculty, Technion-Israel Institute of Technology, 3200003 Haifa, Israel
e-mail: yaely@bm.technion.ac.il;
Edward G. Lakatta, Laboratory of Cardiovascular Science, Biomedical Research Center, Intramural Research Program, National Institute on Aging, NIH, 251 Bayview Blvd, Baltimore, 21224 MD, USA
e-mail: lakattae@grc.nia.nih.gov

The heart's regular electrical activity is initiated by specialized cardiac pacemaker cells residing in the sinoatrial node. The rate and rhythm of spontaneous action potential firing of sinoatrial node cells are regulated by stochastic mechanisms that determine the level of coupling of chemical to electrical clocks within cardiac pacemaker cells. This coupled-clock system is modulated by autonomic signaling from the brain via neurotransmitter release from the vagus and sympathetic nerves. Abnormalities in brain-heart clock connections or in any molecular clock activity within pacemaker cells lead to abnormalities in the beating rate and rhythm of the pacemaker tissue that initiates the cardiac impulse. Dysfunction of pacemaker tissue can lead to tachy-brady heart rate alternation or exit block that leads to long atrial pauses and increases susceptibility to other cardiac arrhythmia. Here we review evidence for the idea that disturbances in the intrinsic components of pacemaker cells may be implemented in arrhythmia induction in the heart.

Keywords: arrhythmias, atrial fibrillation, coupled-clock pacemaker system, heart rate variability, sinus node disease

INTRODUCTION

Normal cardiac impulse initiation and conduction are generated by specialized, self-excitable, pacemaker cells residing in the sinoatrial node (SAN). Defects in these cell-intrinsic capacities to elicit spontaneous action potentials (APs) can lead to disturbances of the rate and rhythm of heart beats, and can induce numerous clinical arrhythmia syndromes: (i) SAN dysfunction has been postulated to be a source of sinus nodal re-entry (i.e., reciprocal beats between SAN and atrium) tachyarrhythmia (Birchfield et al., 1957) which accounts for 2–17% of all arrhythmias (Cossu and Steinberg, 1998). While diagnosis of this arrhythmia is difficult, due to electrocardiographic similarity of the P-wave to the normal sinus rhythm (Gomes et al., 1995), microelectrode studies in isolated rabbit hearts (Han et al., 1968) and later in humans (Childers et al., 1973) indeed demonstrate that SAN is the source that induces re-entry. (ii) Sick sinus syndrome, characterized by symptomatic dysfunction of the SAN (reviewed in Dobrzynski et al., 2007), can be manifested as sinus bradycardia, sinus arrest, or SAN block, and in some cases supraventricular tachyarrhythmias ("tachy-brady" syndrome), atrial flutter or atrial fibrillation. In mice with an inducible phenotype that mimics sick sinus syndrome, heart beating intervals (BIs) were completely irregular both *in vivo* and in the isolated Langendroff perfused model (no brain-heart signaling) (Herrmann et al., 2007). Telemetric ECG recordings revealed a variety of arrhythmias: sino-atrial arrhythmia, sino-atrial pause and supraventricular or ventricular tachycardia. (iii) It has been suggested that abnormal stretch of the rat atria that accompanies many heart diseases (De Jong et al., 2013) and occurs even in transplanted human hearts (Slovut et al., 1998) (no brain-heart connection) induces respiratory sinus arrhythmia.

Here we review evidence for the idea that changes in the membrane and sarcoplasmic reticulum (SR) components of pacemaker cells may be implicated in arrhythmia induction in the heart.

INTRINSIC COUPLED-CLOCK MECHANISMS TO PACEMAKER CELLS CONTROL THE HEART RATE AND RHYTHM

To understand abnormal SAN function it is essential to first understand the normal function of intrinsic properties of pacemaker cells and their modulation by brain-heart signaling. Experimental and theoretical data over the past two decades indicate that pacemaker cells residing in the SAN entrain their AP BI variability (BIV) by regulation of intracellular electric and mechanical coupling (reviewed in Yaniv et al., 2013a).

The coupled-clock system (Yaniv et al., 2013b; Maltsev et al., 2014) that controls the pacemaker cell beating rate and rhythm consists of an intracellular "Ca^{2+} clock" and "M clock." The sarcoplasmic reticulum Ca^{2+} pump and ryanodine channels act as a "Ca^{2+} clock," discharging local Ca^{2+} releases (LCRs) close to the cell surface membrane; LCRs activate membrane electrogenic clock molecules ("M clock"), mainly the Na^+/Ca^{2+} exchanger. Na^+-Ca^{2+} exchange current, the f-channel current, and K^+ channel current, other components of the M clock, concurrently drive the diastolic membrane depolarization to ignite the next AP. The Ca^{2+} and M clocks entrain each other through electrical and chemical signaling: Ca^{2+} activation of calmodulin -adenylyl cyclase (AC)-dependent protein kinase A (PKA) and Ca^{2+}/calmodulin-dependent protein kinase II (CaMKII). Both of these signaling pathways affect phosphorylation of proteins of both clocks [i.e., phospholamban (PLB) and ryanodine receptors (Ca^{2+} clock) and L type and K^+ channels (M clock)]. Additionally, cAMP positively shifts the f-channel activation curve. Based on the coupled-clock theory, a change in the activity or in the quantity of every molecule within the M or the Ca^{2+} clock or a change in the chemical coupling signaling of both clocks will perturb the function of the other clock, and thus alter the degree of entrainment between them. For example, in rabbit pacemaker cells, reduction in I_f activity or in Ca^{2+} clock proteins leads to reduction in the coupled-clock phosphorylation activity and LCR signal (Yaniv et al., 2014b). Thus, a reduction of internal signaling within one clock can lead to a reduction in the degree of clock coupling and changes in the function of the other clock that change automaticity.

Even under normal conditions, spontaneous AP BIs of mammals including human pacemaker cells are not constant, but vary around the average AP BI, due to stochastic properties of intrinsic mechanisms of the coupled-clock system (Verheijck et al., 1998; Rocchetti et al., 2000; Zaza and Lombardi, 2001; Monfredi et al., 2013; Papaioannou et al., 2013; Yaniv et al., 2014b). The degree of AP BIV is related to variability in both the timing of LCR occurrence during the diastolic depolarization, and to the ensemble LCR Ca^{2+} signal: an increase in LCR variability is associated with a reduced ensemble LCR Ca^{2+} signal that occurs later in diastole (i.e., prolonging the next AP ignition). Based on the coupled-clock theory, the stochasticity of LCR periods (i.e., the times of LCR occurrences following the prior AP) not only depends upon stochasticity of spontaneous RyR activation, but also upon stochastic sarcolemmal ion channel openings and closings that regulate the cell Ca^{2+} balance. The amplitude and timing of LCR Ca^{2+} signals to M clock proteins report the efficiency of clock coupling, i.e., a weaker LCR signal to M clock proteins that occurs later in time reports less-efficient clock coupling. Consequently, changes in the steady-state AP BI and the BIV embody contributions of both clocks. Reduction in the degree of synchronization between the clocks disturbs the ability to maintain the basal average AP BI, leading not only to a reduction in the average AP BI, but also to an increase in variability around the prolonged average AP BI.

Autonomic neural input can entrain the rate and rhythm of electrical impulses that are generated by SAN tissue of mammals (Difrancesco, 1993; Boyett et al., 2000; Monfredi et al., 2014; Yaniv et al., 2014a). The balance between sympathetic to parasympathetic stimulation has a role in synchronizing intrinsic clock periods of individual pacemaker cells. β adrenergic receptor stimulation increases synchronization of intrinsic clock mechanisms leading to a decrease of both BI and BIV of pacemaker cells (**Figures 1B,C**). Moreover, β adrenergic receptor stimulation of a single pacemaker cell increases the probability that the beating intervals exhibit fractal-like behavior. Cholinergic receptor stimulation of pacemaker cells, on the other hand, decreases synchronization of intrinsic clock mechanisms, leading to an increase of both the average BI and BIV (**Figures 1B,C**).

SYNCHRONIZATION OF ACTIVITY ACROSS THE POPULATION OF CELLS CAN IMPACT ON THE HEART RATE AND RHYTHM

Although we have focused here upon synchronization of mechanisms intrinsic to pacemaker cells, cell-to-cell interactions (electrotonic and mechanical) of pacemaker cells residing in SAN tissue also entrain the rate and rhythm of electrical impulses that emanate from the SAN (Jalife, 1984; Watanabe et al., 1995). These interactions have a role in synchronizing the intrinsic clock periods of individual cells (Sheikh et al., 2013), because the average range of basal AP BI and AP BIV of single isolated pacemaker cells is well above their range when they reside in rabbit SAN tissue (Yaniv et al., 2014a) (**Figure 1A**). When pacemaker cells are embedded within SAN tissue, those with the shortest AP BI create a primary pacemaker area within the SAN, leading to the origin of an electrotonic force that spreads to other SAN cells, resulting in the emanation of an electric impulse that excites the rest of the heart (Anumonwo et al., 1991). This impulse controls the heart rate and rhythm. When rabbit pacemaker cells are isolated from SAN tissue, their beating interval entropy increases dramatically compared to that when these cells reside in SAN tissue (**Figure 1B**), and fractal-like behavior of AP BIs, a feature that characterizes AP BI of SAN tissue, is absent in isolated single pacemaker cells (Yaniv et al., 2014a).

CHANGES IN HEART RATE VARIABILITY INDEXES AND THE PRESENCE OF ARRHYTHMIA

An increase in pacemaker cells AP BIV, or in mathematical terms coupled-clock-system entropy, above a certain threshold leads to abnormal impulse generation by the SAN that is defined as arrhythmia. Two regimes of heart rate variability (HRV) are analyzed in patients with arrhythmogenic events: during the events when the entropy of the system increases (Costa et al., 2008), and before the occurrence of arrhythmia. The occurrence of major arrhythmic events in patients with right ventricular cardiomyopathy is associated with a reduced BIV (Battipaglia et al., 2012). Interestingly, heart rate variability indexes decrease just prior to an arrhythmogenic event (Postolache et al., 2011). As we summarized here, the degree of synchronization of intrinsic mechanisms to pacemaker cells and the degree of synchronization among pacemaker cells within the SAN are determinants of the heart rate and rhythm. Autonomic receptors on pacemaker cells respond to the imbalances of autonomic impulses associated with cardiac diseases. Specifically, autonomic receptor stimulation of single pacemaker cells alters their beat-to-beat variability. Thus, intrinsic pacemaker mechanisms may contribute to HRV *in vivo*. Although mechanisms of HRV may vary from one patient to another, documentation of the relationship between HRV and different arrhythmias in human patients (**Table 1**) is an important initial step to conceptually link intrinsic pacemaker mechanisms to arrhythmogenic events. Note, that this sort of evidence, however, does not prove that altered synchronization of pacemaker clock mechanisms residing within the SAN are the sole cause of all patient arrhythmias that may be linked to changes in HRV.

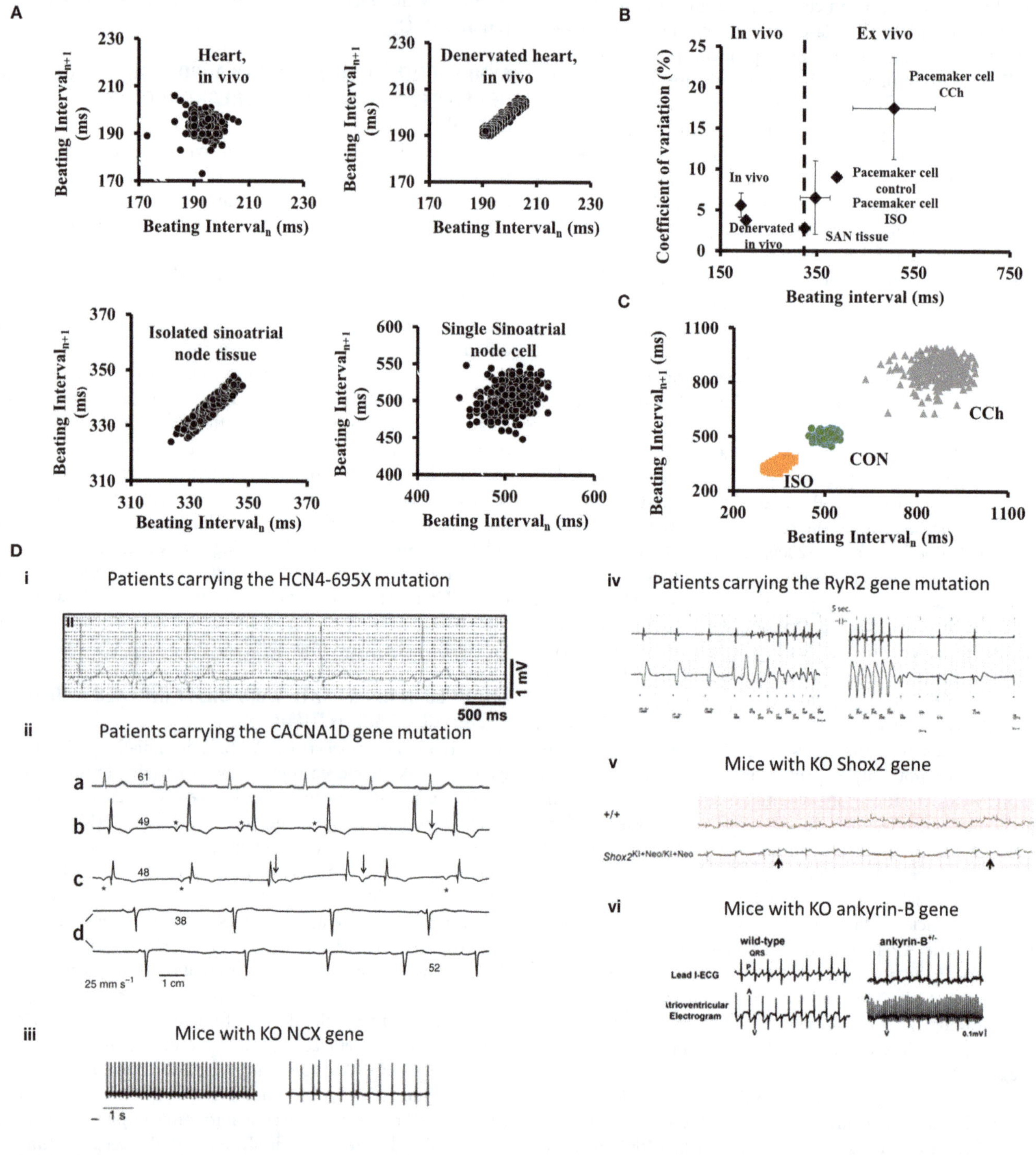

FIGURE 1 | (A) Poincaré plots of the beating interval at different levels of integration from the heart *in vivo* to single isolated pacemaker cells. (B) The relationship between beating intervals and coefficients of variation at different levels of integration from the heart *in vivo* to single pacemaker cells in isolation. **(C)** Poincaré plots of the beating interval variability in single SANC under control (CON), β-adrenergic receptor stimulation (ISO) or cholinergic receptor stimulation (CCh). Modified from Yaniv et al. (2014a). **(D)** Examples of arrhythmias associated with changes in intrinsic clock mechanisms recorded *in vivo*: (i) in patients carrying the HCN4-695X mutation (adapted from Schweizer et al., 2010); (ii) (a–d) ECG recordings from an unaffected person (a) and three individuals who are homozygous for the CACNA1D mutation (b–d) (adapted from Baig et al., 2011); (iii) Cardiac arrhythmias in freely moving NCX KO mice (adapted from Herrmann et al., 2013); (iv) A rapid and presumably polymorphic ventricular tachycardia in patents with mutation in RyR2 (adapted from Bhuiyan et al., 2007); (v) ECG recording demonstrate the occurrence of arrhythmia in Shox2 KO mice (adapted from Liu et al., 2011); (vi) ECG recording from ankyrin-B KO mice (adapted from Cunha et al., 2011).

Table 1 | Summary of primary studies assessing the changes of heart rate variability when arrhythmia occurs.

Type of arrhythmia	Number of patients	Findings	Study
AF	27	Decreased pNN50 was an independent predictor of AF relapse	Akyurek et al., 2003
AF	784	Impaired LF spectral component predicted new-onset AF	Perkiomaki et al., 2014
AF	83	Time and frequency indices attenuated when the treatments failed	Seaborn et al., 2014
PSVT	64	HR increased, HRV and HF power decreased after catheter ablation for PSVT	Kocovic et al., 1993
Sick sinus syndrome	30	Poincare plot often showed random-like pattern; Beta coefficient* of fractal increased toward 0 in sinoatrial node dysfunction	Bergfeldt and Haga, 2003
Sick sinus syndrome	181	Decreased SDNN and rMSSD after pulmonary vein isolation	Wang et al., 2013
VF	24	HRV indices consistently did not change before VF	Vybiral et al., 1993
VF	15	VF patients had lower DFA alpha (0.64 vs. 1.05) and fractal beta coefficient* (−1.63 vs. −1.31) than control	Makikallio et al., 1999
VT	40	All power spectra of HRV decreased before the onset of sustained VT compared to before nonsustained VT	Huikuri et al., 1993
VF/AVB	25	V-shaped trough appeared in the curve of ln(LF/HF) and ln(HF) prior to VF and AVB, respectively	Osaka et al., 2010
VF/AVB	292	Beta coefficient* < −1.5 was the most powerful predictor of VF	Gang et al., 2011
VT/VF	312 after myocardial infraction	Decreased SDNN, VLF, HF, DFA alpha1 predicted VT/VF	Huikuri et al., 2009
VT/VF	28	Decreased scattering in Poincare plot before arrhythmic event	Rozen et al., 2013

*PSVT, Paroxysmal supraventricular tachycardia; VF, Ventricular fibrillation; VT, Ventricular tachycardia; AF, atrial fibrillation; AVB, atrioventricular block; DFA, Detrended fluctuation analysis; pNN50, the number of pairs of successive beats that differ by more than 50 ms; SDNN, standard deviation of the average beating intervals; rMSSD, root mean square of successive differences; HF, high frequency; LF, low frequency; VLF, very low frequency. *Beta coefficient is the slope between power spectra and VLF in log-log scale.*

DIRECT PHARMACOLOGICAL INHIBITION OF COUPLED-CLOCK PROTEINS OF PACEMAKER CELLS CAUSES CHANGES IN RATE AND RHYTHM

Direct pharmacological inhibition of coupled-clock proteins can induce arrhythmias. For example: (i) caging of intracellular Ca^{2+} by NP-EGTA in isolated rabbit pacemaker cells induces an increase in LCR variability and AP BI bradycardia together with arrhythmic events (Yaniv et al., 2011). (ii) A sudden increase in stochastic ryanodine receptor open probability, elicited by caffeine spritz in isolated rabbit pacemaker cells, induces tachycardia, together with arrhythmic events (Yaniv et al., 2013d). (iii) Specific PKA inhibitors (Younes et al., 2008) or CaMKII inhibitors (Yaniv et al., 2013c) superfused onto isolated rabbit pacemaker cells induce AP BI bradycardia together with arrhythmic events. (iv) Perturbing clock coupling in rabbit pacemaker cells by directly inhibiting either the M (ivabradine, an I_f inhibitor) or Ca^{2+} clock (cyclopiazonic acid, a SR Ca^{2+} pump inhibitor) produces increases in AP BI and AP BIV that are related to increases in LCR period and LCR period variability (Yaniv et al., 2014b). These results provide evidence that supports the coupled-clock theory, demonstrating the ability of the LCR Ca^{2+} signal to report the degree of synchronization between the two clocks, and how changes in the degree of synchronization lead to changes in AP BI and AP BIV.

REDUCED EFFICIENCY OF INTRINSIC COUPLED-CLOCK PACEMAKER MECHANISMS AND ARRHYTHMIA

Similar to direct pharmacological inhibitors of coupled-clock proteins, mutation and genetically induced gene deletion of different components of the coupled-clock system are associated with arrhythmias *in vivo*.

HCN GENE

The hyperpolarization-activated channel (I_f) consists of three HCN members (HCN1, HCN2, and HCN4) (Ludwig et al., 1998). HCN4 comprises the major fraction (70–80%) of SAN I_f. Various mutations of human HCN4 channels are associated with arrhythmias, and with bradycardia in particular (Yeh et al., 2009; Schweizer et al., 2010; Duhme et al., 2013). Interestingly, the spontaneous cardiac beating rate of HCN4-knockout embryos is significantly slower than that of wild-type, but no arrhythmic events are observed. These results are in contrast to the conditional deletion of HCN4 in adult animals, where bradycardia is not evident but sinus pauses are detected (Stieber et al., 2004; Herrmann et al., 2007; Yeh et al., 2009) (**Figure 1D**). Other HCN transcripts that compose funny current channel in the mouse are HCN2, and a low level of HCN1. HCN2-deficient mice display mild cardiac dysrhythmia, both in the presence and absence of autonomic control of the heart rate (Stieber et al., 2004; Herrmann et al., 2007). Similarly, HCN1-deficient mice exhibit sinus dysrhythmia *in vivo* and in single isolated cells (Fenske et al., 2013). Interestingly, HCN1-deficient mice exhibit high beat-to-beat dispersion (quantified by Poincaré plots) that is typically observed in SAN dysfunction (Fenske et al., 2013). Therefore, HCN4 apparently is required to protect the heart from severe bradycardia and HCN2 and HCN1 are required to prevent arrhythmias.

Ivabradine is a specific I_f blocker that reduces the heart rate in patients, specifically patients with inappropriate sinus tachycardia to eliminate arrhythmia (Cappato et al., 2012). However, a recent study in isolated rabbit pacemaker cells demonstrated that ivabradine, even at a concentration that specifically inhibits I_f, but does not directly suppress L-type current, SR Ca^{2+} cycling and other surface membrane ion channels, indirectly suppresses intracellular Ca^{2+} cycling (Yaniv et al., 2012, 2013b). The reduction in arrhythmic events is therefore likely due to drug effect on synchronization of functions within the coupled-clock system, and not simply to I_f inhibition, *per se* (Yaniv and Lakatta, 2013).

$Ca_v1.3$

Voltage-gated Ca_v1 channels ($Ca_v1.2$ and $Ca_v1.3$) mediate L-type Ca^{2+} channels that play distinct roles in mediating Ca^{2+} balance in the pacemaker cell. Both $Ca_v1.2$ and $Ca_v1.3$ channels are expressed in SAN, and $Ca_v1.3$ expression in the atria and SAN cells is higher than in ventricular myocytes (Marger et al., 2011). $Ca_v1.3$ current is activated faster and at more negative voltages than $Ca_v1.2$ current and, therefore, in mice can contribute earlier during the diastolic depolarization (Christel et al., 2012). Bradycardia and arrhythmia are particularly prominent in $Ca_v1.3$ knockout mouse pacemaker cells (Mangoni et al., 2003). Loss of function of $Ca_v1.3$ both in mice and humans causes sick sinus syndrome (see above) and is characterized by severe bradycardia (Platzer et al., 2000; Baig et al., 2011). Moreover, patients with a mutation in the CACNA1D gene, which encodes the pore-forming α_1 subunit of $Ca_v1.3$, experience pronounced bradycardia in 12–24-h ECG recordings, and their HRV time-domain indices are increased (Baig et al., 2011) (**Figure 1D**). Note that functional significance of $Ca_v1.3$ in large mammals has yet to be demonstrated.

NCX1

The Na^+/Ca^{2+} exchanger has two important roles in pacemaker cells: it not only maintains the cell Ca^{2+} balance by matching Ca^{2+} efflux to Ca^{2+} influx through the L-type Ca^{2+} current, but also contributes to diastolic depolarization (Maltsev et al., 2014). Specific knockout of SAN Na^+/Ca^{2+} exchanger mice induces bradycardia and increases BIV in the proportion of mycoytes that express arrhythmic AP BI compared to control mice (Herrmann et al., 2013) (**Figure 1D**). Interestingly, numerical model simulations predict that only a reduction in Na^+/Ca^{2+} exchanger density to below a specific threshold is accompanied by arrhythmic AP BI (Maltsev et al., 2013).

TRPM4

TRPM4 is a monovalent nonselective cation channel permeable to Na^+, K^+, and Li^+, but not to Ca^{2+} (Launay et al., 2002). Activation of TRPM4 channels that exist in murine pacemaker cells is achieved by both membrane depolarization and by a rise in intracellular Ca^{2+} (Hof et al., 2013). Although TRPM4 KO mice have heart rates similar to those of their controls, they exhibit a higher incidence of sinus pauses (Hof et al., 2013).

RYANODINE CHANNELS

The stochasticity of spontaneous RyR activation determines the diastolic LCR Ca^{2+} signal and therefore the degree of synchronization of intracellular function of the coupled-clock system. A mutation in RyR, exon-3, in patients with catecholaminergic polymorphic ventricular tachycardia, is associated with arrhythmias (Bhuiyan et al., 2007) (**Figure 1D**). Isolated pacemaker cells from mice that express this mutation have a prolonged average AP BI with pauses between AP BIs together with an impaired chronotropic response to β adrenergic stimulation (Neco et al., 2012). Similarly, in inducible, heart tissue-specific RyR2 knockout mice, both *in vivo* ECG telemetry and *in vitro* isolated perfused heart, demonstrated bradycardic BI and arrhythmia (Bround et al., 2012).

Shox2 AND OTHER TRANSCRIPTION FACTORS

The Shox2 transcriptional factor has been identified as a key regulator in pacemaker formation and differentiation (Liu et al., 2011). Shox2 gene KO mice have a significantly reduced heart beat rate and increased number of arrhythmic events (Liu et al., 2011) (**Figure 1D**). Moreover, deficient Shox2 transcription factor during development may cause abnormal of mouse SAN development associated with severe arrhythmias (Hoffmann et al., 2013). Therefore, the Shox2 gene also appears to be critical for normal pacemaking function. Other transcription factors than Shox2 are involved in pacemaker function. In this regard, expression of Tbx18 in guinea pig has been shown as an essential gene whose expression can convert quiescent cardiomyocytes to pacemaker cells (Kapoor et al., 2013), therefore, increasing the pacemaker-induced spontaneous beating rate of the cells and decreasing their BIV. Interestingly, Tbx18 transduction to the guinea pig embryonic cell lineage inhibits Cx43 expression, leading to significant electrical uncoupling (Kapoor et al., 2011).

ANKYRIN-B

Ankyrins are adaptor proteins that are required for targeting channels and transporters in pacemaker cells to the membranes in which they function. Human patients with ankyrin-B-deficiency have highly penetrant sinus node dysfunction coupled with increased susceptibility to spontaneous and inducible atrial fibrillation (Le Scouarnec et al., 2008). Interestingly, ankyrin-B -deficient mice also have reduced expression of Na^+/Ca^{2+} exchanger and Na^+/K^+ ATPase (Le Scouarnec et al., 2008). Finally, cells isolated from ankyrin-B-deficient mice have increased BIV (Cunha et al., 2011) (**Figure 1D**). Thus, down regulation of ankyrin-B induces abnormal membrane organization that is implicated in a reduced efficiency of pacemaker clock coupling that causes abnormal electrical activity within SAN.

CELL-TO-CELL UNCOUPLING MECHANISMS

As described above, the BIs of pacemaker cells residing in the SAN become entrained by electrotonic and mechanical cell-to-cell interactions within the tissue (Jalife, 1984; Watanabe et al., 1995). Numerical model simulations predict that cardiac arrhythmias can occur when normal coupling between pacemaker cells in SAN tissue is perturbed (Ostborn et al., 2001). Cardiac diseases, and specifically sick sinus syndrome, are associated with reduction in cell-cell junctional proteins (Dobrzynski et al., 2007). ECG of mice with a cardiac conduction-specific knockout of desmoplakin, a protein that affects mechanical cell-to-cell interaction in the cardiac conduction system, exhibits sinus arrhythmias characterized by a strikingly increased number of sinus pauses compared to wild-type mice (Sheikh et al., 2013).

PASSIVE MECHANISMS

Although connexin43 is absent in the center of the pacemaker tissue, it is expressed in the peripheral area. A reduction in connexin 43 in aged guinea pig SAN is associated with a reduction in heart rate and an increase in arrhythmogenic events (Jones et al., 2004). Moreover, pacemaker tissue contains functional gap junctions and connecting cardiac fibroblasts (Camelliti et al., 2004). Because an increase in fibroblasts expression can slow the generation of pacemaker excitability, it may be involved in bradycardia and sick sinus syndrome (for review see Kohl et al., 2005). A detailed review of the role of passive pacemaker tissue properties on its electrical conductance is present in this issue (Unudurthi et al., 2014).

REDUCED EFFICIENCY OF SYNCHRONIZATION OF ACTIVITY ACROSS POPULATIONS OF CELLS AND ARRHYTHMIA

High-resolution optical mapping of SAN tissue has helped to resolve how reduced synchronization of activity across populations of cells within the SAN can induce arrhythmia. In this regard, different intrinsic mechanisms can be involved in tachy-brady heart-rate alteration and exit block that leads to long sinus pauses and increases susceptibility to cardiac arrhythmias: (i) an increase in adenosine level in human SAN tissue, an endogenous metabolite of the heart, through adenosine A1 receptor upregulating, can lead to SAN dysfunction (Lou et al., 2013, 2014); (ii) an increase in B-type and C-type natriuretic peptides increase the mice SAN conduction velocity and shift the initial exit site (Azer et al., 2014). (iii) Mutation in Ca^{2+}-binding protein calsequestrin 2 is associated with different cardiac diseases. In calsequestrin knockout mice the SAN exhibits bradycardia, conduction abnormalities and increase beat-to-beat variability (Glukhov et al., 2013). (iv) Ganglion nerve plexi can stimulate the intrinsic cardiac nervous system. In mice pulmonary vein ganglia stimulation shifts the origin of SAN discharges and decreases the heart rate (Zarzoso et al., 2013). (v) Impaired SR function in canine failing hearts results in an impaired shift in the location of the pacemaker site in response to β-AR stimulation (Shinohara et al., 2010).

SUMMARY

Changes in heart rate and rhythm are harbingers of the appearance of arrhythmogenic events. Reduction in the degree of synchronization of any intrinsic clock functions of pacemaker cells or in the synchronization among pacemaker cells residing in the SAN can be associated with arrhythmia occurrence. The extent to which restoring normal synchronization of intrinsic clock periods within pacemaker cells and among pacemaker cells can prevent arrhythmogenic events awaits further elucidation. In our opinion, future work requires a focus on the connection between dysfunction of inherent intrinsic mechanisms associated with different cardiac diseases and cardiac arrhythmias. This connection can be explored in genetically manipulated mouse models, in animals like rabbit, dog and sheep with heart failure or atrial fibrillation, and in human-derived cardiomyocytes or human SAN. This knowledge will contribute greatly to our understanding of cardiac impulse initiation in health and in cardiac disease.

ACKNOWLEDGMENTS

This research was partially supported by the Intramural Research Program of the NIH, National Institute on Aging, by Technion VPR Fund –Krbling Biomedical Engineering Research Fund (YY) and by NSFC-ISF joint research program, No. 398/14 (YY).

REFERENCES

Akyurek, O., Diker, E., Guldal, M., and Oral, D. (2003). Predictive value of heart rate variability for the recurrence of chronic atrial fibrillation after electrical cardioversion. *Clin. Cardiol.* 26, 196–200. doi: 10.1002/clc.4960260411

Anumonwo, J. M., Delmar, M., Vinet, A., Michaels, D. C., and Jalife, J. (1991). Phase resetting and entrainment of pacemaker activity in single sinus nodal cells. *Circ. Res.* 68, 1138–1153. doi: 10.1161/01.RES.68.4.1138

Azer, J., Hua, R., Krishnaswamy, P. S., and Rose, R. A. (2014). Effects of natriuretic peptides on electrical conduction in the sinoatrial node and atrial myocardium of the heart. *J. Physiol.* 592, 1025–1045. doi: 10.1113/jphysiol.2013.265405

Baig, S. M., Koschak, A., Lieb, A., Gebhart, M., Dafinger, C., Nurnberg, G., et al. (2011). Loss of Ca(v)1.3 (CACNA1D) function in a human channelopathy with bradycardia and congenital deafness. *Nat. Neurosci.* 14, 77–84. doi: 10.1038/nn.2694

Battipaglia, I., Scalone, G., Macchione, A., Pinnacchio, G., Laurito, M., Milo, M., et al. (2012). Association of heart rate variability with arrhythmic events in patients with arrhythmogenic right ventricular cardiomyopathy/dysplasia. *Circ. J.* 76, 618–623. doi: 10.1253/circj.CJ-11-1052

Bergfeldt, L., and Haga, Y. (2003). Power spectral and Poincare plot characteristics in sinus node dysfunction. *J. Appl. Physiol. (1985).* 94, 2217–2224. doi: 10.1152/japplphysiol.01037.2002

Bhuiyan, Z. A., Van Den Berg, M. P., Van Tintelen, J. P., Bink-Boelkens, M. T., Wiesfeld, A. C., Alders, M., et al. (2007). Expanding spectrum of human RYR2-related disease: new electrocardiographic, structural, and genetic features. *Circulation* 116, 1569–1576. doi: 10.1161/CIRCULATIONAHA.107.711606

Birchfield, R. I., Menefee, E. E., and Bryant, G. D. (1957). Disease of the sinoatrial node associated with bradycardia, asystole, syncope, and paroxysmal atrial fibrillation. *Circulation* 16, 20–26. doi: 10.1161/01.CIR.16.1.20

Boyett, M. R., Honjo, H., and Kodama, I. (2000). The sinoatrial node, a heterogeneous pacemaker structure. *Cardiovasc. Res.* 47, 658–687. doi: 10.1016/S0008-6363(00)00135-8

Bround, M. J., Asghari, P., Wambolt, R. B., Bohunek, L., Smits, C., Philit, M., et al. (2012). Cardiac ryanodine receptors control heart rate and rhythmicity in adult mice. *Cardiovasc. Res.* 96, 372–380. doi: 10.1093/cvr/cvs260

Camelliti, P., Green, C. R., Legrice, I., and Kohl, P. (2004). Fibroblast network in rabbit sinoatrial node: structural and functional identification of homogeneous and heterogeneous cell coupling. *Circ. Res.* 94, 828–835. doi: 10.1161/01.RES.0000122382.19400.14

Cappato, R., Castelvecchio, S., Ricci, C., Bianco, E., Vitali-Serdoz, L., Gnecchi-Ruscone, T., et al. (2012). Clinical efficacy of ivabradine in patients with inappropriate sinus tachycardia: a prospective, randomized, placebo-controlled, double-blind, crossover evaluation. *J. Am. Coll. Cardiol.* 60, 1323–1329. doi: 10.1016/j.jacc.2012.06.031

Childers, R. W., Arnsdorf, M. F., De La Fuente, D. J., Gambetta, M., and Svenson, R. (1973). Sinus nodal echoes. Clinical case report and canine studies. *Am. J. Cardiol.* 31, 220–231. doi: 10.1016/0002-9149(73)91035-7

Christel, C. J., Cardona, N., Mesirca, P., Herrmann, S., Hofmann, F., Striessnig, J., et al. (2012). Distinct localization and modulation of Cav1.2 and Cav1.3 L-type Ca^{2+} channels in mouse sinoatrial node. *J. Physiol.* 590, 6327–6342. doi: 10.1113/jphysiol.2012.239954

Cossu, S. F., and Steinberg, J. S. (1998). Supraventricular tachyarrhythmias involving the sinus node: clinical and electrophysiologic characteristics. *Prog. Cardiovasc. Dis.* 41, 51–63. doi: 10.1016/S0033-0620(98)80022-4

Costa, M. D., Peng, C. K., and Goldberger, A. L. (2008). Multiscale analysis of heart rate dynamics: entropy and time irreversibility measures. *Cardiovasc. Eng.* 8, 88–93. doi: 10.1007/s10558-007-9049-1

Cunha, S. R., Hund, T. J., Hashemi, S., Voigt, N., Li, N., Wright, P., et al. (2011). Defects in ankyrin-based membrane protein targeting pathways underlie atrial fibrillation. *Circulation* 124, 1212–1222. doi: 10.1161/CIRCULATIONAHA.111.023986

De Jong, A. M., Maass, A. H., Oberdorf-Maass, S. U., De Boer, R. A., Van Gilst, W. H., and Van Gelder, I. C. (2013). Cyclical stretch induces structural changes in atrial myocytes. *J. Cell. Mol. Med.* 17, 743–753. doi: 10.1111/jcmm.12064

Difrancesco, D. (1993). Pacemaker mechanisms in cardiac tissue. *Annu. Rev. Physiol.* 55, 455–472. doi: 10.1146/annurev.ph.55.030193.002323

Dobrzynski, H., Boyett, M. R., and Anderson, R. H. (2007). New insights into pacemaker activity: promoting understanding of sick sinus syndrome. *Circulation* 115, 1921–1932. doi: 10.1161/CIRCULATIONAHA.106.616011

Duhme, N., Schweizer, P. A., Thomas, D., Becker, R., Schroter, J., Barends, T. R., et al. (2013). Altered HCN4 channel C-linker interaction is associated with familial tachycardia-bradycardia syndrome and atrial fibrillation. *Eur. Heart J.* 34, 2768–2775. doi: 10.1093/eurheartj/ehs391

Fenske, S., Krause, S. C., Hassan, S. I., Becirovic, E., Auer, F., Bernard, R., et al. (2013). Sick sinus syndrome in HCN1-deficient mice. *Circulation* 128, 2585–2594. doi: 10.1161/CIRCULATIONAHA.113.003712

Gang, U. J., Jons, C., Jorgensen, R. M., Abildstrom, S. Z., Messier, M. D., Haarbo, J., et al. (2011). Risk markers of late high-degree atrioventricular block in patients with left ventricular dysfunction after an acute myocardial infarction: a CARISMA substudy. *Europace* 13, 1471–1477. doi: 10.1093/europace/eur165

Glukhov, A. V., Kalyanasundaram, A., Lou, Q., Hage, L. T., Hansen, B. J., Belevych, A. E., et al. (2013). Calsequestrin 2 deletion causes sinoatrial node dysfunction and atrial arrhythmias associated with altered sarcoplasmic reticulum calcium cycling and degenerative fibrosis within the mouse atrial pacemaker complex. *Eur. Heart J.* doi: 10.1093/eurheartj/eht452. [Epub ahead of print].

Gomes, J. A., Mehta, D., and Langan, M. N. (1995). Sinus node reentrant tachycardia. *Pacing Clin. Electrophysiol.* 18, 1045–1057. doi: 10.1111/j.1540-8159.1995.tb04747.x

Han, J., Malozzi, A. M., Moe, G. K. (1968). Sino-atrial reciprocation in the isolated rabbit heart. *Circ. Res.* 22, 355–362.

Herrmann, S., Lipp, P., Wiesen, K., Stieber, J., Nguyen, H., Kaiser, E., et al. (2013). The cardiac sodium-calcium exchanger NCX1 is a key player in the initiation and maintenance of a stable heart rhythm. *Cardiovasc. Res.* 99, 780–788. doi: 10.1093/cvr/cvt154

Herrmann, S., Stieber, J., Stockl, G., Hofmann, F., and Ludwig, A. (2007). HCN4 provides a 'depolarization reserve' and is not required for heart rate acceleration in mice. *EMBO J.* 26, 4423–4432. doi: 10.1038/sj.emboj.7601868

Hof, T., Simard, C., Rouet, R., Salle, L., and Guinamard, R. (2013). Implication of the TRPM4 nonselective cation channel in mammalian sinus rhythm. *Heart Rhythm* 10, 1683–1689. doi: 10.1016/j.hrthm.2013.08.014

Hoffmann, S., Berger, I. M., Glaser, A., Bacon, C., Li, L., Gretz, N., et al. (2013). Islet1 is a direct transcriptional target of the homeodomain transcription factor Shox2 and rescues the Shox2-mediated bradycardia. *Basic Res. Cardiol.* 108, 339. doi: 10.1007/s00395-013-0339-z

Huikuri, H. V., Raatikainen, M. J., Moerch-Joergensen, R., Hartikainen, J., Virtanen, V., Boland, J., et al. (2009). Prediction of fatal or near-fatal cardiac arrhythmia events in patients with depressed left ventricular function after an acute myocardial infarction. *Eur. Heart J.* 30, 689–698. doi: 10.1093/eurheartj/ehn537

Huikuri, H. V., Valkama, J. O., Airaksinen, K. E., Seppanen, T., Kessler, K. M., Takkunen, J. T., et al. (1993). Frequency domain measures of heart rate variability before the onset of nonsustained and sustained ventricular tachycardia in patients with coronary artery disease. *Circulation* 87, 1220–1228. doi: 10.1161/01.CIR.87.4.1220

Jalife, J. (1984). Mutual entrainment and electrical coupling as mechanisms for synchronous firing of rabbit sino-atrial pace-maker cells. *J. Physiol.* 356, 221–243. doi: 10.1113/jphysiol.1984.sp015461

Jones, S. A., Lancaster, M. K., and Boyett, M. R. (2004). Ageing-related changes of connexins and conduction within the sinoatrial node. *J. Physiol.* 560, 429–437. doi: 10.1113/jphysiol.2004.072108

Kapoor, N., Galang, G., Marban, E., and Cho, H. C. (2011). Transcriptional suppression of connexin43 by TBX18 undermines cell-cell electrical coupling in postnatal cardiomyocytes. *J. Biol. Chem.* 286, 14073–14079. doi: 10.1074/jbc.M110.185298

Kapoor, N., Liang, W., Marban, E., and Cho, H. C. (2013). Direct conversion of quiescent cardiomyocytes to pacemaker cells by expression of Tbx18. *Nat. Biotechnol.* 31, 54–62. doi: 10.1038/nbt.2465

Kocovic, D. Z., Harada, T., Shea, J. B., Soroff, D., and Friedman, P. L. (1993). Alterations of heart rate and of heart rate variability after radiofrequency catheter ablation of supraventricular tachycardia. Delineation of parasympathetic pathways in the human heart. *Circulation* 88, 1671–1681. doi: 10.1161/01.CIR.88.4.1671

Kohl, P., Camelliti, P., Burton, F. L., and Smith, G. L. (2005). Electrical coupling of fibroblasts and myocytes: relevance for cardiac propagation. *J. Electrocardiol.* 38, 45–50. doi: 10.1016/j.jelectrocard.2005.06.096

Launay, P., Fleig, A., Perraud, A. L., Scharenberg, A. M., Penner, R., and Kinet, J. P. (2002). TRPM4 is a Ca^{2+}-activated nonselective cation channel mediating cell membrane depolarization. *Cell* 109, 397–407. doi: 10.1016/S0092-8674(02)00719-5

Le Scouarnec, S., Bhasin, N., Vieyres, C., Hund, T. J., Cunha, S. R., Koval, O., et al. (2008). Dysfunction in ankyrin-B-dependent ion channel and transporter targeting causes human sinus node disease. *Proc. Natl. Acad. Sci. U.S.A.* 105, 15617–15622. doi: 10.1073/pnas.0805500105

Liu, H., Chen, C. H., Espinoza-Lewis, R. A., Jiao, Z., Sheu, I., Hu, X., et al. (2011). Functional redundancy between human SHOX and mouse Shox2 genes in the regulation of sinoatrial node formation and pacemaking function. *J. Biol. Chem.* 286, 17029–17038. doi: 10.1074/jbc.M111.234252

Lou, Q., Glukhov, A. V., Hansen, B., Hage, L., Vargas-Pinto, P., Billman, G. E., et al. (2013). Tachy-brady arrhythmias: the critical role of adenosine-induced sinoatrial conduction block in post-tachycardia pauses. *Heart Rhythm* 10, 110–118. doi: 10.1016/j.hrthm.2012.09.012

Lou, Q., Hansen, B. J., Fedorenko, O., Csepe, T. A., Kalyanasundaram, A., Li, N., et al. (2014). Upregulation of adenosine A1 receptors facilitates sinoatrial node dysfunction in chronic canine heart failure by exacerbating nodal conduction abnormalities revealed by novel dual-sided intramural optical mapping. *Circulation* 130, 315–324. doi: 10.1161/CIRCULATIONAHA.113.007086

Ludwig, A., Zong, X., Jeglitsch, M., Hofmann, F., and Biel, M. (1998). A family of hyperpolarization-activated mammalian cation channels. *Nature* 393, 587–591. doi: 10.1038/31255

Makikallio, T. H., Koistinen, J., Jordaens, L., Tulppo, M. P., Wood, N., Golosarsky, B., et al. (1999). Heart rate dynamics before spontaneous onset of ventricular fibrillation in patients with healed myocardial infarcts. *Am. J. Cardiol.* 83, 880–884. doi: 10.1016/S0002-9149(98)01068-6

Maltsev, A. V., Yaniv, Y., Stern, M. D., Lakatta, E. G., and Maltsev, V. A. (2013). RyR-NCX-SERCA local cross-talk ensures pacemaker cell function at rest and during the fight-or-flight reflex. *Circ. Res.* 113, e94–e100. doi: 10.1161/CIRCRESAHA.113.302465

Maltsev, V. A., Yaniv, Y., Maltsev, A. V., Stern, M. D., and Lakatta, E. G. (2014). Modern perspectives on numerical modeling of cardiac pacemaker cell. *J. Pharmacol. Sci.* 125, 6–38. doi: 10.1254/jphs.13R04CR

Mangoni, M. E., Couette, B., Bourinet, E., Platzer, J., Reimer, D., Striessnig, J., et al. (2003). Functional role of L-type Cav1.3 Ca^{2+} channels in cardiac pacemaker activity. *Proc. Natl. Acad. Sci. U.S.A.* 100, 5543–5548. doi: 10.1073/pnas.0935295100

Marger, L., Mesirca, P., Alig, J., Torrente, A., Dubel, S., Engeland, B., et al. (2011). Functional roles of Ca(v)1.3, Ca(v)3.1 and HCN channels in automaticity of mouse atrioventricular cells: insights into the atrioventricular pacemaker mechanism. *Channels (Austin)* 5, 251–261. doi: 10.4161/chan.5.3.15266

Monfredi, O., Lyashkov, A. E., Johnsen, A. B., Inada, S., Schneider, H., Wang, R., et al. (2014). Biophysical characterization of the underappreciated and important relationship between heart rate variability and heart rate. *Hypertension* 64, 1334–1343. doi: 10.1161/HYPERTENSIONAHA.114.03782

Monfredi, O., Maltseva, L. A., Spurgeon, H. A., Boyett, M. R., Lakatta, E. G., and Maltsev, V. A. (2013). Beat-to-beat variation in periodicity of local calcium releases contributes to intrinsic variations of spontaneous cycle length in isolated single sinoatrial node cells. *PLoS ONE* 8:e67247. doi: 10.1371/journal.pone.0067247

Neco, P., Torrente, A. G., Mesirca, P., Zorio, E., Liu, N., Priori, S. G., et al. (2012). Paradoxical effect of increased diastolic $Ca^{(2+)}$ release and decreased sinoatrial node activity in a mouse model of catecholaminergic polymorphic ventricular tachycardia. *Circulation* 126, 392–401. doi: 10.1161/CIRCULATIONAHA.111.075382

Osaka, M., Watanabe, E., Murata, H., Fuwamoto, Y., Nanba, S., Sakai, K., et al. (2010). V-shaped trough in autonomic activity is a possible precursor of life-threatening cardiac events. *Circ. J.* 74, 1906–1915. doi: 10.1253/circj.CJ-09-0935

Ostborn, P., Wohlfart, B., Ohlén, G. (2001). Arrhythmia as a result of poor intercellular coupling in the sinus node: a simulation study. *J. Theor. Biol.* 211, 201–217. doi: 10.1006/jtbi.2001.2339

Papaioannou, V. E., Verkerk, A. O., Amin, A. S., and De Bakker, J. M. (2013). Intracardiac origin of heart rate variability, pacemaker funny current and their possible association with critical illness. *Curr. Cardiol. Rev.* 9, 82–96. doi: 10.2174/157340313805076359

Perkiomaki, J., Ukkola, O., Kiviniemi, A., Tulppo, M., Ylitalo, A., Kesaniemi, Y. A., et al. (2014). Heart rate variability findings as a predictor of atrial fibrillation in middle-aged population. *J. Cardiovasc. Electrophysiol.* 25, 719–724. doi: 10.1111/jce.12402

Platzer, J., Engel, J., Schrott-Fischer, A., Stephan, K., Bova, S., Chen, H., et al. (2000). Congenital deafness and sinoatrial node dysfunction in mice lacking class D L-type Ca^{2+} channels. *Cell* 102, 89–97. doi: 10.1016/S0092-8674(00)00013-1

Postolache, G., Oliveira, M., Rocha, I., Girao, P. S., and Postolache, O. (2011). New insight into arrhythmia onset using HRV and BPV analysis. *Conf. Proc. IEEE Eng. Med. Biol. Soc.* 2011, 2691–2694. doi: 10.1109/IEMBS.2011.6090739

Rocchetti, M., Malfatto, G., Lombardi, F., and Zaza, A. (2000). Role of the input/output relation of sinoatrial myocytes in cholinergic modulation of heart rate variability. *J. Cardiovasc. Electrophysiol.* 11, 522–530. doi: 10.1111/j.1540-8167.2000.tb00005.x

Rozen, G., Kobo, R., Beinart, R., Feldman, S., Sapunar, M., Luria, D., et al. (2013). Multipole analysis of heart rate variability as a predictor of imminent ventricular arrhythmias in ICD patients. *Pacing Clin. Electrophysiol.* 36, 1342–1347. doi: 10.1111/pace.12180

Schweizer, P. A., Duhme, N., Thomas, D., Becker, R., Zehelein, J., Draguhn, A., et al. (2010). cAMP sensitivity of HCN pacemaker channels determines basal heart rate but is not critical for autonomic rate control. *Circ. Arrhythm. Electrophysiol.* 3, 542–552. doi: 10.1161/CIRCEP.110.949768

Seaborn, G. E., Todd, K., Michael, K. A., Baranchuk, A., Abdollah, H., Simpson, C. S., et al. (2014). Heart rate variability and procedural outcome in catheter ablation for atrial fibrillation. *Ann. Noninvasive Electrocardiol.* 19, 23–33. doi: 10.1111/anec.12098

Sheikh, F., Mezzano, V., Wright, A., Zanella, F., Lyon, R. S., Gu, Y., et al. (2013). A novel role for mechanical cell-cell junction proteins in sinus node function. *J. Mol. Cell. Cardiol.* 65.

Shinohara, T., Park, H. W., Han, S., Shen, M. J., Maruyama, M., Kim, D., et al. (2010). Ca^{2+} clock malfunction in a canine model of pacing-induced heart failure. *Am. J. Physiol. Heart Circ. Physiol.* 299, H1805–H1811. doi: 10.1152/ajpheart.00723.2010

Slovut, D. P., Wenstrom, J. C., Moeckel, R. B., Wilson, R. F., Osborn, J. W., and Abrams, J. H. (1998). Respiratory sinus dysrhythmia persists in transplanted human hearts following autonomic blockade. *Clin. Exp. Pharmacol. Physiol.* 25, 322–330. doi: 10.1111/j.1440-1681.1998.tb02358.x

Stieber, J., Hofmann, F., and Ludwig, A. (2004). Pacemaker channels and sinus node arrhythmia. *Trends Cardiovasc. Med.* 14, 23–28. doi: 10.1016/j.tcm.2003.09.006

Unudurthi, S. D., Wolf, R. M., and Hund, T. J. (2014). Role of sinoatrial node architecture in maintaining a balanced source-sink relationship and synchronous cardiac pacemaking. *Front. Physiol.* 5:446. doi: 10.3389/fphys.2014.00446

Verheijck, E. E., Wilders, R., Joyner, R. W., Golod, D. A., Kumar, R., Jongsma, H. J., et al. (1998). Pacemaker synchronization of electrically coupled rabbit sinoatrial node cells. *J. Gen. Physiol.* 111, 95–112. doi: 10.1085/jgp.111.1.95

Vybiral, T., Glaeser, D. H., Goldberger, A. L., Rigney, D. R., Hess, K. R., Mietus, J., et al. (1993). Conventional heart rate variability analysis of ambulatory electrocardiographic recordings fails to predict imminent ventricular fibrillation. *J. Am. Coll. Cardiol.* 22, 557–565. doi: 10.1016/0735-1097(93)90064-8

Wang, K., Chang, D., Chu, Z., Yang, Y., Gao, L., Zhang, S., et al. (2013). Denervation as a common mechanism underlying different pulmonary vein isolation strategies for paroxysmal atrial fibrillation: evidenced by heart rate variability after ablation. *Sci. World J.* 2013:569564. doi: 10.1155/2013/569564

Watanabe, E. I., Honjo, H., Anno, T., Boyett, M. R., Kodama, I., and Toyama, J. (1995). Modulation of pacemaker activity of sinoatrial node cells by electrical load imposed by an atrial cell model. *Am. J. Physiol.* 269, H1735–H1742.

Yaniv, Y., Ahmet, I., Liu, J., Lyashkov, A. E., Guiriba, T. R., Okamoto, Y., et al. (2014a). Synchronization of sinoatrial node pacemaker cell clocks and its autonomic modulation impart complexity to heart beating intervals. *Heart Rhythm* 11, 1210–1219. doi: 10.1016/j.hrthm.2014.03.049

Yaniv, Y., and Lakatta, E. G. (2013). Pacemaker gene mutations, bradycardia, arrhythmias and the coupled clock theory. *J. Cardiovasc. Electrophysiol.* 24, E28–E29. doi: 10.1111/jce.12236

Yaniv, Y., Lyashkov, A. E., and Lakatta, E. G. (2013a). The fractal-like complexity of heart rate variability beyond neurotransmitters and autonomic receptors: signaling intrinsic to sinoatrial node pacemaker cells. *Cardiovasc. Pharmacol.* 2:111. doi: 10.4172/2329-6607.1000111

Yaniv, Y., Lyashkov, A. E., Sirenko, S., Okamoto, Y., Guiriba, T. R., Ziman, B. D., et al. (2014b). Stochasticity intrinsic to coupled-clock mechanisms underlies beat-to-beat variability of spontaneous action potential firing in sinoatrial node pacemaker cells. *J. Mol. Cell. Cardiol.* 77, 1–10. doi: 10.1016/j.yjmcc.2014.09.008

Yaniv, Y., Maltsev, V. A., Escobar, A. L., Spurgeon, H. A., Ziman, B. D., Stern, M. D., et al. (2011). Beat-to-beat $Ca^{(2+)}$-dependent regulation of sinoatrial nodal pacemaker cell rate and rhythm. *J. Mol. Cell. Cardiol.* 51, 902–905. doi: 10.1016/j.yjmcc.2011.08.029

Yaniv, Y., Maltsev, V. A., Ziman, B. D., Spurgeon, H. A., and Lakatta, E. G. (2012). The "Funny" current inhibition by ivabradine at membrane potentials encompassing spontaneous depolarization in pacemaker cells. *Molecules* 17, 8241–8254. doi: 10.3390/molecules17078241

Yaniv, Y., Sirenko, S., Ziman, B. D., Spurgeon, H. A., Maltsev, V. A., and Lakatta, E. G. (2013b). New evidence for coupled clock regulation of the normal automaticity of sinoatrial nodal pacemaker cells: bradycardic effects of ivabradine are linked to suppression of intracellular $Ca^{(2)(+)}$ cycling. *J. Mol. Cell. Cardiol.* 62, 80–89. doi: 10.1016/j.yjmcc.2013.04.026

Yaniv, Y., Spurgeon, H. A., Ziman, B. D., and Lakatta, E. G. (2013c). $Ca^{(2)+}$/calmodulin-dependent protein kinase II (CaMKII) activity and sinoatrial nodal pacemaker cell energetics. *PLoS ONE* 8:e57079. doi: 10.1371/journal.pone.0057079

Yaniv, Y., Stern, M. D., Lakatta, E. G., and Maltsev, V. A. (2013d). Mechanisms of beat-to-beat regulation of cardiac pacemaker cell function by $Ca^{(2)(+)}$ cycling dynamics. *Biophys. J.* 105, 1551–1561. doi: 10.1016/j.bpj.2013.08.024

Yeh, Y. H., Burstein, B., Qi, X. Y., Sakabe, M., Chartier, D., Comtois, P., et al. (2009). Funny current downregulation and sinus node dysfunction associated with atrial tachyarrhythmia: a molecular basis for tachycardia-bradycardia syndrome. *Circulation* 119, 1576–1585. doi: 10.1161/CIRCULATIONAHA.108.789677

Younes, A., Lyashkov, A. E., Graham, D., Sheydina, A., Volkova, M. V., Mitsak, M., et al. (2008). $Ca^{(2+)}$ -stimulated basal adenylyl cyclase activity localization in membrane lipid microdomains of cardiac sinoatrial nodal pacemaker cells. *J. Biol. Chem.* 283, 14461–14468. doi: 10.1074/jbc.M707540200

Zarzoso, M., Rysevaite, K., Milstein, M. L., Calvo, C. J., Kean, A. C., Atienza, F., et al. (2013). Nerves projecting from the intrinsic cardiac ganglia of the pulmonary veins modulate sinoatrial node pacemaker function. *Cardiovasc. Res.* 99, 566–575. doi: 10.1093/cvr/cvt081

Zaza, A., and Lombardi, F. (2001). Autonomic indexes based on the analysis of heart rate variability: a view from the sinus node. *Cardiovasc. Res.* 50, 434–442. doi: 10.1016/S0008-6363(01)00240-1

6

Dynamics of propagation of premature impulses in structurally remodeled infarcted myocardium: A computational analysis

Candido Cabo[1,2]*

[1] Department of Computer Systems, New York City College of Technology, City University of New York, New York, NY, USA
[2] Doctoral Program in Computer Science, Graduate Center, City University of New York, New York, NY, USA

Correspondence:
Candido Cabo, Department of Computer Systems, New York City College of Technology, City University of New York, 300 Jay Street, Brooklyn, New York, NY 11201, USA
e-mail: ccabo@citytech.cuny.edu

Initiation of cardiac arrhythmias typically follows one or more premature impulses either occurring spontaneously or applied externally. In this study, we characterize the dynamics of propagation of single (S2) and double premature impulses (S3), and the mechanisms of block of premature impulses at structural heterogeneities caused by remodeling of gap junctional conductance (*Gj*) in infarcted myocardium. Using a sub-cellular computer model of infarcted tissue, we found that $|I_{Na,max}|$, prematurity (coupling interval with the previous impulse), and conduction velocity (CV) of premature impulses change dynamically as they propagate away from the site of initiation. There are fundamental differences between the dynamics of propagation of S2 and S3 premature impulses: for S2 impulses $|I_{Na,max}|$ recovers fast, prematurity decreases and CV increases as propagation proceeds; for S3 impulses low values of $|I_{Na,max}|$ persist, prematurity could increase, and CV could decrease as impulses propagate away from the site of initiation. As a consequence it is more likely that S3 impulses block at sites of structural heterogeneities causing source/sink mismatch than S2 impulses block. Whether premature impulses block at *Gj* heterogeneities or not is also determined by the values of *Gj* (and the space constant λ) in the regions proximal and distal to the heterogeneity: when λ in the direction of propagation increases >40%, premature impulses could block. The maximum slope of CV restitution curves for S2 impulses is larger than for S3 impulses. In conclusion: (1) The dynamics of propagation of premature impulses make more likely that S3 impulses block at sites of structural heterogeneities than S2 impulses block; (2) Structural heterogeneities causing an increase in λ (or CV) of >40% could result in block of premature impulses; (3) A decrease in the maximum slope of CV restitution curves of propagating premature impulses is indicative of an increased potential for block at structural heterogeneities.

Keywords: premature impulses, cell-to-cell conductance, structural remodeling, conduction velocity restitution curve, infarction, computer model

INTRODUCTION

Many cardiac arrhythmias have a reentrant mechanism, a pattern of excitation in which a wave rotates around an anatomical or functional obstacle (Wit and Janse, 1993). It is well-established that reentrant arrhythmias require a "trigger," which, in combination with a suitable "substrate," creates the conditions for initiation of a reentrant wave (i.e., a wave break) (Wit and Janse, 1993). One of the conditions for initiation of reentrant arrhythmias is the creation of a region of unidirectional block, which, by allowing propagation of the impulse in some directions but not in others, leads to the creation of wave breaks (Kleber and Rudy, 2004). Unidirectional block can occur in homogeneous tissue (Frazier et al., 1989; Quan and Rudy, 1990), in tissues with spatial heterogeneities in cell properties (refractory period, membrane excitability) (Janse and Kleber, 1981; Gough et al., 1985; Coronel, 1994) or in tissues with discontinuities in the microstructure (cell size, gap junction conductance) (Toure and Cabo, 2012) or the macrostructure (muscle bundle branches, narrow isthmuses, pivot points, tissue expansions) (Joyner, 1981; Spach et al., 1982; Cabo et al., 1994, 1996; Fast and Kleber, 1995).

In experimental and clinical cardiac electrophysiology, the conditions for unidirectional block are created by external electrical stimulation using sequences of closely coupled (i.e., premature) impulses (the "trigger"). Premature impulses can also occur spontaneously in healthy and diseased hearts as a result of reentry, abnormal automaticity or triggered activity (Peters et al., 2000). In healthy hearts, premature impulses are often benign (i.e., do not result in unidirectional block and arrhythmias) but, the structural and/or membrane remodeling caused by heart disease may lead to the creation of a suitable "substrate" such that premature impulses may result in unidirectional block and the initiation of arrhythmias (Nattel et al., 2007).

Structural remodeling following heart disease can cause local heterogeneities in the tissue microstructure, like an increase in cell size (hypertrophy) (Nattel et al., 2007) and remodeling of connexin43 (Cx43) (Severs et al., 2008). Myocardial infarction results in a reduction of the amount of Cx43 with the consequent decrease in gap junction conductance and conduction velocity (Cabo et al., 2006). Regions of heterogeneous Cx43 expression and gap junction conductance have been described in infarcted (Cabo et al., 2006) and failing hearts (Poelzing and Rosenbaum, 2004; Akar et al., 2007). In an earlier computational study, we showed that, under conditions of uniform reduced excitability, heterogeneities in gap junction conductance could result in unidirectional block of non-premature impulses (Toure and Cabo, 2012). However, in cardiac patients, the areas of unidirectional block that lead to arrhythmias likely result from the interaction of spontaneously generated premature impulses and a substrate created by the remodeling of cell membrane properties and/or tissue structure (Baba et al., 2005; Cabo et al., 2006). In particular, the mechanisms of conduction and block of premature impulses in regions of heterogeneous gap junction conductance have not been fully characterized.

Our objective is to characterize the dynamics of propagation of premature impulses in the healing infarcted heart, and how those dynamics may result in unidirectional block in structurally remodeled myocardium with heterogeneities in gap junction conductance. To simulate the remodeling in cell membrane properties occurring after myocardial infarction, we use a previously developed ionic model of the action potential of cells from the canine epicardial border zone (Cabo and Boyden, 2003). To study the dynamics of propagation of the action potential, we use a sub-cellular computer model (Spach and Heidlage, 1995), which provides a realistic representation of the tissue microstructure including the natural variability in cell morphology and electrical connections through gap junctions. Sub-cellular models have been used to investigate the effect of cell size, gap junction remodeling, and myofibroblast proliferation on cardiac wave propagation (Hubbard et al., 2007; Cabo and Boyden, 2009; Toure and Cabo, 2010, 2012; Baum et al., 2012).

METHODS

NUMERICAL METHODS

We performed all simulations in a 2D monodomain model with governing equation: $\nabla \cdot ((1/(S_v R_i C_m))\nabla V_m) = (I_{ion}/C_m) + \partial V_m/\partial t$, where V_m is the transmembrane potential (in mV), I_{ion} is the ionic current ($\mu A/cm^2$), R_i is the resistivity of the intracellular space, S_v is the surface to volume ratio (2000 cm^{-1}), and C_m is the specific capacitance ($1\,\mu F/cm^2$). Neumann (non-flow) boundary conditions were used. Membrane dynamics (I_{ion}) were formulated by an ionic model of the action potential of canine epicardial infarcted border zone cell (IZ cell dynamics) (Cabo and Boyden, 2003). The density and kinetics of several ionic currents of IZ cells are markedly different from cells from non-infarcted canine epicardium (Cabo and Boyden, 2003). Earlier results indicate that I_{Na} density is a major determinant of propagation (or block) at sites of microstructural discontinuities (Toure and Cabo, 2012). When compared to cells from normal epicardium, IZ cells have a reduced I_{Na} density that results in a slower conduction velocity and a delayed recovery from inactivation of the Na channel that results in post-repolarization refractoriness.

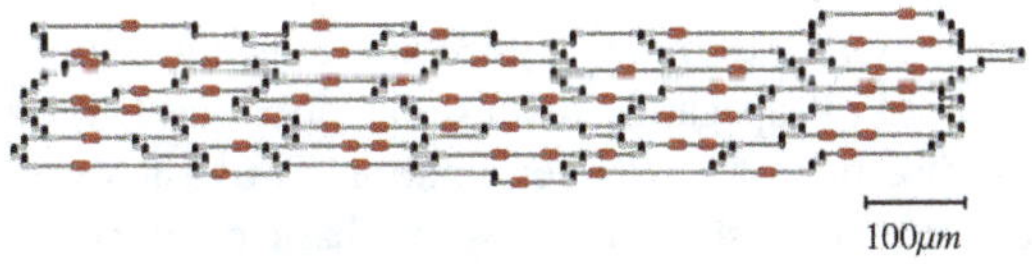

FIGURE 1 | Basic unit of the tissue architecture showing natural variability in cell size and shape as well as the location of gap junctions (Spach and Heidlage, 1995). Different types of gap junctions are shown on the cell membrane: plicate (black), interplicate (gray), and combined plicate (red).

We used the tissue architecture in **Figure 1** as the basis to create other architectures with different cell-to-cell gap junctional conductance (*Gj*) (Spach and Heidlage, 1995). The basic unit in **Figure 1** was replicated to create preparations of any size. That tissue architecture is a realistic representation of the natural variability in cell size and shape as well as the location of gap junctions. Each myocyte was electrically connected to neighboring myocytes only at the gap junctions. Three different types of gap junctions were simulated in the model: plicate (0.5 μS), interplicate (0.33 μS) and combined plicate gap junctions (0.062 μS) (**Figure 1**) (Spach and Heidlage, 1995). Plicate gap junctions, which are located in the plicate region of the intercalated disks, were simulated by resistors connecting cells electrically in the direction of the fiber orientation (longitudinally). Interplicate gap junctions, which are located in the interplicate region of the intercalated disks, were simulated by resistors connecting cells electrically in the direction transverse to the fiber orientation. Combined plicate gap junctions, which represent small intercalated disks located on the lateral membrane, between the larger intercalated disks containing the plicate and interplicate gap junctions, were simulated by resistors connecting cells electrically in the direction transverse to the fiber orientation. To study the effect of *Gj* heterogeneities on propagation, we used the basic tissue architecture, with different regions having different cell-to-cell *Gj* while the location of gap junctions was preserved. The regions with different cell-to-cell *Gj* were created by modifying the original conductance of the three types of gap junctions in the same proportion. The resistivity of the cytoplasm was 150 Ω *cm*. Cells were discretized with a space step of $10\,\mu m$ in both longitudinal and transverse directions. Each discretized cell element consisted of two square membrane surfaces, each one having a surface area of $100\,\mu m^2$, separated by a depth of $10\,\mu m$, with a volume of $1000\,\mu m^3$. Those values result in a surface to volume ratio (S_v) of $0.2\,\mu m^{-1}$ ($= 2000\,cm^{-1}$). In all simulations S_v was kept constant. The governing equation was integrated using the semi-implicit Crank-Nicholson method with a time step of 5 μs.

SIMULATION PROTOCOLS

We studied the dynamics of propagation of premature impulses in uniform preparations having the same average cell-to-cell *Gj* and in preparations with a structural discontinuity having different average cell-to-cell *Gj* in the region proximal to the discontinuity and in the region distal to the discontinuity. Flat wave fronts were initiated at the boundary of the proximal region of the preparation by an externally applied stimulus current (2x diastolic threshold). Propagation in all simulations was longitudinal, i.e., in the direction of the fiber orientation. The basic stimulation train consisted of 10 stimuli (S1) with a basic cycle length (BCL or S1S1) of 250 ms, after which single (S2), and double premature (S3) impulses with different coupling intervals were applied. The size of the preparations was 10 mm × 2.5 mm, and 7.5 mm × 2.5 mm, obtained by replication of the basic unit in **Figure 1** to the appropriate size.

We also calculated λ for tissue architectures with different cell-to-cell *Gj*. λ was calculated from the spatial decay of V_m, five membrane time constants (40 ms) after one end of the preparation was clamped at $-65\ mV$.

RESULTS

PROPAGATION OF SINGLE PREMATURE IMPULSES (S2) IN THE INFARCTED HEART

It is well-known that the conduction velocity (CV) of premature impulses decreases with the coupling interval between the premature impulse and the last impulse of the basic train (S1S2). **Figure 2A** shows the CV restitution curve for single premature impulses after a basic train with a S1S1 coupling interval of 250 ms in a computer model of the infarcted heart with average cell-to-cell coupling $Gj = 0.41\ \mu S$. The average CV of the most premature impulse that propagates (S1S2 = 198 ms) is 0.30 m/s, while the average CV of the basic impulse (S1S1 = 250 ms) is 0.48 m/s.

The CV of single premature impulses is not constant but it increases as the premature impulse propagates away from the stimulation site. **Figure 2B** shows the local CVs of premature impulses with S1S2 coupling intervals ranging from 198 ms (the shortest coupling interval that elicits a propagated response) to 250 ms. For S1S2 = 198 ms, CV varies from 0.12 m/s close to the stimulation site ($x = 0$ mm in **Figure 2B**) to 0.45 m/s 10 mm away from the stimulation site ($x = 10$ mm in **Figure 2B**). As the coupling interval of the premature impulses increases the changes in CV during propagation decrease. For example for the basic impulse in the train (S1S1 = 250 ms; thick black line in **Figure 2B**), CV close to the stimulation site is 0.47 m/s, and CV 10 mm away from the stimulation site is 0.49 m/s.

The changes in CV of premature impulses are caused by the dynamics of recovery from inactivation of the sodium channel. **Figure 3** shows how the absolute value of the peak I_{Na} current changes ($|I_{Na,max}|$), along a line in the center of the preparation, as the premature impulse propagates away from the stimulation site ($x = 0$ mm in **Figure 3**) for different coupling intervals. For S1S2 = 198 ms, $|I_{Na,max}|$ first decreases to reach a minimum of about 36 pA/pF about 2.5 mm (~2.5 λ) away from the stimulation site and then increases steadily as the premature impulse propagates. This minimum identifies the location where the premature impulse is more vulnerable to block. The fact that the minimum $|I_{Na,max}|$ occurs about 2.5 λ from the stimulation site will have some implications for the conditions for block at sites of structural remodeling (see below). The steady increase in $|I_{Na,max}|$ (after having reached a minimum) correlates well with the increase in local CV as propagation proceeds shown in **Figure 2B**. Note in **Figure 3** that the boundaries of the preparation have an effect on the value of $|I_{Na,max}|$: the initiation of a propagating impulse by an external electrical stimulus affects the values of $|I_{Na,max}|$ within ~0.5 mm of the site of initiation ($x = 0$ mm); the rapid decrease of $|I_{Na,max}|$ at the end of the preparation ($x = 10$ mm) is a consequence of the rapid increase in V_m caused by the collision of the propagating wave with the sealed boundary preventing I_{Na} from full activation (Spach and Kootsey, 1985).

An important consequence of the dynamics of propagation of single premature impulses shown in **Figures 2, 3** is that as single premature impulses propagate away from the site of initiation, they become less and less premature. **Figure 4** shows the coupling interval of premature impulses with respect to the last impulse of the basic train (V1V2) as propagation proceeds away from the stimulation site ($x = 0$ mm). For example, a premature impulse initiated with a coupling interval of S1S2 = 200 ms at the simulation site, will have a V1V2 coupling interval of 206 ms at a distance of 5 mm from the stimulation site, and 208 ms at a distance of 10 mm from the stimulation site. This is a consequence of the difference in CV between the premature and the last basic impulse (**Figure 2**). Note also that premature impulses initiated

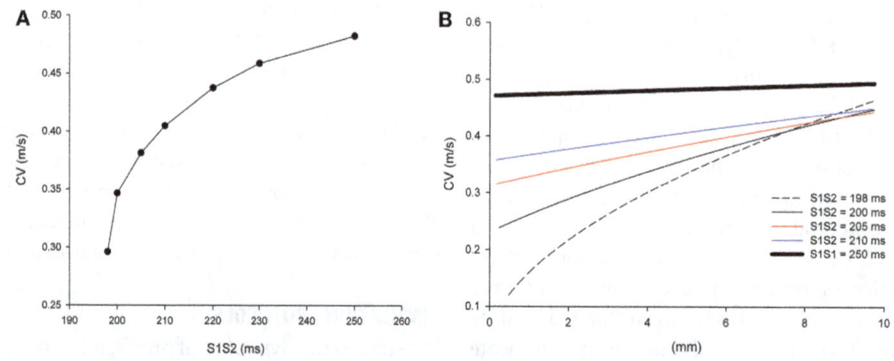

FIGURE 2 | Longitudinal conduction velocity (CV) of single premature impulses with different coupling intervals (S1S2) in a uniform infarcted myocardium preparation with average cell-to-cell coupling $Gj = 0.41\ \mu S$. **(A)** Average longitudinal CV in the preparation for different coupling intervals. **(B)** Local longitudinal CV as the impulse propagates away from the stimulation site ($x = 0$ mm). Size of the preparation: 10 × 2.5 mm.

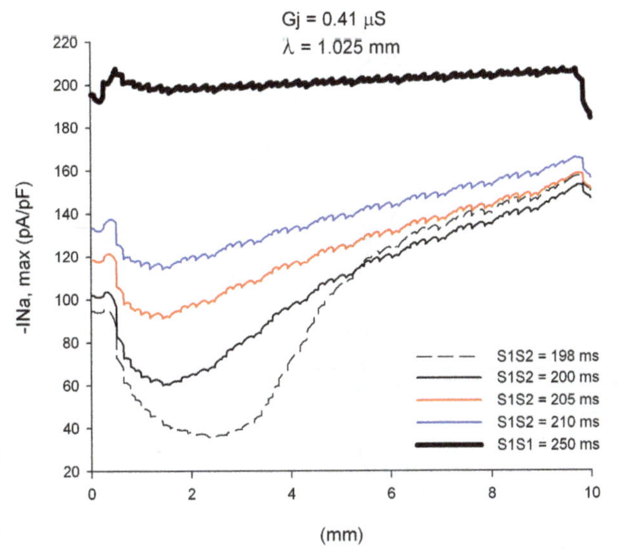

FIGURE 3 | Changes in I_{Na} current peak for single premature impulses, with different coupling intervals (S1S2), as the impulses propagate away from the stimulation site ($x = 0$ mm), in a uniform preparation with average cell-to-cell coupling $Gj = 0.41\ \mu$S. The dashed plot (S1S2 = 198 ms) is the shortest coupling that resulted in a propagated response. Size of the preparation: 10 × 2.5 mm.

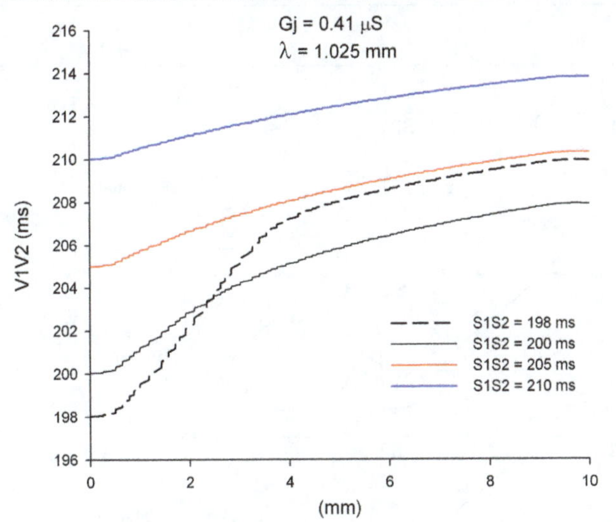

FIGURE 4 | Change in coupling interval between single premature impulses and the last impulse of the basic train (V1V2), for different coupling intervals (S1S2), as premature impulses propagate away from the stimulation site ($x = 0$ mm). The dashed plot (S1S2 = 198 ms) is the shortest coupling that resulted in a propagated response. Uniform preparation with average cell-to-cell coupling $Gj = 0.41\ \mu$S. Size of the preparation: 10 × 2.5 mm.

with a very short coupling interval (S1S2 = 198 ms in **Figure 4**) can result in a longer V1V2 coupling interval far away from the stimulation site (compare V1V2 for S1S2 = 198 ms and S1S2 = 200 ms).

EFFECT OF STRUCTURAL REMODELING ON PROPAGATION OF SINGLE PREMATURE IMPULSES (S2)

We have reported earlier that, in normal myocardium, under conditions of reduced excitability (70% reduction in maximum sodium channel conductance), propagation of action potentials blocks at sites where the space constant in the direction of propagation increases by >40% (Toure and Cabo, 2012). Therefore, we analyzed the dynamics of propagation of premature impulses through heterogeneities in gap junctional conductance which result in increases of space constant of more than 40% in the direction of propagation. **Figure 5** shows $|I_{Na,max}|$ during propagation of premature impulses through a heterogeneity in gap junctional conductance ($\lambda_{distal}/\lambda_{proximal} = 1.49$ or an increase of 49% in the direction of propagation) which is identified in **Figure 5A** by the vertical dashed line. The refractory period is 197 ms (a premature with S1S2 = 197 ms fails to propagate in the proximal side of the heterogeneity). Note in **Figures 5A,B** that all premature impulses (S2) that propagate in the proximal side (S1S2 ≥ 198 ms), also propagate through the heterogeneity (propagation initiated at $x = 0$ mm). The effect of the heterogeneity is to reduce $|I_{Na,max}|$ by ~30 pA/pF for the more premature impulses and by ~20 pA/pF for the basic impulse of the stimulating train (S1S1 = 250 ms). At the interface, as the downstream impedance decreases in tissue with higher cell-to-cell coupling, the stimulatory efficacy of the wave front head decreases due to current dissipation, a phenomenon known as source/sink mismatch. The drop in the absolute value of peak I_{Na} caused by the heterogeneity is not sufficient to bring $|I_{Na,max}|$ below the value that is necessary to block propagation, and that is why all premature impulses propagate through the heterogeneity. For example, for S1S2 = 198 ms, after the premature impulses reaches a minimum $|I_{Na,max}|$ of 34 pA/pF 2.5 mm away from the stimulation site, $|I_{Na,max}|$ increases to ~ 86 pA/pF as the premature impulse propagates, which is reduced by the source/sink mismatch at the heterogeneity to ~ 58 pA/pF, a value which is still sufficient to sustain propagation.

If the initiation of premature impulses occurs closer to the heterogeneity, premature impulses block for a range of coupling intervals (**Figure 6**). In **Figure 6** initiation of premature impulses occurs 2.5 mm (~ 2.5 λ) away from the same heterogeneity in gap junction conductance shown in **Figure 5**. Premature impulses initiated with coupling intervals S1S2 of 198–200 ms block at the heterogeneity (the window of vulnerability to block is 2–3 ms) (**Figures 6A,B**). Note that premature impulses at those same coupling intervals do not block when the premature impulses are initiated 5 mm (~ 5 λ) away from the heterogeneity (**Figure 5**). The mechanism of block relates to the dynamics of propagation of premature impulses shown in **Figure 3**. Premature impulses show a minimum $|I_{Na,max}|$, and are more susceptible to block, at a distance ~ 2 mm from the stimulation site (**Figures 3, 5**); as propagation proceeds, $|I_{Na,max}|$ increases. The heterogeneity in gap junction conductance that results in a sudden increase in space constant in the direction of propagation causes a drop in $|I_{Na,max}|$ (**Figure 5A**). If that drop occurs when the premature impulse is more vulnerable, the value of $|I_{Na,max}|$ may decrease below the value that is necessary to sustain propagation,

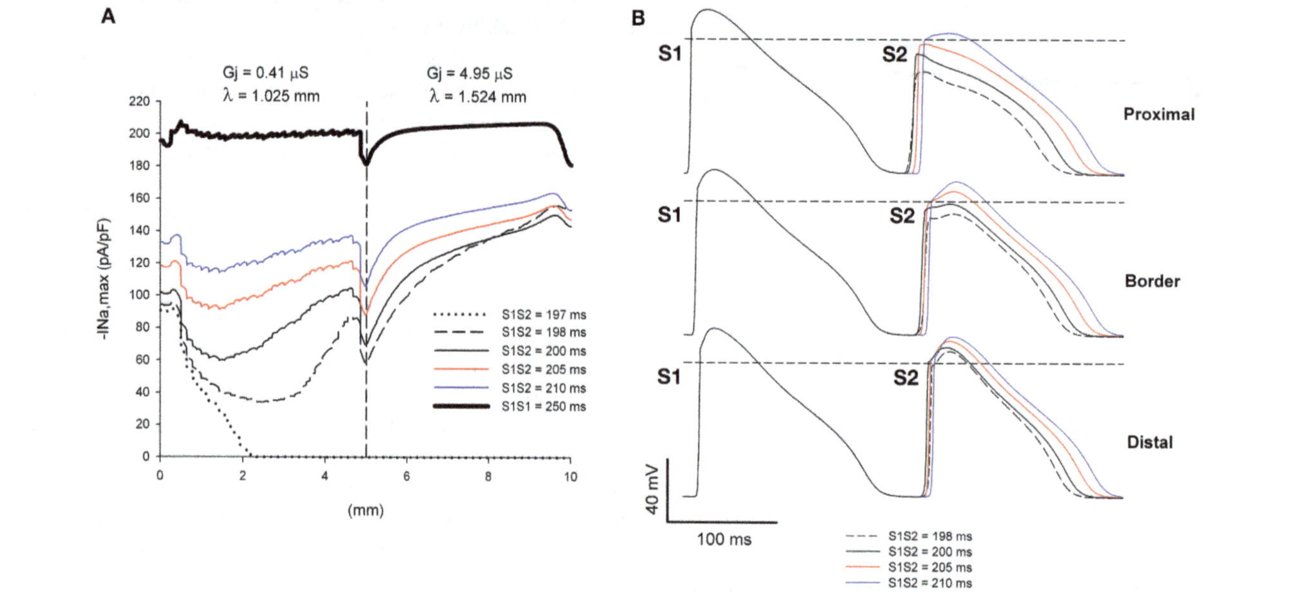

FIGURE 5 | Single premature impulses propagate through a structural heterogeneity when initiated far (5 mm away) from the heterogeneity. **(A)** Changes in I_{Na} current peak for single premature impulses, with different coupling intervals (S1S2), as the impulses propagate away from the stimulation site ($x = 0$ mm), in a preparation with a structural heterogeneity with average cell-to-cell coupling $Gj = 0.41\,\mu S$ in the proximal side and $Gj = 4.95\,\mu S$ in the distal side. The dashed vertical line indicates the location of the heterogeneity. **(B)** Action potentials calculated in the proximal side (2.5 mm from the border), at the border and in the distal side (2.5 mm from the border). Horizontal dashed line indicates a transmembrane potential of 0 mV. The dashed plot (S1S2 = 198 ms) is the shortest coupling that resulted in a propagated response. Size of the preparation: 10 × 2.5 mm (proximal side: 5 mm; distal side: 5 mm). Note that all single premature impulses propagate through the structural heterogeneity.

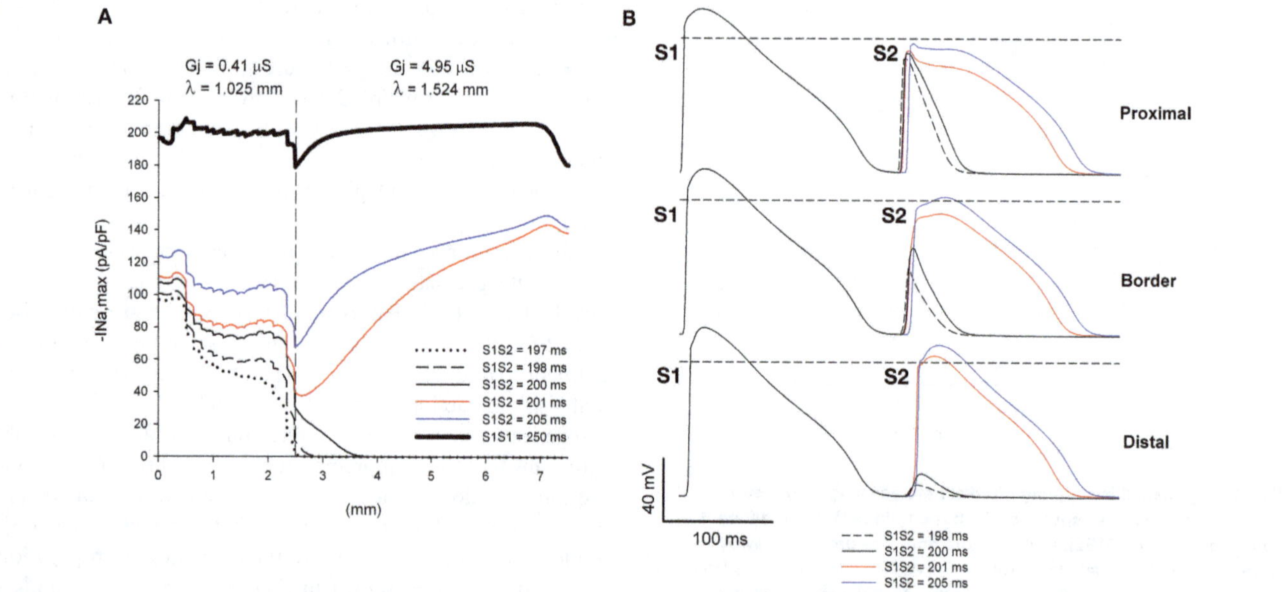

FIGURE 6 | Single premature impulses may block at a structural heterogeneity when initiated close (2.5 mm away) to the heterogeneity. **(A)** Changes in I_{Na} current peak for single premature impulses, with different coupling intervals (S1S2), as the impulses propagate away from the stimulation site ($x = 0$ mm), in a preparation with a structural heterogeneity with average cell-to-cell coupling $Gj = 0.41\,\mu S$ in the proximal side and $Gj = 4.95\,\mu S$ in the distal side. The dashed vertical line indicates the location of the heterogeneity. **(B)** Action potentials calculated in the proximal side (1.5 mm from the border), at the border and in the distal side (2.5 mm from the border). Horizontal dashed line indicates a transmembrane potential of 0 mV. The dashed plot (S1S2 = 198 ms) is the shortest coupling that resulted in a propagated response (in the proximal side). Size of the preparation: 7.5 × 2.5 mm (proximal side: 2.5 mm; distal side: 5 mm). Note that single premature impulses with S1S2 = 198–200 ms block at the structural heterogeneity.

and the premature impulse may block (S1S2 = 198–200 ms in **Figure 6A**). The critical value of $|I_{Na,max}|$ for propagation is ~ 40 pA/pF (the minimum for S1S2 = 201 ms in **Figure 6A**). If the drop occurs when $|I_{Na,max}|$ has partially recovered from its minimum, the drop is not sufficient to bring $|I_{Na,max}|$ below the critical value for propagation, and the premature impulse propagates through the heterogeneity (S1S2 = 198 ms and 200 ms in **Figure 5A**).

The window of vulnerability to block increases when the difference in *Gj* between the distal and proximal sides of the heterogeneity (and consequently the ratio of the space constants) increases. **Figure 7** shows the dynamics of propagation of premature impulses through a heterogeneity with $\lambda_{distal}/\lambda_{proximal}$ = 1.62. The increase in the source/sink mismatch results in a larger drop in $|I_{Na,max}|$ at the heterogeneity (compare **Figure 7A** with **Figure 6A**). Premature impulses with coupling intervals S1S2 = 198–202 ms block at the heterogeneity increasing the window of vulnerability to block to 4–5 ms (which is larger than in **Figure 6**). Note the latency in the recovery of $|I_{Na,max}|$ for S1S2 = 203 ms, which indicates that the premature impulse hovers around the threshold of $|I_{Na,max}|$ necessary for propagation in the distal side (~ 24 pA/pF). For the *Gj* heterogeneity in **Figure 7**, when initiation of premature impulses occurred 5 mm away from the heterogeneity, similarly to what occurred in **Figure 5**, all premature impulses propagated through the heterogeneity (not shown).

PROPAGATION OF DOUBLE PREMATURE IMPULSES (S3) IN THE INFARCTED HEART

Figure 8A shows the CV of double premature impulses (S3) initiated after a first premature (S2) with a coupling interval S1S2 = 200 ms with different S2S3 coupling intervals. As expected, and similarly to what occurred for single premature impulses (**Figure 2A**), average CV decreases with S2S3 coupling interval. **Figure 8B** shows the local CV as the S3 impulse propagate away from the stimulation site. CVs change less as the S3 premature propagates (**Figure 8B**) than when S2 impulses propagate (**Figure 2B**). Compare for example the changes in CV occurring when the S2 impulse with coupling interval S1S2 = 200 ms propagates (thick black line in **Figure 8B**) with the changes occurring when a S3 impulse with a coupling interval S2S3 = 166 ms propagates (black dashed line in **Figure 8B**). In contrast to what occurred during propagation of single premature impulses that show a monotonic increase in CV with propagation, during propagation of double premature impulses (S3) CV can decrease as the wave front propagates (coupling interval S2S3 = 180 ms in **Figure 8B**). For comparison purposes, **Figure 8C** shows both the CV restitution curves for single (S2) and double (S3) premature impulses. The maximum slope of the CV restitution curve for S3 is smaller than for S2, and for all diastolic intervals (DI), the CV for S3 premature impulses is smaller than for S2 premature impulses. However, the CV of a S3 impulse with a big DI is larger than the CV of a S2 impulse with a small DI (see below). For

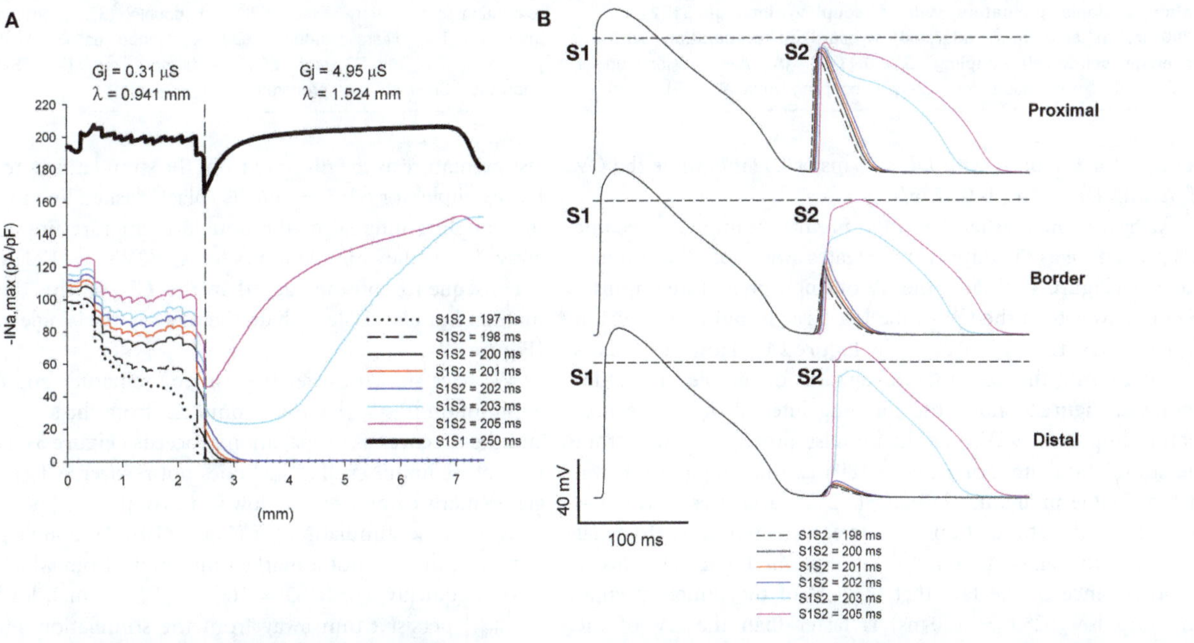

FIGURE 7 | Increasing the discontinuity in *Gj* at the heterogeneity increases the range of coupling intervals for which single premature impulses block at a structural heterogeneity when initiated close (2.5 mm away) to the heterogeneity. (A) Changes in I_{Na} current peak for single premature impulses, with different coupling intervals (S1S2), as the impulses propagate away from the stimulation site ($x = 0$ mm), in a preparation with a structural heterogeneity with average cell-to-cell coupling *Gj* = 0.31 μS in the proximal side and *Gj* = 4.95 μS in the distal side. The dashed vertical line indicates the location of the heterogeneity. **(B)** Action potentials calculated in the proximal side (1.5 mm from the border), at the border and in the distal side (2.5 mm from the border). Horizontal dashed line indicates a transmembrane potential of 0 mV. The dashed plot (S1S2 = 198 ms) is the shortest coupling that resulted in a propagated response (in the proximal side). Size of the preparation: 7.5 × 2.5 mm (proximal side: 2.5 mm; distal side: 5 mm). Note that single premature impulses with S1S2 = 198–202 ms block at the structural heterogeneity.

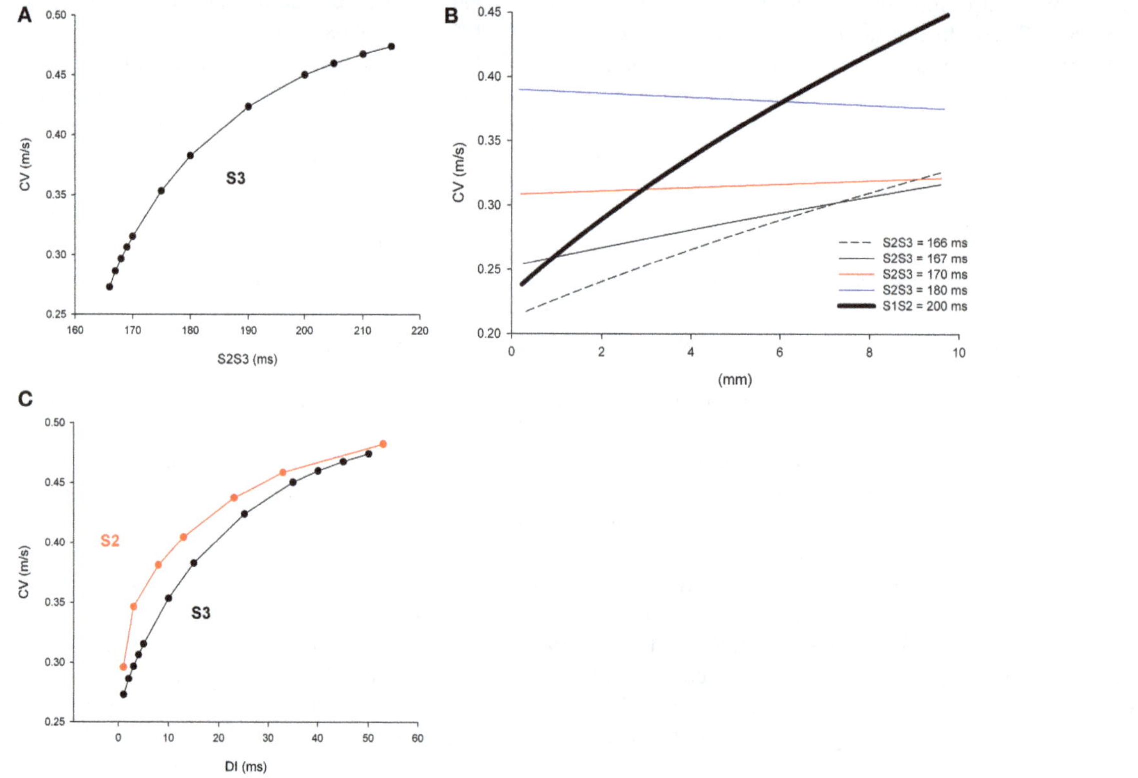

FIGURE 8 | Longitudinal conduction velocity (CV) of double premature impulses with different coupling intervals (S2S3), after a single premature with a coupling interval S1S2 = 200 ms, in a uniform infarcted myocardium preparation with average cell-to-cell coupling $G_j = 0.41\,\mu S$. (A) Average longitudinal CV in the preparation for different coupling intervals. **(B)** Local longitudinal CV as the impulse propagates away from the stimulation site ($x = 0$ mm). **(C)** Comparison of longitudinal CV restitution curves for single (S2) and double (S3) premature impulses. The diastolic interval (DI) is defined as (S1S2—Refractory period of S1) for S2 and (S2S3—Refractory period of S2) for S3 impulses. Size of the preparation: 10 × 2.5 mm.

example the CV of S3 with $DI = 25$ ms is 0.42 m/s while the CV of S2 with $DI = 3$ ms is 0.35 m/s.

We have shown earlier that single premature impulses become less premature as the impulse propagates away from the stimulation site (**Figure 4**) because the CV of single premature impulses (S2) is slower than the CV of the last basic impulse of the train (S1) (see CV restitution curve in **Figure 2A**). However, this is not necessarily the case for propagation of double premature impulses. **Figure 9** shows the coupling interval of double premature impulses (V2V3) as the impulse propagates away from the stimulation site. For S2S3 = 180 ms, the coupling interval of the double premature impulse (V2V3) decreases as the distance from the stimulation site increases (in contrast to what happened for single premature impulses in **Figure 4**). This is a consequence of the fact that the CV of the double premature impulse (S2S3 = 180 ms) is faster than the CV of the single premature impulse (S1S2 = 200 ms) (**Figures 8A,B**). The average CV for the single premature (S1S2 = 200 ms; $DI =$ 3 ms in S2 plot in **Figure 8B**) is ~0.35 m/s, and the average CV for the double premature (S2S3 = 180 ms; $DI = 15$ ms in S3 plot in **Figure 8B**) is ~0.38 m/s. Note also the differences in CV for single and double premature impulses in **Figure 8B**. Only for double premature impulses with a small S2S3 coupling interval (and small DI) the premature impulse becomes less premature as the distance from the stimulation site increases. For example, for S2S3 = 166 ms (black dashed line in **Figure 9**), the coupling interval of the double premature impulse 10 mm away from the stimulation site is V2V3 = 172 ms; this is a consequence of the fact that the CV of the double premature impulse is less than the CV of the single premature (**Figure 8B**).

We have shown earlier that single premature impulses reach a minimum $|I_{Na,max}|$ about 2 mm (2λ) from the stimulation site and then recover as propagation proceeds (**Figure 3**). For double premature impulses, $|I_{Na,max}|$ does not recover as fast as for single premature impulses and low values of $|I_{Na,max}|$ persist further away from the stimulation site (**Figure 10**). For double premature impulses, there is not a marked minimum from which $|I_{Na,max}|$ recovers quickly. For S2S3 = 166 ms ($DI = 1$ ms), low values of $|I_{Na,max}|$ persist 6 mm away from the stimulation site, and its recovery is very slow. Compare with the dynamics of recovery of S1S2 = 200 ms ($DI = 3$ ms), which is also shown for reference in **Figure 10** (thick black line). For S2S3 = 167, 170, and 180 ms there is no evidence of recovery of $|I_{Na,max}|$ with distance from the stimulation site except when the impulses reach the boundary of the preparation ($x = 10$ mm). In fact, for S2S3 = 170 and 180 ms, $|I_{Na,max}|$ decreases as the impulse propagates away of the simulation site.

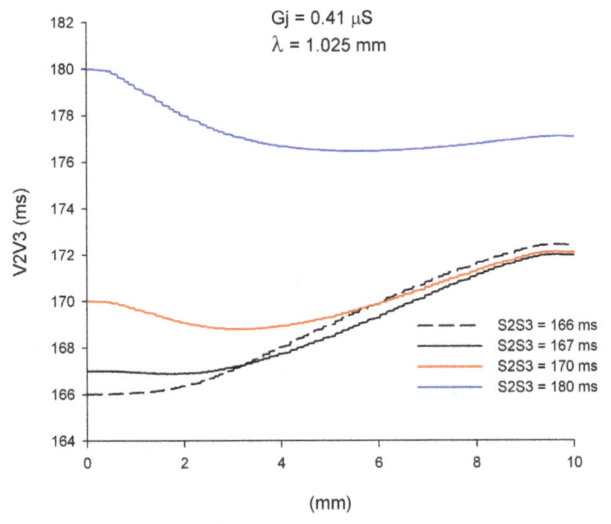

FIGURE 9 | Change in coupling interval between double premature impulses and a single premature with S1S2 = 200 ms (V2V3), for different coupling intervals (S2S3), as double premature impulses propagate away from the stimulation site (x = 0 mm). Uniform preparation with average cell-to-cell coupling Gj = 0.41 μS. Size of the preparation: 10 × 2.5 mm.

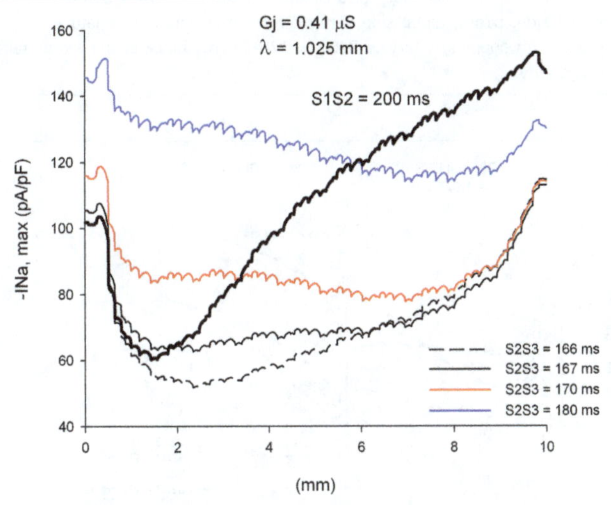

FIGURE 10 | Changes in I_{Na} current peak for double premature impulses with different coupling intervals (S2S3), initiated after a single premature with S1S2 = 200 ms, as the impulses propagate away from the stimulation site (x = 0 mm), in a uniform preparation with average cell-to-cell coupling Gj = 0.41 μS. Also shown for comparison are the changes in I_{Na} current peak for the single premature impulse (S1S2 = 200 ms; thick black line; also shown in **Figure 3**). Size of the preparation: 10 × 2.5 mm.

EFFECT OF STRUCTURAL REMODELING ON PROPAGATION OF DOUBLE PREMATURE IMPULSES (S3)

We have shown earlier that, for a heterogeneity with $\lambda_{distal}/\lambda_{proximal} = 1.49$ (or an increase of 49% in the direction of propagation), single premature impulses with the shortest coupling interval propagate through the heterogeneity when they are initiated far away (5 mm) from the heterogeneity (**Figure 5**). This is a consequence of the recovery of $|I_{Na,max}|$ of single premature impulses as they propagate away from the site of initiation. However, propagating double premature impulses do not show such a recovery in $|I_{Na,max}|$, and low values of $|I_{Na,max}|$ persist far way form the stimulation site (**Figure 10**). As a result, and in contrast to what occur with single premature impulses, double premature impulses initiated 5 mm away from a heterogeneity with $\lambda_{distal}/\lambda_{proximal} = 1.49$ block for a range of S2S3 coupling intervals from 170 to 173 ms (window of vulnerability is 4–5 ms) (**Figure 11**). The mechanism of block is the drop in $|I_{Na,max}|$ caused by the source/sink mismatch at the heterogeneity. For single premature impulses (thick black line in **Figure 11**), the drop occurs after $|I_{Na,max}|$ had recovered and the drop is not sufficient to reduce it below a value that cannot sustain propagation. In contrast, for double premature impulses (with short coupling intervals), $|I_{Na,max}|$ does not recover sufficiently with propagation and the drop in $|I_{Na,max}|$ at the heterogeneity decreases it to a value that cannot sustain propagation.

The window of vulnerability to block decreases when the difference in cell-to-cell Gj between the proximal and the distal side decreases. For $\lambda_{distal}/\lambda_{proximal} = 1.40$, the window of vulnerability decreases to 2–3 ms (**Figure 12A**), and for $\lambda_{distal}/\lambda_{proximal} = 1.3$ there is no block at the heterogeneity for any coupling interval (**Figure 12B**). As the difference in Gj between the proximal and distal side decreases, so does the drop in $|I_{Na,max}|$ caused by the Gj heterogeneity (**Figures 11, 12**).

DISCUSSION

We have shown that $|I_{Na,max}|$, prematurity (i.e., coupling interval with the previous impulse), and CV of premature impulses change dynamically as they propagate away from the site of initiation, and that there are fundamental differences between the dynamics of propagation of single (S2) and double premature impulses (S3). Single premature impulses become less premature, recover their excitability ($|I_{Na,max}|$ increases) and CV increase as propagation proceeds. As a consequence it is unlikely that single premature impulses will block at structural heterogeneities causing source/sink mismatch unless the site of origin of the impulse is close (within 2.5 λ) to the site of the heterogeneity or a transition between thin and thick fibers. In contrast, double premature impulses could become more premature, they do not recover their excitability (low values of $|I_{Na,max}|$ persist far away from the site of initiation) and their CV could decrease as propagation proceeds. Those dynamics make it more likely that double premature impulses block at sites of structural heterogeneities than single premature impulses. While experimental and clinical electrophysiologists have reported for many years that the use of multiple premature impulses during programmed electrical stimulation increases the chances of initiation of ventricular tachycardia (Wit and Janse, 1993), our study provides novel insights into the dynamics of propagation of premature impulses and a mechanistic explanation of the conditions for block at sites of microstructural heterogeneities. The dynamic changes in CV of premature impulses as propagation proceeds away from the site of initiation implies

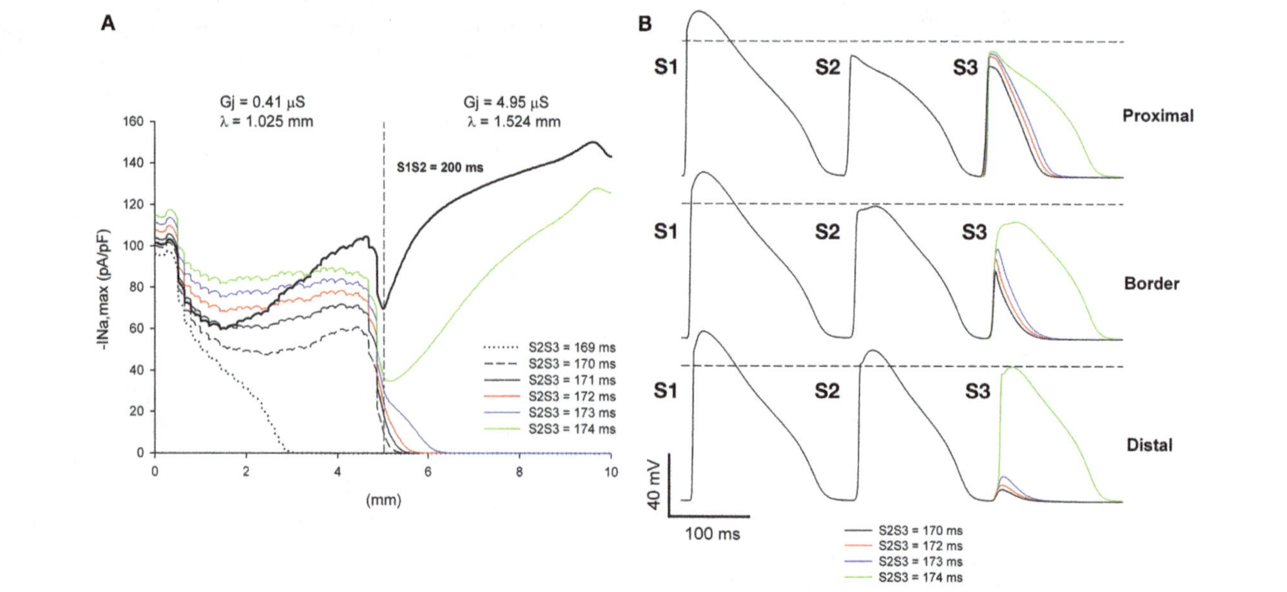

FIGURE 11 | Double premature impulses block at a structural heterogeneity even when initiated far (5 mm away) from the heterogeneity. (A) Changes in I_{Na} current peak for double premature impulses, with different coupling intervals (S2S3), as the impulses propagate away from the stimulation site ($x = 0$ mm), in a preparation with a structural heterogeneity with average cell-to-cell coupling $Gj = 0.41\,\mu S$ in the proximal side and $Gj = 4.95\,\mu S$ in the distal side. Also shown, for reference, are the changes in I_{Na} current peak for the single premature impulse (S1S2 = 200 ms) initiated before the double premature impulses. The dashed vertical line indicates the location of the heterogeneity. **(B)** Action potentials calculated in the proximal side (2.5 mm from the border), at the border and in the distal side (2.5 mm from the border). Horizontal dashed line indicates a transmembrane potential of 0 mV. The dashed plot (S2S3 = 170 ms) is the shortest coupling that resulted in a propagated response in the proximal side. Size of the preparation: 10 × 2.5 mm (proximal side: 5 mm; distal side: 5 mm). Note that double premature impulses with coupling intervals S2S3 = 170–173 ms block at the structural heterogeneity.

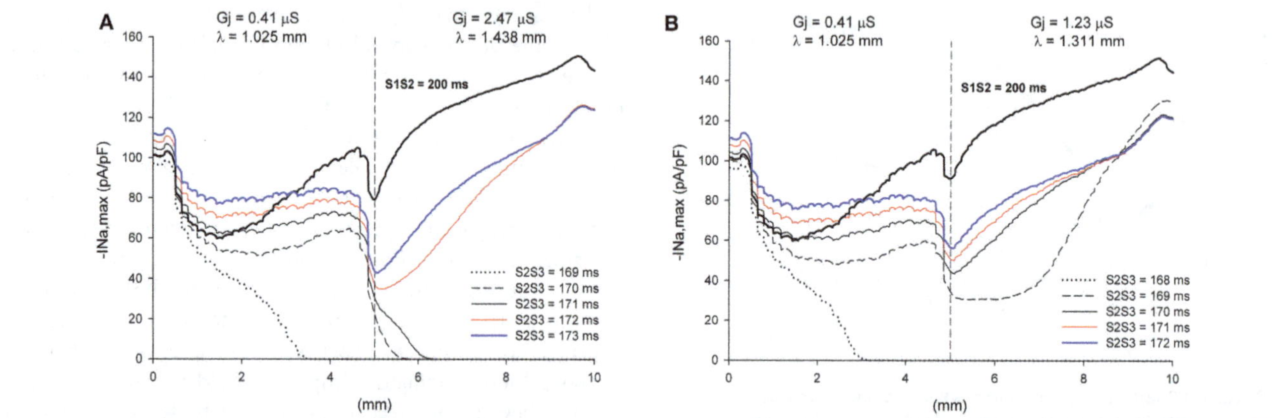

FIGURE 12 | Block at a structural heterogeneity depends on the difference in *Gj* between the proximal and the distal sides of the heterogeneity. Changes in I_{Na} current peak for double premature impulses, with different coupling intervals (S2S3), as the impulses propagate away from the stimulation site ($x = 0$ mm), in a preparation with a structural heterogeneity with average cell-to-cell coupling $Gj = 0.41\,\mu S$ in the proximal side and $Gj = 2.47\,\mu S$ in the distal side ($\lambda_{distal}/\lambda_{proximal} = 1.40$, **A**) and $Gj = 0.41\,\mu S$ in the proximal side and $Gj = 1.23\,\mu S$ in the distal side ($\lambda_{distal}/\lambda_{proximal} = 1.3$, **B**). Also shown, for reference, are the changes in I_{Na} current peak for the single premature impulse (S1S2 = 200 ms) initiated before the double premature impulses. The dashed vertical line indicates the location of the heterogeneity. Note that when $\lambda_{distal}/\lambda_{proximal} = 1.4$ the window of vulnerability is 2–3 ms (S2S3 = 170–171 ms, **A**) and that when $\lambda_{distal}/\lambda_{proximal} = 1.3$ there is no block at the heterogeneity for any S2S3 coupling interval **(B)**.

that measurement techniques that provide local CVs would be more suitable to quantify propagation of premature impulses than techniques that provide global CVs (Linnenbank et al., 2014).

INITIATION OF ARRHYTHMIAS BY EXTERNAL PREMATURE STIMULATION

Regions of heterogeneous Cx43 expression and gap junction conductance have been described in infarcted and failing hearts

(Poelzing and Rosenbaum, 2004; Cabo et al., 2006; Akar et al., 2007), can lead to source/sink mismatch and block of propagation (Kleber and Rudy, 2004), and are likely to provide the "substrate" that leads to initiation of cardiac arrhythmias in diseased hearts. Ventricular tachycardia (VT) can be initiated in clinical electrophysiology laboratories in ~90% of the patients who suffer spontaneous episodes of VT (Wit and Janse, 1993). Several clinical studies (Wit and Janse, 1993) have shown that premature stimulation with a single premature stimulus can induce VT in 20–30% of the patients; two premature stimuli can increase that number by 55%, and the use of three premature impulses can further increase the number by 20%. All in all clinical evidence shows that the use of multiple premature impulses facilitates the initiation of VT. The failure of single premature impulses to initiate arrhythmias is generally explained by their inability to reach the site of the origin of the arrhythmia (Wit and Janse, 1993). Our results explain those experimental and clinical observations by the different dynamics of propagation of S2 and S3 premature impulses. S2 premature impulses may not be able to reach the site of origin of the arrhythmia (possibly a region with heterogeneous cell-to-cell *Gj*) because they recover their excitability relatively close to the stimulation site and they may not be sufficiently premature (**Figure 5**). In contrast, S3 premature impulses do not recover their excitability as fast as S2 impulses, and may be able to reach the site of origin of the arrhythmia with low values of $|I_{Na,max}|$ (**Figure 11**).

The site(s) where premature stimuli are applied during an electrophysiological study may determine whether clinical VTs are initiated or not. It has been reported that one or two premature stimuli initiated on the right ventricle may not induce all clinical VTs (Robertson et al., 1981; Morady et al., 1984). The yield of clinical VTs increases (more clinical VTs induced) when the same protocol is applied to the left ventricle (Robertson et al., 1981; Morady et al., 1984). It is possible that premature impulses are initiated closer to an area with structural heart disease during left ventricular stimulation than during right ventricular stimulation. That would be consistent with the results above demonstrating that single premature impulses may block at structural heterogeneities when the site of origin of the impulse is close to the heterogeneity (**Figures 6, 7**) but not when the site of origin is far away (**Figure 5**).

SPONTANEOUS INITIATION OF ARRHYTHMIAS BY PREMATURE IMPULSES

The patterns of spontaneous initiation of sustained VT in post-myocardial infarction patients can be classified according to the morphology and coupling interval of the premature impulse(s) that precedes the tachycardia (Berger et al., 1988; Roelke et al., 1994). In the first pattern, the premature impulses have a morphology that is similar to that of the VT and a long coupling interval with the last sinus beat. Given the long coupling interval of premature impulses and their morphological similarity to the tachycardia, it has been speculated that those premature impulses could be sinus beats entering an infarcted region, conducting slowly in that region and exiting it before the next sinus beat arrives to excite the rest of the ventricle. In the second pattern, the premature impulses have a morphology that is different from that of the VT and a shorter coupling interval with the last sinus beat.

The success of single premature impulses in spontaneously initiating VT depends on the pattern of initiation. For the first pattern (similar morphology, long coupling), ~70% of VT are initiated by single premature impulses. For the second pattern (different morphology, shorter coupling), only ~16% of VT are initiated by single premature impulses and the rest by double or multiple premature impulses. While, for the first pattern, premature impulses are considered premature because they excite the ventricle prematurely (i.e., before the next sinus beat arrives), the long coupling intervals are much longer than the ventricular refractory period, and the dynamics of propagation of premature impulses described in this study most likely do not apply. However, for the second pattern, the shorter coupling intervals are likely closer to the refractory period, and the dynamics of propagation of premature impulses shown above explain why single premature impulses alone may not be successful in initiating VT, and two or more premature impulses could be necessary.

Microstructural heterogeneities caused by fibrosis can lead to abnormal propagation as a result of source/sink impedance mismatch in explanted hearts from patients with Brugada syndrome (Coronel et al., 2005; Hoogendijk et al., 2010). Even though the cellular mechanism of the heterogeneity in this study (cell-to-cell *Gj* remodeling) is not fibrosis, it is possible that the dynamics of propagation of premature impulses described here may play a role in the initiation of arrhythmias in Brugada syndrome patients.

CELLULAR MECHANISMS OF PROPAGATION AND BLOCK AT SITES OF MICROSTRUCTURAL HETEROGENEITIES CAUSING SOURCE/SINK IMPEDANCE MISMATCH

In an earlier computational study, we found that, in a model of healthy canine epicardium under conditions of reduced excitability (uniform 70% reduction of maximum I_{Na} conductance), heterogeneities in gap junction conductance or cell size (both parameters of the cellular microstructure contribute to λ) cause unidirectional block when λ in the direction of propagation increases by at least 40% (Toure and Cabo, 2012). We have also shown that heterogeneities in myofibroblast density, whose paracrine effect results in heterogeneities in *Gj*, may also create a substrate leading to unidirectional block (Baum et al., 2012). In particular, block of premature impulses occurred at a heterogeneity between an area with a high (50%) density of myofibroblasts ($\lambda \sim 1.02$ mm) and an area without myofibroblasts ($\lambda \sim 1.32$ mm) (Baum et al., 2012). The results presented here are quantitatively consistent with those earlier results (**Figures 11, 12**), indicating that a sharp increase in λ by more than 30–40% in the direction of propagation may lead to block during premature stimulation or under conditions of reduced excitability. It seems that the threshold for block is independent of the cellular mechanism causing the change in space constant (gap junction conductance, cell size, myofibroblast density), and may apply to other situations in which cellular and/or tissue remodeling results in a change of λ. For instance, it may explain the conditions for block at the border between two regions with different fiber alignments (Kudryashova et al., 2014). Block would be expected at a transition from a region where propagation occurs in the direction transverse to the fiber orientation (λ in the direction of propagation = λ_{Trans}) to a region where propagation occurs in the direction longitudinal to the fiber orientation (λ in the direction of propagation = λ_{Long}), if $\lambda_{Long}/\lambda_{Trans} > 1.40$.

The density and kinetics of ionic currents are also important determinants of propagation of the action potential at sites of microstructural heterogeneities. Our results show that source/sink impedance mismatch at the site of the heterogeneity causes a decrease in I_{Na} (**Figures 6, 7, 11, 12**). When the value of I_{Na} at the site of the heterogeneity is close to the value necessary to sustain propagation, the L-type Ca current may determine whether propagation succeeds or not (Joyner et al., 1996; Rohr and Kucera, 1997; Rohr et al., 1997; Shaw and Rudy, 1997; Cabo et al., 2000). Consequently, we expect that modulation of the L-type Ca current will play a crucial role in determining successful propagation of premature impulses through microstructural heterogeneities caused by *Gj* remodeling in infarcted myocardium (Cabo et al., 2000).

RESTITUTION OF THE CONDUCTION VELOCITY OF PREMATURE IMPULSES

The difference in the dynamics of propagation of single (S2) and double premature (S3) impulses is reflected in their CV restitution curves (**Figure 8C**). The pronounced maximum slope of the CV restitution curve for S2 indicates a faster recovery of excitability with diastolic interval and propagation. The smaller maximum slope of the restitution curve for S3 indicates a slower recovery of excitability with diastolic interval and propagation. The cumulative experimental and clinical evidence, as well as the computations presented here, indicate that double premature impulses are more pro-arrhythmic than single premature impulses. Therefore, we can argue that a decrease in the maximum slope in the CV restitution curve of a propagating impulse is indicative of an increased potential for block at structural heterogeneities. This is consistent with other reports demonstrating that less steep CV restitution curves were more likely to cause spiral break up (Qu et al., 1999), and that steep CV restitution curves prevent block in heterogeneous tissues (Sampson and Henriquez, 2001).

REFERENCES

Akar, F. G., Nass, R. D., Hahn, S., Cingolani, E., Shah, M., Hesketh, G. G., et al. (2007). Dynamic changes in conduction velocity and gap junction properties during development of pacing-induced heart failure. *Am. J. Physiol. Heart Circ. Physiol.* 293, H1223–H1230. doi: 10.1152/ajpheart.00079.2007

Baba, S., Dun, W., Cabo, C., and Boyden, P. A. (2005). Remodeling in cells from different regions of the reentrant circuit during ventricular tachycardia. *Circulation* 112, 2386–2396. doi: 10.1161/CIRCULATIONAHA.105.534784

Baum, J., Long, B., Cabo, C., and Duffy, H. S. (2012). Myofibroblasts cause heterogeneous Cx43 reduction and are unlikely to be coupled to myocytes in the healing canine infarct. *Am. J. Physiol. Heart Circ. Physiol.* 302, H790–H800. doi: 10.1152/ajpheart.00498.2011

Berger, M. D., Waxman, H. L., Buxton, A. E., Marchlinski, F. E., and Josephson, M. E. (1988). Spontaneous compared with induced onset of sustained ventricular tachycardia. *Circulation* 78, 885–892. doi: 10.1161/01.CIR.78.4.885

Cabo, C., and Boyden, P. A. (2003). Electrical remodeling of the epicardial border zone in the canine infarcted heart: a computational analysis. *Am. J. Physiol. Heart Circ. Physiol.* 284, H372–H384. doi: 10.1152/ajpheart.00512.2002

Cabo, C., and Boyden, P. A. (2009). Extracellular space attenuates the effect of gap junctional remodeling on wave propagation: a computational study. *Biophys. J.* 96, 3092–3101. doi: 10.1016/j.bpj.2009.01.014

Cabo, C., Pertsov, A. M., Baxter, W. T., Davidenko, J. M., Gray, R. A., and Jalife, J. (1994). Wave-front curvature as a cause of slow conduction and block in isolated cardiac muscle. *Circ. Res.* 75, 1014–1028. doi: 10.1161/01.RES.75.6.1014

Cabo, C., Pertsov, A. M., Davidenko, J. M., Baxter, W. T., Gray, R. A., and Jalife, J. (1996). Vortex shedding as a precursor of turbulent electrical activity in cardiac muscle. *Biophys. J.* 70, 1105–1111. doi: 10.1016/S0006-3495(96)79691-1

Cabo, C., Schmitt, H., and Wit, A. L. (2000). New mechanism of antiarrhythmic drug action: increasing the L-type calcium current prevents reentrant arrhythmias in the infarcted canine heart. *Circulation* 102, 2417–2425. doi: 10.1161/01.CIR.102.19.2417

Cabo, C., Yao, J., Boyden, P. A., Chen, S., Hussain, W., Duffy, H. S., et al. (2006). Heterogeneous gap junction remodeling in reentrant circuits in the epicardial border zone of the healing canine infarct. *Cardiovasc. Res.* 72, 241–249. doi: 10.1016/j.cardiores.2006.07.005

Coronel, R. (1994). Heterogeneity in extracellular potassium concentration during early myocardial ischaemia and reperfusion: implications for arrhythmogenesis. *Cardiovasc. Res.* 28, 770–777. doi: 10.1093/cvr/28.6.770

Coronel, R., Casini, S., Koopmann, T. T., Wilms-Schopman, F. J., Verkerk, A. O., de Groot, J. R., et al. (2005). Right ventricular fibrosis and conduction delay in a patient with clinical signs of Brugada syndrome: a combined electrophysiological, genetic, histopathologic, and computational study. *Circulation* 112, 2769–2777. doi: 10.1161/CIRCULATIONAHA.105.532614

Fast, V. G., and Kleber, A. G. (1995). Cardiac tissue geometry as a determinant of unidirectional conduction block: assessment of microscopic excitation spread by optical mapping in patterned cell cultures and in a computer model. *Cardiovasc. Res.* 29, 697–707. doi: 10.1016/S0008-6363(96)88643-3

Frazier, D. W., Wolf, P. D., Wharton, J. M., Tang, A. S. L., Smith, W. M., and Ideker, R. E. (1989). Stimulus induced critical point. mechanism for electrical initiation of reentry in normal canine myocardium. *J. Clin. Invest.* 83, 1039–1052. doi: 10.1172/JCI113945

Gough, W. B., Mehra, R., Restivo, M., Zeiler, R. H., and el-Sherif, N. (1985). Reentrant ventricular arrhythmias in the late myocardial infarction period in the dog. 13. Correlation of activation and refractory maps. *Circ. Res.* 57, 432–442. doi: 10.1161/01.RES.57.3.432

Hoogendijk, M. G., Potse, M., Linnenbank, A. C., Verkerk, A. O., den Ruijter, H. M., van Amersfoorth, S. C., et al. (2010). Mechanism of right precordial ST-segment elevation in structural heart disease: excitation failure by current-to-load mismatch. *Heart Rhythm* 7, 238–248. doi: 10.1016/j.hrthm.2009.10.007

Hubbard, M. L., Ying, W., and Henriquez, C. S. (2007). Effect of gap junction distribution on impulse propagation in a monolayer of myocytes: a model study. *Europace* 9, Suppl. 6, vi20–vi28. doi: 10.1093/europace/eum203

Janse, M. J., and Kleber, A. G. (1981). Electrophysiological changes and ventricular arrhythmias in the early phase of regional myocardial ischemia. *Circ. Res.* 49, 1069–1081. doi: 10.1161/01.RES.49.5.1069

Joyner, R. W. (1981). Mechanisms of unidirectional block in cardiac tissues. *Biophys. J.* 35, 113–125. doi: 10.1016/S0006-3495(81)84778-9

Joyner, R. W., Kumar, R., Wilders, R., Jongsma, H. J., Verheijck, E., Golod, D. A., et al. (1996). Modulating L-type calcium current affects discontinuous cardiac action potential conduction. *Biophys. J.* 71, 237–245. doi: 10.1016/S0006-3495(96)79220-2

Kleber, A. G., and Rudy, Y. (2004). Basic mechanisms of cardiac impulse propagation and associated arrhythmias. *Physiol. Rev.* 84, 431–488. doi: 10.1152/physrev.00025.2003

Kudryashova, N. N., Teplenin, A. S., Orlova, Y. V., Selina, L. V., and Agladze, K. (2014). Arrhythmogenic role of the border between two areas of cardiac cell alignment. *J. Mol. Cell. Cardiol.* 76, 227–234. doi: 10.1016/j.yjmcc.2014.09.003

Linnenbank, A. C., deBakker, J. M. T., and Coronel, R. (2014). How to measure propagation velocity in cardiac tissue: asimulation study. *Front. Physiol.* 5:267. doi: 10.3389/fphys.2014.00267

Morady, F., DiCarlo, L., Winston, S., Davis, J. C., and Scheinman, M. M. (1984). A prospective comparison of triple extrastimuli and left ventricular stimulation in studies of ventricular tachycardia induction. *Circulation* 70, 52–27. doi: 10.1161/01.CIR.70.1.52

Nattel, S., Maguy, A., Bouter, S. L., and Yeh, Y.-H. (2007). Arrhythmogenic ion-channel remodeling in the heart: heart failure, myocardial infarction, and atrial fibrillation. *Physiol. Rev.* 87, 425–456. doi: 10.1152/physrev.00014.2006

Peters, N., Cabo, C., and Wit, A. L. (2000). "Arrhythmogenic mechanisms: automaticity, triggered activity and reentry," in *Cardiac Electrophysiology: from Cell to Bedside*, eds D. Zipes and J. Jalife (Philadelphia, PA: W. B. Saunders Company), 345–356.

Poelzing, S., and Rosenbaum, D. S. (2004). Altered connexin43 expression produces arrhythmia substrate in heart failure. *Am. J. Physiol. Heart Circ. Physiol.* 287, H1762–H1770. doi: 10.1152/ajpheart.00346.2004

Qu, Z., Weiss, J. N. and Garfinkel, A. (1999). Cardiac electrical restitution properties and stability of reentrant waves: a simulation study. *Am. J. Physiol. Heart Circ. Physiol.* 276, H269–H283.

Quan, W., and Rudy, Y. (1990). Unidirectional block and reentry of cardiac excitation: a model study. *Circ. Res.* 66, 367–382. doi: 10.1161/01.RES.66.2.367

Robertson, J. F., Cain, M. E., Horowitz, L. N., Spielman, S. R., Greenspan, A. M., Waxman, H. L., et al. (1981). Anatomic and electrophysiologic correlates of ventricular tachycardia requiring left ventricular stimulation. *Am. J. Cardiol.* 48, 263–268. doi: 10.1016/0002-9149(81)90606-8

Roelke, M., Garan, H., McGovern, B. A., and Ruskin, J. N. (1994). Analysis of the initiation of spontaneous monomorphic ventricular tachycardia by stored intracardiac electrograms. *J. Am. Coll. Cardiol.* 23, 117–122. doi: 10.1016/0735-1097(94)90509-6

Rohr, S., and Kucera, J. P. (1997). Involvement of the calcium inward current in cardiac impulse propagation: induction of unidirectional conduction block by nifedipine and reversal by Bay K 8644. *Biophys. J.* 72, 754–766 doi: 10.1016/S0006-3495(97)78710-1

Rohr, S., Kucera, J. P., Fast, V. G., and Kleber, A. G. (1997). Paradoxical improvement of impulse conduction in cardiac tissue by partial cellular uncoupling. *Science* 275, 841–844. doi: 10.1126/science.275.5301.841

Sampson, K. J., and Henriquez, C. S. (2001). Simulation and prediction of functional block in the presence of structural and ionic heterogeneity. *Am. J. Physiol. Heart Circ. Physiol.* 281, H2597–H2603.

Severs, N. J., Bruce, A. F., Dupont, E., and Rothery, S. (2008). Remodelling of gap junctions and connexin expression in diseased myocardium. *Cardiovasc. Res.* 80, 9–19. doi: 10.1093/cvr/cvn133

Shaw, R. M., and Rudy, Y. (1997). Ionic mechanisms of propagation in cardiac tissue: roles of the sodium and L-type calcium currents during reduced excitability and decreased gap junction coupling. *Circ. Res.* 81, 727–741. doi: 10.1161/01.RES.81.5.727

Spach, M. S., and Heidlage, J. F. (1995). The stochastic nature of cardiac propagation at a microscopic level. Electrical description of myocardial architecture and its application to conduction. *Circ. Res.* 76, 366–380. doi: 10.1161/01.RES.76.3.366

Spach, M. S., and Kootsey, J. M. (1985). Relating the sodium current and conductance to the shape of transmembrane and extracellular potentials by simulation: effects of propagation boundaries. *IEEE Trans. Biomed. Eng.* 32, 743–755. doi: 10.1109/TBME.1985.325489

Spach, M. S., Miller, W. T., Dolber, P. C., Kootsey, J. M., Sommer, J. R., and Mosher, C. E. (1982). The functional role of structural complexities in the propagation of depolarization in the atrium of the dog. Cardiac conduction disturbances due to discontinuities of effective axial resistivity. *Circ. Res.* 50, 175–191. doi: 10.1161/01.RES.50.2.175

Toure, A., and Cabo, C. (2010). Effect of cell geometry on conduction velocity in a subcellular model of myocardium. *IEEE Trans. Biomed. Eng.* 57, 2107–2114. doi: 10.1109/TBME.2010.2050064

Toure, A., and Cabo, C. (2012). Effect of heterogeneities in the cellular microstructure on propagation of the cardiac action potential. *Med. Biol. Eng. Comput.* 50, 813–825. doi: 10.1007/s11517-012-0934-4

Wit, A. L., and Janse, M. J. (1993). *The Ventricular Arrhythmias of Ischemia and Infarction: Electrophysiological Mechanisms.* Mount Kisco, NY: Futura Publishing Company.

7

Remodeling of cardiac passive electrical properties and susceptibility to ventricular and atrial arrhythmias

Stefan Dhein[1*†], Thomas Seidel[2†], Aida Salameh[3], Joanna Jozwiak[4], Anja Hagen[5], Martin Kostelka[1], Gerd Hindricks[4] and Friedrich-Wilhelm Mohr[1]

[1] *Clinic for Cardiac Surgery, Heart Center Leipzig, University Leipzig, Leipzig, Germany*
[2] *Nora Eccles Harrison Cardiovascular Research and Training Institute, University of Utah, Salt Lake City, UT, USA*
[3] *Clinic for Pediatric Cardiology, Heart Center Leipzig, University Leipzig, Leipzig, Germany*
[4] *Clinic for Cardiology, Heart Center Leipzig, University Leipzig, Leipzig, Germany*
[5] *Hospital for Children and Adolescents, University of Leipzig, Leipzig, Germany*

***Correspondence:**
Stefan Dhein, Clinic for Cardiac Surgery, Heart Center Leipzig, University of Leipzig, Struempellstr. 39, 04289 Leipzig, Germany
e-mail: stefan.dhein@medizin.uni-leipzig.de

†These authors have contributed equally to this work.

Coordinated electrical activation of the heart is essential for the maintenance of a regular cardiac rhythm and effective contractions. Action potentials spread from one cell to the next via gap junction channels. Because of the elongated shape of cardiomyocytes, longitudinal resistivity is lower than transverse resistivity causing electrical anisotropy. Moreover, non-uniformity is created by clustering of gap junction channels at cell poles and by non-excitable structures such as collagenous strands, vessels or fibroblasts. Structural changes in cardiac disease often affect passive electrical properties by increasing non-uniformity and altering anisotropy. This disturbs normal electrical impulse propagation and is, consequently, a substrate for arrhythmia. However, to investigate how these structural changes lead to arrhythmias remains a challenge. One important mechanism, which may both cause and prevent arrhythmia, is the mismatch between current sources and sinks. Propagation of the electrical impulse requires a sufficient source of depolarizing current. In the case of a mismatch, the activated tissue (source) is not able to deliver enough depolarizing current to trigger an action potential in the non-activated tissue (sink). This eventually leads to conduction block. It has been suggested that in this situation a balanced geometrical distribution of gap junctions and reduced gap junction conductance may allow successful propagation. In contrast, source-sink mismatch can prevent spontaneous arrhythmogenic activity in a small number of cells from spreading over the ventricle, especially if gap junction conductance is enhanced. Beside gap junctions, cell geometry and non-cellular structures strongly modulate arrhythmogenic mechanisms. The present review elucidates these and other implications of passive electrical properties for cardiac rhythm and arrhythmogenesis.

Keywords: electrical propagation, passive electrical properties, cardiac tissue, gap junction, connexin, anisotropy, inhomogeneity, cable theory

INTRODUCTION

Although the heart can be considered as a simple mechanical pump, this pump is a highly complex system involving mechanical, electrical, active, passive, and endocrine factors. Many of these factors are subject to remodeling processes in cardiac disease and, thus, are not necessarily constant. This review focuses on remodeling of the passive electrical properties of the heart and its importance for arrhythmogenesis.

Passive electrical properties of cardiac tissue comprise the specific resistance of intracellular and extracellular spaces as well as membrane capacitance. These are strongly influenced by tissue structure. This involves size, shape and arrangement of cardiac cells, including myocytes and non-myocytes, as well as connective tissue, extracellular and intracellular volume conductors and gap junctions. Moreover, anisotropy and inhomogeneities in the spatial (or in some cases temporal) distribution of these factors are of importance.

Electrical anisotropy in the heart refers to differing specific resistances in longitudinal and transverse fiber direction. The elongated shape of myocytes and intercellular coupling mainly at cell poles result in lower longitudinal than transverse resistance. This applies both to the extra- and intracellular space. Spatial inhomogeneities in cardiac tissue, e.g., zones with enhanced deposition of collagen, (fibrosis, which increases with age), lead to a spatial variation of these resistances, which is referred to as non-uniformity. In consequence, cardiac tissue can be considered as non-uniform and anisotropic.

A simple model of the electrical equivalent circuit of cardiac tissue is a cable formed by cells coupled in series via Ohmic resistors. Each cell in this cable represents a resistor with a parallel capacitor (for review see Weidmann, 1990). The change in voltage is a function of distance (x) according to $V_x = V_0 \exp(-x/\lambda)$ with the length constant $\lambda = \sqrt{(r_m/r_i)}$. The membrane resistance, r_m, is expressed in Ωcm, the intracellular longitudinal resistance,

r_i, in Ω/cm. The input resistance at $x = 0$ can be described as $r_{input} = V_0/I = r_i\lambda$. Due to the fiber geometry with radius a, the specific membrane resistance R_m equals $2\ \pi a r_m$ [Ωcm^2] and specific intracellular resistance $R_i = \pi a^2 r_i$ [Ωcm]. The specific membrane capacitance can be described as $C_m = \tau/R_m$ with the time constant τ. In a multicellular preparation with parallel running fibers the longitudinal resistance of the extracellular space r_o also has to be considered. For these conditions λ is reflected by $\lambda = \sqrt{(r_m/(r_i + r_o))}$ and the conduction velocity θ depends on $\theta = \sqrt{(1/(\tau_{foot} C_m(r_i + r_o))}$. This cable theory was originally formulated for nerve axons (Hodgkin and Rushton, 1946) and later on for Purkinje fibers (Weidmann, 1952). It holds true for a continuous cable (**Figure 1**).

However, this is oversimplifying, since the intracellular space of adjacent cells is connected via gap junction channels. A cluster of single gap junction channels forms a gap junction, which connects the cytoplasm of two adjacent cells by the resistance R_{GJ} (see **Figure 2**). The gap junction resistance is higher than the resistance of the cytoplasm. Furthermore, the resistance r_o of the extracellular space is not homogeneous. The resistance R_{cleft} of the extracellular cleft between two cells near intercalated disks (2–5 nm wide) can be assumed to differ significantly from the much wider clefts elsewhere (>20 nm) not only because of its small width, but also because it contains anchoring proteins and gap junction channels. Therefore, the cable necessarily becomes discontinuous (**Figure 2**).

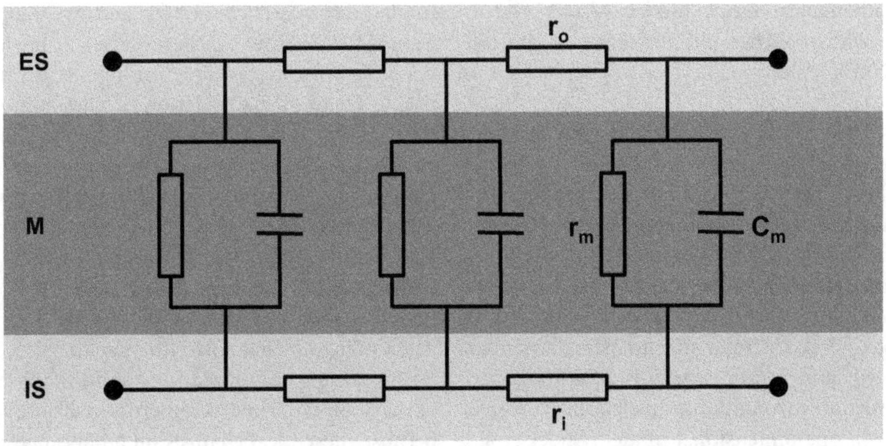

FIGURE 1 | Schematic view of cardiac tissue modeled as a simple cable consisting of intracellular (r_i) and extracellular (r_o) resistors and capacitors (C_m). ES, extracellular space; M, cell membrane; IS, intracellular space.

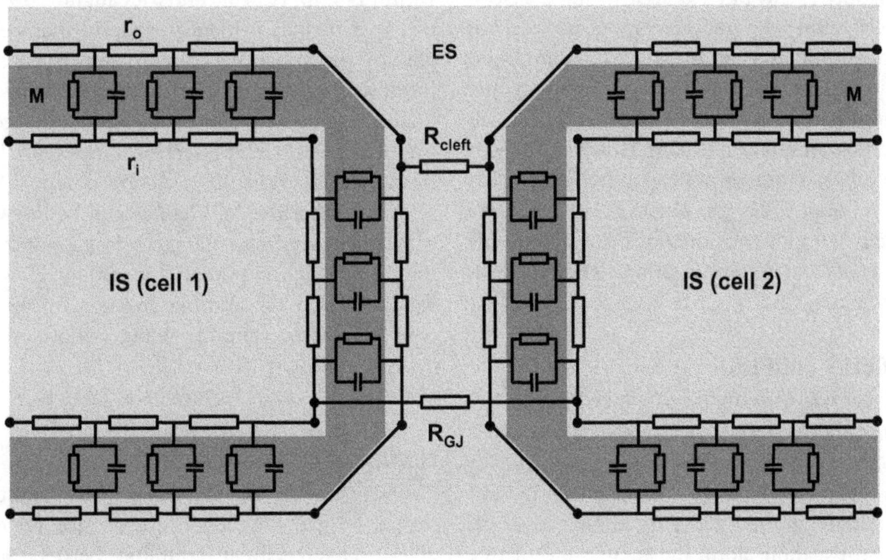

FIGURE 2 | A more realistic scheme of coupled cardiac cells considering discontinuous properties. The cell membrane (M) is represented by a series of resistor-capacitor circuits, connecting the extracellular space (ES) with the intracellular space (IS). They are interconnected within one cell via extracellular (r_o) and intracellular (r_i) resistors. Gap junction resistance (R_{GJ}) connects the intracellular spaces of adjacent cells, while extracellular coupling is realized via the resistance of the extracellular cleft (R_{cleft}).

Fast sodium channels are essential for impulse propagation. Opening of these channels at the beginning of an action potential generates a depolarizing current (I_{Na}), which is responsible for the fast voltage upstroke. Therefore, I_{Na} plays a key role in the propagation of action potentials from cell to cell. It has been shown that these sodium channels are clustered at cell-cell contact zones (Kucera et al., 2002; Maier et al., 2004). This further complicates a correct description of the electrophysiological behavior at cell poles. It also shows that modeling cardiac tissue as a continuum is only reasonable on a macroscopic scale.

Although the equivalent circuit of a discontinuous cable depicted in **Figure 2** is more complex than the simple cable, it remains an oversimplification because it does not reflect the geometrical properties of cells and tissue. Cardiomyocytes are typically not shaped like bricks or regular cylinders—as often assumed in mathematical tissue models—but, instead, are of irregular shape with branches interdigitating at the cell poles (Spach et al., 2000). Additionally, cell size shows some variation.

In this regard, it is important to consider the ratio between the cell surface A_m and the gap junction conductance g_{GJ} (Seidel et al., 2010): increased diameter of the cell can enhance longitudinal propagation velocity θ_L if g_{GJ} is enhanced proportionally to A_m. If g_{GJ} remains constant, however, increased diameter reduces θ_L. This becomes clear when considering that A_m is linearly related to the cell capacitance C_m. Thus, it is important to analyze the ratio of g_{GJ}/A_m in order to understand whether a change in cell size will enhance or reduce θ_L. Furthermore, transverse g_{GJ} may contribute to longitudinal propagation, which cannot be described by a one-dimensional model (Seidel et al., 2010).

Next, we need to consider the three-dimensional nature of the myocardium and the uneven distribution of fibrotic material, mostly collagen fibers, and fibroblasts. Initially, fibroblasts have been considered electrically silent, but research in the past two decades indicates that electrical propagation seems possible. It has been suggested that myofibroblasts can slow conduction (Rohr, 2004, 2012). Furthermore, it has been shown experimentally that impulse propagation along fibroblast inserts was successful over distances up to 300 μm (Gaudesius et al., 2003). However, it needs to be noted that these cells—although not capable of producing action potentials—were coupled via gap junction channels (see below), while HeLa cells without gap junctions did not enable propagation. Thus, it seems that communication-deficient zones will cause propagation failure.

HOW ARE CARDIAC CELLS COUPLED?

Since the discovery of cardiac gap junctions, which form intercellular channels connecting the cytoplasm of adjacent myocytes, it is established that they represent a low-resistance pathway for electrical propagation (Page and Shibata, 1981). However, gap junction resistance is still higher than the cytoplasmic resistance. Accordingly, impulse propagation along the membrane of one cell is faster than over the intercellular gap junction. The time delay at gap junctions is about 0.21–0.27 ms, and ~0.05–0.1 ms at the cell membrane (Fast and Kléber, 1993; Hubbard et al., 2007).

COUPLING WITHOUT GAP JUNCTIONS

If one considers neighbored cells as closely packed capacitors, ephaptic coupling via electrical fields might be possible (Sperelakis, 1979). Electrical field coupling (Sperelakis and Mann, 1977) or ephaptic coupling (Copene and Keener, 2008) refers to the initiation of an action potential in a non-activated downstream cell by the electrical field caused by an activated upstream cell. This kind of impulse propagation does not require cytoplasmic connections via gap junctions. It might occur at the intercalated disks, where the membranes of adjacent cells are only 2–5 nm apart.

Accumulation of K^+ in the junctional extracellular cleft seems necessary to allow sodium channels at the intercalated disk of the upstream cell to fire some microseconds earlier than the channels in the remaining surface membrane. In a theoretical model, this was necessary for effective coupling (Sperelakis and Mann, 1977). However, at present it is unclear whether ephaptic coupling contributes to action potential propagation in normal tissue. Computer simulation studies indicate that, under certain conditions, ephaptic coupling may play a role, but strongly depends on parameters like sodium channel conductance and distribution, and the width of the extracellular cleft at the intercalated disk (Mori et al., 2008; Lin and Keener, 2010). Recent data show that in the perinexus Cx43 gap junctions interact with Na(v)1.5 channels (Rhett et al., 2012). The perinexus has therefore been suggested as the anatomical correlate for ephaptic coupling, the ephapse (Rhett et al., 2013; Veeraraghavan et al., 2014). Local accumulation and shifts of ions may alter local membrane potential. However, there is a lack of experimental evidence, because these local changes on a nanometer scale are difficult to measure. Hence, it remains unclear whether ephaptic coupling significantly contributes to cardiac impulse propagation, especially when considering that, according to the Guoy-Chapman theory, the electrical field near a charged membrane falls to zero within 2–3 nm (Carnie and McLaughlin, 1983).

Experimental evidence suggests that cells need to be coupled by gap junctions to allow the propagation of an electrical impulse: Weingart and Maurer (1988) showed that after manipulating two cells into intimate side-to-side contact, initially there was no transmission of electrotonic potentials or action potentials from one cell to the other. Action potential transfer became possible only after the cells had established new gap junctions. This experiment seems to rule out non-gap junctional mechanisms of intercellular action potential spreading. However, recent evidence was presented for another mechanism of electrical cell-to-cell coupling. Membrane-tunneling nanotubues were suggested as cytosolic bridges between cells (He et al., 2011). This theory, however, still needs further investigation.

CONNEXINS AND GAP JUNCTIONS

Cardiomyocytes and fibroblasts are homocellularly interconnected by gap junction channels (for review see Dhein, 1998, 2004). Heterocellular coupling between cardiomyocytes and fibroblasts, however, has only been shown in cell culture (Goshima and Tonomura, 1969; Gaudesius et al., 2003) or in the sinus node (Camelliti et al., 2004), but not in living ventricular myocardium. Cells can communicate via these gap junction channels. Each channel is about 150 Å long. The membranes of the two cells are separated in this area by a gap of nearly 20 Å, which is spanned by the channel subunits (Beyer et al., 1995). Cardiomyocytes are connected by intercalated disks, which contain three main structures: the fascia adherens, the desmosome (sometimes called macula adherens), and the nexus. While the fascia adherens is composed of two lipid bilayers separated by 200–300 Å, the desmosome is an almost laminated structure formed by the two membranes. At the nexus both cells are in most intimate contact. This zone contains the gap junction channels, which typically are clustered (Gourdie et al., 1990). A gap junction channel comprises of two hemichannels, which are provided by either cell. Each hemichannel is composed of 6 protein subunits, the connexins. Thus, a gap junction channel is a dodecameric channel with a pore in the center (**Figure 3**). Connexins belong to a large protein family with at least 21 isoforms in humans. The connexin protein is a four-transmembrane domain protein with an intracellular N- and C-terminal, 2 extracellular loops, and one intracellular loop. For details see Makowski et al. (1977); Chen et al. (1989); Perkins et al. (1997). The most variant part is the C-terminus, which also serves as binding partner for a number of protein kinases, which can control connexin trafficking, assembly, dis-assembly and single channel conductance by phosphorylation. Connexins are characterized by their molecular weight. For instance, Cx43 refers to the connexin with a molecular weight of 43 kDa. The family of connexins is divided with regard to the amino acid sequences and C-terminal length into five subgroups, i.e., α, β, γ, δ, and ε. The genetic names are composed of a "GJ" followed by the family and a number. Thus, Gjα1 means Cx43 which was the first connexin being characterized from the α-group (see http://www.genenames.org/genefamily/gj.php for reference). For a detailed overview on connexins (see Nielsen et al., 2012).

In the heart the predominant connexin isoform is Cx43, which is found in ventricles and atria. Cx40 is mainly found in atrium and in the specific conduction system. Cx45 is mainly found in early developmental stages, in the conduction system, and between fibroblasts and cardiomyocytes. Connexins are synthesized in the rough endoplasmatic reticulum, folded and transported to the trans Golgi network, where they are oligomerized to hexameric hemichannels (connexons). These hexameres are then transported to the plasma membrane and inserted. It is assumed that they flow with lipid rafts within the membrane and accumulate in areas where N-cadherin and zonula occludens-1 protein (ZO-1) are present. At these sites they dock to other hexameres of the neighboring cell forming the gap junction channel. If the connexins are poly-phosphorylated at certain amino acids of the C-terminal, they can be ubiquitinylated and then degraded. Besides the classical proteosomal degradation lysosomal degradation also has been described.

Regulation of gap junction coupling can be realized by modulating the number of channels, i.e., by influencing synthesis, trafficking docking or degradation, or by changes of the single channel conductance. For a detailed review, see Dhein (2004); Salameh and Dhein (2005); Axelsen et al. (2013). Channel conductance depends on the connexin isoform, the phosphorylation state of the connexin, and on the connexin composition of the channel (e.g., homomeric, heteromeric) (Harris, 2001; Moreno, 2004). Interestingly, besides an open and a closed state a single channel can exhibit several conductance states (Harris, 2001; Bukauskas and Verselis, 2004). Moreover, heterotypic channels consisting of hemichannels of different connexin isoforms can show asymmetric voltage-dependent gating. Asymmetric gating refers to the observation that the conductance-to-voltage relationship depends on the polarity of the transjunctional voltage (see e.g., Bukauskas and Verselis, 2004; Schulte et al., 2008).

ANISOTROPY AND NON-UNIFORMITY (INHOMOGENEITY)

Anisotropy is defined as the property of being directionally dependent. With regard to cardiac tissue the term is mostly used

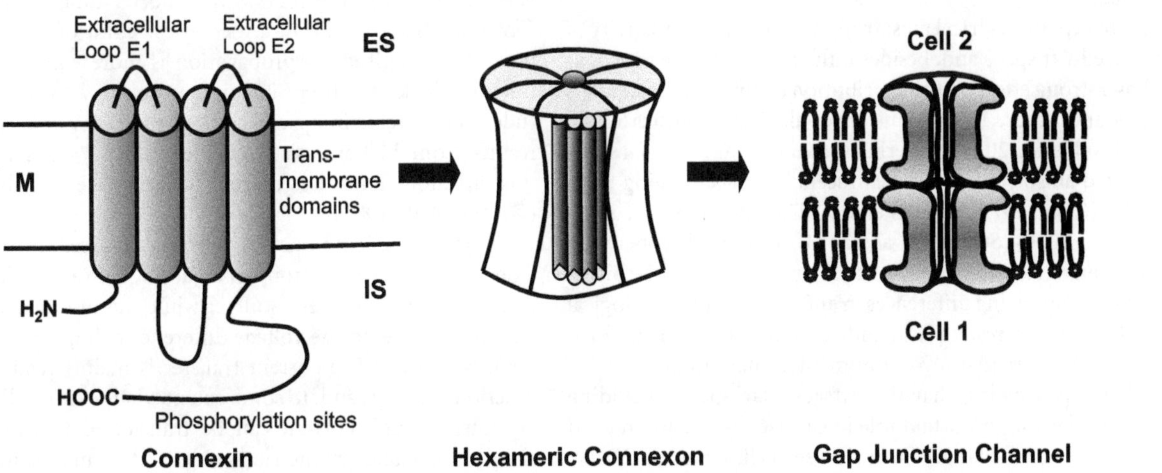

FIGURE 3 | Connexins are four-transmembrane proteins with two extracellular loops and one intracellular loop. They build hexameric connexons (hemichannels), which dock to a connexon of an adjacent cell forming a complete, dodecameric gap junction channel. M, cell membrane; ES, extracellular space; IS, intracellular space.

to describe that specific longitudinal resistivity is lower than transverse resistivity. However, anisotropy values for extracellular and intracellular resistivity differ significantly. Further properties to be taken into account are discontinuity, which means that the fibers are separated by intercalated disks (in contrast to a continuous cable), and non-uniformity, which describes the spatial variation of anisotropy. The latter is due to variations in cellular morphology, cell types (myocytes and non-myocytes) and fibrotic material (collagen) or other non-conducting structures like connective tissue, fat, vessels etc. The difference between uniform and non-uniform anisotropy has many consequences for the pathophysiology of arrhythmia (Spach and Dolber, 1990).

Intracellular resistivity is higher in transverse than in longitudinal direction. Thus, anisotropy in the intracellular space ranges from ~5 to 10 (Clerc, 1976; Roberts and Scher, 1982; Stinstra et al., 2005) and mainly results from cardiomyocyte shape and cellular distribution of connexins. In many cardiac diseases the expression of connexins (Cx43, Cx40, Cx45) is altered. Enhanced levels of Cx43 have been found in cardiac hypertrophy, while in chronic infarction and severe heart failure Cx43 levels are reduced (Severs, 1994; Kostin et al., 2003; Severs et al., 2006). Alterations of Cx43 and Cx40 have been described in atrial fibrillation (Dupont et al., 2001; Polontchouk et al., 2001; Boldt et al., 2003). Since in atrial fibrillation both increased and decreased Cx43 levels have been found, it was suggested that the absolute level may depend not only on the type of arrhythmia but also on the concomitant cardiac pathology (Dhein et al., 2011). In many cardiac pathologies, e.g., chronic atrial fibrillation, cardiac hypertrophy, heart failure and after myocardial infarction, connexins were no longer restricted to cell poles but also expressed at the lateral cell membrane (Polontchouk et al., 2001; Kostin et al., 2002; Cabo et al., 2006). It remained unclear for years whether these lateral gap junctions are functional. In the case of atrial fibrillation, electrophysiological mapping together with immunohistology showed that the lateralization was accompanied by enhanced transverse conduction velocity θ_T (Dhein et al., 2011), suggesting that at least a fraction of these lateral gap junctions is functional.

The concept of electrical anisotropy also applies to resistivity of the extracellular space and, besides influencing impulse propagation, has a strong effect on the distribution of epicardial potentials (Roberts and Scher, 1982; Johnston et al., 2001; Stinstra et al., 2005; Schwab et al., 2013). Experimental and computational studies reported anisotropies in the extracellular space ranging from 1.5 to 3.5 (Clerc, 1976; Roberts et al., 1979; Stinstra et al., 2005; Hand et al., 2009). Schwab et al. (2013) distinguished between the two transverse directions (vertical or parallel to the epicardial surface) suggesting differences in anisotropy and pathological remodeling. Their results also indicate spatially non-uniform anisotropy in ventricular myocardium after infarction.

Evidence is growing that the extracellular space, including fibroblasts, plays an important role in cardiac disease and related electrophysiological changes for review see Pellman et al. (2010); Yue et al. (2011); Weber et al. (2013). This is also reflected in the use of bi-domain or multi-domain models for the simulation of cardiac impulse propagation, taking extracellular conductivity and fibroblasts into account (Jack et al., 1975; Peskoff, 1979; Geselowitz and Miller, 1983; Roberts et al., 2008; Sachse et al., 2009). The group of Veeraraghavan et al. (2012) suggested that the effect of gap junction conductance on impulse propagation is modulated by the fraction of extracellular space. They showed that the percentage of extracellular volume was inversely correlated to conduction velocity. This result is surprising because increased extracellular volume should result in lower extracellular resistivity and, according to cable theory, lead to faster propagation. They found that these effects were especially pronounced in transverse fiber direction. However, to increase extracellular volume they used mannitol, which also reduced cell width. A reduction in cell width, however, can strongly slow transverse velocity (Seidel et al., 2010; Toure and Cabo, 2010). Furthermore, with decreasing velocity the effect of gradual uncoupling (higher gap junction resistance) increases because of a switch from continuous to discontinuous propagation, preferably in transverse fiber direction (Seidel et al., 2010). These results show that effects of intra- and extracellular space on impulse propagation are complex and not easy to predict. It remains challenging to measure extracellular conductance and anisotropy in intact cardiac tissue because due to transmembrane channels the measured current between two electrodes will always contain an intracellular component.

As a result of non-uniformity and anisotropy in cardiac tissue fractionated waveforms develop. These have been interpreted as the reflection of discontinuous propagation where each of the multiple negative peaks represents the activation of a small group of fibers (Spach and Dolber, 1986, 1990). Interestingly, aging leads to a change in the tissue's biophysical properties and is associated with increased non-uniformity. This is due to the deposition of collagen fibers between the cells resulting in predominant uncoupling of side-to-side connections (Spach and Dolber, 1986, 1990; Dhein and Hammerath, 2001).

SOURCE-SINK PROBLEM

When an action potential propagates, the action potential upstroke velocity and amplitude are larger in the case of transverse propagation together with a shorter time constant of the foot potential τ_{foot}. From a theoretical point of view this could mean that longitudinal propagation is more vulnerable to conduction block because of its lower upstroke velocity and amplitude. The increase in upstroke velocity in transverse propagation results from higher resistivity and reduced space constant in this direction. Thus, less current is lost to the neighboring cells (Delmar et al., 1987).

In order to elicit an action potential in a cell, it must receive a depolarizing current from an adjacent, activated cell. The activated cell acts as current source, while the non-activated cell is a current sink with the voltage difference being the driving force for this current. The current transfer is mainly realized via gap junction channels and, to some extent, via the extracellular space. Whether enough current can be transferred to activate a cell is a complex and geometric problem: if a small source (e.g., a tiny strand of activated cardiomyocytes) meets a large sink (e.g., a large area of non-activated cardiomyocytes) the current will flow radially from the activated site to many non-activated sites. Hence, the source current is distributed to many neighboring cells and in each of these the accumulated charge may be too low to trigger an action potential. This will cause conduction failure (Rohr et al., 1997; Rohr, 2004, 2012; Lee and Pogwizd, 2006). In this situation a paradoxical effect can occur: reducing gap junction conductance may preserve conduction by resolving the source-sink mismatch because less current is lost to adjacent sites (Rohr et al., 1997). This is, e.g., realized in the sinus node, where a small current source (sinus node) meets a large sink (atrium). At the sinus node/atrium border there is only little expression of connexins in interdigitating finger-like zones extending from the sinus node into the atrium (Joyner and van Capelle, 1986; Boyett et al., 2006). This reduces the sink because only a small current can flow to a small number of activation sites. In cable theory, this is represented by a smaller space constant leading to a lower capacitive load. On the other hand, if there is high gap junction coupling, the space constant increases leading to a high capacitive load (current sink) and a source-sink mismatch which can evoke conduction failure.

Shaw and Rudy (1997a,b) attempted to describe these phenomena mathematically by the safety factor (SF) of propagation as $SF = Q_c + Q_{out}/Q_{in}$ (=charge produced/charge consumed). If coupling is reduced gradually the safety factor first is enhanced as a result of the smaller space constant. However, if very low levels of coupling are reached, SF decreases until $SF < 1$ and conduction failure occurs. This happens when gap junctions are almost closed or absent, because then not enough current can be transferred to an adjacent cell before the activated cell repolarizes. In contrast, if I_{Na} is reduced this will result in a progressive reduction of SF. However, propagation velocity will be reduced in both situations (Shaw and Rudy, 1997a,b).

Situations with source-sink problems generally occur when the curvature of the propagating wave front is high. Accordingly, they may be found at the end of Purkinje fibers, during propagation through small isthmuses, around obstacles, and during spiral wave re-entry. Furthermore, source-sink mismatch may occur at the border between normal cardiac tissue and an ischemic zone, when depolarizing current flows into the ischemic region. Since this region is usually non-excitable, it will act as a current sink and, consequently, reduce conduction velocity.

ARRHYTHMOGENESIS

Many definitions of arrhythmias are based on comparing a pathological with the normal heart rhythm. Bradyarrhythmia is a rhythm slower than normal, while tachyarrhythmia is faster than normal. Bradyarrhythmias are often caused by a block or delay of conduction within the specific conduction system, i.e., between sinus node and atrium, between atrioventricular node and bundle of His or within the bundles. If in these structures conduction is impaired, e.g., by a scar resulting from infarction, this will lead to delayed ventricular activation. However, the situation can be more complex involving source-sink problems. As described above, the propagation of an action potential from Purkinje fibers to the working myocardium represents a tissue expansion, which is generally prone to conduction block (Rohr et al., 1997). Both high sodium channel conductance and relatively low intercellular coupling increase conduction safety under these conditions. However, pathological changes like gap junction lateralization or cellular hypertrophy (increased sink), and reduced sodium channel availability (decreased source) can lead to unidirectional conduction block (Kléber and Rudy, 2004; Seidel et al., 2010). If unidirectional block occurs in a Purkinje fiber, this will slow ventricular activation and lead to an abnormal activation pattern. This is part of the reason why Purkinje fibers are considered key players in initiation and maintenance of ventricular arrhythmias (for review, see e.g., Boyden et al., 2010). Besides, unidirectional block can lead to reentry circles resulting in ventricular tachycardia or fibrillation. Thus, bradyarrhythmia can evolve into tachyarrhythmia.

REENTRANT ACTIVATION

Reentry happens when the electrical activation follows a circular trajectory and is able to re-activate itself at the point of origin. It is a main cause of tachyarrhythmia. Several mechanisms for reentry are known. One common model is explained as follows: if at a bifurcation of the conducting system (e.g., the bifurcation in the anterior and posterior bundle branch) one branch acts as a unidirectional block, allowing conduction only from the periphery backwards, then activation may propagate along branch 2, thereafter across the ventricular muscle, and finally backwards via branch 1. The unidirectional block in this traditional consideration is thought to be caused by a prolonged refractory period in this area. Another classical example describes reentry as a wave which encircles an electrically inactive obstacle, e.g., a scar. This central zone can also be a permanently refractive area, steadily depolarized by the circulating wave, the "leading circle" (Allessie et al., 1977).

Detachment of the reentry wavefront from the obstacle can lead to spiral wave initiation. In this case, a usually non-stationary rotating source moves along a two- or three-dimensional trajectory. The waves initiated from this source show a typical spiral shape (Cabo et al., 1998). It has been shown that the trajectory of the spiral wave core and whether the wave is stable or not, depends strongly on tissue properties like excitability and non-uniformity (Pertsov et al., 1993).

A certain type of reentrant arrhythmia can originate from a situation in which two closely neighbored obstacles, e.g., collagenous strands or infarct scars, are located transverse to the direction of propagation, with only a small gap of low excitability in between. This structure forces the activation wave to circumvent the obstacles laterally. Behind, the tissue will be activated from both sides causing wavefront collision near the gap. The collision reduces the current sink and increases the source now allowing the activation to propagate through the gap and reactivate the area in front of the obstacles. This kind of reentry has been called "figure-of-eight" reentry mechanisms for ventricular arrhythmias. It may occur in particular when conduction velocity is low (el-Sherif et al., 1987; Lazzara, 1988). See **Figure 4** for illustration.

These explanations illustrate very well the observed phenomena, although underlying mechanisms may be a bit more complicated (see below).

CALCIUM-INDUCED DEPOLARIZATIONS

Under certain pathological conditions like increased adrenergic stimulation or ischemia-reperfusion, cellular calcium overload occurs, leading to spontaneous diastolic calcium waves. These

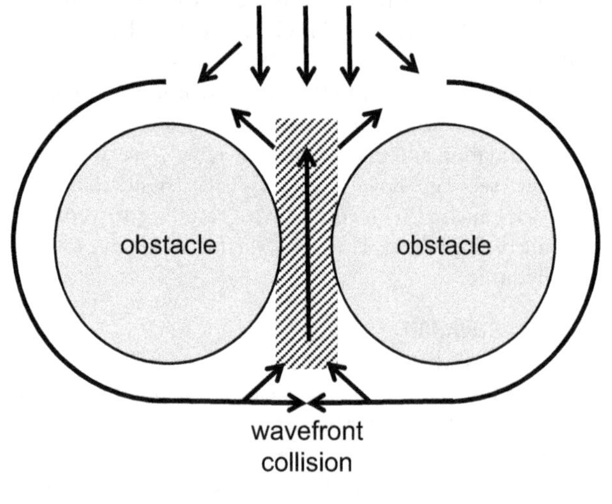

FIGURE 4 | Schematic illustration of a figure-of-eight reentry. A wavefront approaches two obstacles separated by a small gap of low excitability (gray area). Conduction is blocked in front of this gap, separating the wavefront. Behind the obstacles, wavefront collision occurs. This increases the current source while reducing the sink and, thus, allows activation of the area between the obstacles. If conduction is slow enough, this leads to reentry in front of the obstacles as shown by el-Sherif et al. (1987).

waves reflect spontaneous calcium release from the sarcoplasmic reticulum (Kimura et al., 1984; Marban et al., 1986). The sodium-calcium exchanger then operates in the forward mode generating a depolarizing current. The resulting increase of the membrane potential is often referred to as delayed afterdepolarization (DAD). DADs are considered as potential triggers for arrhythmia because, if big enough, they may initiate an action potential and, subsequently, arrhythmogenic ectopic extrasystoles (Lederer and Tsien, 1976; Xie et al., 2010). However, while it has been shown that a DAD can lead to an action potential in isolated cells (Capogrossi et al., 1987), it remains a matter of debate how a DAD in tissue can overcome the obvious source-sink mismatch (Xie et al., 2010; Tveito et al., 2012). A single cardiomyocyte is, on average, coupled to 4–6 adjacent cells. Under normal conditions, it is therefore impossible that an action potential is initiated. Here, the source-sink mismatch protects from arrhythmogenesis. To overcome the mismatch, there must be a reduced sink via uncoupling or an increased source via DAD synchronization between adjacent cells. Both mechanisms have been suggested to appear under conditions of gap-junctional remodeling (Morley et al., 2005) or adrenergic stimulation (Myles et al., 2012), respectively. Following this argumentation, enhanced coupling should increase the sink and may reduce the risk of arrhythmia. Interestingly, it was shown that the antiarrhythmic peptide AAP10 enhanced gap junction conductance and prevented from certain ventricular arrhythmia (Dhein et al., 1994; Müller et al., 1997; Jozwiak and Dhein, 2008; Hagen et al., 2009). This suggests that increasing gap junction conductance via drug therapy might be an effective strategy for certain forms of arrhythmia. Otherwise, closing of gap junctions could be a mechanism of cardiomyocytes to protect neighboring cells from further damage caused, e.g., by acidosis or calcium overload. It has been shown that gap-junction blockers like heptanol decrease the infarct size after myocardial ischemia (Miura et al., 2004). It is, therefore, surprising that the same effect was shown for gap junction openers like rotigaptide (Haugan et al., 2006), while other studies detected no influence on infarct size (Xing et al., 2003). Further research is required in this field to better understand these effects and to develop novel anti-arrhythmic drug therapies.

EFFECTS OF HYPERTROPHY

Cardiac hypertrophy is associated with electrophysiological remodeling and an elevated risk of severe arrhythmia (Tomaselli and Marbán, 1999; Kozhevnikov et al., 2002). This is partly due to changes in cellular electrophysiology like remodeling of potassium channels leading to increased action potential duration and elongated QT intervals (Beuckelmann et al., 1993; Swynghedauw et al., 2003). Whether isolated cellular hypertrophy has pro-arrhythmic effects is, therefore, hard to assess experimentally. However, mathematical models have shown that increased cell capacitance increases capacitive load and the discontinuity of action potential propagation. This steepens the relationship between gap-junction conductance and conduction velocity elevating the risk of conduction block both due to uncoupling and source-sink mismatch (Seidel et al., 2010). Furthermore, hypertrophy leads to increased length or diameter of cardiomyocytes, which has both been shown to influence conduction (McIntyre and Fry, 1997; Spach et al., 2000; Seidel et al., 2010). This suggests that hypertrophy itself, in addition to the associated cardiac disease, can be an arrhythmogenic substrate.

EFFECTS OF GAP JUNCTIONS—LATERALIZATION AND REMODELING

Remodeling of the geometrical distribution of gap junctions occurs in a variety of cardiac diseases (Polontchouk et al., 2001; Kostin et al., 2004; Cabo et al., 2006; Salameh et al., 2009). In most cases the fraction of lateral connexins increases. Provided that these connexins form functional channels, they could contribute to arrhythmogenic alterations in impulse propagation (Cabo et al., 2006; Seidel et al., 2010). However, it is discussed controversially since years whether lateral connexins form fully functional gap junction channels. They might as well form hemichannels, which are assumed to be closed in normal physiological situations, or represent a pool of connexins/hemichannels floating in the membrane until they find anchoring site where they form a complete channel with the hemichannel of a neighboring cell. Pathophysiological situations with lateralized gap junctions comprise atrial fibrillation (Polontchouk et al., 2001; Kostin et al., 2002) cardiomyopathy (Kostin et al., 2003, 2004; Severs et al., 2006; Salameh et al., 2009) or myocardial infarction (Cabo et al., 2006). A study investigating atrial tissue from patients suffering from chronic atrial fibrillation found connexin lateralization accompanied by enhanced transverse conduction velocity. Moreover, in the same study metoprolol treatment led to a lower degree of lateralization and lower transverse conduction velocity (Dhein et al., 2011). This provides evidence that at least parts of these connexins form functional lateral gap junctions, although electrode spacing of 1 mm did not allow to precisely link an activation propagation to a certain cell shape. Direct proof needs

(a) injection of dyes like Lucifer Yellow into cells within a vital layer of atrial tissue (metabolic coupling), and (b) microscopic mapping of electrical activation with a resolution $<10\,\mu m$. This should be complemented with connexin immunohistology and electron microscopy of the mapped area and exact superimposition. Theoretical studies have shown potential effects of gap junction lateralization on action potential propagation and possible arrhythmogenic mechanisms. High side-to-side coupling of cardiomyocytes may favor conduction block due to source-sink mismatches (Seidel et al., 2010), while low side-to-side coupling has been suggested to unmask inhomogeneities (Müller and Dhein, 1993; Seidel et al., 2010).

Non-uniformity and anisotropy in cardiac tissue can cause fractionated waveforms. This is increased by a reduction in gap junction protein expression resulting in progression of irregular activation patterns as shown by de Bakker and van Rijen (2006).

EFFECTS OF FIBROSIS AND ANISOTROPIC INHOMOGENEITY

Fibrosis is a very common process in cardiac remodeling. When cardiomyocytes are impaired by a pathological event and subsequently undergo apoptosis or necrosis, the remnants are eliminated in the context of an inflammatory process. Finally, the area formerly filled by cardiomyocytes is replaced with connective tissue. This includes fibroblasts and extracellular matrix, mainly collagen. This typical repair process helps to maintain cardiac shape and allows maintenance of intracardiac systolic pressures of about 120–150 mmHg. However, a disadvantage is that this replacement tissue is electrically silent, non-contractile and stiffer than normal myocardium. Fibrotic strands typically are between the cardiomyocytes, running parallel to their longitudinal axis (aligned to the fiber axis), thus separating laterally neighbored cardiomyocytes. Occasionally, there will be a remnant connection between cardiomyocytes, so that the activation pattern follows a zig-zag course with reduced transverse conduction velocity. In situations of a longitudinally propagating wavefront, this type of fibrosis will have only little effect. However, if the wavefronts travels transverse to the longitudinal axis, the fibrotic strand will form an obstacle causing "wavefront curvature" because the traveling wavefront will curve around this insulator (Fast and Kléber, 1997). A similar situation can occur at sudden changes in fiber direction (see "Texture of the Heart").

The biophysical properties of the fibrotic cardiac tissue can be described as strongly anisotropic (longitudinal resistance << transverse resistance), discontinuous (cells are separated from each other) and non-uniform (local changes in the anisotropic properties) (de Bakker et al., 1993, 1996). The typical ECG under these conditions of highly discontinuous anisotropic tissue exhibits fractionated QRS complexes with reduced amplitude in the case of reduced myocardial mass (Spear et al., 1979; de Bakker et al., 1988).

Fibroblasts, although non-excitable, may allow electrotonic spread of activation, but with considerable delay. Gaudesius et al. (2003) showed in a strand of cardiomyocytes with an interponate of some fibroblasts successful propagation of the action potential, but with a clear delay at the fibroblast site. They showed that the activation can be successfully transmitted over a distance of up to $300\,\mu m$ filled by fibroblasts. However, it needs to be mentioned that in pathophysiological situations these distances will not be filled with fibroblasts alone but also with a high fraction of collagen. Fibroblasts might couple via gap junctions to cardiomyocytes, which is presumably realized by Cx45 or Cx43, thereby connecting the low-resistance intracellular spaces of fibroblasts and cardiomyocytes. If there is a high fraction of collagen, however, continuous gap junction coupling between myocytes and fibroblasts over long distances becomes very unlikely. Additionally, the ohmic resistance of the extracellular space will be increased. This can lead to conduction failure. It is difficult to estimate the amount of collagenous tissue necessary for electrical isolation, but it will depend on the number of cells in relation to the mass of collagen. Furthermore, it remains unclear whether fibroblast-myocyte coupling occurs *in-vivo* (Kohl and Gourdie, 2014). So far, only one study provides convincing evidence for this possibility in the sinuatrial node (Camelliti et al., 2004), whereas other studies failed to identify heterocellular coupling in the ventricle (Baum et al., 2012).

Different types of fibrosis can be distinguished regarding the texture of collagen deposition: it may be diffuse with small, short, abundant collagenous strands or it may be patchy with larger areas of thick and long collagenous strands. It was shown that the latter type has a higher impact on activation propagation (Kawara et al., 2001). In a computer simulation, discontinuities could be minimized until they vanished when the fibrotic texture was progressively altered from a patchy type to a diffuse type (Pertsov, 1997).

TEXTURE OF THE HEART

Of note, myocardial fiber direction changes from the endocardium to the epicardium by nearly 90° (Greenbaum et al., 1981). In a normal, non-diseased heart this is a gradual change. However, in diseased hearts, e.g., in cardiomyopathy, myocyte disarray has been observed which leads to zones with a sudden change in fiber direction within a short distance. This can result in a sudden change in resistance since a wavefront traveling along the fiber axis suddenly encounters transverse myocyte strands, so that the electrical resistance for the wave changes. This will cause delay of propagation or wavefront curvatures or discontinuities or unidirectional block (Spach et al., 1982). Interestingly, a similar situation of sudden changes in fiber direction was observed in canine and human pulmonary veins. In this area atrial fibrillation is usually initiated, and this structural particularity may contribute to the arrhythmogeneity of this region (Hocini et al., 2002; Arora et al., 2003).

NON-EXCITABLE REGIONS

Beside myocardial fibers, non-excitable tissue components are present in the heart such as connective tissue (see above) or vessels or fat tissue. These non-excitable obstacles "may cause the formation of self-sustained vortices and uncontrolled high-frequency excitation in normal homogeneous myocardium" (Cabo et al., 1998). In this process the wavefront is thought to detach from the obstacle and form a vortex, i.e., spiral waves are initiated. This process of detachment and shedding of vortices is assumed to depend on wavefront curvature (Cabo et al., 1998).

However, there is another characteristic of non-excitable tissue regions: if a wavefront with low curvature propagates, current flows mainly along the potential gradient to the front. Hardly any current is lost to the sides or the area behind the wavefront, because there is no potential gradient. If the wave approaches a non-excitable, electrically insulated obstacle, current flowing to the front will decrease. Thus, in front of an obstacle less current is lost than during normal propagation. As a consequence, the action potential will be prolonged in this area due to the reduced current loss. In contrast, after the wave has surrounded the obstacle it meets unexcited tissue in front and lateral to the wavefront. Thus, current is lost to the sides and the front. As a result, action potential duration will be increased in front and shortened behind the obstacle. It has been shown by epicardial mapping around a coronary vessel that this is indeed the case (Gottwald et al., 1998). For illustration, see **Figure 5**. Interestingly, this study also showed that in ischemic tissue the difference in action potential duration before and behind an obstacle significantly increases due to slowed conduction. This is a consequence of the ischemic depolarization leading to reduced sodium channel availability, prolonging the time during which current can pass from the excited site to the non-excited sites. This will increase the current loss. Similarly, reduction in sodium channel conductance was shown to enhance local dispersion (variance in action potential duration) at zones of reduced gap junction coupling in a computer simulation (Müller and Dhein, 1993). It seems obvious that, in its extreme form, this phenomenon may lead to unidirectional block, which is a potential trigger of arrhythmia.

CHANGES OF THE BIOPHYSICAL PROPERTIES BY MECHANICAL FORCES

Mechanical stimuli will lead to local strain of cells, which means an alteration of cell length and length-to-width ratio. In computer simulations it has been shown that changes in cell geometry have an effect on conduction velocity (Spach et al., 2000; Seidel et al., 2010). A local stretch therefore can alter the local pathways of activation (Dhein et al., 2014). On the other hand, it has been shown that structural heterogeneities can affect stretch-induced ventricular arrhythmia (Seo et al., 2010). Wall thickness can be heterogeneously distributed over the ventricle, which will result in a regional modulation of a mechanical stimulus so that regional strain varies. This strain may activate stretch-activated ion channels thereby eliciting cardiac arrhythmia. It was recently shown that local left ventricular stretch leads to local delays in activation so that early and late activation occur closely beside each other (Dhein et al., 2014).

A sudden mechanical insult, an impact or blow by a small spheroid may induce ventricular fibrillation (Kalin et al., 2011). Such an insult is known as commotio cordis. The impact is thought to induce heterogeneity in repolarization within the wall together with a premature depolarization trigger.

IMPLICATIONS FOR THE CLINICS (AGE)

In the daily clinic we also see the importance of the passive electrical properties as, in particular, elderly patients suffer from cardiac arrhythmia. Age has been described to be associated with cardiac fibrosis (Gottwald et al., 1997) and with disturbances of cardiac conduction velocity and enhanced dispersion of action potential duration (Dhein and Hammerath, 2001). According to the latter study, fibrotic strands aligned to the cardiac myocytes result in reduced transverse propagation velocity and thereby enhanced anisotropy. The authors concluded that reduced lateral gap junction coupling may be a typical feature of aged hearts. In accordance with this assumption, they could show that reduction of gap junction coupling in young hearts could mimic the situation found in aged hearts. They also observed that the extracellular potentials were fractionated in areas where activation spread was particularly inhomogeneous. Thus, age-related fibrosis and the resulting disturbances in activation spreading and repolarization indicate that the biophysical passive properties of the tissue are changed and may help to explain why in elderly patients arrhythmia is more frequent than in the young.

Fibrosis is a key characteristic in atrial fibrillation (Boldt et al., 2004), which can be reduced by angiotensin-converting enzyme inhibitors (Boldt et al., 2006). Fibrosis is, among others, considered a major determinant for the development of atrial fibrillation

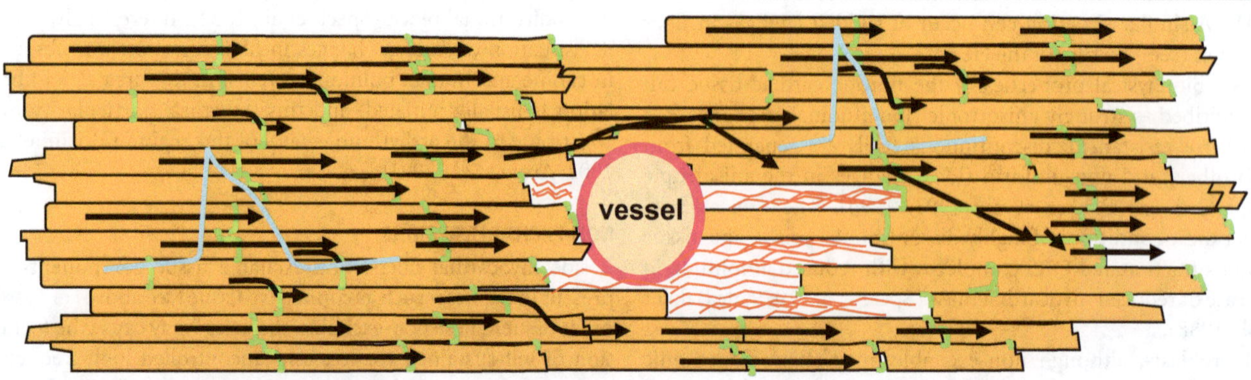

FIGURE 5 | Non-excitable regions like coronary vessels or connective tissue (shown as red strands around the vessel) lead to changes in action potential duration. In front of the non-excitable area, current sink decreases leading to longer action potential duration. In contrast, behind this area current sink is increased, which shortens the action potential. Action potential shapes are illustrated in blue, gap junctions in green, cardiomyocytes in orange. Black arrows indicate impulse propagation.

and may lead to structural uncoupling of fiber strands. Moreover, fibrosis enhances the complexity of atrial fibrillation (Verheule et al., 2013). Since according to the present knowledge fibrosis cannot be reversed, this marks a point of no return for atrial fibrillation. Clinical experience underlines that long-standing persistent atrial fibrillation with dilated atria and fibrotic tissue is unlikely to be successfully converted to sinus rhythm for a longer period.

Chronic pump failure leads to remodeling processes in the heart with hypertrophy of the fibers and lateralization of gap junctions. Clinically, it is known that patients suffering from heart failure, cardiomyopathy or cardiac hypertrophy often die from ventricular arrhythmia rather than from pump failure.

Passive electrical properties of cardiac tissue strongly influence myocardial activation, and thereby importantly contribute to the formation of arrhythmogenic substrates.

FINAL REMARK

There are numerous excellent studies on passive electrical properties, gap junctions, arrhythmia, mechano-electrical feedback and related issues. We seriously apologize to those authors who could not be cited.

REFERENCES

Allessie, M. A., Bonke, F. I., and Schopman, F. J. (1977). Circus movement in rabbit atrial muscle as a mechanism of tachycardia. III. The "leading circle" concept: a new model of circus movement in cardiac tissue without the involvement of an anatomical obstacle. *Circ. Res.* 41, 9–18. doi: 10.1161/01.RES.41.1.9

Arora, R., Verheule, S., Scott, L., Navarrete, A., Katari, V., Wilson, E., et al. (2003). Arrhythmogenic substrate of the pulmonary veins assessed by high-resolution optical mapping. *Circulation* 107, 1816–1821. doi: 10.1161/01.CIR.0000058461.86339.7E

Axelsen, L. N., Calloe, K., Holstein-Rathlou, N. H., and Nielsen, M. S. (2013). Managing the complexity of communication: regulation of gap junctions by post-translational modification. *Front. Pharmacol.* 4:130. doi: 10.3389/fphar.2013.00130

Baum, J. R., Long, B., Cabo, C., and Duffy, H. S. (2012). Myofibroblasts cause heterogeneous Cx43 reduction and are unlikely to be coupled to myocytes in the healing canine infarct. *Am. J. Physiol. Heart Circ. Physiol.* 302, H790–H800. doi: 10.1152/ajpheart.00498.2011

Beuckelmann, D. J., Näbauer, M., and Erdmann, E. (1993). Alterations of K^+ currents in isolated human ventricular myocytes from patients with terminal heart failure. *Circ. Res.* 73, 379–385. doi: 10.1161/01.RES.73.2.379

Beyer, E. C., Veenstra, R. D., Kanter, H. L., and Saffitz, J. E. (1995). "Molecular structure and patterns of expression of cardiac gap junction proteins," in *Cardiac Electrophysiology From cell to Bedside*, 2nd Edn., eds D. Zipes and J. Jalife (Philadelphia: WB Saunders), 31–38.

Boldt, A., Scholl, A., Garbade, J., Resetar, ME., Mohr, F. W., Gummert, J. F., et al. (2006). ACE-inhibitor treatment attenuates atrial structural remodeling in patients with lone chronic atrial fibrillation. *Basic Res. Cardiol.* 101, 261–267. doi: 10.1007/s00395-005-0571-2

Boldt, A., Wetzel, U., Lauschke, J., Weigl, J., Gummert, J., Hindricks, G., et al. (2004). Fibrosis in left atrial tissue of patients with atrial fibrillation with and without underlying mitral valve disease. *Heart* 90, 400–405. doi: 10.1136/hrt.2003.015347

Boldt, A., Wetzel, U., Weigl, J., Garbade, J., Lauschke, J., Hindricks, G., et al. (2003). Expression of angiotensin II receptors in human left and right atrial tissue in atrial fibrillation with and without underlying mitral valve disease. *J. Am. Coll. Cardiol.* 42, 1785–1792. doi: 10.1016/j.jacc.2003.07.014

Boyden, P. A., Hirose, M., and Dun, W. (2010). Cardiac Purkinje cells. *Heart Rhythm* 7, 127–135. doi: 10.1016/j.hrthm.2009.09.017

Boyett, M. R., Inada, S., Yoo, S., Li, J., Liu, J., Tellez, J., et al. (2006). Connexins in the sinoatrial and atrioventricular nodes. *Adv. Cardiol.* 42, 175–197. doi: 10.1159/000092569

Bukauskas, F. F., and Verselis, V. K. (2004). Gap junction channel gating. *Biochim. Biophys. Acta* 1662, 42–60. doi: 10.1016/j.bbamem.2004.01.008

Cabo, C., Pertsov, A. M., Davidenko, J. M., and Jalife, J. (1998). Electrical turbulence as a result of the critical curvature for propagation in cardiac tissue. *Chaos* 8, 116–126. doi: 10.1063/1.166292

Cabo, C., Yao, J., Boyden, P. A., Chen, S., Hussain, W., Duffy, H. S., et al. (2006). Heterogeneous gap junction remodeling in reentrant circuits in the epicardial border zone of the healing canine infarct. *Cardiovasc. Res.* 72, 241–249. doi: 10.1016/j.cardiores.2006.07.005

Camelliti, P., Green, C. R., LeGrice, I., and Kohl, P. (2004). Fibroblast network in rabbit sinoatrial node: structural and functional identification of homogeneous and heterogeneous cell coupling. *Circ. Res.* 94, 828–835. doi: 10.1161/01.RES.0000122382.19400.14

Capogrossi, M. C., Houser, S. R., Bahinski, A., and Lakatta, E. G. (1987). Synchronous occurrence of spontaneous localized calcium release from the sarcoplasmic reticulum generates action potentials in rat cardiac ventricular myocytes at normal resting membrane potential. *Circ. Res.* 61, 498–503. doi: 10.1161/01.RES.61.4.498

Carnie, S., and McLaughlin, S. (1983). Large divalent cations and electrostatic potentials adjacent to membranes. A theoretical calculation. *Biophys. J.* 44, 325–332. doi: 10.1016/S0006-3495(83)84306-9

Chen, L., Goings, G. E., Upshaw-Earley, J., and Page, E. (1989). Cardiac gap junctions and gap junction-associated vesicles: ultrastructural comparison of *in situ* negative staining with conventional positive staining. *Circ. Res.* 64, 501–514. doi: 10.1161/01.RES.64.3.501

Clerc, L. (1976). Directional differences of impulse spread in trabecular muscle from mammalian heart. *J. Physiol.* 255, 335–346.

Copene, E. D., and Keener, J. P. (2008). Ephaptic coupling of cardiac cells through the junctional electric potential. *J. Math. Biol.* 57, 265–284. doi: 10.1007/s00285-008-0157-3

de Bakker, J. M., van Capelle, F. J., Janse, M. J., Tasseron, S., Vermeulen, J. T., de Jonge, N., et al. (1993). Slow conduction in the infarcted human heart. 'Zigzag' course of activation. *Circulation* 88, 915–926. doi: 10.1161/01.CIR.88.3.915

de Bakker, J. M., van Capelle, F. J., Janse, M. J., Tasseron, S., Vermeulen, J. T., de Jonge, N., et al. (1996). Fractionated electrograms in dilated cardiomyopathy: origin and relation to abnormal conduction. *J. Am. Coll. Cardiol.* 27, 1071–1078. doi: 10.1016/0735-1097(95)00612-5

de Bakker, J. M., van Capelle, F. J., Janse, M. J., Wilde, A. A., Coronel, R., Becker, A. E., et al. (1988). Reentry as a cause of ventricular tachycardia in patients with chronic ischemic heart disease: electrophysiologic and anatomic correlation. *Circulation* 77, 589–606. doi: 10.1161/01.CIR.77.3.589

de Bakker, J. M., and van Rijen, H. M. (2006). Continuous and discontinuous propagation in heart muscle. *J. Cardiovasc. Electrophysiol.* 17, 567–573. doi: 10.1111/j.1540-8167.2006.00367.x

Delmar, M., Michaels, D. C., Johnson, T., and Jalife, J. (1987). Effects of increasing intercellular resistance on transverse and longitudinal propagation in sheep epicardial muscle. *Circ. Res.* 60, 780–785. doi: 10.1161/01.RES.60.5.780

Dhein, S. (1998). Gap junction channels in the cardiovascular system: pharmacological and physiological modulation. *Trends Pharmacol. Sci.* 19, 229–241. doi: 10.1016/S0165-6147(98)01192-4

Dhein, S. (2004). Pharmacology of gap junctions in the cardiovascular system. *Cardiovasc. Res.* 62, 287–298. doi: 10.1016/j.cardiores.2004.01.019

Dhein, S., Englert, C., Riethdorf, S., Kostelka, M., Dohmen, P. M., and Mohr, F. W. (2014). Arrhythmogenic effects by local left ventricular stretch: effects of flecainide and streptomycin. *Naunyn Schmiedebergs. Arch. Pharmacol.* 387, 763–775. doi: 10.1007/s00210-014-0988-y

Dhein, S., and Hammerath, S. B. (2001). Aspects of the intercellular communication in aged hearts: effects of the gap junction uncoupler palmitoleic acid. *Naunyn Schmiedebergs. Arch. Pharmacol.* 364, 397–408. doi: 10.1007/s002100100462

Dhein, S., Manicone, N., Müller, A., Gerwin, R., Ziskoven, U., Irankhahi, A., et al. (1994). A new synthetic antiarrhythmic peptide reduces dispersion of epicardial activation recovery interval and diminishes alterations of epicardial activation patterns induced by regional ischemia. A mapping study. *Naunyn Schmiedebergs Arch. Pharmacol.* 350, 174–184. doi: 10.1007/BF00241093

Dhein, S., Rothe, S., Busch, A., Rojas Gomez, D. M., Boldt, A., Reutemann, A., et al. (2011). Effects of metoprolol therapy on cardiac gap junction remodelling and conduction in human chronic atrial fibrillation. *Br. J. Pharmacol.* 164, 607–616. doi: 10.1111/j.1476-5381.2011.01460.x

Dupont, E., Ko, Y., Rothery, S., Coppen, S. R., Baghai, M., Haw, M., et al. (2001). The gap-junctional protein connexin40 is elevated in patients susceptible to postoperative atrial fibrillation. *Circulation* 103, 842–849. doi: 10.1161/01.CIR.103.6.842

el-Sherif, N., Gough, W. B., and Restivo, M. (1987). Reentrant ventricular arrhythmias in the late myocardial infarction period: 14. Mechanisms of resetting, entrainment, acceleration, or termination of reentrant tachycardia by programmed electrical stimulation. *Pacing Clin. Electrophysiol.* 10, 341–371. doi: 10.1111/j.1540-8159.1987.tb05974.x

Fast, V. G., and Kléber, A. G. (1993). Microscopic conduction in cultured strands of neonatal rat heart cells measured with voltage-sensitive dyes. *Circ. Res.* 73, 914–925. doi: 10.1161/01.RES.73.5.914

Fast, V. G., and Kléber, A. G. (1997). Role of wavefront curvature in propagation of cardiac impulse. *Cardiovasc. Res.* 33, 258–271. doi: 10.1016/S0008-6363(96)00216-7

Gaudesius, G., Miragoli, M., Thomas, S. P., and Rohr, S. (2003). Coupling of cardiac electrical activity over extended distances by fibroblasts of cardiac origin. *Circ. Res.* 93, 421–428. doi: 10.1161/01.RES.0000089258.40661.0C

Geselowitz, D. B., and Miller, W. T. (1983). A bidomain model for anisotropic cardiac muscle. *Ann. Biomed. Eng.* 11, 191–206. doi: 10.1007/BF02363286

Goshima, K., and Tonomura, Y. (1969). Synchronized beating of embryonic mouse myocardial cells mediated by FL cells in monolayer culture. *Exp. Cell. Res.* 56, 387–392. doi: 10.1016/0014-4827(69)90029-9

Gottwald, E., Gottwald, M., and Dhein, S. (1998). Enhanced dispersion of epicardial activation-recovery intervals at sites of histological inhomogeneity during regional cardiac ischaemia and reperfusion. *Heart* 79, 474–480.

Gottwald, M., Gottwald, E., and Dhein, S. (1997). Age-related electrophysiological and histological changes in rabbit hearts: age-related changes in electrophysiology. *Int. J. Cardiol.* 62, 97–106. doi: 10.1016/S0167-5273(97)00183-6

Gourdie, R. G., Harfst, E., Severs, N. J., and Green, C. R. (1990). Cardiac gap junctions in rat ventricle: localization using site-directed antibodies and laser scanning confocal microscopy. *Cardioscience* 1, 75–82.

Greenbaum, R. A., Ho, S. Y., Gibson, D. G., Becker, A. E., and Anderson, R. H. (1981). Left ventricular fibre architecture in man. *Br. Heart J.* 45, 248–263. doi: 10.1136/hrt.45.3.248

Hagen, A., Dietze, A., and Dhein, S. (2009). Human cardiac gap-junction coupling: effects of antiarrhythmic peptide AAP10. *Cardiovasc. Res.* 83, 405–415. doi: 10.1093/cvr/cvp028

Hand, P. E., Griffith, B. E., and Peskin, C. S. (2009). Deriving macroscopic myocardial conductivities by homogenization of microscopic models. *Bull. Math. Biol.* 71, 1707–1726. doi: 10.1007/s11538-009-9421-y

Harris, A. L. (2001). Emerging issues of connexin channels: biophysics fills the gap. *Q. Rev. Biophys.* 34, 325–472. doi: 10.1017/S0033583501003705

Haugan, K., Marcussen, N., Kjølbye, A. L., Nielsen, M. S., Hennan, J. K., and Petersen, J. S. (2006). Treatment with the gap junction modifier rotigaptide (ZP123) reduces infarct size in rats with chronic myocardial infarction. *J. Cardiovasc. Pharmacol.* 47, 236–242. doi: 10.1097/01.fjc.0000200990.31611.6e

He, K., Shi, X., Zhang, X., Dang, S., Ma, X., Liu, F., et al. (2011). Long-distance intercellular connectivity between cardiomyocytes and cardiofibroblasts mediated by membrane nanotubes. *Cardiovasc. Res.* 92, 39–47. doi: 10.1093/cvr/cvr189

Hocini, M., Ho, S. Y., Kawara, T., Linnenbank, A. C., Potse, M., Shah, D., et al. (2002). Electrical conduction in canine pulmonary veins: electrophysiological and anatomic correlation. *Circulation* 105, 2442–2448. doi: 10.1161/01.CIR.0000016062.80020.11

Hodgkin, A. L., and Rushton, W. A. (1946). The electrical constants of a crustacean nerve fibre. *Proc. R. Soc. Med.* 134, 444–479. doi: 10.1098/rspb.1946.0024

Hubbard, M. L., Ying, W., and Henriquez, C. S. (2007). Effect of gap junction distribution on impulse propagation in a monolayer of myocytes: a model study. *Europace* 9(Suppl. 6), vi20–vi28. doi: 10.1093/europace/eum203

Jack, J., Noble, D., and Tsien, R. (1975). *Electric Current Flow in Excitable Cells.* Oxford: Clarendon.

Johnston, P. R., Kilpatrick, D., and Li, C. Y. (2001). The importance of anisotropy in modeling ST segment shift in subendocardial ischaemia. *IEEE Trans. Biomed. Eng.* 48, 1366–1376. doi: 10.1109/10.966596

Joyner, R. W., and van Capelle, F. J. (1986). Propagation through electrically coupled cells. How a small SA node drives a large atrium. *Biophys. J.* 50, 1157–1164. doi: 10.1016/S0006-3495(86)83559-7

Jozwiak, J., and Dhein, S. (2008). Local effects and mechanisms of antiarrhythmic peptide AAP10 in acute regional myocardial ischemia: electrophysiological and molecular findings. *Naunyn Schmiedebergs. Arch. Pharmacol.* 378, 459–470. doi: 10.1007/s00210-008-0317-4

Kalin, J., Madias, C., Alsheikh-Ali, A. A., and Link, M. S. (2011). Reduced diameter spheres increases the risk of chest blow-induced ventricular fibrillation (commotio cordis). *Heart Rhythm* 8, 1578–1581. doi: 10.1016/j.hrthm.2011.05.009

Kawara, T., Derksen, R., de Groot, J. R., Coronel, R., Tasseron, S., Linnenbank, A. C., et al. (2001). Activation delay after premature stimulation in chronically diseased human myocardium relates to the architecture of interstitial fibrosis. *Circulation* 104, 3069–3075. doi: 10.1161/hc5001.100833

Kimura, S., Cameron, J. S., Kozlovskis, P. L., Bassett, A. L., and Myerburg, R. J. (1984). Delayed afterdepolarizations and triggered activity induced in feline Purkinje fibers by alpha-adrenergic stimulation in the presence of elevated calcium levels. *Circulation* 70, 1074–1082. doi: 10.1161/01.CIR.70.6.1074

Kléber, A. G., and Rudy, Y. (2004). Basic mechanisms of cardiac impulse propagation and associated arrhythmias. *Physiol. Rev.* 84, 431–488. doi: 10.1152/physrev.00025.2003

Kohl, P., and Gourdie, R. G. (2014). Fibroblast-myocyte electrotonic coupling: does it occur in native cardiac tissue? *J. Mol. Cell. Cardiol.* 70, 37–46. doi: 10.1016/j.yjmcc.2013.12.024

Kostin, S., Dammer, S., Hein, S., Klovekorn, W. P., Bauer, E. P., and Schaper, J. (2004). Connexin 43 expression and distribution in compensated and decompensated cardiac hypertrophy in patients with aortic stenosis. *Cardiovasc. Res.* 62, 426–436. doi: 10.1016/j.cardiores.2003.12.010

Kostin, S., Klein, G., Szalay, Z., Hein, S., Bauer, E. P., and Schaper, J. (2002). Structural correlate of atrial fibrillation in human patients. *Cardiovasc. Res.* 54, 361–379. doi: 10.1016/S0008-6363(02)00273-0

Kostin, S., Rieger, M., Dammer, S., Hein, S., Richter, M., Klövekorn, W. P., et al. (2003). Gap junction remodeling and altered connexin43 expression in the failing human heart. *Mol. Cell. Biochem.* 242, 135–144. doi: 10.1023/A:1021154115673

Kozhevnikov, D. O., Yamamoto, K., Robotis, D., Restivo, M., and El-Sherif, N. (2002). Electrophysiological mechanism of enhanced susceptibility of hypertrophied heart to acquired torsade de pointes arrhythmias: tridimensional mapping of activation and recovery patterns. *Circulation* 105, 1128–1134. doi: 10.1161/hc0902.104711

Kucera, J. P., Rohr, S., and Rudy, Y. (2002). Localization of sodium channels in intercalated disks modulates cardiac conduction. *Circ. Res.* 91, 1176–1182. doi: 10.1161/01.RES.0000046237.54156.0A

Lazzara, R. (1988). Electrophysiological mechanisms for ventricular arrhythmias. *Clin. Cardiol.* 11(3 Suppl. 2), II1–II4.

Lederer, W. J., and Tsien, R. W. (1976). Transient inward current underlying arrhythmogenic effects of cardiotonic steroids in Purkinje fibres. *J. Physiol.* 263, 73–100.

Lee, P. J., and Pogwizd, S. M. (2006). Micropatterns of propagation. *Adv. Cardiol.* 42, 86–106. doi: 10.1159/000092564

Lin, J., and Keener, J. P. (2010). Modeling electrical activity of myocardial cells incorporating the effects of ephaptic coupling. *Proc. Natl. Acad. Sci. U.S.A.* 107, 20935–20940. doi: 10.1073/pnas.1010154107

Maier, S. K., Westenbroek, R. E., McCormick, K. A., Curtis, R., Scheuer, T., and Catterall, W. A. (2004). Distinct subcellular localization of different sodium channel alpha and beta subunits in single ventricular myocytes from mouse heart. *Circulation* 109, 1421–1427. doi: 10.1161/01.CIR.0000121421.61896.24

Makowski, L., Caspar, D. L., Phillips, W. C., and Goodenough, D. A. (1977). Gap junction structures. II. Analysis of the x-ray diffraction data. *J. Cell. Biol.* 74, 629–645. doi: 10.1083/jcb.74.2.629

Marban, E., Robinson, S. W., and Wier, W. G. (1986). Mechanisms of arrhythmogenic delayed and early afterdepolarizations in ferret ventricular muscle. *J. Clin. Invest.* 78, 1185–1192. doi: 10.1172/JCI112701

McIntyre, H., and Fry, C. H. (1997). Abnormal action potential conduction in isolated human hypertrophied left ventricular myocardium. *J. Cardiovasc. Electrophysiol.* 8, 887–894. doi: 10.1111/j.1540-8167.1997.tb00850.x

Miura, T., Ohnuma, Y., Kuno, A., Tanno, M., Ichikawa, Y., Nakamura, Y., et al. (2004). Protective role of gap junctions in preconditioning against myocardial infarction. *Am. J. Physiol. Heart Circ. Physiol.* 286, H214–H221. doi: 10.1152/ajpheart.00441.2003

Moreno, A. P. (2004). Biophysical properties of homomeric and heteromultimeric channels formed by cardiac connexins. *Cardiovasc. Res.* 62, 276–286. doi: 10.1016/j.cardiores.2004.03.003

Mori, Y., Fishman, G. I., and Peskin, C. S. (2008). Ephaptic conduction in a cardiac strand model with 3D electrodiffusion. *Proc. Natl. Acad. Sci. U.S.A.* 105, 6463–6468. doi: 10.1073/pnas.0801089105

Morley, G. E., Danik, S. B., Bernstein, S., Sun, Y., Rosner, G., Gutstein, D. E., et al. (2005). Reduced intercellular coupling leads to paradoxical propagation across the Purkinje-ventricular junction and aberrant myocardial activation. *Proc. Natl. Acad. Sci. U.S.A.* 102, 4126–4129. doi: 10.1073/pnas.0500881102

Müller, A., and Dhein, S. (1993). Sodium channel blockade enhances dispersion of the cardiac action potential duration. A computer simulation study. *Basic Res. Cardiol.* 88, 11–22.

Müller, A., Gottwald, M., Tudyka, T., Linke, W., Klaus, W., and Dhein, S. (1997). Increase in gap junction conductance by an antiarrhythmic peptide. *Eur. J. Pharmacol.* 327, 65–72. doi: 10.1016/S0014-2999(97)89679-3

Myles, R. C., Wang, L., Kang, C., Bers, D. M., and Ripplinger, C. M. (2012). Local β-adrenergic stimulation overcomes source-sink mismatch to generate focal arrhythmia. *Circ. Res.* 110, 1454–1464. doi: 10.1161/CIRCRESAHA.111.262345

Nielsen, M. S., Axelsen, L. N., Sorgen, P. L., Verma, V., Delmar, M., and Holstein-Rathlou, N. H. (2012). Gap junctions. *Compr. Physiol.* 2, 1981–2035. doi: 10.1002/cphy.c110051

Page, E., and Shibata, Y. (1981). Permeable junctions between cardiac cells. *Annu. Rev. Physiol.* 43, 431–441. doi: 10.1146/annurev.ph.43.030181.002243

Pellman, J., Lyon, R. C., and Sheikh, F. (2010). Extracellular matrix remodeling in atrial fibrosis: mechanisms and implications in atrial fibrillation. *J. Mol. Cell. Cardiol.* 48, 461–467. doi: 10.1016/j.yjmcc.2009.09.001

Perkins, G., Goodenough, D., and Sosinsky, G. (1997). Three-dimensional structure of the gap junction connexon. *Biophys. J.* 72(2 Pt 1), 533–544. doi: 10.1016/S0006-3495(97)78693-4

Pertsov, A. (1997). "Scale of geometric structures responsible for discontinuous propagation in myocardial tissue," in *Discontinuous Conduction in the Heart,* eds P. Spooner, R. Joyner, and J. Jalife (New York, NY: Futura Publishing Company Inc.), 273–293.

Pertsov, A. M., Davidenko, J. M., Salomonsz, R., Baxter, W. T., and Jalife, J. (1993). Spiral waves of excitation underlie reentrant activity in isolated cardiac muscle. *Circ. Res.* 72, 631–650. doi: 10.1161/01.RES.72.3.631

Peskoff, A. (1979). Electric potential in three-dimensional electrically syncytial tissues. *Bull. Math. Biol.* 41, 163–181. doi: 10.1007/BF02460876

Polontchouk, L., Haefliger, J. A., Ebelt, B., Schaefer, T., Stuhlmann, D., Mehlhorn, U., et al. (2001). Effects of chronic atrial fibrillation on gap junction distribution in human and rat atria. *J. Am. Coll. Cardiol.* 38, 883–891. doi: 10.1016/S0735-1097(01)01443-7

Rhett, J. M., Ongstad, E. L., Jourdan, J., and Gourdie, R. G. (2012). Cx43 associates with Na(v)1.5 in the cardiomyocyte perinexus. *J. Membr. Biol.* 245, 411–422. doi: 10.1007/s00232-012-9465-z

Rhett, J. M., Veeraraghavan, R., Poelzing, S., and Gourdie, R. G. (2013). The perinexus: sign-post on the path to a new model of cardiac conduction? *Trends Cardiovasc. Med.* 23, 222–228. doi: 10.1016/j.tcm.2012.12.005

Roberts, D. E., Hersh, L. T., and Scher, A. M. (1979). Influence of cardiac fiber orientation on wavefront voltage, conduction velocity, and tissue resistivity in the dog. *Circ. Res.* 44, 701–712. doi: 10.1161/01.RES.44.5.701

Roberts, D. E., and Scher, A. M. (1982). Effect of tissue anisotropy on extracellular potential fields in canine myocardium *in situ*. *Circ. Res.* 50, 342–351. doi: 10.1161/01.RES.50.3.342

Roberts, S. F., Stinstra, J. G., and Henriquez, C. S. (2008). Effect of nonuniform interstitial space properties on impulse propagation: a discrete multidomain model. *Biophys. J.* 95, 3724–3737. doi: 10.1529/biophysj.108.137349

Rohr, S. (2004). Role of gap junctions in the propagation of the cardiac action potential. *Cardiovasc. Res.* 62, 309–322. doi: 10.1016/j.cardiores.2003.11.035

Rohr, S. (2012). Arrhythmogenic implications of fibroblast-myocyte interactions. *Circ. Arrhythm. Electrophysiol.* 5, 442–452. doi: 10.1161/CIRCEP.110.957647

Rohr, S., Kucera, J. P., Fast, V. G., and Kléber, A. G. (1997). Paradoxical improvement of impulse conduction in cardiac tissue by partial cellular uncoupling. *Science* 275, 841–844. doi: 10.1126/science.275.5301.841

Sachse, F. B., Moreno, A. P., Seemann, G., and Abildskov, J. A. (2009). A model of electrical conduction in cardiac tissue including fibroblasts. *Ann. Biomed. Eng.* 37, 874–889. doi: 10.1007/s10439-009-9667-4

Salameh, A., and Dhein, S. (2005). Pharmacology of gap junctions. New pharmacological targets for treatment of arrhythmia, seizure and cancer? *Biochim. Biophys. Acta* 1719, 36–58. doi: 10.1016/j.bbamem.2005.09.007

Salameh, A., Krautblatter, S., Karl, S., Blanke, K., Gomez, D. R., Dhein, S., et al. (2009). The signal transduction cascade regulating the expression of the gap junction protein connexin43 by beta-adrenoceptors. *Br. J. Pharmacol.* 158, 198–208. doi: 10.1111/j.1476-5381.2009.00344.x

Schulte, J. S., Scheffler, A., Rojas-Gomez, D., Mohr, F. W., and Dhein, S. (2008). Neonatal rat cardiomyocytes show characteristics of nonhomotypic gap junction channels. *Cell Commun. Adhes.* 15, 13–25. doi: 10.1080/15419060802014404

Schwab, B. C., Seemann, G., Lasher, R. A., Torres, N. S., Wulfers, E. M., Arp, M., et al. (2013). Quantitative analysis of cardiac tissue including fibroblasts using three-dimensional confocal microscopy and image reconstruction: towards a basis for electrophysiological modeling. *IEEE Trans. Med. Imaging* 32, 862–872. doi: 10.1109/TMI.2013.2240693

Seidel, T., Salameh, A., and Dhein, S. (2010). A simulation study of cellular hypertrophy and connexin lateralization in cardiac tissue. *Biophys. J.* 99, 2821–2830. doi: 10.1016/j.bpj.2010.09.010

Seo, K., Inagaki, M., Nishimura, S., Hidaka, I., Sugimachi, M., Hisada, T., et al. (2010). Structural heterogeneity in the ventricular wall plays a significant role in the initiation of stretch-induced arrhythmias in perfused rabbit right ventricular tissues and whole heart preparations. *Circ. Res.* 106, 176–184. doi: 10.1161/CIRCRESAHA.109.203828

Severs, N. J. (1994). Pathophysiology of gap junctions in heart disease. *J. Cardiovasc. Electrophysiol.* 5, 462–475. doi: 10.1111/j.1540-8167.1994.tb01185.x

Severs, N. J., Dupont, E., Thomas, N., Kaba, R., Rothery, S., Jain, R., et al. (2006). Alterations in cardiac connexin expression in cardiomyopathies. *Adv. Cardiol.* 42, 228–242. doi: 10.1159/000092572

Shaw, R. M., and Rudy, Y. (1997a). Electrophysiologic effects of acute myocardial ischemia. A mechanistic investigation of action potential conduction and conduction failure. *Circ. Res.* 80, 124–138. doi: 10.1161/01.RES.80.1.124

Shaw, R. M., and Rudy, Y. (1997b). Ionic mechanisms of propagation in cardiac tissue. Roles of the sodium and L-type calcium currents during reduced excitability and decreased gap junction coupling. *Circ. Res.* 81, 727–741. doi: 10.1161/01.RES.81.5.727

Spach, M., and Dolber, P. (1990). "Discontinuous anisotropic propagation," in *Cardiac Electrophysiology: A textbook*, eds M. Rosen, M. Janse, and A. Wit (Mount Kisco, NY: Futura Publishing Company Inc.), 517–534.

Spach, M. S., and Dolber, P. C. (1986). Relating extracellular potentials and their derivatives to anisotropic propagation at a microscopic level in human cardiac muscle. Evidence for electrical uncoupling of side-to-side fiber connections with increasing age. *Circ. Res.* 58, 356–371. doi: 10.1161/01.RES.58.3.356

Spach, M. S., Heidlage, J. F., Dolber, P. C., and Barr, R. C. (2000). Electrophysiological effects of remodeling cardiac gap junctions and cell size: experimental and model studies of normal cardiac growth. *Circ. Res.* 86, 302–311. doi: 10.1161/01.RES.86.3.302

Spach, M. S., Miller, W. T., Dolber, P. C., Kootsey, J. M., Sommer, J. R., and Mosher, C. E. (1982). The functional role of structural complexities in the propagation of depolarization in the atrium of the dog. Cardiac conduction disturbances due to discontinuities of effective axial resistivity. *Circ. Res.* 50, 175–191. doi: 10.1161/01.RES.50.2.175

Spear, J. F., Horowitz, L. N., Hodess, A. B., MacVaugh, H., and Moore, E. N. (1979). Cellular electrophysiology of human myocardial infarction. 1. Abnormalities of cellular activation. *Circulation* 59, 247–256. doi: 10.1161/01.CIR.59.2.247

Sperelakis, N. (1979). Propagation mechanisms in heart. *Annu. Rev. Physiol.* 41, 441–457. doi: 10.1146/annurev.ph.41.030179.002301

Sperelakis, N., and Mann, J. E. (1977). Evaluation of electric field changes in the cleft between excitable cells. *J. Theor. Biol.* 64, 71–96. doi: 10.1016/0022-5193(77)90114-X

Stinstra, J. G., Hopenfeld, B., and Macleod, R. S. (2005). On the passive cardiac conductivity. *Ann. Biomed. Eng.* 33, 1743–1751. doi: 10.1007/s10439-005-7257-7

Swynghedauw, B., Baillard, C., and Milliez, P. (2003). The long QT interval is not only inherited but is also linked to cardiac hypertrophy. *J. Mol. Med.* 81, 336–345. doi: 10.1007/s00109-003-0437-8

Tomaselli, G. F., and Marbán, E. (1999). Electrophysiological remodeling in hypertrophy and heart failure. *Cardiovasc. Res.* 42, 270–283. doi: 10.1016/S0008-6363(99)00017-6

Toure, A., and Cabo, C. (2010). Effect of cell geometry on conduction velocity in a subcellular model of myocardium. *IEEE Trans. Biomed. Eng.* 57, 2107–2114. doi: 10.1109/TBME.2010.2050064

Tveito, A., Lines, G. T., Edwards, A. G., Maleckar, M. M., Michailova, A., Hake, J., et al. (2012). Slow Calcium-Depolarization-Calcium waves may initiate fast local depolarization waves in ventricular tissue. *Prog. Biophys. Mol. Biol.* 110, 295–304. doi: 10.1016/j.pbiomolbio.2012.07.005

Veeraraghavan, R., Gourdie, R. G., and Poelzing, S. (2014). Mechanisms of cardiac conduction: a history of revisions. *Am. J. Physiol. Heart Circ. Physiol.* 306, H619–H627. doi: 10.1152/ajpheart.00760.2013

Veeraraghavan, R., Salama, M. E., and Poelzing, S. (2012). Interstitial volume modulates the conduction velocity-gap junction relationship. *Am. J. Physiol. Heart Circ. Physiol.* 302, H278–H286. doi: 10.1152/ajpheart.00868.2011

Verheule, S., Tuyls, E., Gharaviri, A., Hulsmans, S., van Hunnik, A., Kuiper, M., et al. (2013). Loss of continuity in the thin epicardial layer because of endomysial fibrosis increases the complexity of atrial fibrillatory conduction. *Circ. Arrhythm. Electrophysiol.* 6, 202–211. doi: 10.1161/CIRCEP.112.975144

Weber, K. T., Sun, Y., Bhattacharya, S. K., Ahokas, R. A., and Gerling, I. C. (2013). Myofibroblast-mediated mechanisms of pathological remodelling of the heart. *Nat. Rev. Cardiol.* 10, 15–26. doi: 10.1038/nrcardio.2012.158

Weidmann, S. (1952). The electrical constants of Purkinje fibres. *J. Physiol. (Lond).* 118, 348–360.

Weidmann, S. (1990). "Passive properties of cardiac fibers. A textbook," in *Cardiac Electrophysiology,* eds M. Rosen, M. Janse, and A. Wit (Mount Kisco, NY: Futura Publishing Company Inc.), 29–35.

Weingart, R., and Maurer, P. (1988). Action potential transfer in cell pairs isolated from adult rat and guinea pig ventricles. *Circ. Res.* 63, 72–80. doi: 10.1161/01.RES.63.1.72

Xie, Y., Sato, D., Garfinkel, A., Qu, Z., and Weiss, J. N. (2010). So little source, so much sink: requirements for afterdepolarizations to propagate in tissue. *Biophys. J.* 99, 1408–1415. doi: 10.1016/j.bpj.2010.06.042

Xing, D., Kjølbye, A. L., Nielsen, M. S., Petersen, J. S., Harlow, K. W., Holstein-Rathlou, N. H., et al. (2003). ZP123 increases gap junctional conductance and prevents reentrant ventricular tachycardia during myocardial ischemia in open chest dogs. *J. Cardiovasc. Electrophysiol.* 14, 510–520. doi: 10.1046/j.1540-8167.2003.02329.x

Yue, L., Xie, J., and Nattel, S. (2011). Molecular determinants of cardiac fibroblast electrical function and therapeutic implications for atrial fibrillation. *Cardiovasc. Res.* 89, 744–753. doi: 10.1093/cvr/cvq329

8

Fibrosis: A structural modulator of sinoatrial node physiology and dysfunction

Thomas A. Csepe[1], Anuradha Kalyanasundaram[1], Brian J. Hansen[1], Jichao Zhao[2] and Vadim V. Fedorov[1*]

[1] *Department of Physiology and Cell Biology, Davis Heart and Lung Research Institute, The Ohio State University Wexner Medical Center, Columbus, OH, USA*
[2] *Auckland Bioengineering Institute, The University of Auckland, Auckland, New Zealand*

***Correspondence:**
Vadim V. Fedorov, Department of Physiology and Cell Biology, The Ohio State University, Wexner Medical Center, 300A Hamilton Hall, 1645 Neil Avenue, Columbus, OH 43210-1218, USA
e-mail: vadim.fedorov@osumc.edu; fedorov.2@osu.edu

Heart rhythm is initialized and controlled by the Sinoatrial Node (SAN), the primary pacemaker of the heart. The SAN is a heterogeneous multi-compartment structure characterized by clusters of specialized cardiomyocytes enmeshed within strands of connective tissue or fibrosis. Intranodal fibrosis is emerging as an important modulator of structural and functional integrity of the SAN pacemaker complex. In adult human hearts, fatty tissue and fibrosis insulate the SAN from the hyperpolarizing effect of the surrounding atria while electrical communication between the SAN and right atrium is restricted to discrete SAN conduction pathways. The amount of fibrosis within the SAN is inversely correlated with heart rate, while age and heart size are positively correlated with fibrosis. Pathological upregulation of fibrosis within the SAN may lead to tachycardia-bradycardia arrhythmias and cardiac arrest, possibly due to SAN reentry and exit block, and is associated with atrial fibrillation, ventricular arrhythmias, heart failure and myocardial infarction. In this review, we will discuss current literature on the role of fibrosis in normal SAN structure and function, as well as the causes and consequences of SAN fibrosis upregulation in disease conditions.

Keywords: sinoatrial node, fibrosis, sinus node dysfunction, aging, exit block, sinoatrial reentry, atrial fibrillation, heart failure

INTRODUCTION

> "*We might mention also that, in some of the pathological hearts cut by us, sections of this region* (i.e., the sinoatrial node) *appeared to show a definite increase in the amount of fibrous tissue present-a fact of considerable importance...*"
>
> (Keith and Flack, 1907)

In the human heart, cardiac rhythm is initiated and regulated by the primary pacemaker of the heart, the Sinoatrial Node (SAN) (Keith and Flack, 1907; Lewis et al., 1910; James, 1961; Boineau et al., 1988; Opthof, 1988; Boyett et al., 2000; Chandler et al., 2009; Fedorov et al., 2010b). Initiation of heart rhythm occurs within specialized cardiomyocytes of the SAN and is propagated throughout the atria and ventricles by the cardiac conduction system. Sinus Node Dysfunction (SND), also referred to as Sick Sinus Syndrome (SSS), commonly translates into rhythm abnormalities manifested as brady-arrhythmias or tachycardia-bradycardia (tachy-brady) syndrome (Mangrum and DiMarco, 2000), which are frequently associated with cardiac diseases including atrial fibrillation (AF), malignant ventricular arrhythmias, heart failure (HF) and cardiac arrest (Luu et al., 1989; Sumitomo et al., 2007; Faggioni et al., 2013; Hjortshoj et al., 2013; Alonso et al., 2014; Jensen et al., 2014). With the aging population, it is projected that the annual incidence of SND cases in the US will increase from 78,000 in 2012 to 172,000 in 2060 (Jensen et al., 2014). SND is the predominant prognosis for electronic pacemaker implantation (Mangrum and DiMarco, 2000; Packer et al., 2009; Greenspon et al., 2012), emphasizing the important role that the SAN plays in maintaining normal cardiac rhythm and in human arrhythmic diseases.

Since the discovery of the SAN by Keith and Flack in 1907, significant strides in our understanding of SAN pacemaker function (Lakatta and DiFrancesco, 2009) have allowed for new and exciting therapeutic strategies to treat SAN disease, such as the development of Ivabradine as a selective drug against inappropriate SAN tachycardia (Cappato et al., 2012) and artificial biological pacemakers (Miake et al., 2002; Rosen et al., 2004; Rosen, 2014). The heterogeneous distribution of specialized ion channels, intracellular sodium/calcium handling proteins, gap junction channels and receptors within the SAN pacemaker complex are a few of the critical players shown to be involved in SAN pacemaking that have been addressed in recent reviews (Monfredi et al., 2010; Dobrzynski et al., 2013; Wu and Anderson, 2014). In addition to these molecular mechanisms, the passive, structural features of the SAN complex also contributes significantly to its normal functioning.

In contrast to the simplified SAN structure in many textbooks, studies in both human and canine hearts have revealed that the SAN is a complex multi-compartment structure (James, 1961; Opthof, 1988; Boineau et al., 1989; Beau et al., 1995; Boyett et al., 2000; Sanchez-Quintana et al., 2005; Chandler et al., 2009; Fedorov et al., 2009, 2010a). The SAN, in almost all mammalian hearts, is characterized by clusters of specialized cardiomyocytes, enmeshed within strands of connective tissue or fibrosis, mostly a combination of collagen, elastin and fibroblasts (Lev, 1954; Hudson, 1960; Truex et al., 1967; Sanchez-Quintana et al., 2002). This fibrotic matrix provides mechanical protection (Alings et al., 1995) of the SAN and electrically insulates the SAN pacemaker cells from the surrounding atrial myocardium, thereby efficiently regulating normal sinus rhythm. This review will take a more in depth look at the role of fibrosis in normal SAN function, as well as factors involved in unfavorable fibrosis production observed in patients and animal models with cardiac diseases and SND (Liu et al., 2007; de Jong et al., 2011; Nakao et al., 2012; Glukhov et al., 2013, 2015; Alonso et al., 2014; Jensen et al., 2014; Morris and Kalman, 2014).

FIBROSIS IN NORMAL SAN FUNCTION

FIBROSIS DEFINES SAN STRUCTURE AND MAINTAINS FUNCTIONAL INTEGRITY OF THE PACEMAKER COMPLEX

The SAN is anatomically located at the junction of the superior vena cava and right atrium in the mammalian heart (**Figure 1A**). In the normal adult human heart, the SAN is 12–20 mm long and 2–6 mm wide, identified by its ellipsoidal shape that traverses intramurally. The superior part (head) lies about 1 mm beneath the epicardium, separated by a layer of connective tissue and fat (Keith and Flack, 1907; James, 1961; Truex et al., 1967; Matsuyama et al., 2004; Sanchez-Quintana et al., 2005). The SAN spreads from its head inferiorly for 10–20 mm remaining beneath the sulcus terminalis and just above the crista terminalis and has several extensions into the surrounding atrial myocardium, forming the specialized sinoatrial conduction pathways (SACPs) (Lev, 1954; Hudson, 1960; Demoulin and Kulbertus, 1978; Fedorov et al., 2010b) (**Figure 1A**). Importantly, the SAN consists of small clusters of pacemaker myocytes, arranged in parallel rows that frequently anastomose. Dense connective tissue, nerve fibers, and capillaries are interspersed with the SAN pacemaker clusters, creating the SAN pacemaker complex.

A century ago, Keith and Flack's pioneering studies described fibrotic insulation in the human SAN: "In the human heart the fibers (i.e., SAN pacemaker cell clusters) are striated, fusiform, with well-marked elongated nuclei, plexiform in arrangement, and embedded in *densely packed connective tissue*" (Keith and Flack, 1907). Since then, extensive investigations of the human SAN structure by many others (Lev, 1954; Hudson, 1960; James, 1961; Truex et al., 1967; Demoulin and Kulbertus, 1978; Matsuyama et al., 2004) have confirmed the extensive fibrotic pattern within the node. Fibrosis provides an encompassing, honeycomb-like, structural support composed of a network of collagen sheaths of endomysium (Sanchez-Quintana et al., 2002) (**Figure 1B**). These data show that interstitial fibrosis within the normal SAN builds scaffolding to "house" the sophisticated SAN myocytes and may be necessary to maximize electrical insulation and safe propagation in the SAN complex (Davies and Pomerance, 1972; Fedorov et al., 2010b, 2012) (**Figure 1B**). Furthermore, the human SAN is electrically insulated from the surrounding atria by fibrosis and fatty tissue (Lev, 1954; Sanchez-Quintana et al., 2005; Monfredi et al., 2010; Fedorov et al., 2010b) except for distinct SACPs, which electrically connect the SAN to

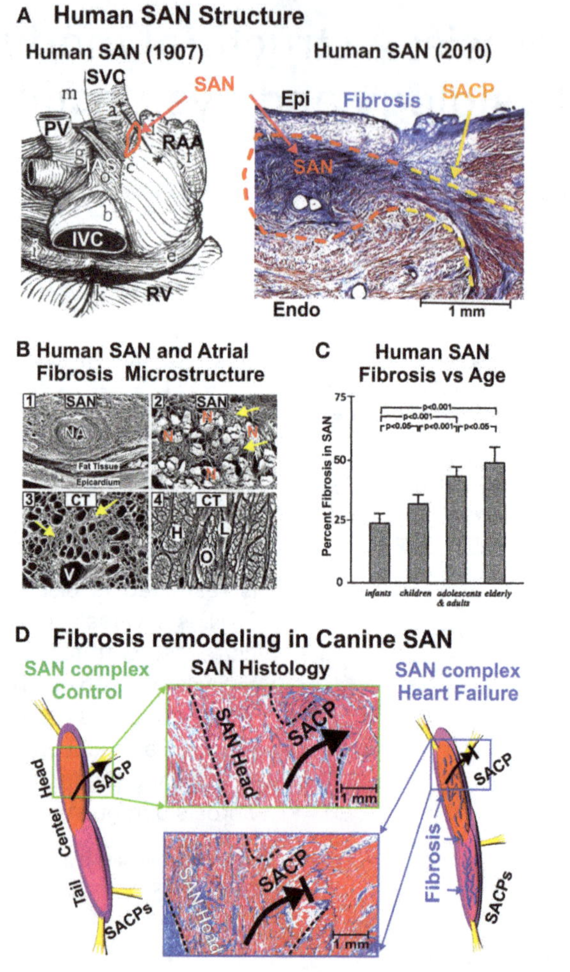

FIGURE 1 | (A) Left: Drawing of the posterior human atrial anatomy from (Keith and Flack, 1907), with SAN outlined in red. Right: Histological cross section of the SAN (red outline) connected to the atria by a SACP (yellow outline). The SAN is seen to be isolated from the atria by sup-epicardial fat and connective tissue. Modified from Fedorov et al. (2010b, 2012) with permission. **(B)** 1—Scanning electron micrograph of the SAN and nodal artery (NA) of a cross section through the CT after digestion of the nodal cells. The collagenous sheaths of endomysial fibrosis formed a complex network in the gaps between the nodal cells, whereas occasional perimysial septums were seen between them. 2—Scanning electron micrograph of non-macerated SAN cells (N), which are encased in dense and coarse endomysial sheaths (yellow arrows) in a specimen from a 75 year old. 3—Scanning electron micrograph of a cross section through the CT, after digestion, from a specimen of 70 years shows a diffuse notable excess of endomysial sheaths (yellow arrows) indicating focal interstitial reactive fibrosis. Vascular space (V) corresponds to a coronary vein. 4—Scanning electron micrograph of non-macerated cross section through the body of the CT shows mainly longitudinal fibers (H) with intermingling oblique (O) or lateral (L) fibers. From Sanchez-Quintana et al. (2002) with permission. **(C)** Graph showing percentage of fibrous connective tissue volume to the total SAN volume, mean value, and standard deviation. From Shiraishi et al. (1992); used with permission. **(D)** Fibrosis in the SAN is increased in HF vs. control dog. Left: A structural model of the control canine SAN complex and SACPs. Middle: histological sections showing upregulated fibrotic and fatty content in SAN complex (black outline) and SACP in HF (bottom, blue box) compared to control (top, green box). Right: A structural model of the heart failure SAN complex and SACPs,

(Continued)

FIGURE 1 | Continued
showing upregulated intranodal fibrosis (blue fibrotic strands). Modified from Lou et al. (2014) with permission. Abbreviations: CT, crista terminalis; Endo, endocardium; Epi, epicardium; HF, heart failure; IAS, interatrial septum; PV, pulmonary veins; RAA, right atrial appendage; RV, right ventricle; SACP, sinoatrial conduction pathway; SAN, sinoatrial node; SVC and IVC, superior and inferior vena cava.

the right atrium (Fedorov et al., 2012). Integral to SAN function, fibrotic and fatty insulation of the SAN prevents the depression of pacemaker automaticity from the hyperpolarizing electrical load of the atrial myocardium (Joyner and van Capelle, 1986).

SAN FIBROSIS INCREASES WITH HEART SIZE AND AGE

Considerable physiological and structural evidence support the generalization that large mammals (including human, dog, pig, yak, horse, etc.) have a more compact and distinct SAN structure than smaller mammals (Keith and Flack, 1907; James, 1961; Opthof et al., 1987; Fedorov et al., 2009, 2012; Duan et al., 2012; Lou et al., 2013, 2014; Glukhov et al., 2015). Histological studies clearly demonstrated that interstitial fibrosis is an inherent component of normal SAN structure and can be traced from newborn hearts (Lev, 1954; Shiraishi et al., 1992; Alings et al., 1995). The size of the heart, as well as its mechanical demands, increases dramatically throughout life and may have a major effect on SAN structure and function. In 1954, Lev published the first detailed study of structural changes of the SAN with age in 54 human SAN samples ranging from 4 months gestation to 90 years of age; this exhaustive investigation revealed that the SAN tissue was already clearly discernable from the atrial tissue at 5 months gestation, particularly due to the greater abundance of fibroblasts and distinctly higher number of collagen fibers (Lev, 1954). Collagen content in the human infant SAN is about 24% and this number climbs to about 70% fibrosis in the adult heart (Shiraishi et al., 1992; Alings et al., 1995) (**Figure 1C**). This natural correlation between aging and increased fibrotic content in the SAN has also been documented in animal models, for example SAN fibrosis in mouse rises from 12–17% at 3 months to 23–25% at 12 months (Hao et al., 2011; Glukhov et al., 2015). The age-induced increase of SAN fibrosis is strongly correlated with slowed intrinsic heart rate as well as slowed SAN conduction in human and mammalian hearts (Kuga et al., 1993; Sanders et al., 1994; Noujaim et al., 2004; Hao et al., 2011; Akoum et al., 2012). The SAN modeling study by Oren and Clancy (2010) is in agreement with a study by Fahrenbach et al. (2007): fibrosis correlates with slowed intrinsic conduction through two mechanisms: (1) heterocellular coupling enables the fibroblast to depolarize the cardiomyocytes (or act as a current sink), (2) fibroblasts physically separate the pacemaker cardiomyocytes, slowing SAN rhythm through a reduction in mutual entrainment (Jalife, 1984).

Apart from aging, a natural size-to-fibrotic content relationship is evidenced in the gradual increase in SAN percent fibrosis as the size of the species increases. The adult mouse SAN is composed of less fibrosis (Hao et al., 2011; Glukhov et al., 2015) than the adult cat SAN, which consists of 27% fibrosis (Alings et al., 1995). The healthy adult canine SAN has a range of 22–30% fibrosis (Glukhov et al., 2013; Lou et al., 2014), while the normal adult human SAN shows roughly 45% fibrosis (Alings et al., 1995). The contribution of increased intranodal fibrosis in large mammals to their functional demands is not completely clear, but as the atrial tissue increases in large vs. small hearts, more insulation around the SAN may be necessary to protect it from the electrical and mechanical load of the atria (Joyner and van Capelle, 1986). Universally, large mammals have slower heart rates vs. smaller animals as established by Noujaim et al.'s multi-species study (Noujaim et al., 2004). Based on the studies discussed above, we suggest that intranodal fibrosis is inversely correlated with intrinsic SAN rhythm and conduction, and directly correlated with age and heart size.

FIBROSIS PROVIDES MECHANICAL PROTECTION FOR THE SAN AND PREVENTS PATHOPHYSIOLOGICAL HEART RATE RESPONSES TO ATRIAL STRETCH AND PRESSURE

In addition to structural scaffolding and electrical insulation from the atria, interstitial fibrosis within the SAN can prevent it from increased interstitial volume changes due to stretch or compression. As the natural growth during the life span or size of the animal increases, the size and thickness of the atria also increases to meet contractile demands (Sanchez-Quintana et al., 2002). Mechanical stretch is a powerful myogenic modulator of SAN function (Brooks and Lange, 1977); in fact, possibly as a local regulator of heart rate, stretch and/or increased intra-atrial pressure can increase SAN rhythm, whereas compression and/or increased arterial pressure in the SAN artery may lead to slowing of SAN rhythm (James and Nadeau, 1962; Lange et al., 1966; Hashimoto et al., 1967). These local responses to stretch and pressure may be carried out through stretch-activated channels in pacemaker cells and SAN fibroblasts, which have been shown to electrically couple with SAN myocytes in some studies (Kohl et al., 1994; Kamkin et al., 2003; Cooper and Kohl, 2005; Fahrenbach et al., 2007; Oren and Clancy, 2010). By providing a relatively tough casing for the compact SAN, fibrosis could prevent the node from overstretching due to the mechanical pressures of the atrial myocardium (Alings et al., 1995).

FIBROSIS IN SAN DYSFUNCTION

INCREASING FIBROSIS WITHIN THE SAN PACEMAKER COMPLEX IS ASSOCIATED WITH SND AND ARRHYTHMIAS

SND is conceptualized as a spectrum of heart rhythm disturbances including bradycardia, sinus pauses/arrest, exit block, "inappropriate" sinus tachycardia and re-entrant arrhythmias, (Alonso et al., 2014; Jensen et al., 2014). It is largely a disease of the elderly and its incidence increases in an exponential manner with age (Mandel et al., 1999; Adan and Crown, 2003; Dobrzynski et al., 2007). Although human SND can be induced by a number of different pathophysiological mechanisms such as drug effects, autonomic imbalances, cardiomyopathy and electrophysiological alterations, SAN structural abnormalities have been commonly observed in these dysfunctions and are significantly associated with HF, SAN ischemia, and inflammatory conditions (Jordan et al., 1978; Adan and Crown, 2003; Sanders et al., 2004; Kottkamp, 2012). In 1907, Keith and Flack saw a "definite increase in the amount of fibrous tissue" present in the SAN from pathological hearts (Keith and Flack, 1907). Later, Hudson emphasized the association of extensive fibrotic lesions in the human SAN with established arrhythmia, especially AF, and suggested that temporary arrhythmias may be associated with minor fibrotic lesions in the SAN (Hudson, 1960). Thery et al. demonstrated a direct correlation between SAN fibrosis and the occurrence of tachy-brady syndrome (Thery et al., 1977). Tachy-brady syndrome, or tachy-brady arrhythmias, have been explained as "the heart rate alternating between too fast and too slow," where termination of paroxysmal tachycardia "may be followed by long atrial pauses lasting several seconds, which can provoke another tachyarrhythmia paroxysm" (**Figure 2A**) (Moss and Davis, 1974; Lou et al., 2013, 2014). While the natural increase in SAN fibrosis observed with aging and heart size is not directly associated with SND, degenerative loss of SAN pacemaker cells and their replacement with fibrosis tissue is frequently evident upon pathologic examination of specimens from patients with SND (Birchfield et al., 1957; Davies and Pomerance, 1972; Thery et al., 1977; Hurle et al., 2006; Yeh et al., 2009).

EXCESSIVE FIBROSIS LEADS TO CONDUCTION BLOCKS AND REENTRY IN THE SAN PACEMAKER COMPLEX

Upregulated interstitial fibrosis may lead to disruption of the continuity of electrically coupled myocytes (Nguyen et al., 2014), which alters the delicate balance between depolarized cells (source) and the resting tissue ahead (sink), thereby disrupting SAN pacemakers' mutual entrainment (Jalife, 1984; Delmar et al., 1986; Michaels et al., 1987). As such, too much fibrosis slows activity of primary pacemaker clusters, as well as enhances beat-to-beat variability and atrial arrhythmias due to competition between multiple primary and subsidiary/latent pacemaker clusters within and outside the SAN pacemaker complex (Glukhov et al., 2013). Increased nodal fibrosis can cause slowed and decremental conduction within the SAN complex, especially in the SACPs (**Figure 1D**), leading to SAN exit block and long pauses, especially after tachycardia termination. Specifically, the atrial tachyarrhythmia or fast pacing depresses conduction/excitability in the structurally remodeled poorly coupled SACP (**Figure 1D**) which enhances source-sink mismatch and leads to exit block from the SAN after tachyarrhythmia termination, which can give rise to tachy-brady syndrome and cardiac arrest (Fedorov et al., 2010a; Glukhov et al., 2010, 2013; Hao et al., 2011; Swaminathan et al., 2011; Froese et al., 2012; Lou et al., 2014). Intramural optical mapping studies integrated with micro-structural analysis directly revealed that fibrosis could also lead to intranodal longitudinal and transverse conduction blocks and cause SAN micro- and macro-reentry (Glukhov et al., 2013; Lou et al., 2014) (**Figures 2B–D**). Interestingly, SAN macro-reentry (where signal travels from the one SACP to the atria and then back to the SAN through another SACP) will lead to tachycardia, but micro-reentry inside the SAN may lead to exit block in the

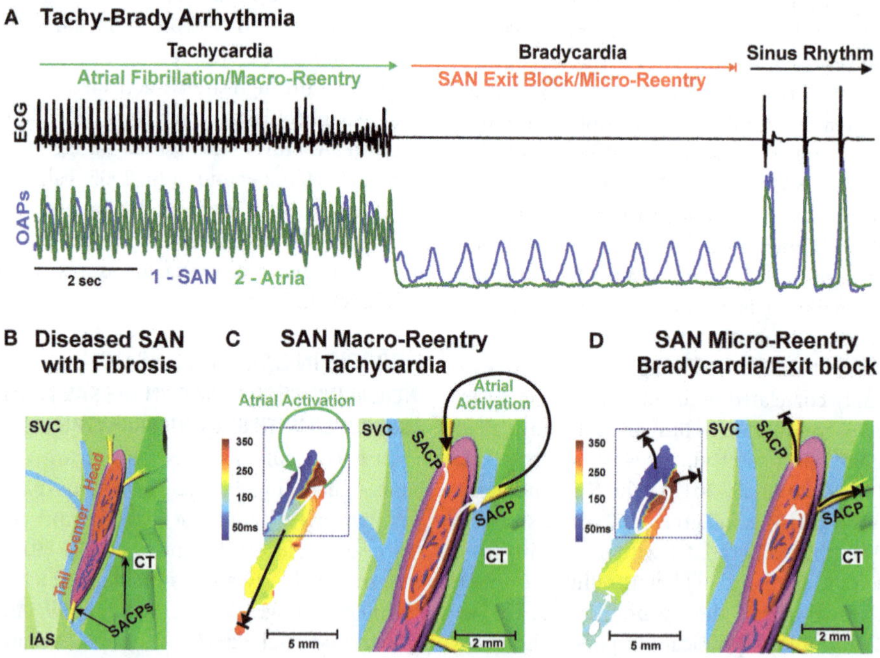

FIGURE 2 | (A) Example of Tachy-Brady arrhythmia often observed in structurally remodeled hearts with upregulated intranodal fibrosis. Atrial Fibrillation or Tachycardia leads to Bradycardia (long pauses) due to SAN exit block, followed by recovery of sinus rhythm or new Tachycardia event. ECG (black) and Optical Action Potentials (green and blue). Modified from Lou et al. (2013) with permission. **(B)** Enlarged epicardial view of 3D canine SAN model based on structural and functional data from optical mapping experiments. The SAN is demarcated from the atrium (green) by 3 bifurcating coronary arteries (light blue) and connective tissue (light purple). The yellow bundles show SACPs that electrically connect the SAN to the atrium. **(C)** Macro-reentry between the SAN and atria that occurred in the structurally remodeled canine heart after cessation of atrial tachypacing. Path of macro-reentry correlated with fibrotic strands within SAN. **(D)** SAN micro-reentry transformed from the previous macro-reentry is shown. Fibrosis strands were the structural substrates anchoring micro-reentry to this area. **(B–D)** modified from Glukhov et al. (2013) with permission. Abbreviations as seen in **Figure 1**.

SACP and severe bradycardia (Glukhov et al., 2013) (**Figure 2**). Histological analysis revealed that these arrhythmias required intranodal fibrotic strands not present in healthy hearts, indicating a critical role of intranodal fibrosis in creating structural substrates for SAN macro- and micro-reentry and atrial arrhythmias (Glukhov et al., 2013; Lou et al., 2014).

Importantly, disease-induced increases in interstitial fibrosis can abnormally insulate latent atrial pacemaker clusters thereby increasing their pacemaking properties (Boineau et al., 1988; Anderson et al., 2009; Atkinson et al., 2013; Dobrzynski et al., 2013). We recently demonstrated this novel mechanism in a mouse model of Calsequestrin 2 knockout, wherein increased pathological fibrosis indeed insulated latent atrial pacemaker clusters that competed with the SAN, causing heterogeneous conduction within the atria and subsequently AF and ventricular tachycardia (Glukhov et al., 2015). However, Verheule et al. found significant depression of atrial conduction and higher inducibility of AF in a mouse model of atria-specific TGF-β1 overexpression but no evidence of SAN dysfunction, indicating upregulation of atrial fibrosis alone may not be sufficient to cause SAN dysfunction (Verheule et al., 2004).

It is not always clear whether fibrosis upregulation always precedes SAN dysfunction, or if fibrosis is generated as a response to SAN dysfunction. However, in SND animal models and recent clinical late-gadolinium MRI studies (Akoum and Marrouche, 2014) where structural remodeling in the SAN was studied, upregulated fibrosis in the SAN pacemaker complex was found (Sakabe et al., 2005; Hao et al., 2011; Herrmann et al., 2011; Swaminathan et al., 2011; Froese et al., 2012; Nakao et al., 2012; Glukhov et al., 2013; Wolf et al., 2013; Lou et al., 2014).

DISEASE-INDUCED FIBROBLAST-MYOCYTE COUPLING

Additionally, some studies have suggested that fibroblast-myocyte coupling (Kohl et al., 1994; Camelliti et al., 2004) can increase during pathological structural remodeling (e.g., MI and HF) (Kamkin et al., 2001, 2002; Vasquez et al., 2010); however, the existence of these electrical connections is still up for debate (Kohl and Gourdie, 2014). Depending on membrane potential, coupling and distribution, the fibroblast-pacemaker cell connections can increase or decrease the source-sink mismatch, thus accelerating or decelerating the pacemaking of the SAN (Fahrenbach et al., 2007). Increased coupling with interspersed fibroblasts may create abnormal cell-to-cell interactions as well as interrupt electrical coupling between SAN myocytes (decreased mutual entrainment) within the SAN complex, which has been shown in modeling (Oren and Clancy, 2010) and cell culture (Fahrenbach et al., 2007) studies. Furthermore, excessive extracellular matrix protein deposition by fibroblasts within the node can increase stiffness, which could impede the normal myogenic response of the SAN to changes in either stretch or arterial pressure, as mentioned above.

MULTIPLE MECHANISMS UPREGULATE FIBROSIS IN THE SAN

Abnormal proliferation of fibroblasts and excessive secretion of ECM proteins have been shown to underlie cardiac fibrosis (Fan et al., 2012). The development of SAN arrhythmias have also been shown to occur in parallel with the loss of pacemaker cells (Hurle et al., 2006; Herrmann et al., 2011; Swaminathan et al., 2011; Wu and Anderson, 2014), leading to activated and reparative fibroblasts that replace dead cardiomyocytes and additional collagen deposition (Davies and Pomerance, 1972; Burstein and Nattel, 2008; Akoum et al., 2012). These deposits may form large, non-compliant areas of collagenous fibrosis devoid of cardiomyocytes, as in myocardial infarction(de Jong et al., 2011), or it may lead to increased intranodal fibrosis, as seen in HF (**Figure 1D**).

From the limited mechanistic studies on fibrosis within the SAN, there are multiple mechanisms believed to upregulate intranodal fibrosis. Myofibroblasts, the activated phenotype of fibroblasts, are known to underlie the excessive deposition of ECM proteins and are more mobile and contractile than fibroblasts (Davis and Molkentin, 2014). Overexpression of myocardial transforming growth factor β1 (TGF-β1) in mice has been shown to selectively increase fibrosis in the atria by causing a cellular transition from fibroblast to the activated myofibroblast phenotype (Nakajima et al., 2000; Vasquez et al., 2011). However, the presence of activated myofibroblasts is yet to be demonstrated in the SAN.

Another mechanism believed to be associated with increased fibrosis is the upregulation of Angiotensin II (Ang II). Circulating Ang II activates NADPH oxidase and increases oxidized calmodulin kinase II, leading to SAN cell apoptosis and fibrosis (Swaminathan et al., 2011). Ox-CaMKII-mediated loss of functional SAN cells contributes to SAN dysfunction and sudden cardiac death (Wu and Anderson, 2014). Recently, we demonstrated that fibrosis is increased within the SAN and could contribute to the slowed heart rate in a mouse model of catecholaminergic polymorphic ventricular tachycardia, a human arrhythmic disease (Glukhov et al., 2015). In this model of abnormal calcium (Ca^{2+}) leak via the ryanodine receptors from the sarcoplasmic reticulum, increased fibrosis could either be due to upregulation of CaMKII secondary to altered Ca^{2+} signaling and/or SAN cell death leading to replacement with connective tissue.

Given the significant role that fibrotic remodeling plays in SND, anti-fibrotic approaches may present therapeutic options for this disease. For example, the ACE inhibitor Enalapril has been shown to reduce SAN fibrosis and SND in a four-week canine model of atrial tachycardia (Sakabe et al., 2005). Corticosteroids have also been shown to reduce TGF-β1 and fibrosis in mouse lungs (Miller et al., 2006), and promising results in patients with complete AV block due to cardiac sarcoidosis have been observed (Selan et al., 2014). These results suggest that corticosteroids may prevent and/or restore fibrosis-induced SAN conduction impairment, but no study has specifically investigated if this approach is feasible.

FUTURE DIRECTIONS AND CONCLUSION

Even after one century of extensive research on the SAN, the lack of understanding of the human SAN complexity remains a critical barrier to the optimal treatment of heart rhythm disorders. Studies on explanted human SAN are necessary to determine its microstructure as well as structural and mechanistic role of fibrosis in normal as well as diseased hearts. Novel imaging techniques such as MRI or microCT (Akoum et al., 2012; Stephenson et al., 2012; Disertori et al., 2014) should be employed in addition to histological analyses to identify the intact structure as well as the contribution of fibrosis to SAN function and dysfunction.

Heterogeneous distribution of fibrosis within and around the SAN pacemaker complex plays a crucial role in proper SAN function by providing (1) structural and functional integrity/stability of the SAN (2) electrical insulation of SAN myocyte clusters and the entire SAN complex, apart from SACPs, preventing depression of pacemaker automaticity from the hyperpolarizing effect of the surrounding atria (3) mechanical protection from pathophysiological heart rate changes due to stretch and pressure from the contractile force of the atria.

The protective role that fibrosis plays in healthy hearts is necessary for proper SAN function, but this role becomes pathophysiological when fibrosis is upregulated in cardiac diseases, leading to (1) slowed SAN rhythm due to fibrosis replacement of pacemaker cells (2) beat-to-beat variability and slowed intranodal conduction due to decreased electrical coupling between SAN myocytes and pacemaker cell clusters (3) long pauses due to source–sink mismatch causing exit block in the SACPs (4) SAN micro- and macro-reentry due to fibrosis-induced conduction dissociation in the SAN. All of these pathological conditions can lead to arrhythmias such as tachy-brady syndrome and AF. By continuing to expand our knowledge of the complex structure that makes up the SAN and exploring the multiple mechanisms involved in fibrosis upregulation, we will come closer to providing new and less invasive treatment options for a growing population of aging patients suffering from SND.

REFERENCES

Adan, V., and Crown, L. A. (2003). Diagnosis and treatment of sick sinus syndrome. *Am. Fam. Physician* 67, 1725–1732.

Akoum, N., and Marrouche, N. (2014). Assessment and impact of cardiac fibrosis on atrial fibrillation. *Curr. Cardiol. Rep.* 16:518. doi: 10.1007/s11886-014-0518-z

Akoum, N., McGann, C., Vergara, G., Badger, T., Ranjan, R., Mahnkopf, C., et al. (2012). Atrial fibrosis quantified using late gadolinium enhancement MRI is associated with sinus node dysfunction requiring pacemaker implant. *J. Cardiovasc. Electrophysiol.* 23, 44–50. doi: 10.1111/j.1540-8167.2011.02140.x

Alings, A. M., Abbas, R. F., and Bouman, L. N. (1995). Age-related changes in structure and relative collagen content of the human and feline sinoatrial node. A comparative study. *Eur. Heart J.* 16, 1655–1667.

Alonso, A., Jensen, P. N., Lopez, F. L., Chen, L. Y., Psaty, B. M., Folsom, A. R., et al. (2014). Association of sick sinus syndrome with incident cardiovascular disease and mortality: the atherosclerosis risk in communities study and cardiovascular health study. *PLoS ONE* 9:e109662. doi: 10.1371/journal.pone.0109662

Anderson, R. H., Yanni, J., Boyett, M. R., Chandler, N. J., and Dobrzynski, H. (2009). The anatomy of the cardiac conduction system. *Clin. Anat.* 22, 99–113. doi: 10.1002/ca.20700

Atkinson, A. J., Logantha, S. J., Hao, G., Yanni, J., Fedorenko, O., Sinha, A., et al. (2013). Functional, anatomical, and molecular investigation of the cardiac conduction system and arrhythmogenic atrioventricular ring tissue in the rat heart. *J. Am. Heart Assoc.* 2:e000246. doi: 10.1161/JAHA.113.000246

Beau, S. L., Hand, D. E., Schuessler, R. B., Bromberg, B. I., Kwon, B., Boineau, J. P., et al. (1995). Relative densities of muscarinic cholinergic and beta-adrenergic receptors in the canine sinoatrial node and their relation to sites of pacemaker activity. *Circ. Res.* 77, 957–963. doi: 10.1161/01.RES.77.5.957

Birchfield, R. I., Menefee, E. E., and Bryant, G. D. (1957). Disease of the sinoatrial node associated with bradycardia, asystole, syncope, and paroxysmal atrial fibrillation. *Circulation* 16, 20–26. doi: 10.1161/01.CIR.16.1.20

Boineau, J. P., Canavan, T. E., Schuessler, R. B., Cain, M. E., Corr, P. B., and Cox, J. L. (1988). Demonstration of a widely distributed atrial pacemaker complex in the human heart. *Circulation* 77, 1221–1237. doi: 10.1161/01.CIR.77.6.1221

Boineau, J. P., Schuessler, R. B., Canavan, T. E., Corr, P. B., Cain, M. E., and Cox, J. L. (1989). The human atrial pacemaker complex. *J. Electrocardiol.* 22(Suppl.), 189–197. doi: 10.1016/S0022-0736(07)80122-1

Boyett, M. R., Honjo, H., and Kodama, I. (2000). The sinoatrial node, a heterogeneous pacemaker structure. *Cardiovasc. Res.* 47, 658–687. doi: 10.1016/S0008-6363(00)00135-8

Brooks, C. M., and Lange, G. (1977). Interaction of myogenic and neurogenic mechanisms that control heart rate. *Proc. Natl. Acad. Sci. U.S.A.* 74, 1761–1762. doi: 10.1073/pnas.74.4.1761

Burstein, B., and Nattel, S. (2008). Atrial fibrosis: mechanisms and clinical relevance in atrial fibrillation. *J. Am. Coll. Cardiol.* 51, 802–809. doi: 10.1016/j.jacc.2007.09.064

Camelliti, P., Green, C. R., LeGrice, I., and Kohl, P. (2004). Fibroblast network in rabbit sinoatrial node: structural and functional identification of homogeneous and heterogeneous cell coupling. *Circ. Res.* 94, 828–835. doi: 10.1161/01.RES.0000122382.19400.14

Cappato, R., Castelvecchio, S., Ricci, C., Bianco, E., Vitali-Serdoz, L., Gnecchi-Ruscone, T., et al. (2012). Clinical efficacy of ivabradine in patients with inappropriate sinus tachycardia: a prospective, randomized, placebo-controlled, double-blind, crossover evaluation. *J. Am. Coll. Cardiol.* 60, 1323–1329. doi: 10.1016/j.jacc.2012.06.031

Chandler, N. J., Greener, I. D., Tellez, J. O., Inada, S., Musa, H., Molenaar, P., et al. (2009). Molecular architecture of the human sinus node: insights into the function of the cardiac pacemaker. *Circulation* 119, 1562–1575. doi: 10.1161/CIRCULATIONAHA.108.804369

Cooper, P. J., and Kohl, P. (2005). Species- and preparation-dependence of stretch effects on sino-atrial node pacemaking. *Ann. N.Y. Acad. Sci.* 1047, 324–335. doi: 10.1196/annals.1341.029

Davies, M. J., and Pomerance, A. (1972). Quantitative study of ageing changes in the human sinoatrial node and internodal tracts. *Br. Heart J.* 34, 150–152. doi: 10.1136/hrt.34.2.150

Davis, J., and Molkentin, J. D. (2014). Myofibroblasts: trust your heart and let fate decide. *J. Mol. Cell. Cardiol.* 70, 9–18. doi: 10.1016/j.yjmcc.2013.10.019

de Jong, S., van Veen, T. A., van Rijen, H. V., and de Bakker, J. M. (2011). Fibrosis and cardiac arrhythmias. *J. Cardiovasc. Pharmacol.* 57, 630–638. doi: 10.1097/FJC.0b013e318207a35f

Delmar, M., Jalife, J., and Michaels, D. C. (1986). Effects of changes in excitability and intercellular coupling on synchronization in the rabbit sino-atrial node. *J. Physiol.* 370, 127–150. doi: 10.1113/jphysiol.1986.sp015926

Demoulin, J. C., and Kulbertus, H. E. (1978). Histopathological correlates of sinoatrial disease. *Br. Heart J.* 40, 1384–1389. doi: 10.1136/hrt.40.12.1384

Disertori, M., Mase, M., Marini, M., Mazzola, S., Cristoforetti, A., Del, G. M., et al. (2014). Electroanatomic mapping and late gadolinium enhancement MRI in a genetic model of arrhythmogenic atrial cardiomyopathy. *J. Cardiovasc. Electrophysiol.* 25, 964–970. doi: 10.1111/jce.12440

Dobrzynski, H., Anderson, R. H., Atkinson, A., Borbas, Z., D'Souza, A., Fraser, J. F., et al. (2013). Structure, function and clinical relevance of the cardiac conduction system, including the atrioventricular ring and outflow tract tissues. *Pharmacol. Ther.* 139, 260–288. doi: 10.1016/j.pharmthera.2013.04.010

Dobrzynski, H., Boyett, M. R., and Anderson, R. H. (2007). New insights into pacemaker activity: promoting understanding of sick sinus syndrome. *Circulation* 115, 1921–1932. doi: 10.1161/CIRCULATIONAHA.106.616011

Duan, D., Yu, S., and Cui, Y. (2012). Morphological study of the sinus node and its artery in yak. *Anat. Rec. (Hoboken).* 295, 2045–2056. doi: 10.1002/ar.22591

Faggioni, M., Hwang, H. S., van der Werf, C., Nederend, I., Kannankeril, P. J., Wilde, A. A., et al. (2013). Accelerated sinus rhythm prevents catecholaminergic polymorphic ventricular tachycardia in mice and in patients. *Circ. Res.* 112, 689–697. doi: 10.1161/CIRCRESAHA.111.300076

Fahrenbach, J. P., Mejia-Alvarez, R., and Banach, K. (2007). The relevance of non-excitable cells for cardiac pacemaker function. *J. Physiol.* 585, 565–578. doi: 10.1113/jphysiol.2007.144121

Fan, D., Takawale, A., Lee, J., and Kassiri, Z. (2012). Cardiac fibroblasts, fibrosis and extracellular matrix remodeling in heart disease. *Fibrogenesis Tissue Repair* 5:15. doi: 10.1186/1755-1536-5-15

Fedorov, V. V., Chang, R., Glukhov, A. V., Kostecki, G., Janks, D., Schuessler, R. B., et al. (2010a). Complex interactions between the sinoatrial node and atrium during reentrant arrhythmias in the canine heart. *Circulation* 122, 782–789. doi: 10.1161/CIRCULATIONAHA.109.935288

Fedorov, V. V., Glukhov, A. V., and Chang, R. (2012). Conduction barriers and pathways of the sinoatrial pacemaker complex: their role in normal rhythm and atrial arrhythmias. *Am. J. Physiol. Heart Circ. Physiol.* 302, H1773–H1783. doi: 10.1152/ajpheart.00892.2011

Fedorov, V. V., Glukhov, A. V., Chang, R., Kostecki, G., Aferol, H., Hucker, W. J., et al. (2010b). Optical mapping of the isolated coronary-perfused human sinus node. *J. Am. Coll. Cardiol.* 56, 1386–1394. doi: 10.1016/j.jacc.2010.03.098

Fedorov, V. V., Schuessler, R. B., Hemphill, M., Ambrosi, C. M., Chang, R., Voloshina, A. S., et al. (2009). Structural and functional evidence for discrete exit pathways that connect the canine sinoatrial node and atria. *Circ. Res.* 104, 915–923. doi: 10.1161/CIRCRESAHA.108.193193

Froese, A., Breher, S. S., Waldeyer, C., Schindler, R. F., Nikolaev, V. O., Rinne, S., et al. (2012). Popeye domain containing proteins are essential for stress-mediated modulation of cardiac pacemaking in mice. *J. Clin. Invest.* 122, 1119–1130. doi: 10.1172/JCI59410

Glukhov, A. V., Fedorov, V. V., Anderson, M. E., Mohler, P. J., and Efimov, I. R. (2010). Functional anatomy of the murine sinus node: high-resolution optical mapping of ankyrin-B heterozygous mice. *Am. J. Physiol. Heart Circ. Physiol.* 299, H482–H491. doi: 10.1152/ajpheart.00756.2009

Glukhov, A. V., Hage, L. T., Hansen, B. J., Pedraza-Toscano, A., Vargas-Pinto, P., Hamlin, R. L., et al. (2013). Sinoatrial node reentry in a canine chronic left ventricular infarct model: the role of intranodal fibrosis and heterogeneity of refractoriness. *Circ. Arrhythm. Electrophysiol.* 6, 984–994. doi: 10.1161/CIRCEP.113.000404

Glukhov, A. V., Kalyanasundaram, A., Lou, Q., Hage, L. T., Hansen, B. J., Belevych, A. E., et al. (2015). Calsequestrin 2 deletion causes sinoatrial node dysfunction and atrial arrhythmias associated with altered sarcoplasmic reticulum calcium cycling and degenerative fibrosis within the mouse atrial pacemaker complex. *Eur. Heart J.* doi: 10.1093/eurheartj/eht452. [Epub ahead of print].

Greenspon, A. J., Patel, J. D., Lau, E., Ochoa, J. A., Frisch, D. R., Ho, R. T., et al. (2012). Trends in permanent pacemaker implantation in the United States from 1993 to 2009: increasing complexity of patients and procedures. *J. Am. Coll. Cardiol.* 60, 1540–1545. doi: 10.1016/j.jacc.2012.07.017

Hao, X., Zhang, Y., Zhang, X., Nirmalan, M., Davies, L., Konstantinou, D., et al. (2011). TGF-beta1-mediated fibrosis and ion channel remodeling are key mechanisms in producing the sinus node dysfunction associated with SCN5A deficiency and aging. *Circ. Arrhythm. Electrophysiol.* 4, 397–406. doi: 10.1161/CIRCEP.110.960807

Hashimoto, K., Tanaka, S., Hirata, M., and Chiba, S. (1967). Responses of the sino-atrial node to change in pressure in the sinus node artery. *Circ. Res.* 21, 297–304. doi: 10.1161/01.RES.21.3.297

Herrmann, S., Fabritz, L., Layh, B., Kirchhof, P., and Ludwig, A. (2011). Insights into sick sinus syndrome from an inducible mouse model. *Cardiovasc. Res.* 90, 38–48. doi: 10.1093/cvr/cvq390

Hjortshoj, S., Riahi, S., Nielsen, J. C., Skjoth, F., Lundbye-Christensen, S., and Andersen, H. R. (2013). Does atrial pacing lead to atrial fibrillation in patients with sick sinus syndrome? insights from the DANPACE trial. *Europace* 16, 241–245. doi: 10.1093/europace/eut306

Hudson, R. E. (1960). The human pacemaker and its pathology. *Br. Heart J.* 22, 153–167. doi: 10.1136/hrt.22.2.153

Hurle, A., Climent, V., and Sanchez-Quintana, D. (2006). Sinus node structural changes in patients with long-standing chronic atrial fibrillation. *J. Thorac. Cardiovasc. Surg.* 131, 1394–1395. doi: 10.1016/j.jtcvs.2006.01.031

Jalife, J. (1984). Mutual entrainment and electrical coupling as mechanisms for synchronous firing of rabbit sino-atrial pace-maker cells. *J. Physiol.* 356, 221–243. doi: 10.1113/jphysiol.1984.sp015461

James, T. N. (1961). Anatomy of the human sinus node. *Anat. Rec.* 141, 109–139. doi: 10.1002/ar.1091410205

James, T. N., and Nadeau, R. A. (1962). Direct perfusion of the sinus node: an experimental model for pharmacologic and electrophysiologic studies of the heart. *Henry Ford Hosp. Med. Bull.* 10, 21–25.

Jensen, P. N., Gronroos, N. N., Chen, L. Y., Folsom, A. R., deFilippi, C., Heckbert, S. R., et al. (2014). Incidence of and risk factors for sick sinus syndrome in the general population. *J. Am. Coll. Cardiol.* 64, 531–538. doi: 10.1016/j.jacc.2014.03.056

Jordan, J. L., Yamaguchi, I., and Mandel, W. J. (1978). "Function and dysfunction of the sinus node clinical studies in the evaluation of sinus node function," in *The Sinus Node*, ed F. I. Bonke (The Hague; Boston; London: Martinus Nijholff Medical Division). 3–22. doi: 10.1007/978-94-009-9715-8_1

Joyner, R. W., and van Capelle, F. J. (1986). Propagation through electrically coupled cells. How a small SA node drives a large atrium. *Biophys. J.* 50, 1157–1164. doi: 10.1016/S0006-3495(86)83559-7

Kamkin, A., Kiseleva, I., Wagner, K. D., Bohm, J., Theres, H., Gunther, J., et al. (2003). Characterization of stretch-activated ion currents in isolated atrial myocytes from human hearts. *Pflugers Arch.* 446, 339–346. doi: 10.1007/s00424-002-0948-0

Kamkin, A., Kiseleva, I., Wagner, K. D., Pylaev, A., Leiterer, K. P., Theres, H., et al. (2002). A possible role for atrial fibroblasts in postinfarction bradycardia. *Am. J. Physiol. Heart Circ. Physiol.* 282, H842–H849. doi: 10.1152/ajpheart.00240.2001

Kamkin, A., Kiseleva, I., Wagner, K. D., Scholz, H., Theres, H., Kazanski, V., et al. (2001). Mechanically induced potentials in rat atrial fibroblasts depend on actin and tubulin polymerisation. *Pflugers Arch.* 442, 487–497. doi: 10.1007/s004240100564

Keith, A., and Flack, M. (1907). The form and nature of the muscular connection between the primary divisions of the vertebrate heart. *J. Anat. Physiol.* 41, 172–189.

Kohl, P., and Gourdie, R. G. (2014). Fibroblast-myocyte electrotonic coupling: does it occur in native cardiac tissue? *J. Mol. Cell. Cardiol.* 70, 37–46. doi: 10.1016/j.yjmcc.2013.12.024

Kohl, P., Kamkin, A. G., Kiseleva, I. S., and Noble, D. (1994). Mechanosensitive fibroblasts in the sino-atrial node region of rat heart: interaction with cardiomyocytes and possible role. *Exp. Physiol.* 79, 943–956. doi: 10.1113/expphysiol.1994.sp003819

Kottkamp, H. (2012). Fibrotic atrial cardiomyopathy: a specific disease/syndrome supplying substrates for atrial fibrillation, atrial tachycardia, sinus node disease, AV node disease, and thromboembolic complications. *J. Cardiovasc. Electrophysiol.* 23, 797–799. doi: 10.1111/j.1540-8167.2012.02341.x

Kuga, K., Yamaguchi, I., and Sugishita, Y. (1993). Age-related changes of sinus node function and autonomic regulation in subjects without sinus node disease–assessment by pharmacologic autonomic blockade. *Jpn. Circ. J.* 57, 760–768. doi: 10.1253/jcj.57.760

Lakatta, E. G., and DiFrancesco, D. (2009). What keeps us ticking: a funny current, a calcium clock, or both? *J. Mol. Cell. Cardiol.* 47, 157–170. doi: 10.1016/j.yjmcc.2009.03.022

Lange, G., Lu, H. H., Chang, A., and Brooks, C. M. (1966). Effect of stretch on the isolated cat sinoatrial node. *Am. J. Physiol.* 211, 1192–1196.

Lev, M. (1954). Aging changes in the human sinoatrial node. *J. Gerontol.* 9, 1–9. doi: 10.1093/geronj/9.1.1

Lewis, T., Oppenheimer, A., and Oppenheimer, B. S. (1910). The site of origin of the mammalian heart beat: the pacemaker in the dog. *Heart* II, 147–169.

Liu, J., Dobrzynski, H., Yanni, J., Boyett, M. R., and Lei, M. (2007). Organisation of the mouse sinoatrial node: structure and expression of HCN channels. *Cardiovasc. Res.* 73, 729–738. doi: 10.1016/j.cardiores.2006.11.016

Lou, Q., Glukhov, A. V., Hansen, B., Hage, L., Vargos-Pinto, P., Billman, G. E., et al. (2013). Tachy-brady arrhythmias: the critical role of adenosine-induced sinoatrial conduction block in post-tachycardia pauses. *Heart Rhythm* 10, 110–118. doi: 10.1016/j.hrthm.2012.09.012

Lou, Q., Hansen, B. J., Fedorenko, O., Csepe, T. A., Kalyanasundaram, A., Li, N., et al. (2014). Upregulation of adenosine A1 receptors facilitates sinoatrial node dysfunction in chronic canine heart failure by exacerbating nodal conduction abnormalities revealed by novel dual-sided intramural optical mapping. *Circulation* 130, 315–324. doi: 10.1161/CIRCULATIONAHA.113.007086

Luu, M., Stevenson, W. G., Stevenson, L. W., Baron, K., and Walden, J. (1989). Diverse mechanisms of unexpected cardiac arrest in advanced heart failure. *Circulation* 80, 1675–1680. doi: 10.1161/01.CIR.80.6.1675

Mandel, W. J., Jordan, J. L., and Karagueuzian, H. S. (1999). Disorders of sinus function. *Curr. Treat. Options Cardiovasc. Med.* 1, 179–186. doi: 10.1007/s11936-999-0021-9

Mangrum, J. M., and DiMarco, J. P. (2000). The evaluation and management of bradycardia. *N. Engl. J. Med.* 342, 703–709. doi: 10.1056/NEJM200003093421006

Matsuyama, T. A., Inoue, S., Kobayashi, Y., Sakai, T., Saito, T., Katagiri, T., et al. (2004). Anatomical diversity and age-related histological changes in the human right atrial posterolateral wall. *Europace* 6, 307–315. doi: 10.1016/j.eupc.2004.03.011

Miake, J., Marban, E., and Nuss, H. B. (2002). Biological pacemaker created by gene transfer. *Nature* 419, 132–133. doi: 10.1038/419132b

Michaels, D. C., Matyas, E. P., and Jalife, J. (1987). Mechanisms of sinoatrial pacemaker synchronization: a new hypothesis. *Circ. Res.* 61, 704–714. doi: 10.1161/01.RES.61.5.704

Miller, M., Cho, J. Y., McElwain, K., McElwain, S., Shim, J. Y., Manni, M., et al. (2006). Corticosteroids prevent myofibroblast accumulation and airway remodeling in mice. *Am. J. Physiol. Lung Cell. Mol. Physiol.* 290, L162–L169. doi: 10.1152/ajplung.00252.2005

Monfredi, O., Dobrzynski, H., Mondal, T., Boyett, M. R., and Morris, G. M. (2010). The anatomy and physiology of the sinoatrial node–a contemporary review. *Pacing Clin. Electrophysiol.* 33, 1392–1406. doi: 10.1111/j.1540-8159.2010.02838.x

Morris, G. M., and Kalman, J. M. (2014). Fibrosis, electrics and genetics. perspectives in sinoatrial node disease. *Circ. J.* 78, 1272–1282. doi: 10.1253/circj.CJ-14-0419

Moss, A. J., and Davis, R. J. (1974). Brady-Tachy syndrome. *Prog. Cardiovasc. Dis.* 16, 439–454. doi: 10.1016/0033-0620(74)90005-X

Nakajima, H., Nakajima, H. O., Salcher, O., Dittie, A. S., Dembowsky, K., Jing, S., et al. (2000). Atrial but not ventricular fibrosis in mice expressing a mutant transforming growth factor-beta(1) transgene in the heart. *Circ. Res.* 86, 571–579. doi: 10.1161/01.RES.86.5.571

Nakao, S., Hirakawa, A., Fukushima, R., Kobayashi, M., and Machida, N. (2012). The anatomical basis of bradycardia-tachycardia syndrome in elderly dogs with chronic degenerative valvular disease. *J. Comp. Pathol.* 146, 175–182. doi: 10.1016/j.jcpa.2011.03.016

Nguyen, T. P., Qu, Z., and Weiss, J. N. (2014). Cardiac fibrosis and arrhythmogenesis: the road to repair is paved with perils. *J. Mol. Cell. Cardiol.* 70, 83–91. doi: 10.1016/j.yjmcc.2013.10.018

Noujaim, S. F., Lucca, E., Munoz, V., Persaud, D., Berenfeld, O., Meijler, F. L., et al. (2004). From mouse to whale: a universal scaling relation for the PR Interval of the electrocardiogram of mammals. *Circulation* 110, 2802–2808. doi: 10.1161/01.CIR.0000146785.15995.67

Opthof, T. (1988). The mammalian sinoatrial node. *Cardiovasc. Drugs Ther.* 1, 573–597. doi: 10.1007/BF02125744

Opthof, T., de Jonge, B., Jongsma, H. J., and Bouman, L. N. (1987). Functional morphology of the pig sinoatrial node. *J. Mol. Cell. Cardiol.* 19, 1221–1236. doi: 10.1016/S0022-2828(87)80532-1

Oren, R. V., and Clancy, C. E. (2010). Determinants of heterogeneity, excitation and conduction in the sinoatrial node: a model study. *PLoS Comput. Biol.* 6:e1001041. doi: 10.1371/journal.pcbi.1001041

Packer, D. L., Prutkin, J. M., Hellkamp, A. S., Mitchell, L. B., Bernstein, R. C., Wood, F., et al. (2009). Impact of implantable cardioverter-defibrillator, amiodarone, and placebo on the mode of death in stable patients with heart failure: analysis from the sudden cardiac death in heart failure trial. *Circulation* 120, 2170–2176. doi: 10.1161/CIRCULATIONAHA.109.853689

Rosen, M. R. (2014). Gene therapy and biological pacing. *N. Engl. J. Med.* 371, 1158–1159. doi: 10.1056/NEJMcibr1408897

Rosen, M. R., Brink, P. R., Cohen, I. S., and Robinson, R. B. (2004). Genes, stem cells and biological pacemakers. *Cardiovasc. Res.* 64, 12–23. doi: 10.1016/j.cardiores.2004.05.012

Sakabe, M., Fujiki, A., Nishida, K., Sugao, M., Nagasawa, H., Tsuneda, T., et al. (2005). Enalapril preserves sinus node function in a canine atrial fibrillation model induced by rapid atrial pacing. *J. Cardiovasc. Electrophysiol.* 16, 1209–1214. doi: 10.1111/j.1540-8167.2005.50100.x

Sanchez-Quintana, D., Anderson, R. H., Cabrera, J. A., Climent, V., Martin, R., Farre, J., et al. (2002). The terminal crest: morphological features relevant to electrophysiology. *Heart* 88, 406–411. doi: 10.1136/heart.88.4.406

Sanchez-Quintana, D., Cabrera, J. A., Farre, J., Climent, V., Anderson, R. H., and Ho, S. Y. (2005). Sinus node revisited in the era of electroanatomical mapping and catheter ablation. *Heart* 91, 189–194. doi: 10.1136/hrt.2003.031542

Sanders, P., Morton, J. B., Kistler, P. M., Spence, S. J., Davidson, N. C., Hussin, A., et al. (2004). Electrophysiological and electroanatomic characterization of the atria in sinus node disease: evidence of diffuse atrial remodeling. *Circulation* 109, 1514–1522. doi: 10.1161/01.CIR.0000121734.47409.AA

Sanders, W. E. J., Sorrentino, R. A., Greenfield, R. A., Shenasa, H., Hamer, M. E., and Wharton, J. M. (1994). Catheter ablation of sinoatrial node reentrant tachycardia. *J. Am. Coll. Cardiol.* 23, 926–934. doi: 10.1016/0735-1097(94)90639-4

Selan, J. C., Michaelson, M., Fanburg, B. L., and Estes, N. A. (2014). Evaluation and management of heart rhythm disturbances due to cardiac sarcoidosis. *Heart Lung Circ.* 23, 1100–1109. doi: 10.1016/j.hlc.2014.07.065

Shiraishi, I., Takamatsu, T., Minamikawa, T., Onouchi, Z., and Fujita, S. (1992). Quantitative histological analysis of the human sinoatrial node during growth and aging. *Circulation* 85, 2176–2184. doi: 10.1161/01.CIR.85.6.2176

Stephenson, R. S., Boyett, M. R., Hart, G., Nikolaidou, T., Cai, X., Corno, A. F., et al. (2012). Contrast enhanced micro-computed tomography resolves the 3-dimensional morphology of the cardiac conduction system in mammalian hearts. *PLoS ONE* 7:e35299. doi: 10.1371/journal.pone.0035299

Sumitomo, N., Sakurada, H., Taniguchi, K., Matsumura, M., Abe, O., Miyashita, M., et al. (2007). Association of atrial arrhythmia and sinus node dysfunction in patients with catecholaminergic polymorphic ventricular tachycardia. *Circ. J.* 71, 1606–1609. doi: 10.1253/circj.71.1606

Swaminathan, P. D., Purohit, A., Soni, S., Voigt, N., Singh, M. V., Glukhov, A. V., et al. (2011). Oxidized CaMKII causes cardiac sinus node dysfunction in mice. *J. Clin. Invest.* 121, 3277–3288. doi: 10.1172/JCI57833

Thery, C., Gosselin, B., Lekieffre, J., and Warembourg, H. (1977). Pathology of sinoatrial node. Correlations with electrocardiographic findings in 111 patients. *Am. Heart J.* 93, 735–740. doi: 10.1016/S0002-8703(77)80070-7

Truex, R. C., Smythe, M. Q., and Taylor, M. J. (1967). Reconstruction of the human sinoatrial node. *Anat. Rec.* 159, 371–378. doi: 10.1002/ar.1091590406

Vasquez, C., Benamer, N., and Morley, G. E. (2011). The cardiac fibroblast: functional and electrophysiological considerations in healthy and diseased hearts. *J. Cardiovasc. Pharmacol.* 57, 380–388. doi: 10.1097/FJC.0b013e31820cda19

Vasquez, C., Mohandas, P., Louie, K. L., Benamer, N., Bapat, A. C., and Morley, G. E. (2010). Enhanced fibroblast-myocyte interactions in response to cardiac injury. *Circ. Res.* 107, 1011–1020. doi: 10.1161/CIRCRESAHA.110.227421

Verheule, S., Sato, T., Everett, T., Engle, S. K., Otten, D., Rubart-von der, L. M., et al. (2004). Increased vulnerability to atrial fibrillation in transgenic mice with selective atrial fibrosis caused by overexpression of TGF-beta1. *Circ. Res.* 94, 1458–1465. doi: 10.1161/01.RES.0000129579.59664.9d

Wolf, R. M., Glynn, P., Hashemi, S., Zarei, K., Mitchell, C. C., Anderson, M. E., et al. (2013). Atrial fibrillation and sinus node dysfunction in human ankyrin-B syndrome: a computational analysis. *Am. J. Physiol. Heart Circ. Physiol.* 304, H1253–H1266. doi: 10.1152/ajpheart.00734.2012

Wu, Y., and Anderson, M. E. (2014). CaMKII in sinoatrial node physiology and dysfunction. *Front. Pharmacol.* 5:48. doi: 10.3389/fphar.2014.00048

Yeh, Y. H., Burstein, B., Qi, X. Y., Sakabe, M., Chartier, D., Comtois, P., et al. (2009). Funny current downregulation and sinus node dysfunction associated with atrial tachyarrhythmia: a molecular basis for tachycardia-bradycardia syndrome. *Circulation* 119, 1576–1585. doi: 10.1161/CIRCULATIONAHA.108.789677

9

Role of the intercalated disc in cardiac propagation and arrhythmogenesis

Andre G. Kleber* and Jeffrey E. Saffitz

Department of Pathology, Beth Israel Medical Center, Harvard Medical School, Boston, MA, USA

***Correspondence:**
Andre G. Kleber, Department of Pathology, Beth Israel Deaconess Medical Center, Harvard Medical School, Dana 752, 330 Brookline Avenue, Boston, MA 02215, USA
e-mail: akleber@bidmc.harvard.edu

This review article discusses mechanisms underlying impulse propagation in cardiac muscle with specific emphasis on the role of the cardiac cell-to-cell junction, called the "intercalated disc." The first part of this review deals with the role of gap junction channels, formed by connexin proteins, as a determinant of impulse propagation. It is shown that, depending on the underlying structure of the cellular network, decreasing the conductance of gap junction channels (so-called "electrical uncoupling") may either only slow, or additionally stabilize propagation and reverse unidirectional propagation block to bidirectional propagation. This is because the safety factor for propagation increases with decreasing intercellular electrical conductance. The role of heterogeneous connexin expression, which may be present in disease states, is also discussed. The hypothesis that so-called ephaptic impulse transmission plays a role in heart and can substitute for electrical coupling has been revived recently. Whereas ephaptic transmission can be demonstrated in theoretical simulations, direct experimental evidence has not yet been presented. The second part of this review deals with the interaction of three protein complexes at the intercalated disc: (1) desmosomal and adherens junction proteins, (2) ion channel proteins, and (3) gap junction channels consisting of connexins. Recent work has revealed multiple interactions between these three protein complexes which occur, at least in part, at the level of protein trafficking. Such interactions are likely to play an important role in the pathogenesis of arrhythmogenic cardiomyopathy, and may reveal new therapeutic concepts and targets.

Keywords: propagation velocity in heart, electrical-cell-to-cell coupling, intercalated disc, cardiac connexins, discontinuous propagation

INTRODUCTION

The observation that the heart is composed of billions of individual cardiac myocytes but functions as a highly coordinated syncytial structure has fascinated scientists since the nineteenth century (Engelmann, 1877). In 1952, Weidmann used classical electrical cable analysis and showed that electrical current injected into a single cell in a Purkinje strand spread along a distance considerably larger than the length of the cell itself, thus suggesting the free movement of electrical charge from one cell to another (Weidmann, 1952). This finding, implicating low resistance pathways between cardiac myocytes, was later confirmed in ventricular muscle (Weidmann, 1966). Since this pioneering work, gap junction channels bridging the cytoplasm of neighboring cells, and forming pathways for cell-to-cell flow of electrical current and small molecules, have been characterized in detail at the genetic, cell biological, and biophysical levels of organization and function (Harris, 2001; Valiunas et al., 2005).

With respect to the physiological role of the cardiac cell-cell interface, the "intercalated disc," the function and role of gap junctions, hosting channels composed of variety of connexins with regional specificity, has been the focus of many experimental and theoretical studies during the past decades (Kleber and Rudy, 2004). While the importance of gap junctions for cardiac function is not disputed, more recent work has shown that the intercalated disc also hosts a number of ion channels, including Na^+ channels and K^+ channels. Together with the proteins forming fascia adherens junctions and desmosomes (which interconnect actin filaments and intermediate filaments of adjacent cells), gap junction channels and ion channels form macromolecular protein complexes in the intercalated disc, each essential for cardiac function (Delmar and Liang, 2012; Delmar and Makita, 2012). Recent experimental studies suggest regulatory interactions between these functional complexes and their involvement in the pathogenesis of important cardiac diseases.

The goal of this review is to discuss (1) the role of gap junction channels and ion channels expressed in the intercalated disc in electrical propagation, and (2) interactions between these functional complexes and their role in disease.

THE CARDIAC CONNEXINS AND ELECTRICAL PROPAGATION

THE CARDIAC CONNEXINS Cx43, Cx40 AND Cx45

In atrial and ventricular myocardium, gap junction channels are formed by three connexins, connexin43 (Cx43), connexin40 (Cx40) and connexin45 (Cx45) (Kanter et al., 1992; Davis et al., 1994). A fourth connexin has been described in the atrioventricular node in mice and humans (Cx30.2 and Cx31.9, respectively)

(Bukauskas et al., 2006). Atrial myocardium gap junctions consist mainly of Cx43 and Cx40, ventricular myocardium of Cx43, and the specific ventricular conducting system of Cx40. Cx45 is present in the sinus and the atrio-ventricular nodes, and in small amounts in the atria and ventricles. Knowledge about the functional roles of Cx43, Cx40, and Cx45 in the cardiac intercalated disc has been derived mainly from experiments in heterologous cell systems and some questions remain unresolved. Common to all cardiac gap junction channels is the apposition and non-covalent binding of two juxtaposed connexons (each expressed in the intercalated disc by adjacent cells) to form a complete gap junction channel, and the composition of each connexon by six connexin molecules (Moreno, 2004; Cottrell and Burt, 2005). Pure homotypic and homomeric gap junction channels composed of Cx43 or Cx40 have relatively large electrical conductances (60–120 pS, and 175–210 pS, respectively) whereas Cx45 forms a small conductance channel of 30–40 pS (Moreno, 2004).

While it is often stated that the dominance of Cx43 in the ventricle and of Cx40 in the Purkinje system are responsible for the relatively high propagation velocities observed in these tissues, and that the presence of Cx45 contributes importantly to the low velocity in the atrio-ventricular node (for values see Kleber et al., 2011), the co-existence of Cx43 and Cx45 in the ventricles, and of Cx40, Cx43 and Cx45 in the atria, likely creates more complex biological interactions in which a connexin species present in relatively low amounts may have an important effect on conduction or modulate other aspects of cell-cell communication. For example, Cx45 has been shown to form heteromeric connexons with Cx43 (Moreno, 2004), and probably Cx40 (Desplantez et al., 2012) thereby reducing the unitary conductance of the channels. It has also been postulated that although Cx45 may not contribute much to intercellular electrical conductance by forming homomeric/homotypic channels, it could function as a modulator of gap junction size (Grikscheit et al., 2008).

In atrial myocardium Cx40 and Cx43 co-localize in the intercalated disc, but the role of mixed Cx43/Cx40 gap junction channels has not been clarified. In heterologous expression systems, it has been shown that Cx43 and Cx40 chemically aggregate, but the question of whether heteromeric connexons and heteromeric/heterotypic Cx43/Cx40 gap junction channels contribute significantly to intercellular current flow in heart remains disputed (Beyer et al., 2001; Cottrell and Burt, 2005). Another question of functional importance is whether expression and/or trafficking of Cx43 and Cx40 are coordinately regulated in atrial tissue. In human atrial tissue, for example, local expression levels of Cx43 and Cx40 affect local propagation velocity; high levels of Cx40 relative to Cx43 are inversely correlated with propagation velocity, whereas high levels of Cx43 relative to Cx40 correlate directly with local propagation velocity (Kanagaratnam et al., 2004). These results are in line with findings in cultured mouse atrial myocytes, in which genetic ablation of Cx40 is associated with *increased* propagation velocity and more Cx43 immmunosignal at the intercalated disc, whereas ablation of Cx43 leads to a decrease of propagation velocity and a concomitant reduction in Cx40 and Cx45 signal (Beauchamp et al., 2006; Desplantez et al., 2012). A further indication that atrial connexins are coordinately regulated comes from analysis of intercellular conductances in cells transfected with mutant Cx43 (Thibodeau et al., 2010). In this situation, co-expression of mutated Cx43 with wild type Cx43, or co-expression of mutated Cx43 with wild type Cx43 and wild type Cx40 produced a transdominant negative effect of the mutated Cx43 on intercellular conductance, indicating interactions between mutated Cx43 and wild type Cx43 and Cx40, possibly at the level of trafficking. Although basic mechanisms of connexin forward and retrograde trafficking have been defined recently (Smyth et al., 2010, 2012, 2014; Smyth and Shaw, 2012a,b), interactions between Cx43 and Cx40 and the resultant effects in cardiac disease remain largely unclarified.

THE EFFECT ON PROPAGATION OF CONNEXIN COMPARTMENTATION AT THE CELL SURFACE

Immediately after birth ventricular myocytes have a spindle-like shape and gap junction plaques are distributed at more or less regular intervals around the cell perimeter (Beauchamp et al., 2004). During development of the adult phenotype, gap junctions become concentrated at the cell border, and fewer junctions (~30%) are located in the lateral cell membrane (Hoyt et al., 1989). In an elegant theoretical study specifically addressing the effect of gap junction distribution on propagation (Spach et al., 2000), the authors compared *two real cell types*, small neonatal canine ventricular myocytes with neonatal gap junction pattern and large adult canine ventricular myocytes with typical adult end-to-end gap junction distribution pattern, to *two virtual cell types*, small neonatal myocytes with the adult gap junction distribution pattern and large adult myocytes with the neonatal pattern. This approach enabled the authors to separate the effects of cell size from the effects of gap junction distribution on propagation. The surprising result was that the pattern of gap junction distribution exerts only a minor influence on propagation, while cell size (as expected) has a strong influence on propagation velocity.

THE PRINCIPLE OF ELECTRICAL CELL-TO-CELL COUPLING AND CARDIAC PROPAGATION

Insights into the roles of gap junctions and pathways of low electrical resistance between adjacent cells in propagation were derived originally from theories established in nerve (Hodgkin and Rushton, 1946). For propagation in a linear excitable structure with a homogeneous "intracellular electrical medium," the square root of propagation velocity is proportional to the electrical resistance of the intracellular medium (so-called "square root relationship") (Hodgkin, 1954; Tasaki and Hagiwara, 1957). In heart, the intracellular electrical medium is not homogeneous. Rather, the resistance of the cytoplasm is lower than the resistance of the gap junctions, and cytoplasmic propagation shows a finite conduction time (Fast and Kleber, 1993; Spach and Heidlage, 1995). Yet, for normal electrical coupling in heart and for small deviations thereof, the square root relationship is an approximate predictor of conduction behavior. At medium to high levels of electrical uncoupling, when the resistance of the intercellular barrier increases, the propagation behavior becomes discontinuous (Rudy and Quan, 1987). Discontinuous propagation in a linear strand of cells with uniform electrical uncoupling is resistant to propagation block, and a more than 100-fold increase in gap

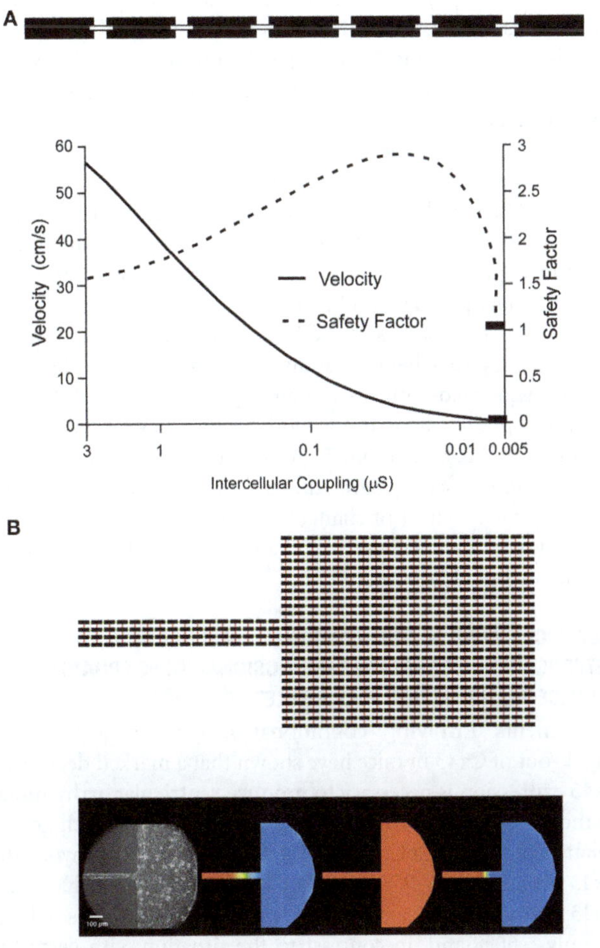

FIGURE 1 | Effect of cell-to-cell coupling on linear (A) vs. discontinuous (B) propagation: (A) depicts schematically a linearly conducting chain of cells coupled by resistors representing the gap junctions (top). The lower part shows the dependence of propagation velocity and safety factor of propagation on cell-to-cell coupling, expressed as conductance in nS. For explanation see text. Reproduced from Shaw and Rudy (1997) with permission. **(B)** The equivalent electrical circuit of a discontinuous tissue structure is illustrated on top. Black rectangles correspond to cells linked by resistors in the x-axis direction (green) and y-axis direction (red). The bottom (left most part) shows experimentally determined propagation in a engineered cell culture of the shape depicted on top (neonatal rat ventricular myocytes). Right of the cell culture picture three propagation maps are coded in color: activation (presence of action potential) is coded in red, resting cells are coded in blue. Normal propagation (left color map) from the strand to the bulk of cells is blocked in the strand, because of source-sink mismatch. Partial uncoupling of the cells restores propagation across the strand and into the bulk (middle color map), whereas as full gap junction uncoupling of the bulk cells produces block at the expansion (right color map). From Rohr et al. (1997) with permission.

junction resistance may be needed for block to occur (**Figure 1A**). This behavior, demonstrated in theoretical studies, was confirmed in engineered strands of neonatal rat ventricular myocytes uncoupled by palmitoleic acid (Rohr et al., 1998), and in strands with complete (i.e., germ-line) genetic ablation of Cx43, in which only a low degree of residual electrical coupling is present due to Cx45 (Beauchamp et al., 2004).

For simple multicellular structures represented, for instance, by a linear strand of cardiac myocytes, this behavior can be explained by the effect of the coupling resistance on the so-called safety factor of propagation (Shaw and Rudy, 1997). The safety factor (SF) can be defined as the ratio of the electrical charge produced by an excited cell and the charge needed to depolarize the same cell. As long as the charge produced by excitation is greater than the charge needed for excitation (SF > 1), propagation is successful. The electrical charge produced by excitation (numerator in the SF formalism) must fulfill two functions which balance one another: it must change the charge at the membrane capacitance and thus produce the action potential, and it must drive the flow of electrical current across cell borders to excite cells downstream of the propagating wavefront. Importantly, increasing cell-to-cell electrical resistance homogeneously will slow propagation, but it will also enhance propagation safety (Shaw and Rudy, 1997) by limiting axial current being dissipated into the downstream cells. It will thus change the balance between the amount of charge flowing into the membrane capacitance and the amount of axial current flow, thereby promoting a higher and faster charge of the capacity and, accordingly, faster action potential upstroke (increase of $dV/dt_{\max}$ of the action potential). The fact that electrical uncoupling slows propagation (initially, as aforementioned with an increased propagation safety) is related to the decrease in axial current exciting the downstream cells. Initially this decrease causes slowing of the charge flowing into the membrane capacitance downstream and conduction slowing. Only when the degree of uncoupling becomes extreme does propagation safety decrease and block occurs (Shaw and Rudy, 1997).

While the safety factor principle, as defined by Shaw and Rudy, is very useful for understanding the general dependence of propagation on electrical coupling and the change in ion channel function (not discussed here) in linear structures, two further complexities warrant discussion: the discontinuous nature of cardiac architecture, and the effects of heterogeneity in expression of cardiac connexins with concomitant heterogeneity in electrical coupling.

THE INTERACTION BETWEEN THE MICRO-STRUCTURE OF THE MYOCARDIAL CELLULAR NETWORK AND PROPAGATION

Normal cardiac myocardium shows a laminar arrangement of myocardial "sheet-like" structures wrapped around the left ventricle and bridged by small trabeculae at regular intervals (Legrice et al., 1995; Pope et al., 2008). These structural discontinuities of the myocardial network occur at a scale similar to the wavelength of electrical excitation (approximately 1 mm) and are predicted to affect the behavior of the electrical waves. Moreover, additional structural changes, caused for instance by fibrosis in pathological settings or with aging (Dolber and Spach, 1987), may enhance this interaction. In the context of this review, it is important to discuss the role of cell-to-cell coupling as modulator of propagation at structural discontinuities, as shown by several theoretical and experimental studies. The ability to pattern 2-dimensional multicellular cardiac structures in culture to produce distinct and reproducible geometrical shapes offers the opportunity to study the effect of cellular network structure on propagation, and to unveil the biophysical behavior of such structures in theoretical studies using equivalent simulated tissue shapes (Rohr et al., 1991).

A typical engineered structure is represented by a small fiber emerging from, or leading into, a large bulk of tissue (so-called "geometrical expansion"). The structural mismatch between the small fiber and the large bulk leads to a corresponding asymmetrical mismatch in electrical propagation. When the small fiber leads into a large bulk, axial current produced by the small amount of cells in the strand has to excite the large bulk. The expansion between the strand and the large mass causes axial electrical current to disperse (current sink), thus, causing current density to decrease. This dispersion causes a local delay in propagation and, in the extreme case, propagation block (Fast and Kleber, 1995a,b; Rohr et al., 1997). In the opposite direction, propagation remains safe, because the large bulk of tissue has only to excite the small mass of cells in the narrow fiber. Thus, the geometrical expansion causes propagation block to be unidirectional. Unidirectional block has been recognized as a prerequisite for initiation of circus movement and re-entry since the beginning of the last century (Mines, 1913). Similar phenomena occur at other types of structural discontinuities such as pivot points and isthmuses, and obey the same biophysical principles (Cabo et al., 1996, 1998; Fast et al., 1996; Kleber and Rudy, 2004).

Importantly, discontinuities in propagation, as described above, are very sensitive to the function of ion currents responsible for excitation and to the state of underlying electrical cell-to-cell coupling. Partial uncoupling of cells at a geometrical expansion produces resistance to dissipation of local current at this site and to a decrease in the current sink (**Figure 1B**). Reduced dispersion of axial current protects the impulse from being blocked at the expansion, a phenomenon that has been demonstrated in experimental and theoretical studies (Fast and Kleber, 1995a,b; Rohr et al., 1997). As a consequence, application of agents causing partial uncoupling of cells can reverse the unidirectional block and allow bidirectional propagation. In whole tissue this is predicted to decrease the probability of initiation of re-entry. In addition to the state of electrical cell-to-cell coupling, the state of the ion channels is an additional player affecting propagation at geometrical expansions, pivot points, and isthmuses. For example, the fact that impulses are delayed locally changes the contributions of the two charge carriers in excitation, the Na^+ inward current and the L-type Ca^{2+} inward current, to successful propagation. At a geometrical expansion the downstream cells are excited with a delay relative to the upstream cells. Accordingly the upstroke of the downstream action potential may occur at a time when the upstroke of the upstream action potential is nearly or fully complete. As a consequence the inward Na^+ current of the upstream cells is "too fast" to excite the downstream cells, and the excitatory charge is delivered instead by the slower L-type Ca^{2+} current. In other words, with increasing discontinuity the flow of L-type Ca^{2+} current becomes increasingly more important as the charge carrier for excitation (Shaw and Rudy, 1997). Proof of this behavior, which has been shown in several theoretical studies (Kleber and Rudy, 2004), is given by the observation, shown in **Figure 1**, that anterograde propagation across a geometrical expansion can be blocked by a Ca^{2+} channel blocker, depending on whether the source-to-sink mismatch is large enough and leads to a local delay >2 ms (Rohr and Kucera, 1997). This effect depends on the underlying state of cell-to-cell coupling, because partial uncoupling will decrease the degree of source-to-sink mismatch for a given structural discontinuity.

Taken together, these observations demonstrate that (1) microscopic tissue structure, (2) expression of ion channels and associated flow of depolarizing currents (Na^+ current and L-type Ca^{2+} current), and (3) cell-to-cell electrical coupling interact to affect local propagation and define local propagation and risk of unidirectional propagation block in tissues with a discontinuous structure such as occurs in the heart. Since microscopic cardiac structure may vary between individuals and may be affected by fibrosis associated with disease and age, it becomes difficult to accurately predict arrhythmogenesis and its prevention by drugs in any individual situation. Experimental and theoretical studies offer more of a general understanding, and the potential arrhythmogenic effect of changes in cell-to-cell coupling cannot be considered independently of changes in the other variables in this highly interactive system.

ELECTRICAL IMPULSE PROPAGATION IN PRESENCE OF VERY LOW AND HETEROGENEOUS CONNEXIN IMMUNOSIGNAL: DOES EPHAPTIC IMPULSE TRANSMISSION PLAY A ROLE?

Experiments involving conditional cardiac myocyte-specific knock-out of Cx43 in mice have shown that a marked decrease in Cx43 expression is necessary to produce ventricular arrhythmias. In the first such study (Gutstein et al., 2001a), in which genetic ablation of Cx43 by a Cre/loxP system decreased total myocardial Cx43 protein by 86–95% associated with a marked reduction in Cx43 immunosignal, electrical propagation velocity was reduced by only ~50% and, in contrast to the situation with germ-line knock-out of Cx43, mortality was delayed by 15–30 days. In two subsequent studies, cardiac myocyte-specific genetic approaches were used to produce a progressive decrease in Cx43 expression with age (Danik et al., 2004) or to create a mosaic of ventricular tissues showing either normal or absent Cx43 expression (Gutstein et al., 2001b). In the first model, significant propagation slowing occurred only when the amount of Cx43 immunosignal decreased by ≥50%, and malignant ventricular arrhythmias were initiated if Cx43 immunosignal was ≤18%. In the second model, mosaic expression caused much more irregular electrical excitation patterns and marked arrhythmogenesis, suggesting that not only the average degree of ventricular Cx43 expression but also the distribution patterns and scale of heterogeneity might be important. In a subsequent study, intercellular conductance measured by dual whole cell voltage clamp in pairs of adult rat ventricular myocytes with genetic Cx43 ablation was dramatically reduced from 588 to 10 nS (Yao et al., 2003). Since impulse propagation was reduced by only 50% in tissue composed of the same cells (with conditional cardiac-specific Cx43 knockout associated with a marked decrease of Cx43 immunosignal), these observations raised the question of whether propagation of the cardiac impulse could occur in the absence of electrical cell-to-cell coupling. In fact, this phenomenon, so-called ephaptic impulse transmission, due to local circuit current at the intercalated disc, had been postulated in the 1960s (Sperelakis et al., 1960) and proposed as an alternative to the role of gap junction channels (Weidmann, 1993).

Theoretical studies have investigated the possible role of ephaptic impulse transmission (also termed "field effect transmission") in myocardium using computer models that take into account the presence of Na^+ channels at the intercalated disc (Kucera et al., 2002; Mori et al., 2008; Veeraraghavan et al., 2014). The key difference in modeling an electrical equivalent circuit for ephaptic transmission relative to earlier models is the focus on the pool of Na^+ channels located within the intercalated disc, which in biophysical terms, represents a narrow cleft with an electrical resistance higher than the normal extracellular resistance. As a consequence, excitation of the upstream cell by inward flow of Na^+ current establishes a voltage gradient between the cleft space and the normal extracellular space, which acts to depolarize the cleft space and the Na^+ channels in the downstream cell facing the cleft. The excitatory effect on the downstream cell, which theoretically may occur in the absence of resistive coupling by gap junctions, depends critically on the cleft width (determining cleft resistance) and the extent to which Na^+ channels are clustered in the intercalated disc. These models also suggest that Na^+ ions accumulate with narrowing cleft width, a phenomenon that decreases the electrochemical gradient for Na^+ and is, therefore, expected to decrease Na^+ current (Kucera et al., 2002; Mori et al., 2008).

The hypothesis that ephaptic transmission occurs in the heart under conditions of marked cell-to-cell uncoupling was put forward as an alternative idea to explain why propagation velocity is only moderately reduced when Cx43 levels are apparently very low, such as occurs in mouse hearts following conditional cardiac myocyte-specific knockout of Cx43. However, its existence has never been proven experimentally. In pairs of cultured neonatal myocytes the existence of ephaptic transmission has been ruled out (Beauchamp et al., 2004). In pairs of ventricular myocytes with germline genetic ablation of Cx43 (i.e., not dependent on the action of Cre recombinase) there is residual electrical coupling (about 5% of normal) due to the presence of gap junction channels formed by Cx45. If these cells are chemically uncoupled, electrical impulse transfer is immediately and reversibly interrupted, while the cells remain excitable by field stimulation, demonstrating that in this setting ephaptic transmission cannot substitute for resistive coupling by gap junctions (Beauchamp et al., 2004).

An attempt to experimentally elucidate the mechanism of impulse propagation in ventricular tissue with inhomogeneous reduction in connexin distribution has been made by (1) quantifying the relationship between the amount of Cx43 at the intercalated disc (as measured by immunohistochemistry) and intercellular electrical conductance across the intercalated disc (McCain et al., 2012), and (2) engineering strands of neonatal mouse ventricular myocytes composed of fixed mixtures of wild type myocytes and cells with genetic Cx43 ablation (Beauchamp et al., 2012). Using this approach, it was first shown that the amount of Cx43 quantified immunohistochemically correlates linearly with electrical conductance, but low levels of conductance can be measured under conditions in which Cx43 signal is below the level of detection using conventional indirect immunofluorescence methods (McCain et al., 2012). In other words, the absence of detectable Cx43 immunosignal does not exclude residual electrical coupling and impulse transmission. In another study (Beauchamp et al., 2012), recently supported by theoretical work (Prudat and Kucera, 2014), it was shown that in tissue with heterogeneously distributed Cx43 expression, fast propagation can be maintained by meandering propagation involving cells with higher Cx43 levels (**Figure 2**). Marked propagation slowing is observed only when the proportion of Cx43-null cells falls below 50%. Moreover, the overall amount of apparent Cx43 immunosignal in such tissues markedly underestimates the percentage of cells expressing normal levels of Cx43 because no Cx43 immunofluorescence is detectable at boundaries between Cx43 expressing myocytes and cells with genetically ablated Cx43 expression (Beauchamp et al., 2012). In conclusion, the observation of relatively preserved propagation at low and inhomogeneous levels of Cx43 expression can be accounted for by cell-to-cell impulse transmission solely involving gap junction channels. The existence of ephaptic transmission as an additional modulator of cardiac impulse propagation has yet to be clearly demonstrated experimentally, although it can be simulated theoretically within narrow limits of specific variables. More sophisticated experimental studies will be required to clarify this point.

INTERACTIONS BETWEEN DESMOSOMAL PROTEINS, ION CHANNELS AND CONNEXINS AT THE INTERCALATED DISC

In the previous paragraphs, this review has focused on the role of gap junctions in impulse transmission and propagation. Ion channels were invoked in the discussion insofar as they might theoretically play a role in cell-to-cell transmission of the electrical impulse. Now, we will discuss mutual interactions between (i) desmosomal and fascia adherens proteins, (ii) connexins and (ii) ion channels expressed in the intercalated disc. New insights into such interactions have emerged recently, stimulated in large part by work to understand mechanisms in arrhythmogenic cardiomyopathy. It thus forms an interesting link to translational medicine and is an example how findings in translational science can feed back to the understanding of basic mechanisms of cardiac function. It mostly involves defining the effect of genetic ablation of components of one of these protein complexes or the use of cells transfected with mutant proteins implicated in human disease, and the subsequent association of the findings in animal models with the human phenotype.

An important principle underlying this work is that major classes of ion channels responsible for generating the cardiac action potential are partitioned in different membrane compartments such as the T-tubular invaginations, the (lateral) surface membrane and the intercalated discs (Cohen, 1996; Kucera et al., 2002; Maier et al., 2004; Petitprez et al., 2011; Milstein et al., 2012). The specificity of Na^+ channel partitioning has been further explained by observations that channels in specific locations are associated with specific regulatory proteins. This includes dystrophin in the case of Nav1.5 channels at the lateral membrane, and the MAGUK protein SAP97 for Nav1.5 at the intercalated disc (Petitprez et al., 2011). It has also been shown that SAP97, which has PDZ binding motifs for several ion channels, is an important

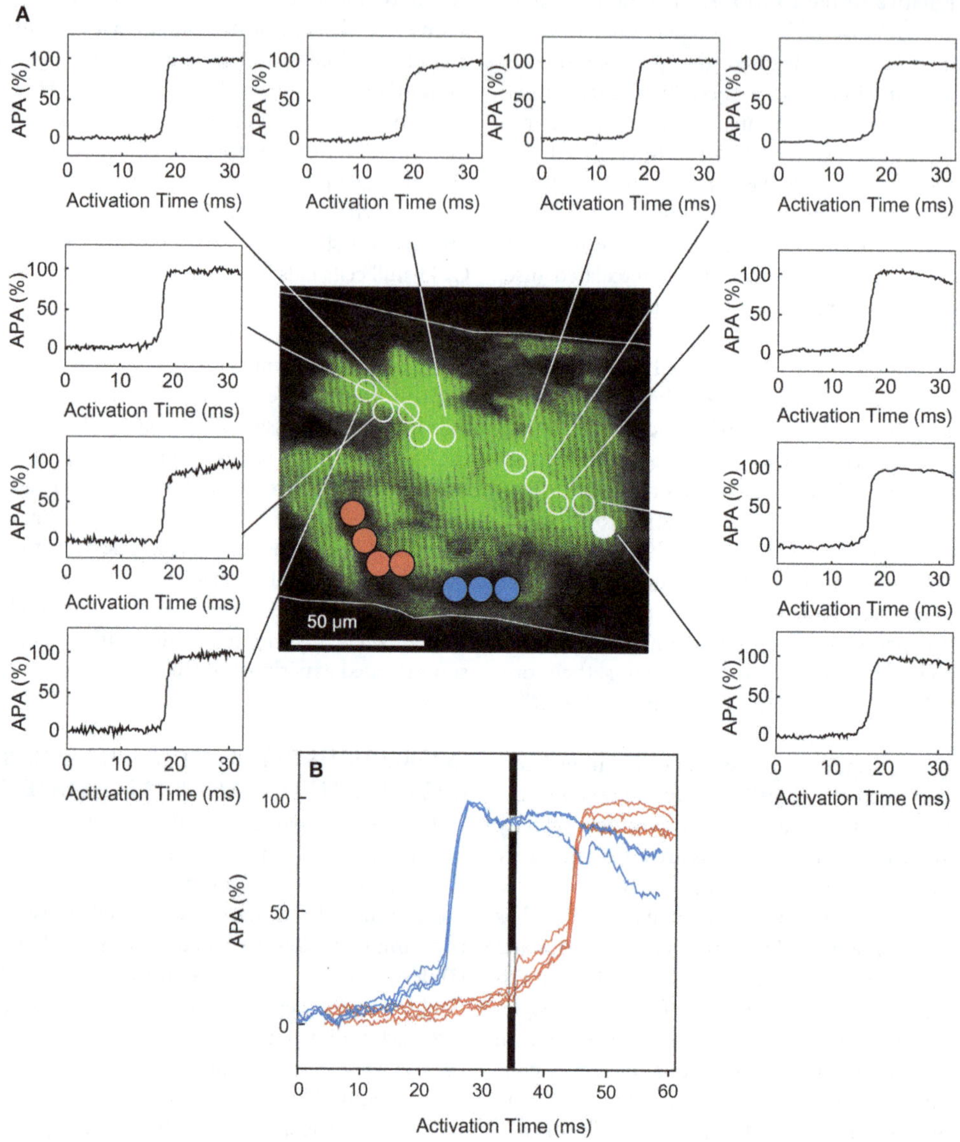

FIGURE 2 | Propagation in engineered cardiac tissue with heterogeneous expression of Cx43. (A) An engineered cardiac strand is produced by 50–50 mixtures of wild type cells (GFP-labeled) and cells with genetic ablation of Cx43 (no GFP-labeling). Electrical stimulation of this strand produces rapid meandering propagation across the Cx43 expressing cell cluster. The action potentials in **(B)** compare excitation of the area with Cx43 deletion (colored action potential) with the first and last action potentials of the Cx43 expressing cluster (which, at this time scale, appear to be nearly superimposed). This comparison illustrates a marked pre-delay and delay in excitation of the areas not expressing Cx43 with respect to the wild type cluster. However, all cells of the strands are eventually excited. From Beauchamp et al. (2012) with permission.

regulator of the intercalated disc fractions of Nav1.5 and Kir2.1 (Milstein et al., 2012). At the same time, recent studies involving knock-in of Nav1.5 channels lacking the PDZ binding motifs have implicated a more complex role for SAP97 involving localization of ion channels at the lateral membrane (Shy et al., 2014). Within the intercalated disc Nav1.5 channels have been shown to closely localize with Cx43 in a region around the gap junction plaque termed the perinexus (Rhett et al., 2012).

Recent studies have identified mechanistic links between proteins of the desmosome, Nav1.5 and Cx43. For example, silencing of plakophilin-2, an armadillo repeat protein contributing to the protein anchor of desmosomal cadherins, leads to a marked decrease in Na^+ inward current via Nav1.5 at the intercalated disc (Sato et al., 2009). Interactions between Cx43 and Nav1.5 expression at the intercalated disc are also suggested by observations that germline ablation of Cx43 in cultured neonatal rat atrial myoctes leads to a nearly 50% decrease in whole cell Na^+ current (Desplantez et al., 2012). Ankyrin-G, a polypeptide involved in surface expression and targeting of membrane channels, has been shown to affect plakophillin-2 and Nav1.5 expression at the intercalated disc (Sato et al., 2011; Makara et al., 2014). The role of ankyrin-G in the regulation of Cx43 is less clear. While silencing of ankyrin-G decreased Cx43 and intercellular electrical conductance (Sato et al., 2011), no effect of cardiospecific knock-out of ankyrin-G on Cx43 was observed (Makara et al., 2014). Taken together, these observations highlight important, although as yet incompletely understood, interactions among regulatory proteins at the intercalated disc, desmosomal proteins, connexins and ion channels (Nav1.5 and probably others) at the intercalated disc which likely play a significant role in human heart disease.

Additional knowledge about these interactions has come from work defining the molecular pathology of arrhythmogenic cardiomyopathy, a disease in which approximately 60% of cases have (mainly dominant) mutations in desmosomal proteins (plakoglobin, desmoplakin, plakophilin-2, desmocollin-2 and desmoglein-2) (Saffitz et al., 2009; Sen-Chowdhry et al., 2010). For reasons not well understood, the majority of these cases are associated with a decrease in the amount of plakoglobin (γ-catenin) in the intercalated disc and a concomitant decrease in Cx43, raising the possibility that plakoglobin might play a central role in disease pathogenesis (Asimaki et al., 2009). Reductions in the levels of desmosomal plakoglobin and Cx43 at the intercalated disc apparently occur in the presence of normal cellular levels of these proteins, thus implicating a protein trafficking defect as an underlying mechanism. Arrhythmogenic cardiomyopathy is also associated with a marked decrease in Nav1.5 expression, as inferred from experiments involving cultures of neonatal rat ventricular myocytes transfected to express mutant forms of plakoglobin or plakophilin-2 known to cause the human disease. In both situations, a $\geq$50% decrease in Na^+ inward current has been observed (Asimaki et al., 2014).

A potentially important insight into the underlying molecular interactions came from discovery of a drug in a high throughput chemical screen in zebrafish. This small molecule, SB216763, annotated as an inhibitor of glycogen synthase kinase-3β (GSK-3β), prevents the development of cardiac failure in a fish model of arrhythmogenic cardiomyopathy and also prevents changes in the cardiac action potential and decreased currents flowing through Nav1.5 and Kir2.1 in isolated zebrafish ventricular myocytes. SB216763 also blocked expression of disease-related changes in cultured neonatal rat myocytes transfected to express known disease alleles (Asimaki et al., 2014). Furthermore, abnormal subcellular distribution of SAP97 is reversed by SB216763 in cardiac myocytes derived from pluripotent stem cells of 2 human probands carrying plakophilin-2 mutations. The exact role of GSK-3β and its inhibition in the disease phenotype is currently under investigation. Nevertheless, our current knowledge of disease mechanisms in arrhythmogenic cardiomyopathy suggests that expression of desmosomal proteins, connexins and at least two important ion channels (Nav1.5 and Kir2.1) are all regulated interactively at the level of trafficking.

SUMMARY: CELL-TO-CELL COUPLING, ARRHYTHMOGENESIS AND PROPAGATION

In the classical literature, the effects of changes in cell-to-cell coupling are mostly discussed using simple models of linear propagation. In such models, a decrease in cell-to-cell coupling will reduce propagation velocity and, accordingly, decrease the wavelength of excitation. As a consequence an increase in the likelihood of re-entry of circulating excitation is to be expected. This review attempts to summarize and discuss both the classical and contemporary literature which, taken together, reveals a much more complex role for cell-to-cell coupling in normal physiology and arrhythmogenesis. These complexities involve heterogeneous expression of connexins, the structure of the cellular network and expression of ion channels in the intercalated disc all being interactively affected by common regulators of expression. Moreover, disease phenotypes are likely to involve changes in multiple proteins affecting electrical propagation. This complexity of the arrhythmogenic substrate makes it difficult to exactly predict the exact impact of changes in cell-to-cell coupling as an event isolated from all other factors. At the extreme—as discussed in this review—electrical uncoupling may weaken the effect of a discontinuous structure and actually stabilize propagation. Theoretical simulation of these complex interactions including the multitude of variables is certainly a means to improve our understanding of the role in arrhythmogenesis.

The fact that a single disease may produce hundreds of changes at the level of functional proteins, which may be arrhythmogenic in concert, also casts doubt on the concept that targeting a single peripheral protein, as only one of the multitude of variables, will effectively reduce arrhythmogenesis. Instead so-called "upstream drugs" targeting an important common pathway of dysregulation and reversing a pathological phenotype are likely to be more effective. The discovery of an apparent GSK-3β inhibitor as a substance globally rescuing the arrhythmogenic cardiomyopathy phenotype supports this concept.

REFERENCES

Asimaki, A., Kapoor, S., Plovie, E., Karin Arndt, A., Adams, E., Liu, Z., et al. (2014). Identification of a new modulator of the intercalated disc in a zebrafish model of arrhythmogenic cardiomyopathy. *Sci. Transl. Med.* 6, 240–274. doi: 10.1126/scitranslmed.3008008

Asimaki, A., Tandri, H., Huang, H., Halushka, M. K., Gautam, S., Basso, C., et al. (2009). A new diagnostic test for arrhythmogenic right ventricular cardiomyopathy. *N. Engl. J. Med.* 360, 1075–1084. doi: 10.1056/NEJMoa0808138

Beauchamp, P., Choby, C., Desplantez, T., de Peyer, K., Green, K., Yamada, K. A., et al. (2004). Electrical propagation in synthetic ventricular myocyte strands from germline connexin43 knockout mice. *Circ. Res.* 95, 170–178. doi: 10.1161/01.RES.0000134923.05174.2f

Beauchamp, P., Desplantez, T., McCain, M. L., Li, W., Asimaki, A., Rigoli, G., et al. (2012). Electrical coupling and propagation in engineered ventricular myocardium with heterogeneous expression of connexin43. *Circ. Res.* 110, 1445–1453. doi: 10.1161/CIRCRESAHA.111.259705

Beauchamp, P., Yamada, K. A., Baertschi, A. J., Green, K., Kanter, E. M., Saffitz, J. E., et al. (2006). Relative contributions of connexins 40 and 43 to atrial impulse propagation in synthetic strands of neonatal and fetal murine cardiomyocytes. *Circ. Res.* 99, 1216–1224. doi: 10.1161/01.RES.0000250607.34498.b4

Beyer, E. C., Gemel, J., Martinez, A., Berthoud, V. M., Valiunas, V., Moreno, A. P., et al. (2001). Heteromeric mixing of connexins: compatibility of partners and functional consequences. *Cell Commun. Adhes.* 8, 199–204. doi: 10.3109/15419060109080723

Bukauskas, F. F., Kreuzberg, M. M., Rackauskas, M., Bukauskiene, A., Bennett, M. V., Verselis, V. K., et al. (2006). Properties of mouse connexin 30.2 and human connexin 31.9 hemichannels: implications for atrioventricular conduction in the heart. *Proc. Natl. Acad. Sci. U.S.A.* 103, 9726–9731. doi: 10.1073/pnas.0603372103

Cabo, C., Pertsov, A. M., Davidenko, J. M., Baxter, W. T., Gray, R. A., and Jalife, J. (1996). Vortex shedding as a precursor of turbulent electrical activity in cardiac muscle. *Biophys. J.* 70, 1105–1111. doi: 10.1016/S0006-3495(96)79691-1

Cabo, C., Pertsov, A. M., Davidenko, J. M., and Jalife, J. (1998). Electrical turbulence as a result of the critical curvature for propagation in cardiac tissue. *Chaos* 8, 116–126. doi: 10.1063/1.166292

Cohen, S. A. (1996). Immunocytochemical localization of rH1 sodium channel in adult rat heart atria and ventricle. Presence in terminal intercalated disks. *Circulation* 94, 3083–3086. doi: 10.1161/01.CIR.94.12.3083

Cottrell, G. T., and Burt, J. M. (2005). Functional consequences of heterogeneous gap junction channel formation and its influence in health and disease. *Biochim. Biophys. Acta* 1711, 126–141. doi: 10.1016/j.bbamem.2004.11.013

Danik, S. B., Liu, F., Zhang, J., Suk, H. J., Morley, G. E., Fishman, G. I., et al. (2004). Modulation of cardiac gap junction expression and arrhythmic susceptibility. *Circ. Res.* 95, 1035–1041. doi: 10.1161/01.RES.0000148664.33695.2a

Davis, L. M., Kanter, H. L., Beyer, E. C., and Saffitz, J. E. (1994). Distinct gap junction protein phenotypes in cardiac tissues with disparate conduction properties. *J. Am. Coll. Cardiol.* 24, 1124–1132. doi: 10.1016/0735-1097(94)90879-6

Delmar, M., and Liang, F. X. (2012). Connexin43 and the regulation of intercalated disc function. *Heart Rhythm* 9, 835–838. doi: 10.1016/j.hrthm.2011.10.028

Delmar, M., and Makita, N. (2012). Cardiac connexins, mutations and arrhythmias. *Curr. Opin. Cardiol.* 27, 236–241. doi: 10.1097/HCO.0b013e328352220e

Desplantez, T., McCain, M. L., Beauchamp, P., Rigoli, G., Rothen-Rutishauser, B., Parker, K. K., et al. (2012). Connexin43 ablation in foetal atrial myocytes decreases electrical coupling, partner connexins, and sodium current. *Cardiovasc. Res.* 94, 58–65. doi: 10.1093/cvr/cvs025

Dolber, P. C., and Spach, M. S. (1987). Thin collagenous septa in cardiac muscle. *Anat. Rec.* 218, 45–55. doi: 10.1002/ar.1092180109

Engelmann, T. (1877). Vergleichende Untersuchungen zur Lehre von den Muskel- und Nervenelektricitat. *Pfluegers Arch.* 15, 116–148. doi: 10.1007/BF01628342

Fast, V. G., Darrow, B. J., Saffitz, J. E., and Kleber, A. G. (1996). Anisotropic activation spread in heart cell monolayers assessed by high-resolution optical mapping. Role of tissue discontinuities. *Circ. Res.* 79, 115–127. doi: 10.1161/01.RES.79.1.115

Fast, V. G., and Kleber, A. G. (1993). Microscopic conduction in cultured strands of neonatal rat heart cells measured with voltage-sensitive dyes. *Circ. Res.* 73, 914–925. doi: 10.1161/01.RES.73.5.914

Fast, V. G., and Kleber, A. G. (1995a). Block of impulse propagation at an abrupt tissue expansion: evaluation of the critical strand diameter in 2- and 3-dimensional computer models. *Cardiovasc. Res.* 30, 449–459. doi: 10.1016/S0008-6363(95)00071-2

Fast, V. G., and Kleber, A. G. (1995b). Cardiac tissue geometry as a determinant of unidirectional conduction block: assessment of microscopic excitation spread by optical mapping in patterned cell cultures and in a computer model. *Cardiovasc. Res.* 29, 697–707. doi: 10.1016/S0008-6363(96) 88643-3

Grikscheit, K., Thomas, N., Bruce, A. F., Rothery, S., Chan, J., Severs, N. J., et al. (2008). Coexpression of connexin 45 with connexin 43 decreases gap junction size. *Cell Commun. Adhes.* 15, 185–193. doi: 10.1080/1541906080 2013943

Gutstein, D. E., Morley, G. E., Tamaddon, H., Vaidya, D., Schneider, M. D., Chen, J., et al. (2001a). Conduction slowing and sudden arrhythmic death in mice with cardiac-restricted inactivation of connexin43. *Circ. Res.* 88, 333–339. doi: 10.1161/01.RES.88.3.333

Gutstein, D. E., Morley, G. E., Vaidya, D., Liu, F., Chen, F. L., Stuhlmann, H., et al. (2001b). Heterogeneous expression of Gap junction channels in the heart leads to conduction defects and ventricular dysfunction. *Circulation* 104, 1194–1199. doi: 10.1161/hc3601.093990

Harris, A. L. (2001). Emerging issues of connexin channels: biophysics fills the gap. *Q. Rev. Biophys.* 34, 325–472. doi: 10.1017/S0033583501003705

Hodgkin, A. L. (1954). A note on conduction velocity. *J. Physiol.* 125, 221–224.

Hodgkin, A. L., and Rushton, W. A. (1946). The electrical constants of a crustacean nerve fibre. *Proc. R. Soc. Med.* 134, 444–479. doi: 10.1098/rspb.1946.0024

Hoyt, R. H., Cohen, M. L., and Saffitz, J. E. (1989). Distribution and three-dimensional structure of intercellular junctions in canine myocardium. *Circ. Res.* 64, 563–574. doi: 10.1161/01.RES.64.3.563

Kanagaratnam, P., Cherian, A., Stanbridge, R. D., Glenville, B., Severs, N. J., and Peters, N. S. (2004). Relationship between connexins and atrial activation during human atrial fibrillation. *J. Cardiovasc. Electrophysiol.* 15, 206–216. doi: 10.1046/j.1540-8167.2004.03280.x

Kanter, H., Saffitz, J., and Beyer, E. (1992). Cardiac myocytes express multiple gap junction proteins. *Circ. Res.* 70, 438–444. doi: 10.1161/01.RES.70.2.438

Kleber, A. G., Janse, M. J., and Fast, V. G. (2011). "Normal and abnormal conduction in the heart," in *Handbook of Physiology, The Cardiovascular System, The Heart*, 455–530. doi: 10.1002/cphy.cp020112

Kleber, A. G., and Rudy, Y. (2004). Basic mechanisms of cardiac impulse propagation and associated arrhythmias. *Physiol. Rev.* 84, 431–488. doi: 10.1152/physrev.00025.2003

Kucera, J. P., Rohr, S., and Rudy, Y. (2002). Localization of sodium channels in intercalated disks modulates cardiac conduction. *Circ. Res.* 91, 1176–1182. doi: 10.1161/01.RES.0000046237.54156.0A

Legrice, I. J., Smaill, B. H., Chai, L. Z., Edgar, S. G., Gavin, J. B., and Hunter, P. J. (1995). Laminar structure of the heart: ventricular myocyte arrangement and connective tissue architecture in the dog. *Am. J. Physiol.* 269, H571–H582.

Maier, S. K., Westenbroek, R. E., McCormick, K. A., Curtis, R., Scheuer, T., and Catterall, W. A. (2004). Distinct subcellular localization of different sodium channel alpha and beta subunits in single ventricular myocytes from mouse heart. *Circulation* 109, 1421–1427. doi: 10.1161/01.CIR.0000121421.61896.24

Makara, M. A., Curran, J., Little, S., Musa, H., Polina, I., Smith, S. A., et al. (2014). Ankyrin-G coordinates intercalated disc signaling platform to regulate cardiac excitability *in vivo*. *Circ. Res.* doi: 10.1161/CIRCRESAHA.115.305154. [Epub ahead of print].

McCain, M. L., Desplantez, T., Geisse, N. A., Rothen-Rutishauser, B., Oberer, H., Parker, K. K., et al. (2012). Cell-to-cell coupling in engineered pairs of rat ventricular cardiomyocytes: relation between Cx43 immunofluorescence and intercellular electrical conductance. *Am. J. Physiol.* 302, H443–H450. doi: 10.1152/ajpheart.01218.2010

Milstein, M. L., Musa, H., Balbuena, D. P., Anumonwo, J. M., Auerbach, D. S., Furspan, P. B., et al. (2012). Dynamic reciprocity of sodium and potassium channel expression in a macromolecular complex controls cardiac excitability and arrhythmia. *Proc. Natl. Acad. Sci. U.S.A.* 109, E2134–E2143. doi: 10.1073/pnas.1109370109

Mines, G. R. (1913). On dynamic equilibrium in the heart. *J. Physiol.* 46, 349–383.

Moreno, A. P. (2004). Biophysical properties of homomeric and heteromultimeric channels formed by cardiac connexins. *Cardiovasc. Res.* 62, 276–286. doi: 10.1016/j.cardiores.2004.03.003

Mori, Y., Fishman, G. I., and Peskin, C. S. (2008). Ephaptic conduction in a cardiac strand model with 3D electrodiffusion. *Proc. Natl. Acad. Sci. U.S.A.* 105, 6463–6468. doi: 10.1073/pnas.0801089105

Petitprez, S., Zmoos, A. F., Ogrodnik, J., Balse, E., Raad, N., El-Haou, S., et al. (2011). SAP97 and dystrophin macromolecular complexes determine two pools of cardiac sodium channels Nav1.5 in cardiomyocytes. *Circ. Res.* 108, 294–304. doi: 10.1161/CIRCRESAHA.110.228312

Pope, A. J., Sands, G. B., Smaill, B. H., and Legrice, I. J. (2008). Three-dimensional transmural organization of perimysial collagen in the heart. *Am. J. Physiol. Heart Circ. Physiol.* 295, H1243–H1252. doi: 10.1152/ajpheart.00484.2008

Prudat, Y., and Kucera, J. P. (2014). Nonlinear behaviour of conduction and block in cardiac tissue with heterogeneous expression of connexin 43. *J. Mol. Cell. Cardiol.* 76C, 46–54. doi: 10.1016/j.yjmcc.2014.07.019

Rhett, J. M., Ongstad, E. L., Jourdan, J., and Gourdie, R. G. (2012). Cx43 associates with Na(v)1.5 in the cardiomyocyte perinexus. *J. Membr. Biol.* 245, 411–422. doi: 10.1007/s00232-012-9465-z

Rohr, S., and Kucera, J. P. (1997). Involvement of the calcium inward current in cardiac impulse propagation: induction of unidirectional conduction block by nifedipine and reversal by Bay K 8644. *Biophys. J.* 72, 754–766. doi: 10.1016/S0006-3495(97)78710-1

Rohr, S., Kucera, J. P., Fast, V. G., and Kleber, A. G. (1997). Paradoxical improvement of impulse conduction in cardiac tissue by partial cellular uncoupling. *Science* 275, 841–844. doi: 10.1126/science.275.5301.841

Rohr, S., Kucera, J. P., and Kleber, A. G. (1998). Slow conduction in cardiac tissue, I: effects of a reduction of excitability versus a reduction of electrical coupling on microconduction. *Circ. Res.* 83, 781–794. doi: 10.1161/01.RES.83.8.781

Rohr, S., Schölly, D. M., and Kleber, A. G. (1991). Patterned growth of neonatal rat heart cells in culture: morphological and electrophysiological characterization. *Circ. Res.* 68, 114–130. doi: 10.1161/01.RES.68.1.114

Rudy, Y., and Quan, W. L. (1987). A model study of the effects of the discrete cellular structure on electrical propagation in cardiac tissue. *Circ. Res.* 61, 815–823. doi: 10.1161/01.RES.61.6.815

Saffitz, J. E., Asimaki, A., and Huang, H. (2009). Arrhythmogenic right ventricular cardiomyopathy: new insights into disease mechanisms and diagnosis. *J. Investig. Med.* 57, 861–864. doi: 10.231/JIM.0b013e3181c5e631

Sato, P. Y., Coombs, W., Lin, X., Nekrasova, O., Green, K. J., Isom, L. L., et al. (2011). Interactions between ankyrin-G, Plakophilin-2, and Connexin43 at the cardiac intercalated disc. *Circ. Res.* 109, 193–201. doi: 10.1161/CIRCRESAHA.111.247023

Sato, P. Y., Musa, H., Coombs, W., Guerrero-Serna, G., Patino, G. A., Taffet, S. M., et al. (2009). Loss of plakophilin-2 expression leads to decreased sodium current and slower conduction velocity in cultured cardiac myocytes. *Circ. Res.* 105, 523–526. doi: 10.1161/CIRCRESAHA.109.201418

Sen-Chowdhry, S., Morgan, R. D., Chambers, J. C., and McKenna, W. J. (2010). Arrhythmogenic cardiomyopathy: etiology, diagnosis, and treatment. *Annu. Rev. Med.* 61, 233–253. doi: 10.1146/annurev.med.052208.130419

Shaw, R. M., and Rudy, Y. (1997). Ionic mechanisms of propagation in cardiac tissue. Roles of the sodium and L-type calcium currents during reduced excitability and decreased gap junction coupling. *Circ. Res.* 81, 727–741. doi: 10.1161/01.RES.81.5.727

Shy, D., Gillet, L., Ogrodnik, J., Albesa, M., Verkerk, A. O., Wolswinkel, R., et al. (2014). PDZ domain-binding motif regulates cardiomyocyte compartment-specific NaV1.5 channel expression and function. *Circulation* 130, 147–160. doi: 10.1161/CIRCULATIONAHA.113.007852

Smyth, J. W., Hong, T. T., Gao, D., Vogan, J. M., Jensen, B. C., Fong, T. S., et al. (2010). Limited forward trafficking of connexin 43 reduces cell-cell coupling in stressed human and mouse myocardium. *J. Clin. Invest.* 120, 266–279. doi: 10.1172/JCI39740

Smyth, J. W., and Shaw, R. M. (2012a). The gap junction life cycle. *Heart* 9, 151–153. doi: 10.1016/j.hrthm.2011.07.028

Smyth, J. W., and Shaw, R. M. (2012b). Visualizing cardiac ion channel trafficking pathways. *Methods Enzymol.* 505, 187–202. doi: 10.1016/B978-0-12-388448-0.00018-8

Smyth, J. W., Vogan, J. M., Buch, P. J., Zhang, S. S., Fong, T. S., Hong, T. T., et al. (2012). Actin cytoskeleton rest stops regulate anterograde traffic of connexin 43 vesicles to the plasma membrane. *Circ. Res.* 110, 978–989. doi: 10.1161/CIRCRESAHA.111.257964

Smyth, J. W., Zhang, S. S., Sanchez, J. M., Lamouille, S., Vogan, J. M., Hesketh, G. G., et al. (2014). A 14-3-3 mode-1 binding motif initiates gap junction internalization during acute cardiac ischemia. *Traffic* 15, 684–699. doi: 10.1111/tra.12169

Spach, M. S., and Heidlage, J. F. (1995). The stochastic nature of cardiac propagation at a microscopic level. Electrical description of myocardial architecture and its application to conduction. *Circ. Res.* 76, 366–380. doi: 10.1161/01.RES.76.3.366

Spach, M. S., Heidlage, J. F., Dolber, P. C., and Barr, R. C. (2000). Electrophysiological effects of remodeling cardiac gap junctions and cell size: experimental and model studies of normal cardiac growth. *Circ. Res.* 86, 302–311. doi: 10.1161/01.RES.86.3.302

Sperelakis, N., Hoshiko, T., and Berne, R. M. (1960). Nonsyncytial nature of cardiac muscle: membrane resistance of single cells. *Am. J. Physiol.* 198, 531–536.

Tasaki, I., and Hagiwara, S. (1957). Capacity of muscle fiber membrane. *Am. J. Physiol.* 188, 423–429.

Thibodeau, I. L., Xu, J., Li, Q., Liu, G., Lam, K., Veinot, J. P., et al. (2010). Paradigm of genetic mosaicism and lone atrial fibrillation: physiological characterization of a connexin 43-deletion mutant identified from atrial tissue. *Circulation* 122, 236–244. doi: 10.1161/CIRCULATIONAHA.110.961227

Valiunas, V., Polosina, Y. Y., Miller, H., Potapova, I. A., Valiuniene, L., Doronin, S., et al. (2005). Connexin-specific cell-to-cell transfer of short interfering RNA by gap junctions. *J. Physiol.* 568, 459–468. doi: 10.1113/jphysiol.2005.090985

Veeraraghavan, R., Poelzing, S., and Gourdie, R. G. (2014). Intercellular electrical communication in the heart: a new, active role for the intercalated disk. *Cell Commun. Adhes.* 21, 161–167. doi: 10.3109/15419061.2014.905932

Weidmann, S. (1952). The electrical constants of Purkinje fibres. *J. Physiol.* 118, 348–360.

Weidmann, S. (1966). The diffusion of radiopotassium across intercalated disks of mammalian cardiac muscle. *J. Physiol.* 187, 323–342.

Weidmann, S. (1993). Cardiac action potentials, membrane currents, and some personal reminiscences. *Annu. Rev. Physiol.* 55, 1–14. doi: 10.1146/annurev.ph.55.030193.000245

Yao, J. A., Gutstein, D. E., Liu, F., Fishman, G. I., and Wit, A. L. (2003). Cell coupling between ventricular myocyte pairs from connexin43-deficient murine hearts. *Circ. Res.* 93, 736–743. doi: 10.1161/01.RES.0000095977.66660.86

10

Na^+ current expression in human atrial myofibroblasts: Identity and functional roles

Jussi T. Koivumäki[1], Robert B. Clark[2], Darrell Belke[2], Colleen Kondo[2], Paul W. M. Fedak[3], Mary M. C. Maleckar[1] and Wayne R. Giles[2*]

1 *Simula Research Laboratory, Center for Biomedical Computing and Center for Cardiological Innovation, Oslo, Norway*
2 *Faculty of Kinesiology, University of Calgary, Calgary, AB, Canada*
3 *Division of Cardiothoracic Surgery, Department of Cardiac Sciences, University of Calgary, Calgary, AB, Canada*

Correspondence:
Wayne R. Giles, Faculty of Kinesiology, University of Calgary, 2500 University Drive NW, Calgary, AB T2N 1N4, Canada
e-mail: wgiles@ucalgary.ca

In the mammalian heart fibroblasts have important functional roles in both healthy conditions and diseased states. During pathophysiological challenges, a closely related myofibroblast cell population emerges, and can have distinct, significant roles. Recently, it has been reported that human atrial myofibroblasts can express a Na^+ current, I_{Na}. Some of the biophysical properties and molecular features suggest that this I_{Na} is due to expression of Na_v 1.5, the same Na^+ channel α subunit that generates the predominant I_{Na} in myocytes from adult mammalian heart. In principle, expression of Na_v 1.5 could give rise to regenerative action potentials in the fibroblasts/myofibroblasts. This would suggest an active as opposed to passive role for fibroblasts/myofibroblasts in both the "trigger" and the "substrate" components of cardiac rhythm disturbances. Our goals in this preliminary study were: (i) to confirm and extend the electrophysiological characterization of I_{Na} in a human atrial fibroblast/myofibroblast cell population maintained in conventional 2-D tissue culture; (ii) to identify key molecular properties of the α and β subunits of these Na^+ channel(s); (iii) to define the biophysical and pharmacological properties of this I_{Na}; (iv) to integrate the available multi-disciplinary data, and attempt to illustrate its functional consequences, using a mathematical model in which the human atrial myocyte is coupled via connexins to fixed numbers of fibroblasts/myofibroblasts in a syncytial arrangement. Our experimental findings confirm that a significant fraction (approximately 40–50%) of these human atrial myofibroblasts can express I_{Na}. However, our data suggest that I_{Na} may be generated by a combination of Na_v 1.9, Na_v 1.2, and Na_v 1.5. Our results, when complemented with mathematical modeling, provide a background for re-evaluating pharmacological management of supraventricular rhythm disorders, e.g., persistent atrial fibrillation.

Keywords: Na^+ current, atrial arrhythmias, mathematical models, fibroblast, myofibroblast

INTRODUCTION

Within approximately the last 10 years, experimental results and clinical data have established that both fibroblast and myofibroblast cell populations in the mammalian heart (including the adult human) can play very important functional roles in physiological and pathophysiological settings, respectively (Nattel, 2002; Baudino et al., 2006; Munoz et al., 2008; Porter and Turner, 2009; Baum and Duffy, 2011; Biernacka and Frangogiannis, 2011). The fibroblast population, when judged in terms of cell numbers, is predominant in all adult mammalian hearts (cf. Baudino et al., 2006). Until quite recently, these fibroblasts were considered to be passive. That is, they were thought to have few, if any primary electrophysiological roles. Rather, both fibroblasts and myofibroblasts were believed to function predominantly in the synthesis, and degradation (homeostasis) of the extracellular matrix, largely as a consequence of their roles in collagen production/breakdown (Weber et al., 1993). However, this view changed after publication of data demonstrating that both fibroblasts and myofibroblasts have the capability of communicating (cell-to-cell) electrically and metabolically through conventional connexins within gap junctions. This connexin-mediated electrotonic communication may also include functional interactions of these fibroblasts/myofibroblasts with adjacent myocytes (Gaudesius et al., 2003; Chilton et al., 2007; Zlochiver et al., 2008; Kakkar and Lee, 2010). It is now apparent that both the fibroblast and the myofibroblast cell populations can serve as a significant source of paracrine substances that, when secreted, act on adjacent cells (Powell et al., 1999; Pedrotty et al., 2009; Rohr, 2011). Both fibroblasts and myofibroblasts can also be regulated by neurotransmitters, co-transmitters, peptides, and circulating hormones (Brilla et al., 1995; Rose et al., 2007; cf. Rose and Giles, 2008). Important early work on isolated fibroblasts also drew attention to the fact that the electrophysiological properties of these cells can be modulated significantly by mechanical perturbations, including both stretch and shear forces. Abramochkin et al. (2014) have recently reviewed this data.

Experimental work, based mainly on co-culture methods, combined with simulations using mathematical models of, e.g., human atrial myocytes and fibroblasts, have drawn attention to the possibility that the fibroblast cell population could significantly modulate the electrophysiological substrate in a number of cardiac tissues. Papers that deal specifically with these interactions in the atria include: (Maleckar et al., 2009a; Ashihara et al., 2012; McDowell et al., 2013) and ventricles (MacCannell et al., 2007; Sachse et al., 2008; McDowell et al., 2011) of the human heart. However, in all cases, these interactions have been assumed to be passive; that is, to not involve any regenerative or propagated responses that originate in the fibroblast/myofibroblast cell population (Gaudesius et al., 2003; Maleckar et al., 2009a; McDowell et al., 2011, 2013).

Important early work on atrial rhythm disturbances by Spach and his colleagues (Spach and Boineau, 1997) drew attention to the ability of "microfibrosis" to alter the electrical substrate in the atrium and thus promote arrhythmias. Spach et al. (2007) also recognized that in the human atrium an important consequence of aging was an increased incidence of supraventricular rhythm disturbances with some fibrosis. Enhanced fibrosis in the setting of healthy aging is now a well-known contributor to atrial flutter/fibrillation (Nattel, 2002; Biernacka and Frangogiannis, 2011; Diness et al., 2011; Guzadhur et al., 2012).

Recently, it has been reported that myofibroblasts derived from explanted human right atrial tissue (the right atrial appendage) can express measurable (and potentially functionally important) Na^+currents. Specifically, Chatelier et al. (2012) have reported that approximately 75% of the myofibroblasts that are isolated from the human right atrial appendage express Na^+ current after being maintained in a primary 2-D cell culture 8–12 days. They observed that 100% of these cells expressed Na^+ current after 13–17 days in culture. These investigators have also provided evidence that this Na^+ current is generated by the same Na^+ channel α subunit, Na_v 1.5 that produces the Na^+ current in the atria and ventricles of the adult human heart.

After the properties of this Na^+-selective integral membrane protein in fibroblasts/myofibroblasts are understood more completely, a paradigm shift concerning the functional properties of human cardiac syncytium in both health and disease may be required. As an example, the expression of Na_v 1.5 in this cell population raises the possibility that the myofibroblast cell population could be the source of ectopic foci. That is, this Na^+ current could provide a significant source of regenerative inward current. In principle, the resulting depolarization could serve both as the trigger and the substrate for supraventricular rhythm disturbances originating in the fibroblast/myofibroblast cell population.

The main focus of our study was to complement and extend the Chatelier et al. (2012) findings by addressing four separate, but related, objectives:

(i) To carry out whole-cell voltage clamp experiments and obtain the additional data that is needed for determining the probability that measurable Na^+ currents, I_{Na}, in fact can be recorded in single myofibroblasts from the human right atrial appendage, in situations where these cells are isolated, purified, and maintained in conventional 2-D culture.

(ii) To further define the functional roles of I_{Na} based on its fundamental biophysical properties, e.g., voltage-dependence of activation and inactivation.

(iii) To make PCR measurements aimed at identifying mammalian Na^+ channel α and β subunits in this myofibroblast cell population.

(iv) To integrate and illustrate the consequences of the Chatelier et al. (2012) findings and compare them with our results, through implementation of current mathematical models of the human atrial myocyte action potential coupled to a defined fibroblast/myofibroblast electrophysiological parameter set, and then to study these interactions *in silico* in selected ratios (myocytes/myofibroblasts) and coupling configurations.

Here, we report our preliminary findings based on conventional whole-cell voltage-clamp measurements of the electrophysiological properties of single myofibroblasts that were isolated from the human right atrial appendage and then placed in conventional 2-D tissue culture for approximately 6 days (2–4 passages). PCR analyses of the expression of a number of α and β subunits of mammalian Na^+ channels are also presented. Our results are compared and contrasted with those in the original paper on this topic (Chatelier et al., 2012). Mathematical models of the human atrial myocyte and/or the fibroblast/myofibroblast are used to explore and illustrate plausible functional consequences of Na^+ current expression in the myofibroblast population.

Taken together, this experimental and theoretical work contributes to ongoing discussions regarding possible functional roles for Na^+ current in human atrial myofibroblasts. These findings also raise interesting possibilities and questions concerning novel molecular targets in the compromised human atrium, e.g., during persistent atrial fibrillation (Benito et al., 2008; Biernacka and Frangogiannis, 2011; Aguilar-Shardonofsky et al., 2012). This class of rhythm disturbance is of importance due to its increased incidence during the healthy aging process (Benito et al., 2008; Aguilar-Shardonofsky et al., 2012; Guzadhur et al., 2012); and because persistent atrial fibrillation can increase the incidence of transient ischemic attack and/or stroke (cf. Bersohn et al., 2012).

METHODS

HUMAN RIGHT ATRIAL APPENDAGE TISSUE

Excised human atrial appendage specimens were obtained after written consent from patients undergoing coronary artery bypass graft surgeries at Foothills Medical Centre. Administrative approval was granted to the Fedak Laboratory by the University of Calgary Conjoint Health Ethics Board. After being transported to the Fedak Laboratory, each preparation was subjected to enzymatic treatment resulting in release of atrial fibroblasts, as described in previous papers from the Fedak Group (cf. Fedak et al., 2012).

CELL CULTURE METHODS

At selected times, (2 days to 2 weeks), populations of these myofibroblasts were transferred to the Giles Laboratory where they were maintained in conventional 2-D culture for an additional 1–2 days. As required, cells were released by enzymatic treatment (trypsinization) and then used for electrophysiological studies on that same day.

ISOLATION OF MYOFIBROBLAST RNA AND TARGETED PCR ANALYSES

Messenger RNA was isolated from these cultured human atrial fibroblasts using a Qiagen RNeasy kit, and transformed into cDNA using Qiagen Quantitect reverse transcriptase kit according to the manufactures protocol. Real time-PCR analysis was performed using Quantitect SYBR Green Master Mix and primer pairs on a BioRad iCycler. Gene expression levels were calculated using the delta-delta CT method with 18s RNA serving as the housekeeping gene. Values represent the mean ± s.e.m. of three individual cell cultures performed in duplicate measurements. The primers for the analysis of human alpha and beta sodium channel subunits were generated at the University of Calgary DNA lab and BLASTed against the human genome to ensure 100% specificity against the targeted genes. To assess the possibility that expression of neonatal isoforms of the cardiac Na^+ channel were upregulated, SCN5A, or $Na_V1.5$, mRNA expression measurements were separated into primers recognizing splice variants 1 and 2, and primers recognizing variants 3 through 6 (see **Table 1**).

ELECTROPHYSIOLOGICAL METHODS

A small piece of coverslip with adherent cells was placed in a 200 μL recording chamber on the stage of an inverted microscope, where it was superfused with a HEPES-buffered solution (see below) at a rate of about 1 ml/min. The temperature was maintained at 20–22°C.

Membrane currents were measured in single human atrial myofibroblasts using whole-cell "patch clamp" techniques. Cells that were isolated from their neighbors, and lacked obvious connections to surrounding cells, were chosen for patch clamp recordings. Patch pipettes were pulled from borosilicate capillaries, and had a d.c. resistance of 4–9 MΩ when filled with pipette solution. Recordings of membrane current were made with a Multi-Clamp 700A amplifier (Molecular Devices; Sunnyvale, CA, USA). At least 75% series resistance compensation was used (series resistance <5 MΩ). When recording Na^+ currents in the absence of K^+ currents, a P/4 subtraction protocol was used to remove leak currents and reduce uncompensated capacity transient currents. Signals were digitized with a 1322A Digi-Data acquisition system (Molecular Devices), stored on a microcomputer and analyzed offline with pClamp v.8. Plots and statistical analysis were done with "Sigmaplot" (Systat Software; San Jose, CA, USA or "Prism" Graphpad Software, La Jolla, CA, USA).

Current-voltage relations for the global transmembrane ionic current expressed in single human atrial myofibroblasts were obtained using a series of 200 ms voltage clamp steps from −120 to +100 mV (see **Figure 1**). For Na^+ currents, a series of 100 ms steps from −50 to +40 mV (see **Figure 2**) were applied at 0.1 Hz. Steady-state inactivation of Na^+ current was determined with a two-step protocol consisting of a 500 ms "conditioning"

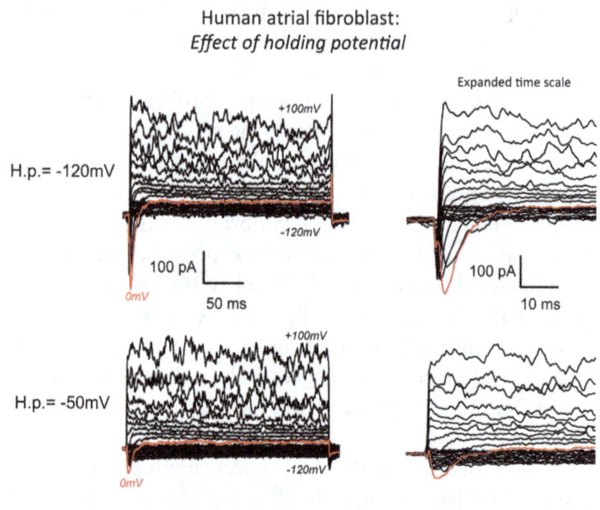

FIGURE 1 | Whole cell patch clamp records of the predominant transmembrane ionic currents recorded from an isolated human atrial myofibroblast using our standard superfusion solution at 22–23°C. The pipette solution in this experiment was "K^+-rich." (See Methods for details of solutions and voltage-clamp protocols). The superimposed current records in the bottom left panel are typical of the data recorded when the voltage clamp "holding potential" (−50 mV) was set near the presumed resting membrane potential of the myofibroblast (approximately −40 mV). As shown, membrane depolarizations in the voltage range from about +20 to 100 mV resulted in a large "noisy" outward current that is likely generated by Ca^{2+}-activated K^+ channels. In this and most other recordings, hyperpolarization from HP −50 mV produced only very small current changes (see Chilton et al., 2007). Note, however, that depolarizing steps did elicit (red trace) a small but distinct transient inward current. The same records at an expanded time scale are shown on the right. The data in the top panel were obtained in response to the same levels of step depolarizations applied from a holding potential of −120 mV. As expected from the fundamental biophysical properties of a voltage-dependent Na^+ (or Ca^{2+}) current this hyperpolarized HP "unmasked" a much more prominent transient inward current (see Results).

Table 1 | Primer sequences for PCR analyses of human atrial myofibroblast Na^+ channel complex transcripts.

Channel	Gene	Forward	Reverse
Na_V 1.1	SCN1A	ctccccacaccagtctttgt	tggtctgactcaggttgctg
Na_V 1.2	SCN2A	gccagcttatcaatcccaaa	tcttctgcaatgcgttgttc
Na_V 1.3	SCN3A	gtagtggtgcattggccttt	gcaccgagttctgagtagcc
Na_V 1.4	SCN4A	ttcacaggcatcttcacagc	ggaaggagcgtagcacagac
Na_V 1.5	SCN5A Var 1,2	cttcaccgccatttacacct	tgcgtaaggctgagacattg
Na_V 1.5	SCN5A Var 3,4,5,6	cttcaccgccatttacacct	aagttcgaagagccgacaaa
Na_V 1.6	SCN8A	tggacatccttttgccttc	ctgcaggaccactgcagata
Na_V 1.7	SCN9A	ccacttcatccaccacctct	actgcactgccttcgagaat
Na_V 1.8	SCN10A	tctttgcagcttcttcagca	acccacacagtcggattagc
Na_V 1.9	SCN11A	cccagcagctgttaaaggag	ctgggacagtcgtttggttt
$Na_V\beta$ 1	SCN1B	tgcgctatgagaatgaggtg	atcttcttgacgacgctggt
$Na_V\beta$ 2	SCN2B	tgacccactctcttccatcc	caccaggtcctctctgaagc
$Na_V\beta$ 3	SCN3B	ccacacacccagacttcctt	tcctgcaaagatgcagtgac
$Na_V\beta$ 4	SCN4B	cccccacagtcttccaagta	gagagcagaggagcaggcta

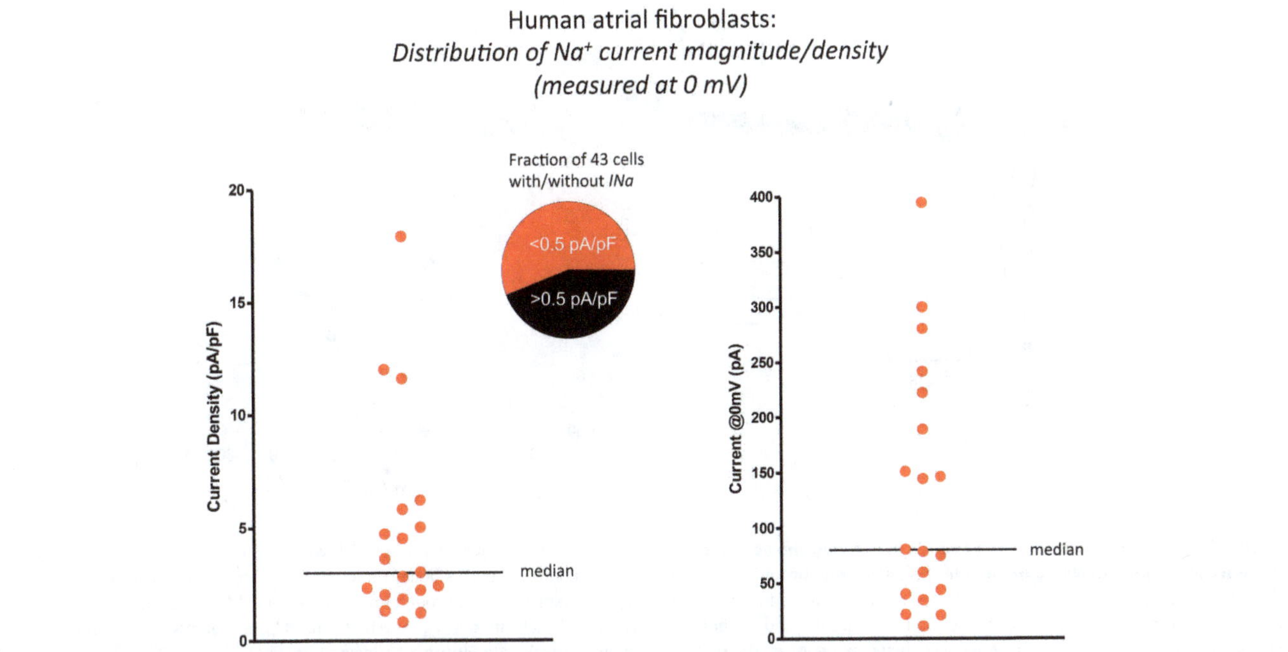

FIGURE 2 | Scatter plots illustrating the significant range of values of functional Na$^+$ current expression in isolated human atrial myofibroblasts ($n = 19$ cells). The data in the left panel summarizes these findings as current densities, i.e., by expressing I_{Na} values (recorded in response to depolarization to 0 mV) normalized for cell (myofibroblast) capacitance (mean ± s.e.m.; 30.8 ± 4.9 pF). The same data set is presented in the right panel as peak I_{Na} at 0 mV. Horizontal bars in both plots indicate the median value of each distribution.

clamp step to −120 mV, followed by a "test" step to −10 mV. Cell capacitance was obtained from the displacement current transient produced by a +10 mV step from the holding potential (HP) −40 mV, which was close to the apparent resting membrane potential of these cells (see Discussion).

Analar grade chemicals (Sigma-Aldrich) were used to make all solutions. "Standard" external solution consisted of (mM): NaCl, 140; KCl, 5; $CaCl_2$, 2; $MgCl_2$, 1; HEPES, 10; glucose, 5.5; mannitol, 15. pH was adjusted to 7.4 with NaOH. K^+-rich "internal" (pipette) solution consisted of (mM): K-aspartate, 100; KCl, 20; $MgCl_2$, 1; Na2ATP, 4; $CaCl_2$, 0.85; EGTA, 5; HEPES, 10. pH was adjusted to 7.2 with KOH. The approximate pCa of the solution was 7.9. Cs^+-rich pipette solution, used to isolate Na$^+$ currents, consisted of Cs-aspartate, 100; CsCl, 30; $MgCl_2$, 1; Na2ATP, 4; $CaCl_2$, 0.85; EGTA, 5; HEPES, 10. pH was adjusted to 7.2 with CsOH.

MATHEMATICAL MODELING OF THE HUMAN ATRIAL ACTION POTENTIAL AND MYOFIBROBLAST/MYOCYTE INTERACTIONS

Mathematical modeling was done using a combination of (i) the Koivumäki et al. model (2011) of the human atrial action potential and intracellular $[Ca^{2+}]_i$ changes, and (ii) the "active" model of the human atrial myofibroblast described in detail in Maleckar et al. (2009a,b). For our simulations, the mathematical expression for the inwardly rectifying background K$^+$ current, I_{K1}, in the fibroblast originally developed by MacCannell et al. (2007) was modified. This was done so that this important non-linear background current, and its contribution to the fibroblast resting potential could be simulated more accurately. Specifically, the equation for I_{K1} in Nygren et al. (Nygren and Giles, 2000) was used, and I_{K1} current density was scaled for the size (capacitance) of the fibroblast. This adjustment required a directly related small change in the size of the Na$^+$/K$^+$ pump current.

Three variants of this myofibroblast/atrial myocyte model were used in the simulations shown in **Figures 6–8:**

- V_o: the original model developed by Maleckar et al. (2009a) with I_{K1} modified as described.
- V_1: V_o with the addition of a Na$^+$ current based on the electrophysiological data shown in **Figures 1–4**.
- V_2: V_o after Na$^+$ current was parameterized based on the *in vitro* data published by Chatelier et al. (2012), as opposed to our data.

The illustrations in **Figures 6–9** were generated by using these myocyte/myofibroblast models, assuming connexin-mediated electrotonic cell-to-cell communication with an assumed gap junctional conductance of 0.5 nS. This value corresponds to the lower end of those measured between fibroblast-myocyte pairs *in vitro* (Maleckar et al., 2009a,b).

In addition to a 1:1 myocyte-myofibroblast coupling scheme, two slightly more complex sets of starting conditions were explored in these simulations. Either 3 or 9 myofibroblasts were connected in series to 1 myocyte. Based on our findings that only approximately 30–50% of the isolated myofibroblasts express a measurable Na$^+$ current, only approximately one third of these myofibroblasts models were programmed to express a Na$^+$ current with the properties in **Figures 1–4** (model variant V_1).

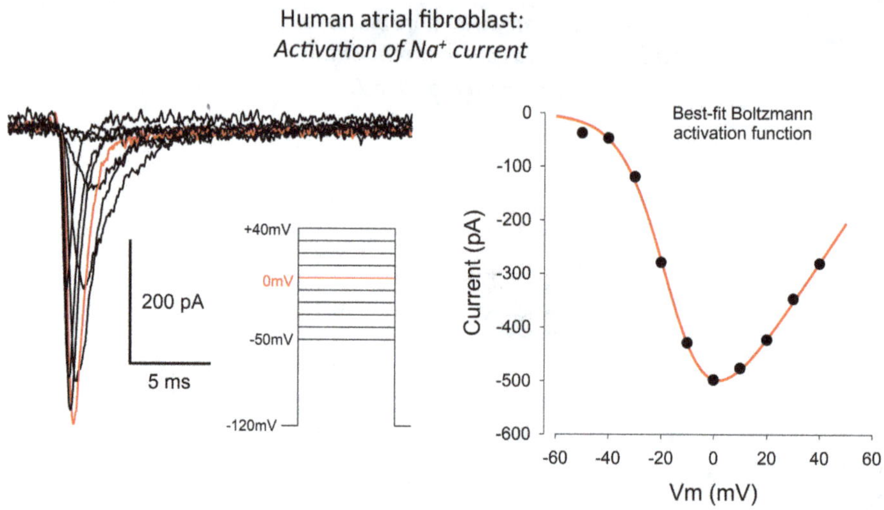

FIGURE 3 | Whole-cell voltage clamp records illustrating the activation of the transient inward Na^+ current in human atrial myofibroblasts. Raw data (10 superimposed current records) elicited by 100 ms depolarizing clamp steps from −50 to +40 mV are shown; the red trace indicates the current elicited at 0 mV. The voltage clamp protocol is shown in the inset. The plot in the right-hand panel is an I–V curve. It was constructed by plotting the peak inward current at each selected voltage clamp depolarization level. The patch pipette solution in this experiment was Cs^+-rich (Methods), to block the large and rapidly activating I_{K-Ca}, which obscured I_{Na} at potentials positive to about +30 mV (see **Figure 1** and text in Results).

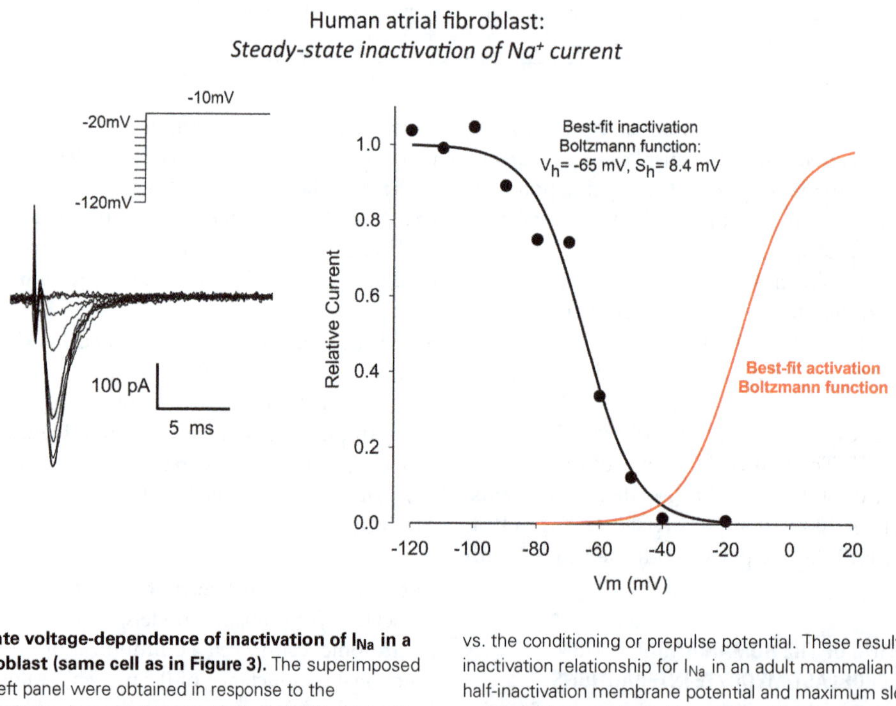

FIGURE 4 | Steady-state voltage-dependence of inactivation of I_{Na} in a human atrial myofibroblast (same cell as in Figure 3). The superimposed current records in the left panel were obtained in response to the conventional two-step voltage clamp protocol that is illustrated in the inset (500 ms "conditioning" step from −120 mV, "test" step to −20 mV). Peak inward I_{Na} values are plotted in the right-hand panel (continuous black curve) vs. the conditioning or prepulse potential. These results reveal a conventional inactivation relationship for I_{Na} in an adult mammalian myocyte with the half-inactivation membrane potential and maximum slope at $V_{1/2}$being −65 and 8.4 mV, respectively. The relationship shown in red—a derived voltage-dependent activation curve—is based on the data in **Figure 2**. See Results for further, more detailed description.

RESULTS

A conventional whole-cell patch clamp method was used to characterize the predominant transmembrane ionic currents in these single isolated human atrial myofibroblasts. Representative families of membrane currents are shown in **Figure 1**. In this myofibroblast and in the majority of others that were studied, voltage clamp depolarizations resulted in rapid activation of a small outward current. Larger depolarizations (in the +60 to +100 mV range) consistently gave rise to large "noisy" transmembrane records, that are characteristic of Ca^{2+}-activated K^+

currents. In contrast, hyperpolarizing clamp steps from the holding potential produced much smaller changes in transmembrane current, similar to the pattern that has been reported in rat ventricular fibroblasts/myofibroblasts (Chilton et al., 2005).

A main focus of this study was to determine whether transient inward Na^+ currents could be detected in these myofibroblasts. For this reason, families of transmembrane currents were generated from two different holding potentials. After each cell was voltage clamped near the resting potential, the holding potential was set to −50 mV, and step depolarizations lasting 100 ms were applied in 10 mV increments covering the range of membrane potentials −120 mV to +100 mV. As shown in the bottom row of **Figure 1**, this protocol produced small but measurable transient inward currents (indicated by the red traces). To enhance the likelihood of detecting Na^+ current, and to attempt to record the maximum transient inward Na^+ current that could be generated by each individual myofibroblast, the holding potential was then set to −120 mV. Transmembrane currents, in response to the same levels of depolarization, were elicited. These families of currents are shown in the top row of **Figure 1**. As expected (as a consequence of the more hyperpolarized holding potential removing inactivation), this maneuver resulted in significantly larger transient inward currents (see red traces). This type of protocol was applied to 40 myofibroblasts in total: the data indicate that approximately 50% of these isolated myofibroblasts express a measurable transient inward current, when the holding potential was −120 mV (see Discussion).

In this series of experiments, it became apparent that there was considerable variability in the expression levels of these Na^+ currents. The scatterplots in **Figure 2** illustrate and summarize this variability. Note that when the transient inward Na^+ current is measured, either in terms of current density (left) in response to a depolarization to 0 mV or plotted as peak current, (right) there is very significant heterogeneity or scatter. The average current density at 0 mV was approximately 3 pA/pF when the holding potential was −120 mV.

The raw data (left) and current-voltage relationship (right) in **Figure 3** provide useful information concerning the peak size, as well as the activation and inactivation kinetics, and the voltage-dependence of this peak inward current in the human atrial myofibroblast, respectively. The family of currents shown in the left panel of **Figure 3** was obtained by applying rectangular voltage clamp depolarizations from a holding potential of −120 mV, as illustrated in the inset. The peak current in response to this step-depolarization to 0 mV is highlighted in red. This current trace provides a point of reference for the summarized data described in **Figure 2**.

A representative peak inward current-voltage relationship is shown in the right panel of **Figure 3**. Note that this inward current first activates at a membrane potential near −50 mV, and that it is maximal near 0 mV. The positive limb of this I–V curve could not be obtained in its entirety due to the rapid activation of a substantial and noisy outward current (see **Figure 1**) at membrane potentials positive to approximately +50 mV. Overall, this pattern of current changes closely resembles families of currents and peak current-voltage relationships that have been published for Na^+ current in cardiac myocytes. This includes myocytes from human atrium (Baba et al., 2006), and data based on heterologous expression, when the α subunit of the cardiac Na^+ channel, Na_v 1.5 is overexpressed in mammalian cell lines, and then studied with conventional patch clamp methods.

The raw data and corresponding analysis shown in **Figure 4** summarize our experimental measurements of the steady-state inactivation characteristics of the Na^+ current in these human atrial myofibroblasts. A conventional two-step voltage clamp protocol was used to progressively inactivate this Na^+ current. From a holding potential of −120 mV, a relatively long "inactivating" prepulse (500 ms) was applied, and this was followed immediately by a second step-depolarization to −10 mV. As expected and as illustrated in the superimposed currents in the left panel, when the prepulse voltage depolarized the cell beyond approximately −40 mV, peak Na^+ current decreased progressively. This voltage-dependent inactivation was characterized over the entire physiological range of membrane potentials, as shown in the plot in the right panel of this Figure. The best-fit parameters for this steady-state inactivation relationship were: membrane potential for half an activation or V_h −65 mV, and maximum slope factor 8.4 mV. In this panel of **Figure 4**, the sigmoid relationship shown in red is a derived relationship depicting voltage-dependent activation for the Na^+ currents shown in **Figure 3** (right).

These electrophysiological findings are somewhat similar to those in the original paper on this topic (Chatelier et al., 2012). Certainly, both data sets reveal the functional expression of Na^+ channels in tissue cultured human atrial myofibroblasts.

Additional molecular evidence for the expression of Na^+ channels in these human atrial myofibroblasts is presented in **Figure 5**. These histograms are based on our PCR analyses of the relative expression levels of a range of human Na^+ channel (SCN-5) α and β subunits. From panel A note the two strongest α subunit signals are for the "nerve" Na^+ channels SCN9A and SCN2A, respectively. However, the predominant (TTX-insensitive) mammalian heart α subunit was also be detected. **Figure 5B** presents analogous PCR data directed toward Na^+ channel β subunits. Here, the β_1 subunit represents the predominant signal (see Discussion).

Our data (**Figures 1–5**) and the Chatelier et al. publication (2012) that first reported functional expression of Na^+ current in human atrial myofibroblasts suggest the possibility that these cells may be able to exhibit regenerative, action potential-like responses when appropriate depolarizing stimuli are applied. **Figures 6–8** illustrate the results of *in silico* tests of this possibility.

For these simulations, two quite different starting conditions were chosen: (i) the myofibroblast was assumed to have a resting membrane potential E_m of −35 mV, and (ii) the myofibroblast E_m values were set at −60 mV. This was done in recognition of the uncertainty of the fibroblast resting potential *in situ* (see Discussion), and because the Na^+ current is inactivated almost completely at −35 mV. In both cases, selected 16 ms de- and hyperpolarizing stimuli were applied intracellularly, as diagrammed in **Figure 6A**.

The results in **Figures 6B,C** illustrate the responses when the myofibroblast was stimulated from a steady membrane

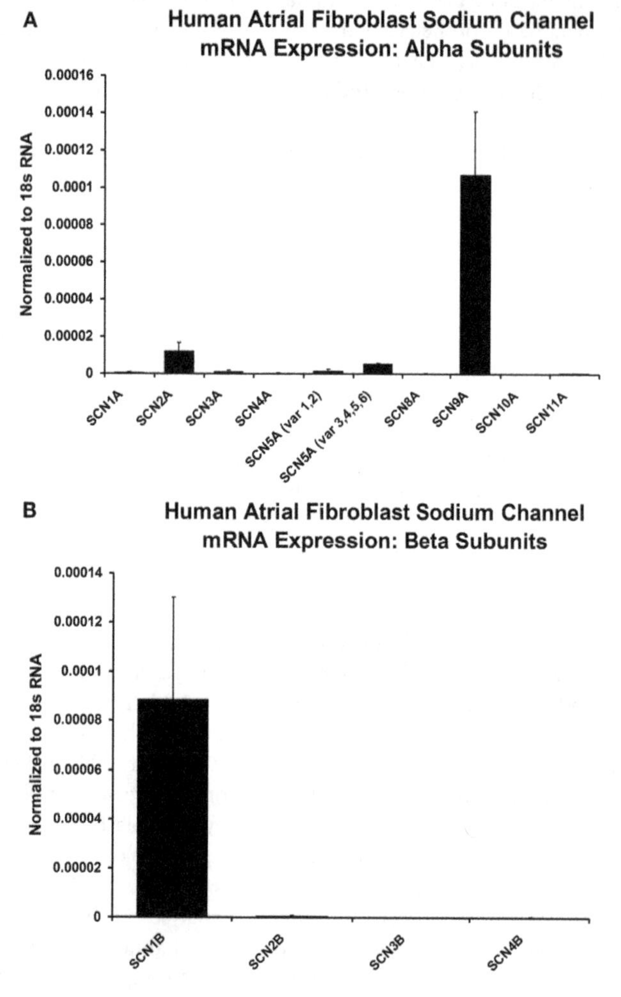

FIGURE 5 | Histograms of normalized data from PCR measurements of relative levels of Na^+ channel α and β subunits, based on RNA derived from populations of isolated human atrial myofibroblasts maintained in 2-D tissue culture. Note from panel **(A)** the predominant α subunits are SCN9A and SCN2A; Panel **(B)** shows that the strongest β subunit signal is for β_1. However, the cardiac isoform of Na^+ current α subunit, SCN5A, also can be detected (see Discussion). Sample size for mRNA measurements are from $n = 3$ individual samples for plated and collagen treated fbs (only plated values are shown). The statistical analysis was based on the difference between plated and collagen treated cells, with a simple unpaired *t*-test to compare gene expression under the two conditions.

potential of −35 mV, and no I_{Na} was introduced/expressed. As expected, the myofibroblast membrane potential responds to small rectangular stimuli with a quasi-exponential electrotonic de- or hyperpolarization, having characteristic time-courses governed approximately by the product of the mean input resistance (3–5 Gigohms) and single cell capacitance (6–10 pF). Note that the original mathematical model of the myofibroblast employed in these simulations (MacCannell et al., 2007) includes a rapidly activating delayed rectifier K^+ current, in accordance with experimental data from rat ventricular myofibroblasts. This K^+ current is activated when E_m depolarizes positive to approximately −30 mV. Indeed, the myofibroblast exhibits a partial repolarization (top trace, panel B) at positive membrane voltages (approximately 0 mV). In addition, a post-stimulus hyperpolarization due to the subsequent deactivation of this K^+ current was observed. The results in **Figure 6D,E** were obtained using the same 4 constant current stimuli (panel A) after the Na^+ current (identified in our study; **Figures 1–4**) was introduced. Note (panel **E**) that there is a tendency for regenerative depolarization in the voltage responses corresponding to all 3 depolarizing stimuli when E_m is set at −65 mV. The data in panels **F** and **G** is analogous to that in panels **D** and **E**, except that in these simulations I_{Na} equations that replicate the Na^+ current described by Chatelier et al. (2012) have been "introduced" into the myofibroblast.

In the next two sets of computational studies, a mathematical model of the human atrial myocyte was combined with the modified mammalian myofibroblast model that is described in Methods. Three sets of computations were done: (i) a fixed number of *in silico* myofibroblasts were coupled to a single human atrial myocyte through a linear resistance corresponding to a conductance of 0.5 nS. These results are shown in the left column, panels **B,E,H** of **Figure 7**. (ii) In the second set of computations, Na^+ current consistent with the biophysical properties depicted in **Figures 1–4** in this paper was introduced into the myofibroblast cell population. These results are shown in the middle column, or panels **C**, **F**, and **I** of **Figure 7**. (iii) Finally, an analogous set of computations was done, this time using the Na^+ current having the biophysical properties reported by Chatelier et al. (2012). In **Figure 7**, these computations are shown in the third column, or panels **D,G,J**. For a reference and starting point, panel **A** shows the atrial myocyte resting potential and action potential waveform (red); and also illustrates the assigned myofibroblast resting potential when these two types of cells are *not* coupled. Overall, this pattern of responses was *not* particularly revealing with respect to Na^+-current dependent patterns of action potential waveforms or the electrotonic responses in the myofibroblast population. Specifically, the expression of Na^+ current in the myofibroblast appeared to have *no* significant effects on the electrotonic waveform.

Note, however, that an important variable was that the myofibroblast resting membrane potential was initially set to that reported for these isolated cells, namely approximately −35 mV. After coupling in the 1:1 (panels **B–D**) and 1:3 (panels **E–G**) cases the fibroblast hyperpolarized and experienced a significant electrotonic depolarization and repolarization driven by the myocyte action potential. In the case of 1:9 ratio coupling (panels **H–J**) the atrial myocyte depolarized significantly and exhibited only a weak regenerative response, which resulted in a small electrotonic depolarization in the myofibroblast(s). We note that when the resting potential in either the myocyte or the fibroblasts is positive to approximately −60 mV, I_{Na} would be strongly inactivated (see **Figure 4**), and thus would not contribute to the membrane voltage profile in the myofibroblast or the immediately adjacent myocyte.

After recognizing that the resting membrane potential of the myofibroblast was a critically important determinant of the size of the peak inward Na^+ current, a second set of computations was carried out with the membrane potential of the myofibroblast set to approximately −65 mV, rather than −35 mV. In **Figure 8**,

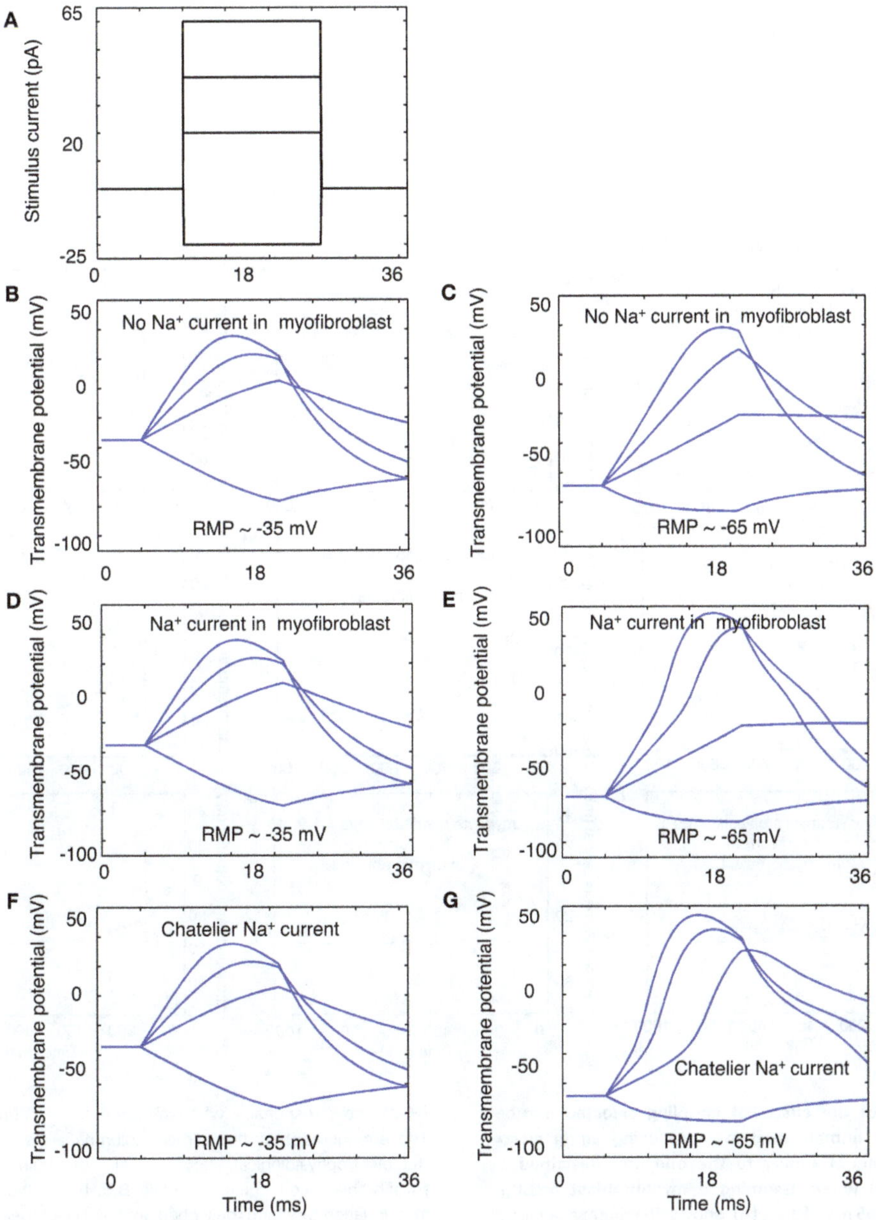

FIGURE 6 | Illustration of "electrotonic" responses in an *in silico* human atrial myofibroblast produced by 16 ms constant current stimuli that progressively depolarize or hyperpolarize the myofibroblast model. The stimulus protocol is shown in panel **(A)**. The superimposed responses in **(B,C)** were obtained using a modified (see Methods) MacCannell et al. (2007) model of an atrial myofibroblast with no Na^+ current added. The families of responses in **(D,E)** were obtained when this model also included equations for the Na^+ current in this paper; or the Na^+ current in the Chatelier et al. paper (2012) **(F,G)**. Note when Na^+ current is included, most of the depolarizing stimuli produce a biphasic response. This may suggest a contribution of Na^+ current activation to the stimulus-induced depolarization (see Discussion).

the presentation of the data is the same as that of data **Figure 7**. Thus, the panels in column 1 (**B,D,E,H**) were based on computations done with no Na^+ current in the myofibroblast cell population, and with coupling ratios of myocyte to myofibroblasts of 1:1, 1:3, and 1:9, respectively. As expected from our previous papers (MacCannell et al., 2007; Maleckar et al., 2009a), the myocyte membrane potential dominates that of the myofibroblast at low myofibroblast/myocyte ratios. In distinction, to when the myofibroblast resting membrane potential is much more depolarized (−35 mV), when the coupling ratio is 1:3 or 1:9, both the myofibroblasts and the myocytes have well-polarized resting membrane potentials. Partly for this reason, the waveform of the voltage change in the myofibroblast also differs substantially. This arises from the fact that more hyperpolarized resting membrane potential removes inactivation from the Na^+ channels. This effect would be expected to be strongly manifested in the computations shown in panels **C,F,I**—as well a **D,G,I**, since the voltage dependence for inactivation of the Na^+ current falls

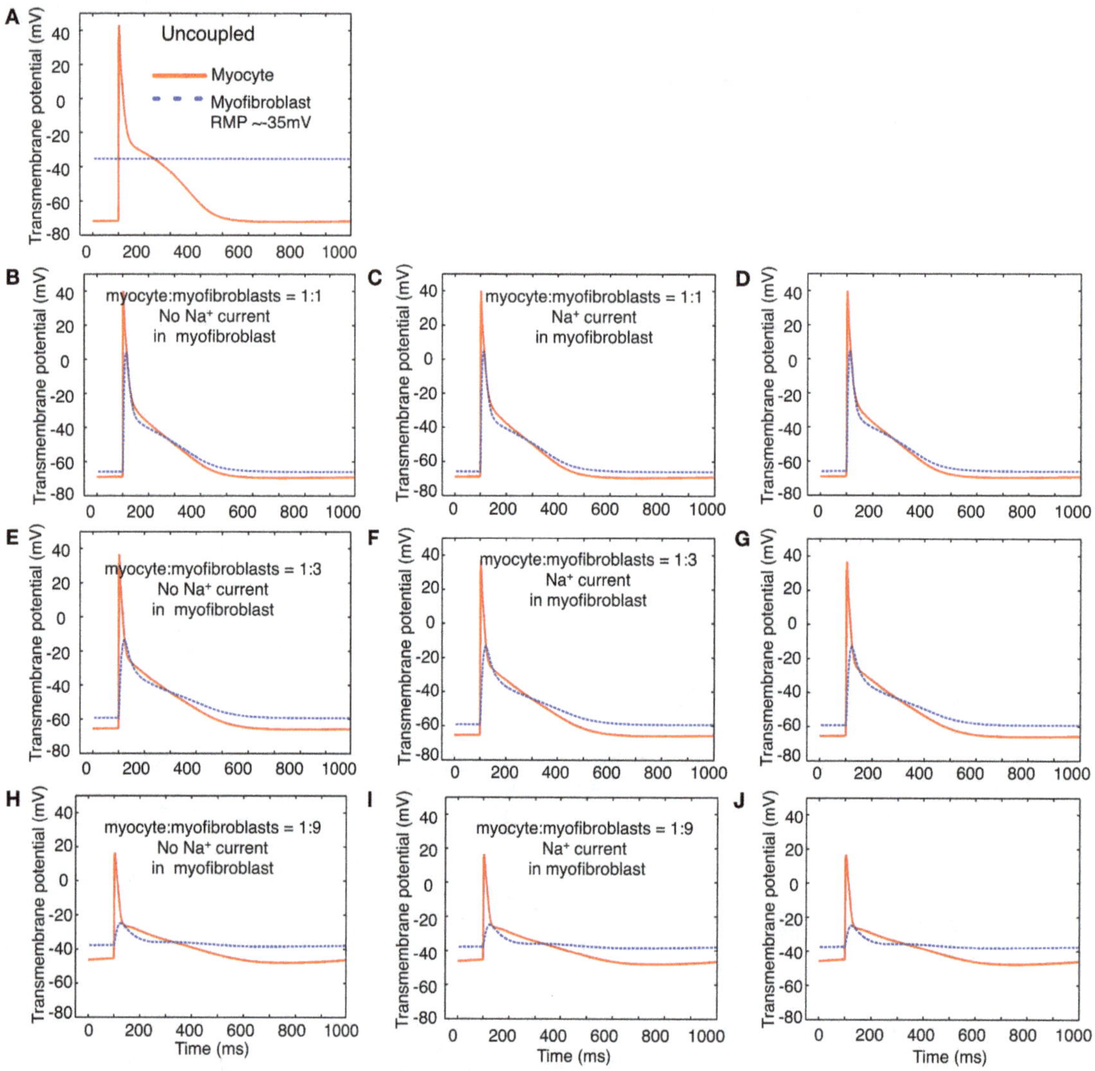

FIGURE 7 | Illustration of the effects of coupling selected numbers of myofibroblasts to 1 human atrial myocyte using an *in silico* hybrid mathematical model similar to the one first described by Maleckar et al. (2009a) when assuming a myofibroblast resting potential of −35 or −65 mV. Panel **(A)** shows the human atrial myocyte action potential (red) and the myofibroblast at a resting potential of −35 mV, prior to these cells being coupled through a linear intercellular conductance of 0.5 nS. The remainder of this Figure is arranged in three rows. Panels **(B–D)** illustrate responses obtained when the myocyte to myofibroblast ratio is 1:1, panels **(E–G)** were computed based on a myocyte to myofibroblast ratio of 1:3; and panels **(H–J)** show responses when myocyte to myofibroblast ratio was 1:9. The arrangement of the vertical columns allow a direct comparison of the electrophysiological effects of (a) there being no Na^+ current in any myofibroblast (left column, panels **B,E,H**); (b) the Na^+ current identified in our laboratory and described in the paper being introduced (panels **C,F,I**); or (c) the Na^+ current reported by Chatelier et al. (2012) being added to each myofibroblast **(D,G,J)**. Note that the myocyte action potential causes a significant electrotonic waveform in each myofibroblast at ratios of 1:1 and 1:3. At a coupling ratio of 1:9, the myofibroblasts exert a pronounced depolarizing influence of the myocyte resting potential in these assumed conditions (see Discussion).

well within the range of the resting membrane potential of the myofibroblast.

Careful inspection of some of the computational results in **Figures 7, 8** may suggest that activation of I_{Na} in the myofibroblast influences the overall "substrate" electrophysiological profile. Thus, in some cases, the membrane potential in the myofibroblast(s) depolarizes, when the atrial myocyte is repolarizing.

The computational results shown in **Figure 9** provide some further insight into this intriguing possibility. All of these computations were done using a 1 myocyte to 1 myofibroblast ratio. Two different values of coupling (intercellular) resistance, either 0.5 nS (top row) or 8 nS (bottom row) were selected for study. As expected, when intercellular resistance is very small, the myocyte action potential produces an electrotonic response in the myofibroblast that is essentially unattenuated.

Note that at both these values of intercellular resistance (panels **C,D**), the current flowing between the "cells" is dominated by the net inward (depolarizing) and outward (repolarizing)

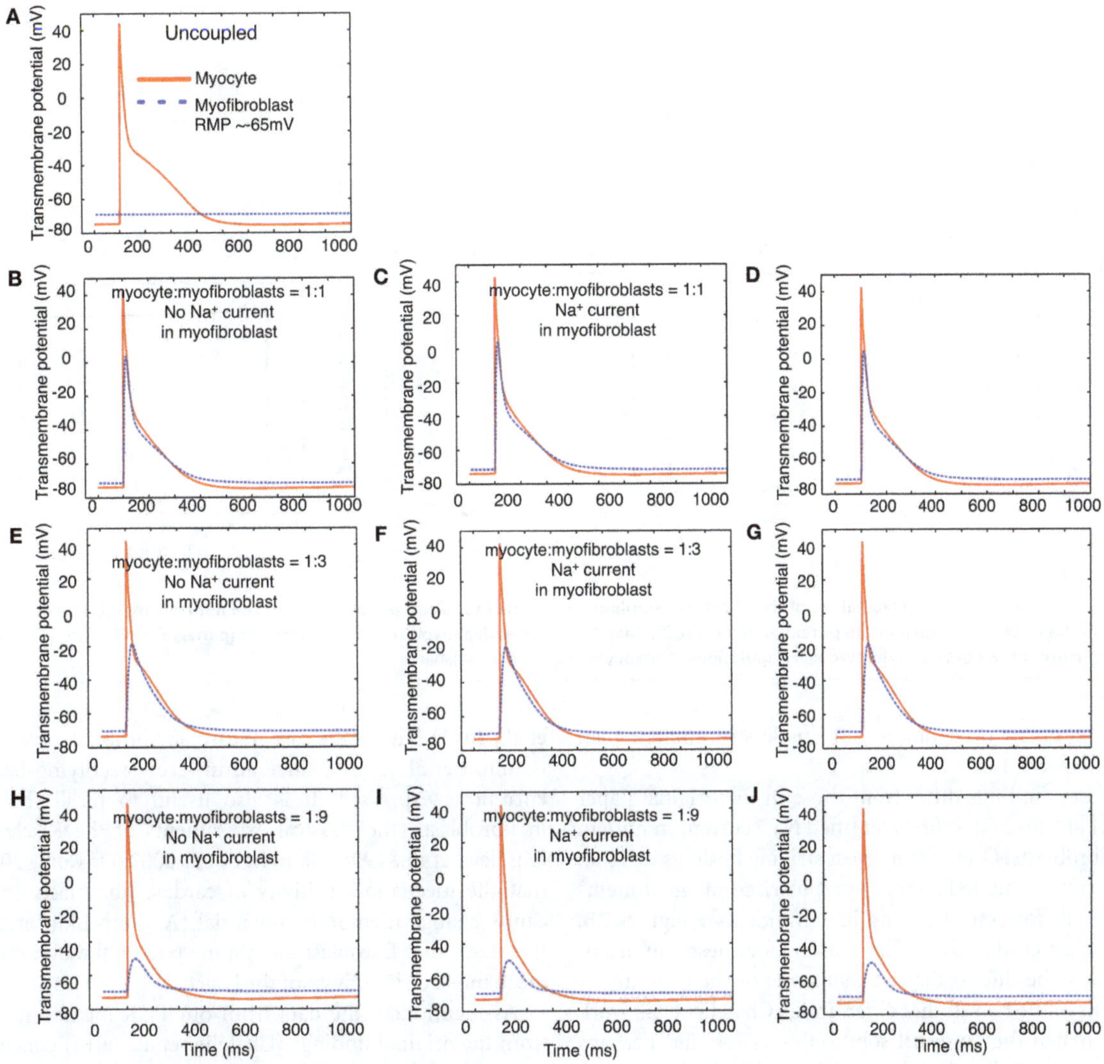

FIGURE 8 | Illustration of the effects of coupling selected numbers of myofibroblasts to 1 human atrial myocyte using an *in silico* hybrid model similar to the one first described by Maleckar et al. (2009a), assuming a myofibroblast resting potential of −65 mV. The layout of this Figure is the same as that of **Figure 7**. Note that two potentially important differences in the patterns of *in silico* responses were obtained: (1) in all situations, the myofibroblast electrotonic responses are larger, (2) the myofibroblasts exert only a minimal depolarizing influence on the resting potential of the atrial myocyte.

currents generated by the *atrial* myocyte. Panels **E** and **F** show the net transmembrane current in the myofibroblast population. Again, the inward, depolarizing current appears to be contributed mainly by the activation of I_{Na} in the *atrial* myocyte(s), as opposed to the myofibroblast(s) (see Discussion).

DISCUSSION

MAIN FINDINGS

The whole-cell voltage clamp measurements shown in **Figures 1–4** confirm that when human atrial fibroblasts are isolated and then placed in conventional 2-D culture, a sizeable fraction (approximately 50%) of these cells (myofibroblasts) express a measurable Na^+ current. A number of electrophysiological and biophysical features of this current are noteworthy. (i) Its peak amplitude (in the range: 0.8–17.9 pA/pF) is sufficient to suggest that the myofibroblast may exhibit a regenerative action potential. (ii) The steady-state voltage dependence of inactivation, and the derived relationship that depicts quasi steady-state voltage dependence of activation, both strongly resemble the analogous biophysical parameters for the Na^+ current recorded in adult human atrial myocytes (Baba et al., 2006). (iii) These findings, in conjunction with the PCR data in **Figure 5**, provide initial evidence that this current is similar to the Na^+ current in an adult human atrial myocyte, as was originally reported by Chatelier et al. (2012). However, we note that our PCR analysis yielded data that identifies two nerve Na^+ channel α subunits, $Na_v1.9$ and $Na_v1.2$, as the predominant transcripts. The cardiac Na^+ channel α subunit was detectable

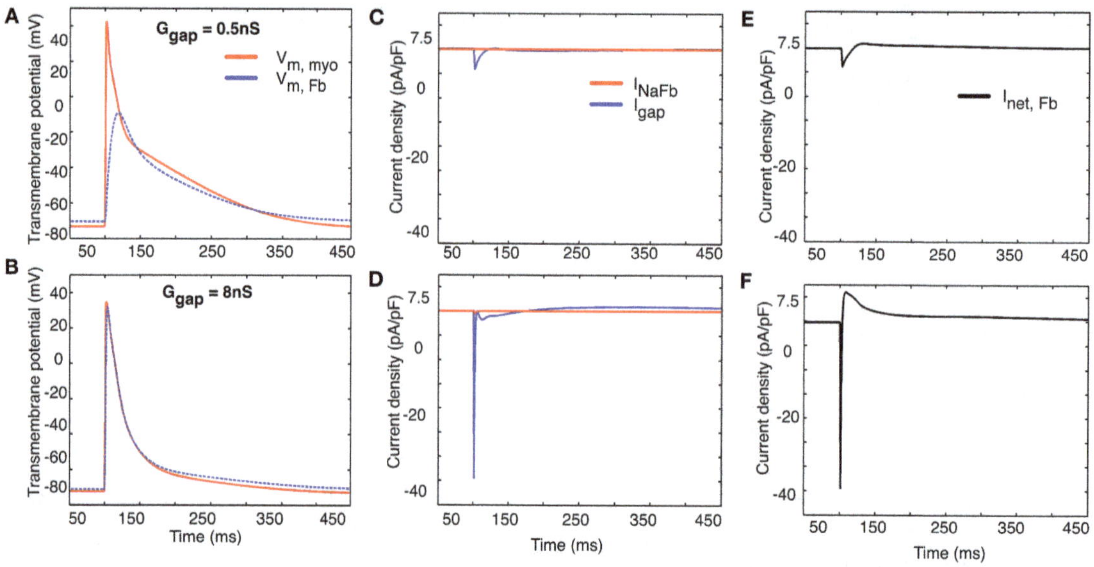

FIGURE 9 | Illustration of two selected values of the effects of coupling resistance on the electrotonic membrane potential (panels A,B), "gap current" and current flow between the two cell populations (1 myocyte: 1 myofibroblast, panels C,D) and the net transmembrane current in the collective myofibroblast population (panels E,F). See text in Results for further explanation.

in our myofibroblast preparation, but was less prominent than either $Na_V1.9$ or $Na_V1.2$.

Some of our findings differ from those in the original paper (Chatelier et al., 2012) that first identified Na^+ current in human atrial myofibroblasts. One of their most striking findings was that this Na^+ current exhibited a very hyperpolarized range of membrane potentials for activation and inactivation (see Figures 2B, 3A, in Chatelier et al., 2012). The reasons for these important differences may be due to the fact that some of the experimental conditions in the two studies differ. In the Chatelier et al. work (2012), the pH of the "internal solution" was 7.4; and perhaps more importantly, CsF rather than CsCl was used in the pipette-filling solution. It is well-known that F^- in the internal solution can cause a pronounced hyperpolarizing shift in Na^+ current gating parameters (Chandler and Meves, 1970). An important consequence of the gating variables for the Na^+ current being shifted in the hyperpolarizing direction in the Chatelier et al. paper (2012) is that the myofibroblast resting potential would need to be negative to −60 mV before this current could be activated. Second, in principle, there could be a substantial non-inactivating or "background/steady" Na^+ influx, when the myofibroblast membrane potential is in the voltage range approximately −90 to −40 mV. This would depolarize the myofibroblast and tend to increase $[Na^+]_i$ and have significant secondary consequences on $[Ca^{2+}]_i$, and $[pH]_i$ homeostasis.

These considerations raise the very important question: what is the resting potential of the human atrial fibroblast/myofibroblast? Values in the range −30 to −50 mV are often reported for isolated single cell mammalian fibroblast/myofibroblast preparations. However, accurate measurement of membrane potential in these small cells is very challenging (Dubois, 2000), especially under conditions, in which a background inwardly rectifying K^+ current is expressed (Wilson et al., 2011). This is the case in cardiac fibroblasts/myofibroblasts (Chilton et al., 2007), since an inwardly rectifying background current is expressed. It is also useful to recall that, as it is in fibroblasts, the classical experiments of the Kiseleva Group (Kiseleva et al., 1998; Kamkin et al., 2002; cf. Kohl, 2003) show that the mechano-sensitivity of cardiac fibroblasts can significantly change membrane potential (Abramochkin et al., 2014). It is likely that fibroblast membrane potential may vary with the mechanoelectric activity of the heart.

As mentioned, the data from our PCR measurements differ from the original findings (Chatelier et al., 2012) concerning the molecular identity of the Na^+ current α subunit(s) in human atrial myofibroblasts (see **Figure 6**). Thus, we suggest that the major α subunits are $Na_V1.9$ and Na_V 1.2, as opposed to Na_V 1.5. Of the four known Na^+ channel β subunits that could, in principle, contribute to the Na^+ channel complex (Abriel and Kass, 2005), the β_1 subunit predominates in the human atrial myofibroblasts in the mammalian heart, as is the case in the corresponding adult myocyte. At present, we cannot explain the significant difference in the pattern of Na^+ channel α subunit expression. However, it is possible that our cell culture preparation is less uniform than that of Chatelier et al. (2012). Our PCR analysis was done using a preparation that had been plated on coverslips only 24–48 h before being studied. However, these myofibroblasts had been passaged a number of times (2–6) before they were "released and plated." In contrast, Chatelier et al. studied myofibroblasts after some 3 weeks in culture, corresponding to approximately passage 9. This difference is an important issue that can only be resolved by a separate, much more extensive study.

Our study did not focus on the molecular pharmacology of the Na^+ currents in the myofibroblast. However, the original paper (Chatelier et al., 2012) reported (**Figure 5**) that tetrodotoxin (TTX) did block this current. In these experiments, the effective concentrations of TTX were in the 10–100 μM range. This further supports its identity as a cardiac myocyte-like Na^+ current, generated by the complex of Na_v 1.5 and the β_1 subunit.

COMPUTATIONAL WORK

It is somewhat surprising that introduction of Na^+ current into the modified MacCannell model of the mammalian fibroblast (MacCannell et al., 2007) did *not* result in any convincing action potential-like regenerative responses (**Figures 6, 7**). With respect to the results shown in **Figure 6**, this may be due to the fact that the relatively depolarized "assigned" resting potential (−35 or −65 mV) of the fibroblasts/myofibroblasts resulted in very significant inactivation of I_{Na}. A second contributing factor may be the incomplete information concerning the kinetics of activation and inactivation of I_{Na} in the human atrial myofibroblast. The high input resistance of these cells (5–10 Gigohms) results in a large intrinsic membrane time constant; and this may contribute to Na^+ current "accommodation"—inactivation developing at a rate similar to activation at membrane potential near the normal firing threshold for I_{Na}.

At this stage of its development, the hybrid modeling illustrated in **Figures 7, 8** does not independently reveal significant new information. Perhaps the most realistic myocyte to myofibroblast ratios that we have explored is the 1:3 case. In this defined starting condition, we confirm that the myocyte action potential produces a significant electrotonic waveform in the connexin-coupled myofibroblasts (MacCannell et al., 2007; Maleckar et al., 2009a). In addition, when large differences in the resting potential of the myofibroblast vs. the myocyte are assumed/assigned, the myofibroblast can significantly depolarize the atrial myocyte. This depolarization would be expected to reduce myocyte excitability and conduction velocity; and may significantly change diastolic Ca^{2+} levels. It is worth noting that these effects could be anticipated to be spatially heterogeneous within the human atrial substrate.

TRANSLATIONAL PERSPECTIVES

The expression of Na^+ current (more specifically the detection of essential components of the Na^+ channel complex) in the myofibroblast, may be important for reasons quite different than the well-known ability of this integral membrane protein to give rise to a transient inward current and thus promote cell and/or substrate excitability. The so-called "non-conducting functions" of the Na^+ channel complex (Kaczmarek, 2006; Brackenbury and Isom, 2011) are gaining increasing attention, for example, in the setting of the metastatic phase of the progression of a number of different solid tumor cancers. During metastasis of solid tumors and during nerve "sprouting," it is very likely that the expression of Na^+ channels result in mechanical stability of the cells in which they are expressed, rather than, or in addition to, a conventional electrophysiological function (Chioni et al., 2009; Fraser et al., 2010). Some Na^+ channel β subunits can covalently link with well-known adhesion molecules. This suggests the possibility that expression of the β subunit, and by implication the entire Na^+ complex (Abriel and Kass, 2005), may have an important adhesion function. It is interesting that Watanabe et al. (2009) have reported alterations in the β1 and β2 subunits of the Na^+ channel in tissue taken from atria that had exhibited persistent fibrillation, a condition often associated with enhanced fibrosis and perhaps with altered cell-matrix dynamics.

It is also known that one aspect of an acute inflammatory response involves binding of emigrated neutrophils to the Na^+ channel complex, and a resulting (very significant) Na^+ influx, due to a "late" Na^+ current. This arises from Na^+ channels opening but then inactivating very slowly (Poon et al., 2001; Ward et al., 2006). Thus, provided that the membrane potential of the myofibroblast is sufficiently negative that even a small fraction of the Na^+ channels could open (see **Figure 2**), the pathophysiological chain events involving substantial leak of Na^+ into the cell through non-inactivating Na^+ channels followed by Ca^{2+} overload may need to be considered in the setting of cytokine or inflammation-induced apoptosis or necrosis.

Quite recently, the so-called "re-programmed" fibroblast has been advanced as the preparation of choice for heterologous introduction into the compromised myocardium or other end-organs in the context of Regenerative Medicine approaches to Chronic Disease Management (Leri and Kajstura, 2012; Palpant and Murry, 2012; Qian et al., 2012; Song et al., 2012; Srivastava and Ieda, 2012; Miki et al., 2013). The fundamental principles of fibroblast isolation and reprogramming appear now to be well understood. However, in the cases of cardiac and vascular pathophysiology, an essential requirement is that these implanted cells must have a stable, quiescent electrophysiological phenotype. For this reason, the expression of Na^+ current in myofibroblast that is the focus of this study needs to be understood fully and perhaps avoided or suppressed. Similar considerations are likely to apply to more preliminary attempts to use reprogrammed fibroblasts in the context of cardiac rhythm control (Yankelson et al., 2008; Cho and Marbán, 2010).

LIMITATIONS

A major limitation of the experimental work presented in this paper is that, as judged by both electrophysiological and PCR methodology, expression of Na^+ channels could be detected only a considerable time period *after seeding* of what were originally human atrial fibroblasts in 2-D tissue culture. This raises the possibility (both with respect to the Chatelier paper and our work) that Na^+ channel expression could be tissue culture specific. Such an epi-phenomenon would have little if any physiological or pathophysiological significance. Perhaps the strongest argument against this possibility is that, although ion channel expression is known to change in tissue culture, under most circumstances the expression levels are *reduced* (Banyasz et al., 2008). In addition, and as noted in Methods, although the enzymatic isolation of fibroblasts from the human atrial right appendage was somewhat similar in these two studies, in fact, post-isolation treatment of the resulting fibroblast/myofibroblast cell populations differed quite significantly. In our work [consistent with the previous work and ongoing investigations in the Fedak Laboratory (Fedak et al., 2012)], these cells are maintained and held in a 3D-substrate for most of the post-isolation period, i.e., to being released for study by conventional electrophysiological or PCR methods.

The results based on mathematical modeling (**Figures 6–9**) are preliminary, in part because the experimental data is incomplete. This part of this paper is limited by a lack of information with respect to (i) the extent of the electrotonic coupling between myofibroblasts, and/or (ii) among single or multi-cellular groups of myofibroblasts and the immediately adjacent human atrial myocytes. It would seem implausible that this coupling ratio could be 1:1. Other, more likely possibilities are illustrated in the computations in **Figures 7** and **8**. It is clear, however, that more extensive and detailed experimental data and more refined computations are needed to further evaluate myocyte/fibroblast electrotonic interactions in defined starting conditions that are directed toward a defined myocyte/fibroblast ratio.

In addition, future work will need to consider the influence of tonic effects of autonomic transmitters and/or paracrine substances. Success based on these improvements may provide the possibility that within the extracellular matrix of the atrium, a "double hit" approach can be developed to modulate Na^+ channel activity, and thus achieve improved anti-arrhythmic therapy (Maingret et al., 2008).

AUTHOR CONTRIBUTIONS

Doctors Robert Clark and Darrell Belke were responsible for the experimental work shown in **Figures 1–4** and **5**, respectively. Doctors Jussi Koivumäki and Mary Maleckar produced the simulation results in **Figures 6–9**. Doctor Wayne Giles planned and wrote draft #1 of this manuscript. All authors read and provided comments on the original and revised manuscripts.

ACKNOWLEDGMENTS

An Alberta Innovates—Health Solutions Scientist Award (WRG), an AI-HS Starter Grant, the Canadian Institutes of Health Research, and the Heart and Stroke Foundation of Alberta supported the experimental work and mathematical model development in the Giles Laboratory. Jussi T. Koivumäki and Mary M. C. Maleckar gratefully acknowledge support via partnership in the Center for Cardiological Innovation at Oslo University Hospital and by a Center of Excellence grant from the Research Council of Norway to the Center for Biomedical Computing at Simula Research Laboratory. We are grateful to the Fedak Laboratory and Division of Cardiothoracic Surgery at the University of Calgary for supply of right atrial appendage tissue. Ms. Colleen Kondo prepared and maintained the tissue cultures and was responsible for project management.

REFERENCES

Abramochkin, D. V., Lozinsky, I. T., and Kamkin, A. (2014). Influence of mechanical stress on fibroblast-myocyte interactions in mammalian heart. *J. Mol. Cell. Cardiol.* 70C, 27–36. doi: 10.1016/j.yjmcc.2013.12.020

Abriel, H., and Kass, R. S. (2005). Regulation of the voltage-gated cardiac sodium channel Nav 1.5 by interacting proteins. *Trends Cardiovasc. Med.* 15, 35–40. doi: 10.1016/j.tcm.2005.01.001

Aguilar-Shardonofsky, M., Vigmond, E. J., Nattel, S., and Comtois, P. (2012). *In silico* optimization of atrial fibrillation—selective sodium channel blocker pharmacodynamics. *Biophys. J.* 102, 951–960. doi: 10.1016/j.bpj.2012.01.032

Ashihara, T., Haraguchi, R., Nakazawa, K., Namba, T., Ikeda, T., Nakazawa, Y., et al. (2012). The role of fibroblasts in complex fractionated electrograms during persistent/permanent atrial fibrillation: implications for electrogram-based catheter ablation. *Circ. Res.* 110, 275–284. doi: 10.1161/CIRCRESAHA.111.255026

Baba, S., Dun, W., Hirose, M., and Boyden, P. A. (2006). Sodium current function in adult and aged canine atrial cells. *Am. J. Physiol. Heart Circ. Physiol.* 291, H756–H761. doi: 10.1152/ajpheart.00063.2006

Banyasz, T., Lozinskiy, I., Payne, C. E., Edelmann, S., Norton, B., Chen, B., et al. (2008). Transformation of adult rat cardiac myocytes in primary culture. *Exp. Physiol.* 93, 370–382. doi: 10.1113/expphysiol.2007.040659

Baudino, T. A., Carver, W., Giles, W., and Borg, T. K. (2006). Cardiac fibroblasts: friend or foe? *Am. J. Physiol. Heart Circ. Physiol.* 291, H1015–H1026. doi: 10.1152/ajpheart.00023.2006

Baum, J., and Duffy, H. S. (2011). Fibroblasts and myofibroblasts: what are we talking about? *J. Cardiovasc. Pharmacol.* 57, 376–379. doi: 10.1097/FJC.0b013e3182116e39

Benito, B., Brugada, R., Perich, R. M., Lizotte, E., Cinca, J., Mont, L., et al. (2008). A mutation in the sodium channel is responsible for the association of long QT syndrome and familial atrial fibrillation. *Heart Rhythm* 5, 1434–1440. doi: 10.1016/j.hrthm.2008.07.013

Bersohn, M. M., Waldo, A. L., and Halperin, J. L. (2012). Subclinical atrial fibrillation and the risk of stroke. *N. Engl. J. Med.* 366, 1352.

Biernacka, A., and Frangogiannis, N. G. (2011). Aging and cardiac fibrosis. *Aging Disease* 2, 158–173.

Brackenbury, W. J., and Isom, L. L. (2011). Na channel beta subunits: overachievers of the ion channel family. *Front. Pharmacol.* 2:53. doi: 10.3389/fphar.2011.00053

Brilla, C., Maisch, B., Zhou, G., and Weber, K. (1995). Hormonal regulation of cardiac fibroblast function. *Eur. Heart J.* 16, 45–50. doi: 10.1093/eurheartj/16.suppl_C.45

Chandler, W. K., and Meves, H. (1970). Slow changes in membrane permeability and long-lasting action potentials in axons perfused with fluoride solutions. *J. Physiol.* 211, 707–728.

Chatelier, A., Mercier, A., Tremblier, B., Thériault, O., Moubarak, M., Benamer, N., et al. (2012). A distinct de novo expression of Navl. 5 sodium channels in human atrial fibroblasts differentiated into myofibroblasts. *J. Physiol.* 590, 4307–4319. doi: 10.1113/jphysiol.2012.233593

Chilton, L., Giles, W. R., and Smith, G. L. (2007). Evidence of intercellular coupling between co-cultured adult rabbit ventricular myocytes and myofibroblasts. *J. Physiol.* 583, 225–236. doi: 10.1113/jphysiol.2007.135038

Chilton, L., Ohya, S., Freed, D., George, E., Drobic, V., Shibukawa, Y., et al. (2005). K+ currents regulate the resting membrane potential, proliferation, and contractile responses in ventricular fibroblasts and myofibroblasts. *Am. J. Physiol. Heart Circ. Physiol.* 288, H2931–H2939. doi: 10.1152/ajpheart.01220.2004

Chioni, A. M., Brackenbury, W. J., Calhoun, J. D., Isom, L. L., and Djamgoz, M. B. (2009). A novel adhesion molecule in human breast cancer cells: voltage-gated Na+ channel beta1 subunit. *Int. J. Biochem. Cell Biol.* 41, 1216–1227. doi: 10.1016/j.biocel.2008.11.001

Cho, H. C., and Marbán, E. (2010). Biological therapies for cardiac arrhythmias: can genes and cells replace drugs and devices? *Circ. Res.* 106, 674–685. doi: 10.1161/CIRCRESAHA.109.212936

Diness, J. G., Skibsbye, L., Jespersen, T., Bartels, E. D., Sørensen, U. S., Hansen, R. S., et al. (2011). Effects on atrial fibrillation in aged hypertensive rats by Ca2+-activated K+ channel inhibition. *Hypertension* 57, 1129–1135. doi: 10.1161/HYPERTENSIONAHA.111.170613

Dubois, J.-M. (2000). What is the true resting potential of small cells? *Gen. Physiol. Biophys.* 19, 3–7.

Fedak, P. W. M., Bai, L. P., Turnbull, J., Ngu, J., Narine, K., and Duff, H. J. (2012). Cell therapy limits myofibroblast differentiation and structural cardiac remodeling: basic fibroblast growth factor-mediated paracrine mechanism. *Circulation Heart Fail.* 5, 349–356. doi: 10.1161/CIRCHEARTFAILURE.111.965889

Fraser, S. P., Ozerlat-Gunduz, I., Onkal, R., Diss, J. K., Latchman, D. S., and Djamgoz, M. B. (2010). Estrogen and non-genomic upregulation of voltage-gated Na(+) channel activity in MDA-MB-231 human breast cancer cells: role in adhesion. *J. Cell. Physiol.* 224, 527–539. doi: 10.1002/jcp.22154

Gaudesius, G., Miragoli, M., Thomas, S. P., and Rohr, S. (2003). Coupling of cardiac electrical activity over extended distances by fibroblasts of cardiac origin. *Circ. Res.* 93, 421–428. doi: 10.1161/01.RES.0000089258.40661.0C

Guzadhur, L., Jiang, W., Pearcey, S. M., Jeevaratnam, K., Duehmke, R. M., Grace, A. A., et al. (2012). The age-dependence of atrial arrhythmogenicity in Scn5a+/- murine hearts reflects alterations in action potential propagation and recovery. *Clin. Exp. Pharmacol. Physiol.* 39, 518–527. doi: 10.1111/j.1440-1681.2012.05706.x

Kaczmarek, L. K. (2006). Non-conducting functions of voltage-gated ion channels. *Nat. Rev. Neurosci.* 7, 761–771. doi: 10.1038/nrn1988

Kakkar, R., and Lee, R. T. (2010). Intramyocardial fibroblast myocyte communication. *Circ. Res.* 106, 47–57. doi: 10.1161/CIRCRESAHA.109.207456

Kamkin, A., Kiseleva, I., Wagner, K.-D., Pylaev, A., Leiterer, K. P., Theres, H., et al. (2002). A possible role for atrial fibroblasts in postinfarction bradycardia. *Am. J. Physiol. Heart Circ. Physiol.* 282, H842–H849.

Kiseleva, I., Kamkin, A., Pylaev, A., Kondratjev, D., Leiterer, K. P., Theres, H., et al. (1998). Electrophysiological properties of mechanosensitive atrial fibroblasts from chronic infarcted rat heart. *J. Mol. Cell. Cardiol.* 30, 1083–1093. doi: 10.1006/jmcc.1998.0673

Kohl, P. (2003). Heterogeneous cell coupling in the heart: an electrophysiological role for fibroblasts. *Circ. Res.* 93, 381–383. doi: 10.1161/01.RES.0000091364.90121.0C

Koivumäki, J. T., Korhonen, T., and Tavi, P. (2011). Impact of sarcoplasmic reticulum calcium release on calcium dynamics and action potential morphology in human atrial myocytes: a computational study. *PLoS Comput. Biol.* 7:e1001067. doi: 10.1371/journal.pcbi.1001067

Leri, A., and Kajstura, J. (2012). Created equal? The many facets of cell reprogramming. *Circ. Res.* 111, 152–155. doi: 10.1161/CIRCRESAHA.112.272526

MacCannell, K. A., Bazzazi, H., Chilton, L., Shibukawa, Y., Clark, R. B., and Giles, W. R. (2007). A mathematical model of electrotonic interactions between ventricular myocytes and fibroblasts. *Biophys. J.* 92, 4121–4132. doi: 10.1529/biophysj.106.101410

Maingret, F., Coste, B., Padilla, F., Clerc, N., Crest, M., Korogod, S. M., et al. (2008). Inflammatory mediators increase Nav1.9 current and excitability in nociceptors through a coincident detection mechanism. *J. Gen. Physiol.* 131, 211–225. doi: 10.1085/jgp.200709935

Maleckar, M. M., Greenstein, J. L., Giles, W. R., and Trayanova, N. A. (2009a). Electrotonic coupling between human atrial myocytes and fibroblasts alters myocyte excitability and repolarization. *Biophys. J.* 97, 2179–2190. doi: 10.1016/j.bpj.2009.07.054

Maleckar, M. M., Greenstein, J. L., Giles, W. R., and Trayanova, N. A. (2009b). K+ current changes account for the rate dependence of the action potential in the human atrial myocyte. *Am. J. Physiol. Heart Circ. Physiol.* 297, H1398–H1410. doi: 10.1152/ajpheart.00411.2009

McDowell, K. S., Arevalo, H. J., Maleckar, M. M., and Trayanova, N. A. (2011). Susceptibility to arrhythmia in the infarcted heart depends on myofibroblast density. *Biophys. J.* 101, 1307–1315. doi: 10.1016/j.bpj.2011.08.009

McDowell, K. S., Vadakkumpadan, F., Blake, R., Blauer, J., Plank, G., MacLeod, R. S., et al. (2013). Mechanistic inquiry into the role of tissue remodeling in fibrotic lesions in human atrial fibrillation. *Biophys. J.* 104, 2764–2773. doi: 10.1016/j.bpj.2013.05.025

Miki, K., Yoshida, Y., and Yamanaka, S. (2013). Making steady progress on direct cardiac reprogramming toward clinical application. *Circ. Res.* 113, 13–15. doi: 10.1161/CIRCRESAHA.113.301788

Munoz, V., Campbell, K., and Shibayama, J. (2008). Fibroblasts: modulating the rhythm of the heart. *J. Physiol.* 586, 2423–2424. doi: 10.1113/jphysiol.2008.153387

Nattel, S. (2002). New ideas about atrial fibrillation 50 years on. *Nature* 415, 219–226. doi: 10.1038/415219a

Nygren, A., and Giles, W. R. (2000). Mathematical simulation of slowing of cardiac conduction velocity by elevated extracellular [K^+] in a human atrial strand. *Ann. Biomed. Eng.* 28, 951–957. doi: 10.1114/1.1308489

Palpant, N. J., and Murry, C. E. (2012). Regenerative medicine: reprogramming the injured heart. *Nature* 485, 585–586. doi: 10.1038/485585a

Pedrotty, D. M., Klinger, R. Y., Kirkton, R. D., and Bursac, N. (2009). Cardiac fibroblast paracrine factors alter impulse conduction and ion channel expression of neonatal rat cardiomyocytes. *Cardiovasc. Res.* 83, 688–697. doi: 10.1093/cvr/cvp164

Poon, B. Y., Ward, C. A., Cooper, C. B., Giles, W. R., Burns, A. R., and Kubes, P. (2001). α4-Integrin mediates neutrophil-induced free radical injury to cardiac myocytes. *J. Cell Biol.* 152, 857–866. doi: 10.1083/jcb.152.5.857

Porter, K. E., and Turner, N. A. (2009). Cardiac fibroblasts: at the heart of myocardial remodeling. *Pharmacol. Ther.* 123, 255–278. doi: 10.1016/j.pharmthera.2009.05.002

Powell, D., Mifflin, R., Valentich, J., Crowe, S., Saada, J., and West, A. (1999). Myofibroblasts. I. Paracrine cells important in health and disease. *Am. J. Physiol. Cell Physiol.* 277, C1–C19. doi: 10.1111/j.1469-7793.1999.001af.x

Qian, L., Huang, Y., Spencer, C. I., Foley, A., Vedantham, V., Liu, L., et al. (2012). *In vivo* reprogramming of murine cardiac fibroblasts into induced cardiomyocytes. *Nature* 485, 593–598. doi: 10.1038/nature11044

Rohr, S. (2011). Cardiac fibroblasts in cell culture systems: myofibroblasts all along? *J. Cardiovasc. Pharmacol.* 57, 389–399. doi: 10.1097/FJC.0b013e3182137e17

Rose, R., Hatano, N., Ohya, S., Imaizumi, Y., and Giles, W. (2007). C-type natriuretic peptide activates a non-selective cation current in acutely isolated rat cardiac fibroblasts via natriuretic peptide C receptor-mediated signalling. *J. Physiol.* 580, 255–274. doi: 10.1113/jphysiol.2006.120832

Rose, R. A., and Giles, W. R. (2008). Natriuretic peptide C receptor signalling in the heart and vasculature. *J. Physiol.* 586, 353–366. doi: 10.1113/jphysiol.2007.144253

Sachse, F. B., Moreno, A. P., and Abildskov, J. A. (2008). Electrophysiological modeling of fibroblasts and their interaction with myocytes. *Ann. Biomed. Eng.* 36, 41–56. doi: 10.1007/s10439-007-9405-8

Song, K., Nam, Y.-J., Luo, X., Qi, X., Tan, W., Huang, G. N., et al. (2012). Heart repair by reprogramming non-myocytes with cardiac transcription factors. *Nature* 485, 599–604. doi: 10.1038/nature11139

Spach, M. S., and Boineau, J. P. (1997). Microfibrosis produces electrical load variations due to loss of side–to–side cell connections; a major mechanism of structural heart disease arrhythmias. *Pacing Clin. Electrophysiol.* 20, 397–413. doi: 10.1111/j.1540-8159.1997.tb06199.x

Spach, M. S., Heidlage, J. F., Dolber, P. C., and Barr, R. C. (2007). Mechanism of origin of conduction disturbances in aging human atrial bundles: experimental and model study. *Heart Rhythm* 4, 175–185. doi: 10.1016/j.hrthm.2006.10.023

Srivastava, D., and Ieda, M. (2012). Critical factors for cardiac reprogramming. *Circ. Res.* 111, 5–8. doi: 10.1161/CIRCRESAHA.112.271452

Ward, C. A., Bazzazi, H., Clark, R. B., Nygren, A., and Giles, W. R. (2006). Actions of emigrated neutrophils on Na(+) and K(+) currents in rat ventricular myocytes. *Prog. Biophys. Mol. Biol.* 90, 249–269. doi: 10.1016/j.pbiomolbio.2005.07.003

Watanabe, H., Darbar, D., Kaiser, D. W., Jiramongkolchai, K., Chopra, S., Donahue, B. S., et al. (2009). Mutations in sodium channel β1-and β2-subunits associated with atrial fibrillation. *Circulation* 2, 268–275. doi: 10.1161/CIRCEP.108.779181

Weber, K. T., Brilla, C. G., and Janicki, J. S. (1993). Myocardial fibrosis: functional significance and regulatory factors. *Cardiovasc. Res.* 27, 341–348. doi: 10.1093/cvr/27.3.341

Wilson, J. R., Clark, R. B., Banderali, U., and Giles, W. R. (2011). Measurement of the membrane potential in small cells using patch clamp methods. *Channels (Austin)* 5, 530–537. doi: 10.4161/chan.5.6.17484

Yankelson, L., Feld, Y., Bressler-Stramer, T., Itzhaki, I., Huber, I., Gepstein, A., et al. (2008). Cell therapy for modification of the myocardial electrophysiological substrate. *Circulation* 117, 720–731. doi: 10.1161/CIRCULATIONAHA.106.671776

Zlochiver, S., Munoz, V., Vikstrom, K. L., Taffet, S. M., Berenfeld, O., and Jalife, J. (2008). Electrotonic myofibroblast-to-myocyte coupling increases propensity to reentrant arrhythmias in two-dimensional cardiac monolayers. *Biophys. J.* 95, 4469–4480. doi: 10.1529/biophysj.108.136473

11

Stem cells can form gap junctions with cardiac myocytes and exert pro-arrhythmic effects

***Nicoline W. Smit*[1]* and Ruben Coronel*[1,2]**

[1] Department of Clinical and Experimental Cardiology, Heart Centre, Academic Medical Centre, University of Amsterdam, Amsterdam, Netherlands
[2] L'Institut de RYthmologie et modélisation Cardiaque, Université Bordeaux Segalen, Bordeaux, France

Correspondence:
Nicoline W. Smit, Heart Center, Department of Experimental Cardiology, Academic Medical Center, University of Amsterdam, K2-113, Meibergdreef 9, 1105 AZ Amsterdam, Netherlands
e-mail: n.w.smit@amc.uva.nl

Stem cell therapy has been suggested to be a promising option for regeneration of injured myocardium, for example following a myocardial infarction. For clinical use cell-based therapies have to be safe and applicable and are aimed to renovate the architecture of the heart. Yet for functional and coordinated activity synchronized with the host myocardium stem cells have to be capable of forming electrical connections with resident cardiomyocytes. In this paper we discuss whether stem cells are capable of establishing functional electrotonic connections with cardiomyocytes and whether these may generate a risk for arrhythmias. Application of stem cells in the clinical setting with outcomes concerning arrhythmogenic safety and future perspectives will also briefly be touched upon.

Keywords: stem cells, cardiomyocytes, electrotonic connections, arrhythmias, clinical trials

INTRODUCTION

Electrical remodeling and loss of working myocardium after a myocardial infarction (MI) remains a major health challenge (McMurray and Pfeffer, 2005). Both processes disrupt the coordinated activation and repolarization of the heart. A theoretical remedy would be to replace the injured tissue with new cardiomyocytes (CM) that are capable of integrating and forming a functional network with the resident cardiomyocytes.

Stem cells have an unlimited proliferation ability and are capable of differentiating into multiple cell types (Wagers and Weissman, 2004). These two properties explain why so much time and energy has been put in making cell therapy effective for regeneration of the myocardium. Yet for proper functional integration within the host's myocardium there are several prerequisites including safety (the absence of adverse effects), a suitable delivery mode and proper timing of delivery. Although many questions concerning stem cells and their mechanism of actions remain, numerous clinical trials have been performed, with varying results.

The Myoblast Autologous Grafting in Ischemic Cardiomyopathy (MAGIC) trial, a multicenter randomized double blind and placebo-controlled study, was the first human trial concerning regenerative stem cell therapy involving skeletal myoblasts. Patients ($n = 90$) with prior MI, left ventricular dysfunction [left ventricular ejection fraction (LVEF) < 35%] and indications for coronary surgery received intra-myocardial injections of autologous myoblasts (low dose: 4×10^8 or high dose: 8×10^8) or placebo solutions. No changes were seen at 6 months in either global or regional left ventricular (LV) function between placebo treated patients and those treated with autologous skeletal myoblast (Eisen, 2008; Menasche et al., 2008). Arrhythmias were documented throughout the 6 months, although there was a higher occurrence in the pooled treatment group this was not significantly different from the control group, most likely owing to the small number of subjects.

In the CADUCEUS trial, cardio-sphere derived stem cells (CDC) were used, which were infused (low dose: 12.5×10^6 or high dose: 25×10^6) into the coronary artery of patients with LV dysfunction at 1.5–3 months post MI. The study was designed to assess safety. At 6 and 12 months follow-up period, despite the reduction in scar size and increase in viable myocardium in the group receiving CDC, no differences in ejection fraction were seen between the control and intervention groups (Makkar et al., 2012; Pompilio et al., 2012). Similar to the MAGIC trial non-sustained ventricular tachycardia (VT) occurred numerically more often in the CDC treated group. However, this was not statistically significant, again due to the small number of patients (17 patients in CDC group, 8 control patients).

The investigators of the SCIPIO and BOOST trials used C-kit$^+$ cardiac derived stem cells and autologous bone marrow stem cells, respectively, and did show functional improvements (Wollert et al., 2004; Bolli et al., 2011). The SCIPIO trial enrolled and randomized post MI patients with left ventricular dysfunction (LVEF $\leq$ 40%) before coronary artery bypass surgery into either the treatment (16 patients) or control group (7 patients) (Bolli et al., 2011). At 4 months post-surgery 16 patients received intracoronary infusion of stem cells (1×10^6). At 6 months post infusion, global improvement in left ventricular ejection fraction (LVEF) by approximately 8.2 $\pm$ 2.0 LVEF units was seen. LVEF increased by 12.3 $\pm$ 2.0 LVEF units at 1 year post treatment

(Bolli et al., 2011). In the BOOST trial, patients who had undergone successful percutaneous coronary intervention for (acute) ST-segment elevation MI were randomly assigned to the intracoronary bone-marrow transfer (30 patients) or to the control infusion (30 control patients). Patients showed increased global LVEF (about 6%) at 6 months post intracoronary infusion, which is similar to the SCIPIO trial. The effects observed in the BOOST trial, however, were not long-lasting and at 18 months and 5 years follow-up no difference was detected between the cell treated and non-cell treated groups. At 12 months post treatment the positive hemodynamic effects of the SCIPIO trial were maintained. However, that was the last follow-up point and hence it remains unknown whether the positive effects are long lasting or are only maintained up to 12 months post treatment as was seen in the BOOST trial. The SCIPIO trial investigators reported no occurrence of adverse arrhythmogenic events due to cell therapy such as (ventricular) arrhythmias but did not provide a definition of ventricular arrhythmias (Chugh et al., 2012). The BOOST trial reported that there was no difference in occurrence of adverse event, including arrhythmias, between treatment group and control group. However, also in this trial report, arrhythmias were not defined (e.g., duration of VT) and only mentioned as occurrence of VT (Meyer et al., 2006). In addition, similar to the MAGIC and CADUCEUS trial a limited number of patients were involved.

The clinical trials show that delivery of stem cells (either by intracoronary or intra-myocardial injection) is feasible and safe. However, whether the applied stem cells did differentiate and contribute to long-term functional improvements and safety remains questionable. The main reasons for this uncertainty are methodological differences between the trials and the low number of patients involved. Moreover, electrophysiological safety has not been extensively addressed and the electrophysiological variables investigated vary per study. This makes comparison between the studies difficult (Bursac et al., 2010).

Recently two meta-analyzes on stem cell based therapies in (i) chronic ischemic heart disease and congestive heart failure (Fisher et al., 2014) and (ii) acute MI (de Jong et al., 2014) were published. Each study included more than 20 randomized clinical trials adding up to more than 1200 patients. In the first meta-analysis concerning heart failure patients (without MI) there is moderate evidence that stem cells improve LVEF and that it has potential beneficial clinical outcome in terms of performance status (at least 1 year) and mortality (Fisher et al., 2014). The authors do underline the fact that the conclusions are still of low quality as the studies used are small and aimed at safety and feasibility. The second meta-analysis involving cell based therapies in patients with acute MI noted that there was a reasonable improvement in LVEF, which were explained by reduction in scar size and sustained LV end systole volume. Unlike the meta-analysis on heart failure no effects on clinical outcomes were found (de Jong et al., 2014). Similar to the other meta-analysis is that the studies included were only targeted at feasibility and safety.

Not only must cell therapy be delivered in a safe manner and at the right time, the cells should also be capable of making electrotonic connections with CM so that they can integrate and be properly functional within the host's myocardium. Currently, a number of different stem cell types are known, and although these are believed to behave differently from each other, this paper will evaluate studies that have used cardiomyocytes and stem cells, without focusing on one specific type/regardless of the type. The following questions will be addressed: (i) Are stem cells capable of forming functional intercellular connections with cardiomyocytes? and (ii) can pro-arrhythmic effects results from the interaction between stem cells and cardiomyocytes?

INTERCELLULAR CONNECTIONS

Gap junctions are specialized intercellular channels found in the membranes of neighboring cardiomyocytes, and allow exchange of ions and small molecules between cells (Kanno and Saffitz, 2001). These specialized regions are composed of two hexameric hemichannels, one in each neighboring CM. Each hemichannel, or connexon, in turn consists of 6 subunits called connexins (Kanno and Saffitz, 2001; Dhein, 2004). The gap junctional channels allow propagation of the action potential from one cell to the next. In normal healthy cardiomyocytes gap junctions are predominantly found at the intercalated disks, allowing the action potential to spread predominantly along the fiber's axis, resulting in faster conduction along the fiber than across the fiber direction (anisotropy) (Kanno and Saffitz, 2001).

The properties of these gap junctions play an important role in the determination of conduction velocity, and the electrical activation of the heart. Several cardiac connexin isoforms have been identified, each with a different channel conductance; the most predominantly expressed gap junction in ventricular myocytes is connexin43 (Cx43) (van Kempen et al., 1995). The lack of or loss of Cx43 is associated with diminished electrical coupling and formation of arrhythmias (de Groot et al., 2003; de Diego et al., 2008; Procida et al., 2009). Heart failure models show that decreased Cx43 coupling leads to an increase in conduction heterogeneity and to an increase in the inducibility of arrhythmias (Wiegerinck et al., 2008). The relation between uncoupling and conduction velocity is non-linear implying that a relatively large degree of loss of gap junctions is required to cause conduction slowing (Jongsma and Wilders, 2000). Furthermore, reduced intercellular coupling causes increased heterogeneity of repolarization and can contribute to a pro-arrhythmic substrate (Wiegerinck et al., 2008).

Because gap junctions are of crucial importance for the electrical activation and repolarization of the heart, alteration in gap junctions can lead to fundamental changes in the electrical activity of the heart. Stem cells must therefore be not only capable of coupling with CM but also do this with a sufficiently high gap junctional conductance.

ELECTROTONIC INTERACTIONS BETWEEN STEM CELLS AND CARDIOMYOCYTES

IN VITRO STUDIES

Various *in vitro* studies employing immunofluorescence staining have shown that gap junctions containing Cx43 exist between mesenchymal stem cells (MSC) and neonatal rat cardiomyocytes (NRCM) (Beeres et al., 2005; Chang et al., 2006; Pijnappels et al., 2006). Beeres et al. and Chang et al. additionally have proved, through the use of dye transfer, that these gap junctions were functional (Beeres et al., 2005; Chang et al., 2006).

The question therefore remains whether the gap junctions between MSC and cardiomyocytes also have (adverse) electrophysiological consequences. Electrophysiological functionality can be confirmed in *in vitro* studies with uncoupling substances such as gap junction blockers. Intercellular uncoupling or blocking of the formation of electrotonic connections can be used to detect both potential pro-arrhythmic as anti- arrhythmic consequences of the interconnections between the cell types. Using Tetrodotoxin in an *in vitro* co-culture of NRCM and human MSC, Askar et al. demonstrated that hetero-cellular coupling was the predominant mechanism for the observed conduction slowing in these preparations (Askar et al., 2013). Beeres et al. showed that electrotonic coupling with human MSC was needed to join two asynchronously beating fields of cardiomyocytes (Beeres et al., 2005). When carbenoxolene, a potent gap junctional uncoupling agent (de Groot et al., 2003), was added to these cultures the synchronized beating of the two fields was lost (Beeres et al., 2005; Pijnappels et al., 2006).

Another approach to establish functionality of connections between CM and stem cells is via genetic modification. In the *in vitro* model used by Beeres and Pijnappels, Cx43 knockdown in human MSC led to failure of synchronization of two asynchronously beating cardiomyocyte fields (Pijnappels et al., 2006). Co-cultures of skeletal myoblasts and NRCM demonstrated a decrease in conduction velocity and easily inducible re-entry, both of which could be attenuated when skeletal myoblasts were modified to overexpress Cx43 (Abraham et al., 2005; Tolmachov et al., 2006; Roell et al., 2007). More efficient coupling therefore appears to be beneficial whereas incomplete coupling is potentially arrhythmogenic.

IN VIVO STUDIES

Demonstrating functional coupling between stem cells and resident cardiomyocytes in *in vivo* studies is challenging. The implanted cells are usually not directly accessible and the lack of high-resolution functional measurements in a beating heart hampers direct assessment of functional coupling between stem cells and endogenous cardiomyocytes. Post mortem histological analyses may demonstrate successful engraftment of stem cells but not functional coupling.

Autologous stem cells engraftment has also been established in various studies through labeling stem cells with a cross-linkable membrane dye (Dye IL) (Price et al., 2006), transfection with GFP labeled lenti-virus (Valina et al., 2007; Mazo et al., 2011), or transfected *E. Coli* lac Z encoding B-gal (Rigol et al., 2010). Species-specific antibodies can determine the engraftment when xenografted cells are applied (Chong et al., 2014). However, in histological sections the electrophysiological interaction due to functional gap junctions cannot be demonstrated.

Alternative techniques to establish functional coupling *in vivo* is through calcium transients. Rubart et al. transplanted GFP expressing fetal cardiomyocytes into adult mice hearts (Rubart et al., 2003). Imaging of calcium transients in the intact heart of both host and donor cells showed that they were identical, encouraging the concept that cells can functionally couple to host cells (Rubart et al., 2003). Recently, this same concept was used to confirm functional coupling of human embryonic stem cell derived cardiomyocytes in a non-human primate myocardium (Chong et al., 2014). This last study convincingly supported the idea that stem cells can form a functional and synchronized network with the host myocardium. It has to be noted though that the cells used in this study are cardiomyocytes created from embryonic stem cells. This is where stem cell derived cardiomyocytes are purified and cryopreserved before application.

Kehat et al. performed *in vitro* electrophysiological analysis of hES that had formed spontaneous beating embryoid bodies. He demonstrated that hES had both structural and electrical features that resembled those of CM (Kehat et al., 2001). These hES were not grown together with myocytes and therefore it is not possible to state whether electrical coupling would form. Nevertheless, the fact that these cells obtained structural features specific for cardiomyocytes is attractive, because for proper integration within the myocardium the current generated in the host cell must not only pass through gap junctions to depolarize the transplanted cell, these cells must also have the appropriate excitation-contraction coupling properties.

PRO-ARRHYTHMIC EFFECTS OF ELECTROTONIC CONNECTIONS

Although engraftment of stem cells may occur, it does not imply that the engrafted cells are functionally and electrically coupled to resident cardiomyocytes. In addition, if these cells do couple electrically it is not self-evident that these interactions can contribute to the synchronized network of endogenous cardiomyocytes without any risks or side effects. It has been suggested that stem cells are capable of influencing the electrophysiological properties of cardiomyocytes, resulting in the formation of a pro-arrhythmic substrate (Chang et al., 2006; Askar et al., 2013). Proposed mechanisms including depolarization, anatomical block, abnormal automaticity and triggered activity are discussed and are schematically shown in **Figure 1**.

DEPOLARIZATION AND REFRACTORY PERIOD

The membrane potential of MSC has been shown to be around −35 mV (Heubach et al., 2004; Valiunas et al., 2004; Sundelacruz et al., 2008). After electrical coupling, depolarization of the resting membrane of CM is anticipated (Xie et al., 2009). The magnitude of depolarization depends on the membrane potential of the connected stem cell, but also to the extent of the intercellular coupling between the two cells (the coupling resistance) and the size of the cells (Tan and Joyner, 1990; Henriquez et al., 2001).

If depolarization of the resting membrane is severe (by more than 30 mV) the excitability of the cells is reduced; the voltage gated sodium channels are inactivated, resulting in reduction in upstroke velocity and conduction velocity (Shaw and Rudy, 1997; Kléber and Rudy, 2004; Hubbard et al., 2007). Also, the plateau phase is expected to be shorter while the action potential duration is expected to be prolonged **Figure 1A**. Action potential prolongation can lead to (unidirectional) block at tissue level and may facilitate re-entrant arrhythmias (de Bakker et al., 1993; Coronel et al., 2013).

Electrotonic connections between stem cells and cardiomyocytes can also lead to the "current sink" or "current

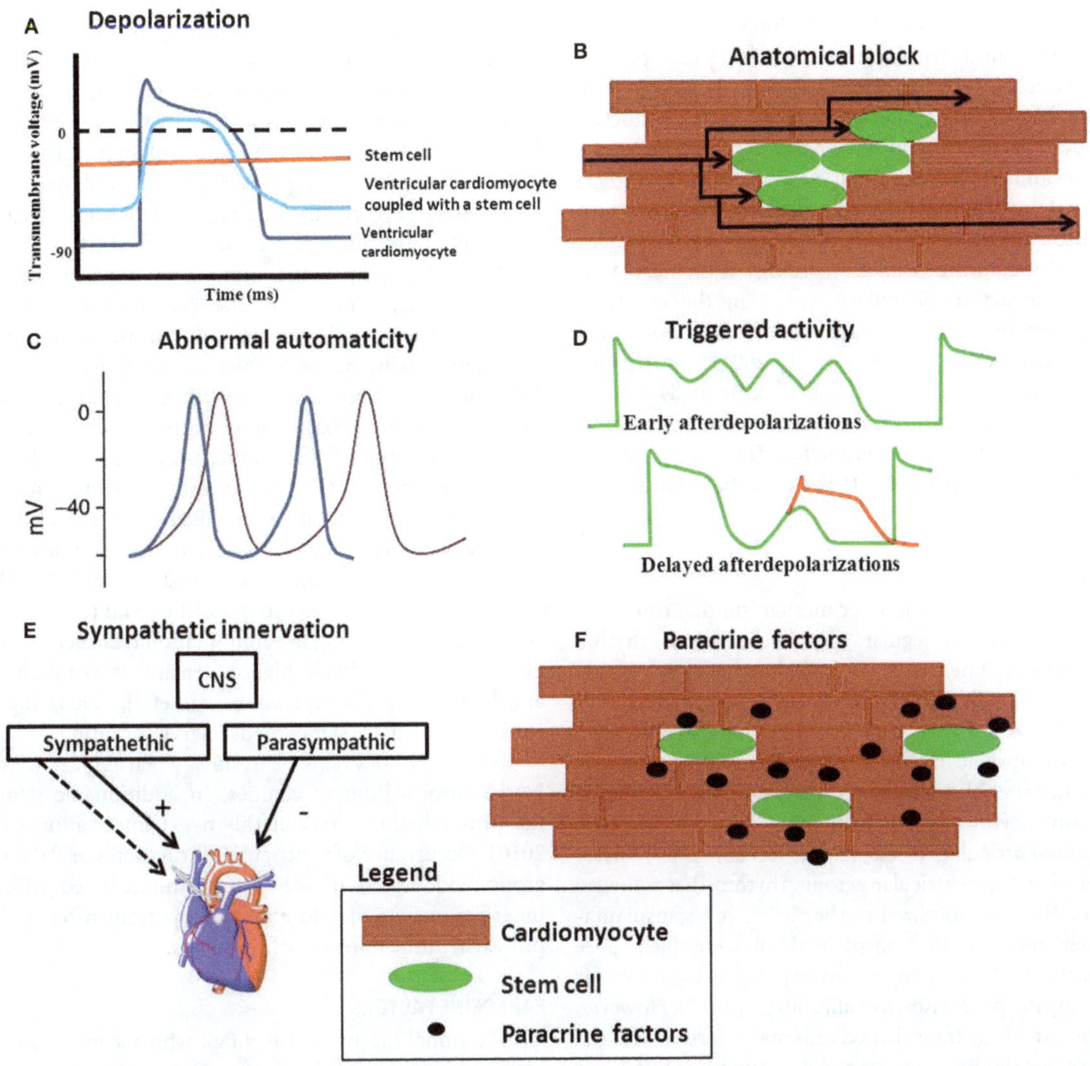

FIGURE 1 | Possible mechanisms of stem cell induced arrhythmias. **(A)** Depolarization of cardiomyocytes reduces the upstroke velocity and conduction velocity. **(B)** Clusters of stem cells can create an anatomical block and force the electrical pathway to find a different (and longer) route. **(C)** Stem cells can be spontaneously beating and may compete with the hosts own automaticity when engrafted. Stem cells may also be capable of inducing arrhythmias via triggered activity **(D)**. **(E)** Increased sympathetic innervation induced by stem cells can give an unbalance in the sympathetic and parasympathetic equilibrium. **(F)** Paracrine factors released by stem cells may effect electrophysiology of cardiomyocytes.

source" phenomenon (Rohr, 2004). This occurs when the load of an excited region supplying the depolarization current is not matched to the amount of current needed to excite the region ahead; current to load mismatch (Rohr, 2004). Stem cells depolarize cardiomyocytes, suggesting that the regions where stem cells are applied are more depolarized and that the depolarizing current coming from these hetero-cellular areas is not enough to excite the regions, consisting of endogenous cardiomyocytes, around it.

Depolarization of cardiomyocytes can thus lead to a reduction in upstroke velocity and conduction velocity but also affect the duration and shape of an action potential. These properties are all related to refractoriness and restitution properties (Hondeghem et al., 2001). Alterations in restitution properties and the effective refractory period (ERP) may lead to arrhythmias (Qu et al., 1999; Tran et al., 2007). The ERP plays an important role, together with conduction slowing and unidirectional block, in facilitating re-entry arrhythmias at a multicellular level. In a porcine MI model administration of MSC shortened ERP and resulted in steeper ERP restitution curves (Price et al., 2006), both indicators of electrical instability.

ANATOMICAL BLOCK

Cells used for cell-based regenerative therapies do not necessarily have to couple functionally to generate potential threatening situations for the formations of arrhythmias. Cells injected into the myocardium can integrate in such a way that they nestle themselves between CM causing resident CM to uncouple or prevent the coupling of CM (Duffy, 2008). Islands of uncoupled cells can cause anatomical block, forcing the electrical wave front to find an alternative route, resulting in a possible increased activation time over a specific region (de Bakker et al., 1993) (Figure 2A). If this results in heterogeneous conduction slowing it could facilitate unidirectional block and re-entrant arrhythmias (Lammers et al., 1990; de Bakker et al., 1993). In infarcted rat myocardium the transplanted myoblasts were functionally isolated from the resident cardiomyocytes (Leobon et al., 2003). Although intracellular recordings in the heart were obtained and the action potentials evoked in the myotubes were accompanied by (local) contractions, these did not spread out over the myocardium (Leobon et al., 2003). Information on conduction heterogeneity and local (fractionated) electrograms were not present in this publication. Both factors could have indicated discontinuous conduction (de Bakker et al., 1993; de Bakker and Wittkampf, 2010) a potential indicator for arrhythmogenesis.

ABNORMAL AUTOMATICITY

Abnormal automaticity is yet another mechanism that can evoke arrhythmias. The normal regular spontaneous sinus rhythm can be lost because other excitable cells have a higher spontaneous activity than the original endogenous pacemaker cells (**Figure 1C**). This could hold true for human embryonic stem cells that form embryoid bodies of spontaneously beating cardiomyocytes. Kehat et al. transplanted clusters of spontaneously beating cardiomyocytes (derived from hES) into a swine with complete atrio-ventricular block (Kehat et al., 2004). They demonstrated that the ventricular ectopic rhythm that followed the transplantation was localized at the site of cell transplantation. The observation that the transplanted cells were able to pace the entire heart at first glance appears to be positive, especially for bio-pace making purposes (Rosen et al., 2007; Li, 2012). However, the pacing rhythm of the transplanted cells may interfere with the animal's own sinus rhythm. In a recent paper published by Chong et al. human embryonic stem cell derived cardiomyocytes were injected into a non-human primate model of myocardial ischemia and reperfusion. The animals showed an usual high number of non-lethal arrhythmias (Chong et al., 2014). Compared to small animal models (Laflamme et al., 2007; Shiba et al., 2012), in which the same human embryonic cells were also used, the high number of non-lethal arrhythmias seen in the non-primate model may be explained by graft automaticity. These animals have lower heart rates compared to the smaller animals (mice and rats) used prior (Chong et al., 2014).

TRIGGERED ACTIVITY

Triggered activity initiated by (delayed or early) after depolarizations, may also be involved in arrhythmogenesis caused by stem cell therapy (**Figure 1D**).

Although a scarce number of studies concerning human embryonic stem cell derived CM (Jonsson et al., 2011) and induced pluripotent stem cell derived CM (Knollmann, 2013) have been performed to look at pro-arrhythmic potential, no conclusion can be drawn yet to associated stem cells directly with early after depolarizations or delayed after depolarizations.

SYMPATHETIC HYPER-INNERVATION

Stimulation of sympathetic nerve sprouting is an alternative mechanism of stem cells that promote arrhythmogenesis (Pak et al., 2003; Kim et al., 2010). Although this process does not require the formation of gap junctions it is important to keep in mind when evaluating the safety of stem cells. The heart is innervated by both the parasympathetic and sympathetic nervous system (**Figure 1E**), whereby the latter has a higher density in de sub-epicardium and central conduction system (Kawano et al., 2003). Sympathetic stimulation leads to acceleration of the heart rate, contractility and can improve cardiac output. However, it has also been shown that disturbed innervation can cause lethal arrhythmias (Cao et al., 2000). Pak et al. stated that MSC induce cardiac nerve sprouting in a large animal model of MI (Pak et al., 2003). One month post MI induction, swines received injections of either a mixture of MSC and bone marrow cells, bone marrow cells alone or only the culture medium. One month later the animals were killed and immunofluorescence staining was performed on tissue samples. Samples were stained for nerve sprouting (growth-associated protein; GAP-43), sympathetic nerves (tyrosine hydroxylase; TH) and for tenascin expression. Animals receiving the combination treatment showed more GAP43-positive nerves, higher density of sympathetic nerves and higher tenascin expression (Pak et al., 2003) suggesting an increase in cardiac (sympathetic) nerve sprouting.

Kim et al. saw similar results when MSCs were injected in the myocardium of canines. In addition, he demonstrated the pro-arrhythmic risk of this hyper-innervation (Kim et al., 2010). Occurrence of ventricular fibrillation was 0% in the sham group and 33.3% in the group who received MSC. Hyper-innervation may therefore be an important mechanism for the pro-arrhythmic potential of stem cells.

PARACRINE FACTORS

An additional mechanism through which stem cells can be pro-arrhythmic is the influence of secreted paracrine factors or factors released once these cells are connected to cardiomyocytes (**Figure 1F**). Although the "paracrine hypothesis" (Gnecchi et al., 2008) is suggested to be an indirect mechanism behind improvement in left ventricular (LV) function, changes in scar properties, angiogenesis induction and/or improvement in survival of endogenous cardiomyocytes, several studies have documented pro-arrhythmic effects of paracrine factors (Pedrotty et al., 2009; Askar et al., 2013). However, the actual factor(s) and mechanism behind these observed results still need to be identified.

CONCLUSION

After nearly two decades of research in stem cell based therapies for cardiac regeneration the search for the "perfect" stem cell—based therapy for cardiac tissue regeneration continues as there are still many questions left that remain unanswered.

Stem cells have the ability to couple electrically to cardiomyocytes via gap junctions. Formations of functional intercellular connections influence the electrical properties of cardiomyocytes and are associated with pro-arrhythmic effects. Depolarization of resting membrane, heterogeneous conduction slowing, and electrical instability are factors that can occur after electrotonic connections between stem cells and cardiomyocytes are formed. Depending on the magnitude of effect these factors can contribute to the formation of arrhythmias.

Future studies should not only be aimed at efficacy and long-term effects but also in making clinical trials similar so that factors (e.g., different in/exclusion criteria, cells dose/type, timing, and route of cell infusion) contributing to conflicting data can be limited and a provide solid framework for the safe application of stem cells without arrhythmogenic side effects.

ACKNOWLEDGMENTS

We would like to thank Veronique M. F. Meijborg for her valuable input and suggestions.

REFERENCES

Abraham, M. R., Henrikson, C. A., Tung, L., Chang, M. G., Aon, M., Xue, T., et al. (2005). Antiarrhythmic engineering of skeletal myoblasts for cardiac transplantation. *Circ. Res.* 97, 159–167. doi: 10.1161/01.RES.0000174794.22491.a0

Askar, S. F., Ramkisoensing, A. A., Atsma, D. E., Schalij, M. J., de Vries, A. A., and Pijnappels, D. A. (2013). Engraftment patterns of human adult mesenchymal stem cells expose electrotonic and paracrine proarrhythmic mechanisms in myocardial cell cultures. *Circ. Arrhythm. Electrophysiol.* 6, 380–391. doi: 10.1161/CIRCEP.111.000215

Beeres, S. L., Atsma, D. E., van der Laarse, A., Pijnappels, D. A., van Tuyn, J., Fibbe, W. E., et al. (2005). Human adult bone marrow mesenchymal stem cells repair experimental conduction block in rat cardiomyocyte cultures. *J. Am. Coll. Cardiol.* 46, 1943–1952. doi: 10.1016/j.jacc.2005.07.055

Bolli, R., Chugh, A. R., D'Amario, D., Loughran, J. H., Stoddard, M. F., Ikram, S., et al. (2011). Cardiac stem cells in patients with ischaemic cardiomyopathy (SCIPIO): initial results of a randomised phase 1 trial. *Lancet* 378, 1847–1857. doi: 10.1016/S0140-6736(11)61590-0

Bursac, N., Kirkton, R. D., McSpadden, L. C., and Liau, B. (2010). Characterizing functional stem cell-cardiomyocyte interactions. *Regen. Med.* 5, 87–105. doi: 10.2217/rme.09.69

Cao, J. M., Chen, L. S., Kenknight, B. H., Ohara, T., Lee, M. H., Tsai, J., et al. (2000). Nerve sprouting and sudden cardiac death. *Circ. Res.* 86, 816–821. doi: 10.1161/01.RES.86.7.816

Chang, M. G., Tung, L., Sekar, R. B., Chang, C. Y., Cysyk, J., Dong, P., et al. (2006). Proarrhythmic potential of mesenchymal stem cell transplantation revealed in an *in vitro* coculture model. *Circulation* 113, 1832–1841. doi: 10.1161/CIRCULATIONAHA.105.593038

Chong, J. J., Yang, X., Don, C. W., Minami, E., Liu, Y. W., Weyers, J. J., et al. (2014). Human embryonic-stem-cell-derived cardiomyocytes regenerate non-human primate hearts. *Nature* 510, 273–277. doi: 10.1038/nature13233

Chugh, A. R., Beache, G. M., Loughran, J. H., Mewton, N., Elmore, J. B., Kajstura, J., et al. (2012). Administration of cardiac stem cells in patients with ischemic cardiomyopathy: the SCIPIO trial: surgical aspects and interim analysis of myocardial function and viability by magnetic resonance. *Circulation* 126(11 Suppl. 1), S54–S64. doi: 10.1161/CIRCULATIONAHA.112.092627

Coronel, R., Wilders, R., Verkerk, A. O., Wiegerinck, R. F., Benoist, D., and Bernus, O. (2013). Electrophysiological changes in heart failure and their implications for arrhythmogenesis. *Biochim. Biophys. Acta* 1832, 2432–2441. doi: 10.1016/j.bbadis.2013.04.002

de Bakker, J. M., van Capelle, F. J., Janse, M. J., Tasseron, S., Vermeulen, J. T., de Jonge, N., et al. (1993). Slow conduction in the infarcted human heart. 'Zigzag' course of activation. *Circulation* 88, 915–926. doi: 10.1161/01.CIR.88.3.915

de Bakker, J. M., and Wittkampf, F. H. (2010). The pathophysiologic basis of fractionated and complex electrograms and the impact of recording techniques on their detection and interpretation. *Circ. Arrhythm. Electrophysiol.* 3, 204–213. doi: 10.1161/CIRCEP.109.904763

de Diego, C., Pai, R. K., Chen, F., Xie, L. H., De, L. J., Weiss, J. N., et al. (2008). Electrophysiological consequences of acute regional ischemia/reperfusion in neonatal rat ventricular myocyte monolayers. *Circulation* 118, 2330–2337. doi: 10.1161/CIRCULATIONAHA.108.789149

de Groot, J. R., Veenstra, T., Verkerk, A. O., Wilders, R., Smits, J. P., Wilms-Schopman, F. J., et al. (2003). Conduction slowing by the gap junctional uncoupler carbenoxolone. *Cardiovasc. Res.* 60, 288–297. doi: 10.1016/j.cardiores.2003.07.004

de Jong, R., Houtgraaf, J. H., Samiei, S., Boersma, E., and Duckers, H. J. (2014). Intracoronary stem cell infusion after acute myocardial infarction: a meta-analysis and update on clinical trials. *Circ. Cardiovasc. Interv.* 7, 156–167. doi: 10.1161/CIRCINTERVENTIONS.113.001009

Dhein, S. (2004). Pharmacology of gap junctions in the cardiovascular system. *Cardiovasc. Res.* 62, 287–298. doi: 10.1016/j.cardiores.2004.01.019

Duffy, H. S. (2008). Cardiac connections–the antiarrhythmic solution? *N. Engl. J. Med.* 358, 1397–1398. doi: 10.1056/NEJMcibr0708922

Eisen, H. J. (2008). Skeletal myoblast transplantation: no MAGIC bullet for ischemic cardiomyopathy. *Nat. Clin. Pract. Cardiovasc. Med.* 5, 520–521. doi: 10.1038/ncpcardio1299

Fisher, S. A., Brunskill, S. J., Doree, C., Mathur, A., Taggart, D. P., and Martin-Rendon, E. (2014). Stem cell therapy for chronic ischaemic heart disease and congestive heart failure. *Cochrane Database Syst. Rev.* 4:CD007888. doi: 10.1002/14651858.CD007888

Gnecchi, M., Zhang, Z., Ni, A., and Dzau, V. J. (2008). Paracrine mechanisms in adult stem cell signaling and therapy. *Circ. Res.* 103, 1204–1219. doi: 10.1161/CIRCRESAHA.108.176826

Henriquez, A. P., Vogel, R., Muller-Borer, B. J., Henriquez, C. S., Weingart, R., and Cascio, W. E. (2001). Influence of dynamic gap junction resistance on impulse propagation in ventricular myocardium: a computer simulation study. *Biophys. J.* 81, 2112–2121. doi: 10.1016/S0006-3495(01)75859-6

Heubach, J. F., Graf, E. M., Leutheuser, J., Bock, M., Balana, B., Zahanich, I., et al. (2004). Electrophysiological properties of human mesenchymal stem cells. *J. Physiol.* 554(Pt 3), 659–672. doi: 10.1113/jphysiol.2003.055806

Hondeghem, L. M., Carlsson, L., and Duker, G. (2001). Instability and triangulation of the action potential predict serious proarrhythmia, but action potential duration prolongation is antiarrhythmic. *Circulation* 103, 2004–2013. doi: 10.1161/01.CIR.103.15.2004

Hubbard, M. L., Ying, W., and Henriquez, C. S. (2007). Effect of gap junction distribution on impulse propagation in a monolayer of myocytes: a model study. *Europace* 9 Suppl. 6, vi20–vi28. doi: 10.1093/europace/eum203

Jongsma, H. J., and Wilders, R. (2000). Gap junctions in cardiovascular disease. *Circ. Res.* 86, 1193–1197. doi: 10.1161/01.RES.86.12.1193

Jonsson, M. K., Wang, Q. D., and Becker, B. (2011). Impedance-based detection of beating rhythm and proarrhythmic effects of compounds on stem cell-derived cardiomyocytes. *Assay Drug Dev. Technol.* 9, 589–599. doi: 10.1089/adt.2011.0396

Kanno, S., and Saffitz, J. E. (2001). The role of myocardial gap junctions in electrical conduction and arrhythmogenesis. *Cardiovasc. Pathol.* 10, 169–177. doi: 10.1016/S1054-8807(01)00078-3

Kawano, H., Okada, R., and Yano, K. (2003). Histological study on the distribution of autonomic nerves in the human heart. *Heart Vessels* 18, 32–39. doi: 10.1007/s003800300005

Kehat, I., Kenyagin-Karsenti, D., Snir, M., Segev, H., Amit, M., Gepstein, A., et al. (2001). Human embryonic stem cells can differentiate into myocytes with structural and functional properties of cardiomyocytes. *J. Clin. Invest.* 108, 407–414. doi: 10.1172/JCI200112131

Kehat, I., Khimovich, L., Caspi, O., Gepstein, A., Shofti, R., Arbel, G., et al. (2004). Electromechanical integration of cardiomyocytes derived from human embryonic stem cells. *Nat. Biotechnol.* 22, 1282–1289. doi: 10.1038/nbt1014

Kim, S. K., Pak, H. N., Park, J. H., Fang, Y. F., Kim, G. I., Park, Y. D., et al. (2010). Cardiac cell therapy with mesenchymal stem cell induces cardiac nerve sprouting, angiogenesis, and reduced connexin43-positive gap junctions, but concomitant electrical pacing increases connexin43-positive gap junctions in canine heart. *Cardiol. Young* 20, 308–317. doi: 10.1017/S1047951110000132

Kléber, A. G., and Rudy, Y. (2004). Basic mechanisms of cardiac impulse propagation and associated arrhythmias. *Physiol. Rev.* 84, 431–488. doi: 10.1152/physrev.00025.2003

Knollmann, B. C. (2013). Induced pluripotent stem cell-derived cardiomyocytes: boutique science or valuable arrhythmia model? *Circ. Res.* 112, 969–976. doi: 10.1161/CIRCRESAHA.112.300567

Laflamme, M. A., Chen, K. Y., Naumova, A. V., Muskheli, V., Fugate, J. A., Dupras, S. K., et al. (2007). Cardiomyocytes derived from human embryonic stem cells in pro-survival factors enhance function of infarcted rat hearts. *Nat. Biotechnol.* 25, 1015–1024. doi: 10.1038/nbt1327

Lammers, W. J., Schalij, M. J., Kirchhof, C. J., and Allessie, M. A. (1990). Quantification of spatial inhomogeneity in conduction and initiation of reentrant atrial arrhythmias. *Am. J. Physiol.* 259(4 Pt 2), H1254–H1263.

Leobon, B., Garcin, I., Menasche, P., Vilquin, J. T., Audinat, E., and Charpak, S. (2003). Myoblasts transplanted into rat infarcted myocardium are functionally isolated from their host. *Proc. Natl. Acad. Sci. U.S.A.* 100, 7808–7811. doi: 10.1073/pnas.1232447100

Li, R. A. (2012). Gene- and cell-based bio-artificial pacemaker: what basic and translational lessons have we learned? *Gene Ther.* 19, 588–595. doi: 10.1038/gt.2012.33

Makkar, R. R., Smith, R. R., Cheng, K., Malliaras, K., Thomson, L. E., Berman, D., et al. (2012). Intracoronary cardiosphere-derived cells for heart regeneration after myocardial infarction (CADUCEUS): a prospective, randomised phase 1 trial. *Lancet* 379, 895–904. doi: 10.1016/S0140-6736(12)60195-0

Mazo, M., Gavira, J. J., Pelacho, B., and Prosper, F. (2011). Adipose-derived stem cells for myocardial infarction. *J. Cardiovasc. Transl. Res.* 4, 145–153. doi: 10.1007/s12265-010-9246-y

McMurray, J. J., and Pfeffer, M. A. (2005). Heart failure. *Lancet* 365, 1877–1889. doi: 10.1016/S0140-6736(05)66621-4

Menasche, P., Alfieri, O., Janssens, S., McKenna, W., Reichenspurner, H., Trinquart, L., et al. (2008). The Myoblast Autologous Grafting in Ischemic Cardiomyopathy (MAGIC) trial: first randomized placebo-controlled study of myoblast transplantation. *Circulation* 117, 1189–1200. doi: 10.1161/CIRCULATIONAHA.107.734103

Meyer, G. P., Wollert, K. C., Lotz, J., Steffens, J., Lippolt, P., Fichtner, S., et al. (2006). Intracoronary bone marrow cell transfer after myocardial infarction: eighteen months' follow-up data from the randomized, controlled BOOST (BOne marrOw transfer to enhance ST-elevation infarct regeneration) trial. *Circulation* 113, 1287–1294. doi: 10.1161/CIRCULATIONAHA.105.575118

Pak, H. N., Qayyum, M., Kim, D. T., Hamabe, A., Miyauchi, Y., Lill, M. C., et al. (2003). Mesenchymal stem cell injection induces cardiac nerve sprouting and increased tenascin expression in a Swine model of myocardial infarction. *J. Cardiovasc. Electrophysiol.* 14, 841–848. doi: 10.1046/j.1540-8167.2003.03124.x

Pedrotty, D. M., Klinger, R. Y., Kirkton, R. D., and Bursac, N. (2009). Cardiac fibroblast paracrine factors alter impulse conduction and ion channel expression of neonatal rat cardiomyocytes. *Cardiovasc. Res.* 83, 688–697. doi: 10.1093/cvr/cvp164

Pijnappels, D. A., Schalij, M. J., van Tuyn, J., Ypey, D. L., de Vries, A. A., van der Wall, E. E., et al. (2006). Progressive increase in conduction velocity across human mesenchymal stem cells is mediated by enhanced electrical coupling. *Cardiovasc. Res.* 72, 282–291. doi: 10.1016/j.cardiores.2006.07.016

Pompilio, G., Capogrossi, M. C., Leone, A. M., and Crea, F. (2012). The SCIPIO and CADUCEUS studies. *G. Ital. Cardiol. (Rome).* 13, 777–782. doi: 10.1714/1188.13160

Price, M. J., Chou, C. C., Frantzen, M., Miyamoto, T., Kar, S., Lee, S., et al. (2006). Intravenous mesenchymal stem cell therapy early after reperfused acute myocardial infarction improves left ventricular function and alters electrophysiologic properties. *Int. J. Cardiol.* 111, 231–239. doi: 10.1016/j.ijcard.2005.07.036

Procida, K., Jorgensen, L., Schmitt, N., Delmar, M., Taffet, S. M., Holstein-Rathlou, N. H., et al. (2009). Phosphorylation of connexin43 on serine 306 regulates electrical coupling. *Heart Rhythm* 6, 1632–1638. doi: 10.1016/j.hrthm.2009.07.043

Qu, Z., Weiss, J. N., and Garfinkel, A. (1999). Cardiac electrical restitution properties and stability of reentrant spiral waves: a simulation study. *Am. J. Physiol.* 276(1 Pt 2), H269–H283.

Rigol, M., Solanes, N., Farre, J., Roura, S., Roque, M., Berruezo, A., et al. (2010). Effects of adipose tissue-derived stem cell therapy after myocardial infarction: impact of the route of administration. *J. Card. Fail.* 16, 357–366. doi: 10.1016/j.cardfail.2009.12.006

Roell, W., Lewalter, T., Sasse, P., Tallini, Y. N., Choi, B. R., Breitbach, M., et al. (2007). Engraftment of connexin 43-expressing cells prevents post-infarct arrhythmia. *Nature* 450, 819–824. doi: 10.1038/nature06321

Rohr, S. (2004). Role of gap junctions in the propagation of the cardiac action potential. *Cardiovasc. Res.* 62, 309–322. doi: 10.1016/j.cardiores.2003.11.035

Rosen, M. R., Brink, P. R., Cohen, I. S., and Robinson, R. B. (2007). Biological pacemakers based on I(f). *Med. Biol. Eng. Comput.* 45, 157–166. doi: 10.1007/s11517-006-0060-2

Rubart, M., Pasumarthi, K. B., Nakajima, H., Soonpaa, M. H., Nakajima, H. O., and Field, L. J. (2003). Physiological coupling of donor and host cardiomyocytes after cellular transplantation. *Circ. Res.* 92, 1217–1224. doi: 10.1161/01.RES.0000075089.39335.8C

Shaw, R. M., and Rudy, Y. (1997). Electrophysiologic effects of acute myocardial ischemia. A mechanistic investigation of action potential conduction and conduction failure. *Circ. Res.* 80, 124–138. doi: 10.1161/01.RES.80.1.124

Shiba, Y., Fernandes, S., Zhu, W. Z., Filice, D., Muskheli, V., Kim, J., et al. (2012). Human ES-cell-derived cardiomyocytes electrically couple and suppress arrhythmias in injured hearts. *Nature* 489, 322–325. doi: 10.1038/nature11317

Sundelacruz, S., Levin, M., and Kaplan, D. L. (2008). Membrane potential controls adipogenic and osteogenic differentiation of mesenchymal stem cells. *PLoS ONE* 3:e3737. doi: 10.1371/journal.pone.0003737

Tan, R. C., and Joyner, R. W. (1990). Electrotonic influences on action potentials from isolated ventricular cells. *Circ. Res.* 67, 1071–1081. doi: 10.1161/01.RES.67.5.1071

Tolmachov, O., Ma, Y. L., Themis, M., Patel, P., Spohr, H., MacLeod, K. T., et al. (2006). Overexpression of connexin 43 using a retroviral vector improves electrical coupling of skeletal myoblasts with cardiac myocytes *in vitro*. *BMC Cardiovasc. Disord.* 6:25. doi: 10.1186/1471-2261-6-25

Tran, D. X., Yang, M. J., Weiss, J. N., Garfinkel, A., and Qu, Z. (2007). Vulnerability to re-entry in simulated two-dimensional cardiac tissue: effects of electrical restitution and stimulation sequence. *Chaos* 17:043115. doi: 10.1063/1.2784387

Valina, C., Pinkernell, K., Song, Y. H., Bai, X., Sadat, S., Campeau, R. J., et al. (2007). Intracoronary administration of autologous adipose tissue-derived stem cells improves left ventricular function, perfusion, and remodelling after acute myocardial infarction. *Eur. Heart J.* 28, 2667–2677. doi: 10.1093/eurheartj/ehm426

Valiunas, V., Doronin, S., Valiuniene, L., Potapova, I., Zuckerman, J., Walcott, B., et al. (2004). Human mesenchymal stem cells make cardiac connexins and form functional gap junctions. *J. Physiol.* 555(Pt 3), 617–626. doi: 10.1113/jphysiol.2003.058719

van Kempen, M. J., ten Velde, I., Wessels, A., Oosthoek, P. W., Gros, D., Jongsma, H. J., et al. (1995). Differential connexin distribution accommodates cardiac function in different species. *Microsc. Res. Tech.* 31, 420–436. doi: 10.1002/jemt.1070310511

Wagers, A. J., and Weissman, I. L. (2004). Plasticity of adult stem cells. *Cell* 116, 639–648. doi: 10.1016/S0092-8674(04)00208-9

Wiegerinck, R. F., van Veen, T. A., Belterman, C. N., Schumacher, C. A., Noorman, M., de Bakker, J. M., et al. (2008). Transmural dispersion of refractoriness and conduction velocity is associated with heterogeneously reduced connexin43 in a rabbit model of heart failure. *Heart Rhythm* 5, 1178–1185. doi: 10.1016/j.hrthm.2008.04.026

Wollert, K. C., Meyer, G. P., Lotz, J., Ringes-Lichtenberg, S., Lippolt, P., Breidenbach, C., et al. (2004). Intracoronary autologous bone-marrow cell transfer after myocardial infarction: the BOOST randomised controlled clinical trial. *Lancet* 364, 141–148. doi: 10.1016/S0140-6736(04)16626-9

12

The role of inhibitory G proteins and regulators of G protein signaling in the *in vivo* control of heart rate and predisposition to cardiac arrhythmias

Richard Ang[1], Aaisha Opel[1] and Andrew Tinker[2]*

[1] *Centre for Clinical Pharmacology, Division of Medicine, University College London, London, UK*
[2] *William Harvey Heart Centre, Barts and The London School of Medicine and Dentistry, London, UK*

Correspondence:
Andrew Tinker, William Harvey Heart Centre, Barts and The London School of Medicine and Dentistry, Room 1.02, Charterhouse Square, London EC1M 6BQ, UK.
e-mail: a.tinker@qmul.ac.uk

Inhibitory heterotrimeric G proteins and the control of heart rate. The activation of cell signaling pathways involving inhibitory heterotrimeric G proteins acts to slow the heart rate via modulation of ion channels. A large number of Regulators of G protein signalings (RGSs) can act as GTPase accelerating proteins to inhibitory G proteins and thus it is important to understand the network of RGS\G-protein interaction. We will review our recent findings on *in vivo* heart rate control in mice with global genetic deletion of various inhibitory G protein alpha subunits. We will discuss potential central and peripheral contributions to the phenotype and the controversies in the literature.

Keywords: inhibitory G protein, regulators of G protein signaling, heart, arrhythmia

INTRODUCTION

The pacemaker in the sinoatrial node (SAN) of the heart has an intrinsic rate independent of autonomic innervation and this leads to a measurement of "intrinsic" heart rate that is determined in practice by pharmacologically inhibiting the sympathetic and parasympathetic systems. At the molecular level this self-regenerating electrical activity arises from a membrane clock and\or a calcium clock dependent on intracellular calcium release events (Lakatta and DiFrancesco, 2009). This pacemaker activity can be modulated: increased sympathetic activity leads to an increase in rate and an increase in vagal tone to a decrease. The release of noradrenaline from sympathetic nerve endings or the release of adrenaline from the adrenal medulla into the circulation modulates SAN cells by binding to β-adrenoreceptors. The stimulatory G protein is activated and this leads to stimulation of adenylate cyclase and the generation of cyclic adenosine monophosphate (cAMP). Increased cAMP can directly modulate the hyperpolarization-activated cation currents (I_h/I_f) leading to increased pacemaker depolarization and rate. However, increased cAMP can also activate protein kinase A (PKA), which can modulate intracellular calcium-handling proteins such as phospholamban and the ryanodine receptor to modulate rate.

However, the main focus of this review is on the inhibitory events typified by the negative chronotropic response in the SAN to vagal nerve efferent activation. Acetylcholine (ACh) released from the vagus nerve binds to the muscarinic (M2) receptor, leading to the activation, and dissociation of inhibitory G protein heterotrimers. The resulting βγ-dimer directly activates the G protein coupled inward rectifying potassium (GIRK) channel to cause membrane hyperpolarization, slowing pacemaker depolarization, and sinus rate. Furthermore, the activation of the inhibitory Gα subunit will inhibit adenylate cyclase and thus modulate I_h/I_f as detailed above. Regulators of G protein signaling (RGS) proteins interact with the inhibitory Gα subunit to switch off this pathway through GTPase accelerating protein (GAP) activity and allow the heterotrimer to reform. This process is summarized in **Figure 1**.

It has emerged from the SHIFT trial using ivabradine, an inhibitor of I_h/I_f, in addition to standard therapy that heart rate *per se* may be an important risk factor in chronic heart failure (Swedberg et al., 2010). Furthermore, autonomic precipitants are well known for common arrhythmias such as atrial fibrillation (AF) and ventricular tachyarrhythmia (see below). Thus the focus in this review is an attempt to link physiological and pathophysiological function in the control of heart rate and rhythm with the known molecular isoforms of the inhibitory G proteins and RGSs. These proteins are widely distributed in the heart thus we will consider not only their effects on heart rate but also what electrical processes they might modulate in the atria, atrioventricular node (AVN), and ventricles. One of the key approaches is the use of genetically modified mice. However, these often have global knockout of the relevant gene and this will mean deletion of the signaling molecule in central circuits and peripheral nerves of the autonomic nervous system. Thus we review the role of inhibitory G proteins in the central circuits and peripheral limbs of the autonomic nervous system, consider the limited information available and experimental approaches by which this might be investigated.

THE MOLECULAR NUTS AND BOLTS

We initially discuss this from a cardiac perspective but the role of the nervous system is obviously important and this is addressed in another section.

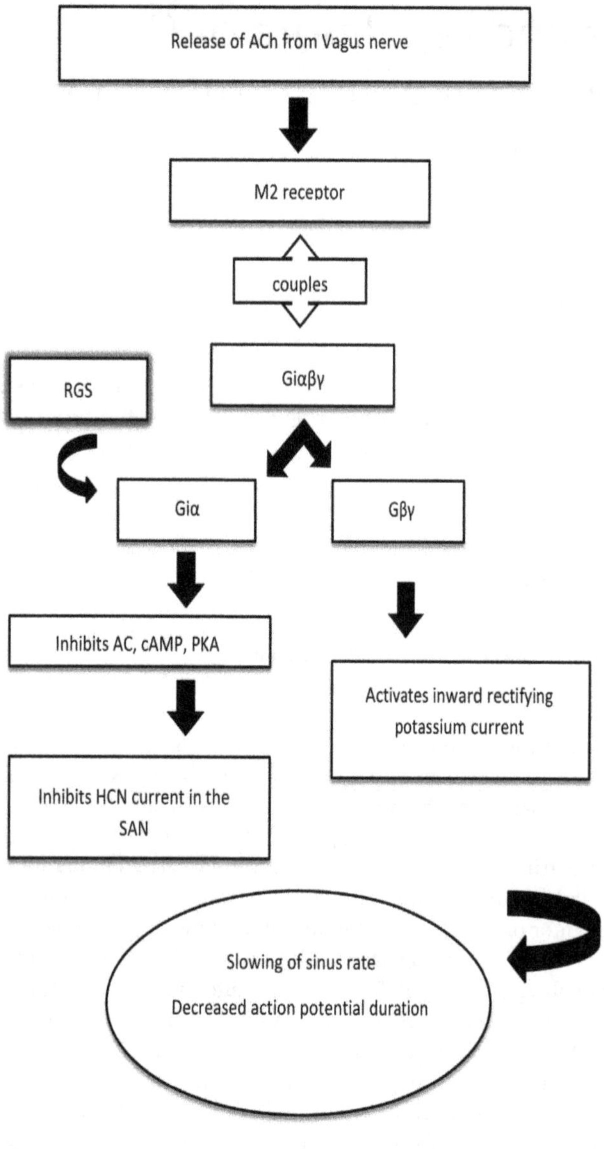

FIGURE 1 | A simplified schematic for the mechanism of heart rate regulation by inhibitory G proteins. Acetylcholine released from the vagus nerve binds to the muscarinic (M2) receptor, which is coupled to the inhibitory G protein. The βγ-dimer activates the G protein coupled inward rectifying potassium (GIRK) channel to slow the sinus rate, decrease the action potential duration and allow arrhythmia generation. Regulators of G protein signaling (RGS) interact with the α-subunit to switch off this pathway through GTPase accelerating protein activity and allow the heterotrimer to reform. AC, adenylyl cyclase; cAMP, cyclic AMP; PKA, protein kinase A; HCN, hyperpolarization-activated cyclic nucleotide-gated channel.

INHIBITORY G PROTEINS

There are four families of G proteins namely $G\alpha_{i/o}$, $G\alpha_s$, $G\alpha_{q/11}$, $G\alpha_{12/13}$. The inhibitory G proteins ($G\alpha_{i/o}$) are the most highly expressed and predominant class followed by $G\alpha_s$, $G\alpha_{q/11}$ then $G\alpha_{12/13}$. The inhibitory G proteins themselves have multiple isoforms: $G\alpha_{i1}$, $G\alpha_{i2}$, $G\alpha_{i3}$, and $G\alpha_o$. The $G\alpha_o$ ("other") isoform has two splice variants $G\alpha_{oA}$ and $G\alpha_{oB}$. $G\alpha_o$ is the predominant isoform in the brain whereas $G\alpha_{i1}$, $G\alpha_{i2}$, $G\alpha_{i3}$ are highly homologous and widely distributed in many tissues (Wettschureck and Offermanns, 2005). The inhibitory G proteins characteristically inhibit adenylate cyclase activity and lower the concentration of cAMP (Wong et al., 1991; Rudolph et al., 1996), however they also activate PI-3 kinase activity and directly regulate ion channel activity (see below).

REGULATORS OF G PROTEIN SIGNALING

Regulators of G protein signaling proteins act to effectively inhibit G protein signaling; they interact with the α-subunit and accelerate GTPase activity. Characteristically this family have a 120 amino acid conserved RGS domain, flanked by variable length N- and C-terminals. Six main subfamilies of mammalian RGSs are distinguished: R4, R7, R12, RA, RL, and RZ. The vast majority of RGSs are GAPs for inhibitory G proteins but some have activity to the $G_{q/11}$ family as well. They may also have other roles in signaling (Hollinger and Hepler, 2002). There are more than 20 mammalian RGS isoforms and many of these are expressed to some extent in the heart (Kardestuncer et al., 1998; Doupnik et al., 2001; Owen et al., 2001; Wieland and Mittmann, 2003). For both $G\alpha_{i/o}$ and RGSs the pattern of expression in conducting tissues, atria, and ventricles and in specific cell types such as myocytes and fibroblasts is not well delineated.

KEY ION CHANNELS

The current paradigm for the mechanism underlying SAN automaticity involves a complex interaction between activity of the voltage gated ion channels/exchangers in the plasma membrane and the sarcoplasmic reticulum (SR) (Lakatta and DiFrancesco, 2009). The key membrane ion channel thought to be involved in pacemaker setting is the I_h/I_f channel (DiFrancesco, 2010), and pacemaker activity is further modulated by K^+, Na^+, and Ca^{2+} currents. In addition, recent studies suggest that rhythmic local calcium releases from the SR modulated by PKA also contribute to pacemaker activity by activating inward Na^+/Ca^{2+} exchanger currents during late diastolic depolarization (Maltsev and Lakatta, 2008).

The hyperpolarization-activated cyclic nucleotide (HCN) gated cation current (I_h), also known as the "funny" current (I_f), is a non-specific cation conductance. Hyperpolarization and the binding of cAMP mediate activation of the channel. Thus inhibition of adenylate cyclase can reduce the current and slow pacemaker depolarization and heart rate. HCN4 is the major isoform present in the heart and it is present solely in conducting tissues in the healthy heart. There is not complete consensus on the relative roles of I_h/I_f and GIRK, but it is thought about half the negative chronotropic effect of muscarinic receptor activation is due to each mechanism (Wickman et al., 1998; Gehrmann et al., 2002).

GIRK channels (Kir3.x) are part of the family of inwardly rectifying K^+ channels. The subfamily has five members (Kir3.1–3.5) with a heterotetramer of Kir3.1 and 3.4 constituting the cardiac channel and is present in the atria and conducting tissues but has little if any expression in the ventricle (Karschin et al., 1994; Krapivinsky et al., 1995). The channel is characteristically activated by ACh binding to muscarinic (M2) receptors leading to the common designation as I_{KACh}. The increase in channel activity occurs because of a direct interaction of the G$\beta\gamma$ dimer, released from the inhibitory G protein heterotrimer, with specific domains in the N- and C-termini of the channel and as such is a paradigm for $\beta\gamma$ subunit mediated signaling (Logothetis et al., 1987). The current is also stimulated via adenosine, sphingosine-1-phosphate, and endothelin-A receptors in the heart (Ono et al., 1994, 2001; Bösche et al., 2003; Ochi et al., 2006).

The L-type calcium current is the most prominent calcium current in mammalian ventricular heart cells. The alpha subunit is $Ca_V1.2$ (also known as α1C). It is classically regulated by phosphorylation by PKA and thus will be modulated by variations in G protein coupled receptor pathways involving $G\alpha_s$ and $G\alpha_{i/o}$. For example, the activation of β1-adrenoreceptors by agonists leads to up to a fourfold increase in current and shifts the voltage dependence of activation and inactivation to more hyperpolarized potentials (McCleskey et al., 1986; Hirayama and Hartzell, 1997). Although ACh has no effect upon basal L-type calcium currents, it antagonizes their increase on application of a catecholamine (Fischmeister and Hartzell, 1986).

Other membrane and sarcolemmal ion currents modulated via the cAMP/PKA pathway can also play a role in modulation of pacemaker activity. For example, isoprenaline reduced action potential duration (APD) and increased spontaneous action potential firing rate in rabbit SAN cells by increasing the amplitude and causing a negative shift in the activation of the total delayed rectifier K^+ current (I_K) in a PKA-dependent manner (Lei et al., 2000).

REDUNDANCY IN FUNCTION

It is clear then that there are a number of isoforms of inhibitory G proteins and RGSs expressed in the heart and other tissues, which have potentially overlapping functions. Thus the question is do specific isoforms carry out unique physiological roles or does the system have significant redundancy? For example, inhibitory G proteins are characterized by their sensitivity to pertussis toxin, which ADP ribosylates the proteins and uncouples them from receptors. It is possible to engineer $G\alpha_{i/o}$ isoforms that are resistant to the toxin and thus design experimental strategies in which the isoforms can be selectively investigated. In our own work using *in vitro* cellular systems, we were able to show that only rarely would there be an absolute preference of a receptor for an inhibitory G protein isoform: most G protein coupled receptors couple well with a number of isoforms (Leaney and Tinker, 2000).

THE ROLE OF $G\alpha_{i/o}$ AND RGSS IN CONTROLLING HEART RATE

We studied the question of which inhibitory G protein isoform *in vivo* governs heart rate modulation and dynamics using mice with global KO of $G\alpha_{i2}$, $G\alpha_{i1}$, and $G\alpha_{i3}$ combined and $G\alpha_o$ (Zuberi et al., 2008). We analyzed heart rate dynamics in the time and frequency domain with implanted telemetry probes in awake and mobile mice. The influence of the autonomic system can be measured indirectly by the beat-to-beat variation of heart rate ("heart rate variability," HRV). In man R–R interval shows characteristic patterns of variability with a low frequency (LF) component (>6 s cycle length) determined by sympathetic and parasympathetic drive and a high frequency (HF) component (2.5–6 s cycle length) governed by parasympathetic input (Stauss, 2003). Such analysis has also been applied to the mouse but there is less agreement on the contribution of the different arms of the autonomic nervous system to the frequency components (Thireau et al., 2007). We found that $G\alpha_{i2}$ deficient mice were generally tachycardic with preservation of diurnal variation, had loss of HF power in HRV analysis similar to that seen with GIRK channel blocker TertiapinQ and with the muscarinic receptor blocker atropine and an attenuated bradycardic response to the muscarinic agonist carbachol. Mice with global deficiency in $G\alpha_{i1,3}$ were similar to WT but $G\alpha_o$ showed a different phenotype that is discussed below. There is one conflicting study suggesting $G\alpha_o$ and not $G\alpha_{i2}$ is necessary in muscarinic mediated parasympathetic activity which may be due to methodological issues as the mice were studied very early after probe implantation (Duan et al., 2007). In keeping with our observations, mice with a G184S knockin point mutation in the switch I region of $G\alpha_{i2}$, preventing the binding of RGS proteins and deactivation of $G\alpha_{i2}$, had marked enhancement of muscarinic agonist mediated bradycardia (Fu et al., 2007).

$G\alpha_{i2}$ and $G\alpha_o$ signaling has also been implicated in the muscarinic inhibition of β-adrenoreceptor activated voltage gated L-type calcium channels in the heart. Using ventricular myocytes isolated from global $G\alpha_{i2}$ and $G\alpha_{i3}$ knockout mice, Nagata et al. (2000) demonstrated reduced calcium channel currents with carbachol following isoproterenol stimulation in $G\alpha_{i3}$ knockout mice and littermate controls but not in $G\alpha_{i2}$ knockout mice. Using a similar experimental strategy in $G\alpha_o$ knockout mice, Valenzuela et al. (1997) demonstrated similar impaired muscarinic regulation of L-type calcium channels in ventricular myocytes lacking $G\alpha_o$ but no difference in potassium current compared to wild type controls.

Differential coupling of G protein subtypes to adenosine A1 and muscarinic M2 receptor mediated heart rate slowing was also demonstrated *in vitro* using RGS insensitive $G\alpha_o$ and $G\alpha_{i2}$ ES derived cardiomyocytes (Fu et al., 2006). The RGS insensitive $G\alpha_o$ homozygous knockin cells demonstrated enhanced adenosine A1 and muscarinic M2 receptor mediated bradycardic responses. In contrast, RGS insensitive $G\alpha_{i2}$ homozygous knockin cells showed enhanced responses to M2 but not A1 receptors. Blocking GIRK channels largely abolished the mutation-induced enhancement of the M2 receptor mediated response but had a minimal effect on A1 responses.

Taken together, the evidence suggests that M2 mediated GIRK channel activation is coupled preferentially to the $G\alpha_{i2}$ subunit whereas coupling to voltage gated L-type calcium channel appears to be less specific with both $G\alpha_o$ and $G\alpha_{i2}$ implicated.

There are two studies asking which individual RGS might be important for heart rate control. Cifelli et al. (2008) suggested RGS4 is likely to be the predominant RGS in the SAN. RGS4 mRNA levels were found to be higher in the SAN compared to the atrium, conscious RGS4 null mice showed an increased bradycardic response to carbachol and isolated sinus node myocytes from these mice have modified M2 receptor mediated K_{ACh} currents. More recently, RGS6 has been found to be highly expressed in the heart, in particular in the SAN and AVN. Conscious and anesthetized RGS6 null mice also show an increased bradycardic response to carbachol. Perfused hearts demonstrated a similar phenomenon, together with the inhibition of spontaneous action potential firing rates in the SAN, as well as atrioventricular block (Yang et al., 2010). RGS6 deficient mice show impaired desensitization and slower deactivation of the GIRK current in atrial myocytes in response to agonist application (Posokhova et al., 2010), confirming that RGS6 has GAP activity. Taken together, the results indicate that RGS4 and RGS6 have an important parasympathetic modulatory role in the SAN, preventing severe bradycardia and that there is very little redundancy. It would be interesting to know if the combined knockout has a more severe phenotype.

ATRIAL FIBRILLATION

Atrial fibrillation is the most common cardiac arrhythmia and affects at least 10% of the octogenarian population (Ho et al., 1993; Benjamin et al., 1998). It is characterized by rapid, irregular, and chaotic electrical excitation of the atria, where these can beat 300 times per minute in the human. The AVN has decremental properties and prevents every beat from being conducted to the ventricle. Despite this, the ventricular rate can still be rapid resulting in symptoms of palpitations, shortness of breath, and dizziness and it can precipitate overt heart failure. There have been several proposed mechanisms of AF. Classically, it has been suggested that AF arises due to an atrial ectopic focus, a single re-entry circuit, or multiple re-entrant circuits (Nattel, 2002). A more modern variant of these mechanisms for AF involves the concept of rotors and spiral waves (Jalife, 2003). A rotor is a stable rotating pattern around a pivot point. This gives rise to a spiraling wavefront (spiral waves) into the surrounding tissue. Such a rotor is thought to be present at the pulmonary vein-left atrial junction, with spiral waves emanating into the atria, giving fibrillation. Catheter ablation producing anatomical block between the pulmonary veins and left atrium can terminate AF supporting this hypothesis (Haissaguerre et al., 1998).

It has been said that "AF begets AF" (Wijffels et al., 1995). This statement is an illustration of the remodeling that occurs once AF has commenced. Indeed permanent AF is often preceded by paroxysmal AF. Remodeling can take two forms: electrical, which occurs as a result of AF itself and structural, which is associated with congestive cardiac failure and other cardiac and extracardiac diseases predisposing to fibrosis. An increase in rate caused by AF results in increased cellular calcium loading, which threatens cell viability. Subsequently, the density of the L-type calcium channel is reduced with a corresponding increase in the inward rectifying potassium currents, leading to a decreased APD and effective refractory period (ERP). This, in turn, promotes and perpetuates the induction and maintenance of AF through multiple re-entrant circuits. These calcium-handling abnormalities impair atrial contractility and can cause atrial dilatation, which also promotes AF (Nattel et al., 2008). In contrast, patients with congestive cardiac failure are thought to develop AF secondary to a change in atrial architecture due to fibrosis, which interferes with electrical conductance. Profibrotic signaling pathways have been identified and these include angiotensin II, transforming growth factor-β_1 and platelet derived growth factor. Extracardiac disease, such as diabetes, obesity, and sleep apnea, may also be responsible for an increased risk of AF through fibrosis. Atrial stretch, which can occur secondary to mitral valve disease, is also a known trigger. Genetic factors may contribute to remodeling; gain-of-function mutations in the potassium channels and loss-of-function mutations in the L-type calcium channel can promote AF. Moreover, single nucleotide polymorphisms alongside genes contributing to atrial integrity have been associated with AF, for example, angiotensin-converting enzyme and *PITX2* (Wakili et al., 2011).

An imbalance in the autonomic system may increase the propensity to AF. In 18 subjects with paroxysmal AF, vagal overactivity was described as the precipitating factor. Here, each paroxysm was preceded by atrial coupling followed by a pause and accompanied by slowing of the sinus rate (Coumel et al., 1978). Changes in autonomic tone through the study of HRV has been assessed in 77 patients with paroxysmal AF (Bettoni and Zimmermann, 2002). This study showed that at least 20 min prior to the onset of paroxysmal AF, there was an initial increase in adrenergic drive followed by a shift in autonomic tone such that increased vagal tone dominated immediately before the onset of paroxysmal AF. The effects of both cholinergic and β-adrenergic stimulation and blockade were studied in the intact dog heart (Sharifov et al., 2004). ACh and catecholamines, individually and in combination, were infused into the heart via the sinus node artery. No electrical stimulation was performed. Cholinergic stimulation was found to be the main factor responsible for spontaneous AF initiation. Adrenergic tone, however, was involved in modulating the initiation and maintenance of cholinergically mediated AF. Further evidence for the role of a vagal mechanism in paroxysmal AF was demonstrated in patients undergoing circumferential pulmonary vein ablation in whom complete vagal denervation was also performed (Pappone et al., 2004). These patients had greater freedom from AF.

Activation of GIRK current results in membrane hyperpolarization, and shortening of APD and ERP. The change in atrial ERP may predispose to the induction and maintenance of AF. Thus any increased activity in inhibitory G protein signaling may predispose to AF. There is surprisingly little data mapping specific genetic modifications in this pathway to experimental supraventricular tachyarrhythmia. It is possible to induce non-sustained AF in the mouse using programmed electrical stimulation (Kovoor et al., 2001). Patch clamp studies utilizing atrial cardiomyocytes from humans (Dobrev et al., 2005) and dogs (Voigt et al., 2008) illustrate that the GIRK channel is constitutively active in AF. Furthermore, the Kir3.4 knockout mouse is resistant to AF (Kovoor et al., 2001). Overexpression of $G\alpha_{i2}$ using a viral vector has also been tried as a therapeutic strategy (Bauer et al., 2004). Injection of the construct into the AVN of animals slowed the heart rate in AF (Bauer et al., 2004). The delivery of cell penetrating peptides to the posterior left atrium to disrupt M2-$G\alpha_i$ coupling prolonged refractoriness in the left atrium and suppressed vagally induced AF (Aistrup et al., 2009). It is interesting to note that it was necessary to target both $G\alpha_{i2}$ and $G\alpha_{i3}$ here. Furthermore, it has been shown that in $G\alpha_{i2}$ knockout mice, where the hearts are studied *ex vivo*, pacemaking occurs from the atria not the SAN and there is no impairment of muscarinic receptor mediated heart rate slowing (Boknik et al., 2009). This suggests that there may be differences in the coupling profile between the M2 receptor and

GIRK channel in the atria and SAN. Once again there is little information on which RGSs might be important in the atria. Of those studied functionally, RGS6 but not RGS4 is expressed there and RGS10 mediates β-adrenergic receptor effects on the GIRK current in rat atrial cells (Bender et al., 2008). There is one report showing inducible AF in the RGS2 knockout mouse (Tuomi et al., 2010).

VENTRICULAR ARRHYTHMIA

Ventricular cardiac arrhythmias, namely ventricular tachycardia (VT) and ventricular fibrillation (VF), cause sudden cardiac death (SCD). SCD poses a significant clinical burden with an estimated 300 000 cases per year recorded in the USA (Noseworthy and Newton-Cheh, 2008). This highlights the importance in predicting risk of SCD, although precise calculation of such a risk remains challenging. Drug therapy, as in AF, can be limited by modest efficacy, significant toxicity, and can be proarrhythmic. ICDs have proven benefit but are complicated by inappropriate shocks, the need for a generator and possible lead changes and complications at the time of insertion, for example infection. Catheter ablation is invasive and is suitable for only modest numbers of patients. Therefore, there is a need to understand the molecular mechanisms responsible for VT initiation and maintenance, in order to develop successful treatments.

The etiology of VT/VF can be broadly divided into those occurring in patients with structurally normal or abnormal hearts. Normal heart VT/VF has traditionally been considered a primary electrical problem, caused by "channelopathies" including the long QT (LQT) syndromes and Brugada syndrome. In some cases, the cause of VT/VF is unknown and hence diagnosed as idiopathic VT. Structurally abnormal hearts causing VT/VF can be due to inherited conditions such as hypertrophic cardiomyopathy (HCM) and arrhythmogenic right ventricular cardiomyopathy (ARVC) or acquired cardiomyopathies, the most common of which is ischemic cardiomyopathy.

Autonomic precipitants to VT/VF is well recognized clinically. Both increased sympathetic and parasympathetic tone can lead to VT/VF depending on etiology and the underlying electrical abnormalities. For example, LQT 1 and 2 are precipitated by an increase in sympathetic tone whereas in LQT 3, it is protective (Moss and Kass, 2005). In Brugada syndrome, vagotonic agents and β adrenergic blockers can precipitate VT/VF (Kasanuki et al., 1997). In patients with idiopathic VT/VF and short coupled variant of torsades des pointes, HRV was significantly depressed prior to the onset of ventricular tachyarrhythmia suggesting vagal precipitant (Leenhardt et al., 1994). The arrhythmogenic substrate is thought to be due to the amplification of spatial dispersion of repolarization by the underlying autonomic tone, causing abnormal re-entry, or triggered activity (Verrier and Antzelevitch, 2004).

Bradycardia itself *per se* may precipitate polymorphic VT by causing prolongation of APD and development of early afterdepolarizations, leading to triggered activity in the form of ventricular premature beats (El-Sherif et al., 1988). Hence any perturbation of $G\alpha_{i/o}$ signaling in the conduction system which leads to bradycardia could in theory increase susceptibility to ventricular arrhythmia.

In patients with ischemic cardiomyopathy induced VT/VF and heart failure, the picture is somewhat different. Sympathetic nervous system activation is beneficial acutely in heart failure but detrimental in the long term. Such a mechanism promotes apoptosis of cardiac myocytes, ion channel remodeling, and is proarrhythmic (DeGeorge et al., 2008). Cardiac $G\alpha_{i/o}$ signaling pathways may counteract this process (Zheng et al., 2005). Indeed, in chronic heart failure, β_1-adrenoceptors are downregulated whereas $G\alpha_{i2}$ is significantly increased (Eschenhagen et al., 1992). Overexpression of β_1-adrenoceptors in transgenic mice results in a dilated cardiomyopathy but a more modest phenotype is seen with β_2-adrenoceptor overexpression. β_2-adrenoceptors are coupled to $G\alpha_{i/o}$ and $G\alpha_s$, suggesting a cardioprotective role for $G\alpha_{i/o}$ (Foerster et al., 2003; DeGeorge et al., 2008).

In heart failure patients with ICDs, a loss in HRV was noted immediately before an episode of VT and this was found to be an independent predictor of SCD (Pruvot et al., 2000). Parasympathetic activation can terminate VT and increase VF threshold whereas increases in sympathetic activation can precipitate ventricular arrhythmias (Kolman et al., 1975; Waxman and Wald, 1977; Brack et al., 2007). Taken together, there is good evidence that increased vagal tone protects against the development of heart failure and VT/VF precipitated by ischemic cardiomyopathy. Certainly β-blocker therapy improves prognosis in those with heart failure (Poole-Wilson et al., 2003).

To explore the role of $G\alpha_{i2}$ and predisposition to cardiac ventricular arrhythmias, we performed *in vivo* cardiac electrophysiological studies on global $G\alpha_{i2}$ knockout mice and compared them with wild type littermates and combined $G\alpha_{i1}$ and $G\alpha_{i3}$ knockout controls (Zuberi et al., 2010). Mice with global genetic deletion of $G\alpha_{i2}$ were found to have a reduced ventricular effective refractive period and propensity for VT induced with programmed electrical stimulation compared to controls. Conscious $G\alpha_{i2}$ knockout mice had a prolonged QT interval and single ventricular myocytes studied with patch clamping showed a steep restitution curve but prolonged APD. Increased levels of message for the L-type calcium channel was found on gene expression studies, with confirmation of an increase in this current on patch clamping. No structural heart disease was noted on histology or echocardiography. These findings suggest that the absence of $G\alpha_{i2}$ is a substrate for VT. Interestingly, Dizayee et al. (2011) studied ventricular myocytes isolated from $G\alpha_{i2}$ and $G\alpha_{i3}$ knockout mice and found reduced L-type calcium channel current density in $G\alpha_{i2}$ knockouts compared to littermate controls but increased in $G\alpha_{i3}$ knockouts where there was a compensatory increase in $G\alpha_{i2}$ expression. The differences between our results and theirs may be accounted for by strain differences in the mice (129\Sv versus C57\Black) Clinically, pravastatin, given to patients in order to lower cholesterol, selectively upregulates $G\alpha_{i2}$ and increases HF power in HRV analysis (Welzig et al., 2003).

REGULATION OF THE HEART BY THE AUTONOMIC NERVOUS SYSTEM

The autonomic nervous system maintains homeostasis and coordinates physiological responses in the body via its two functional limbs: the sympathetic and parasympathetic nervous systems. The

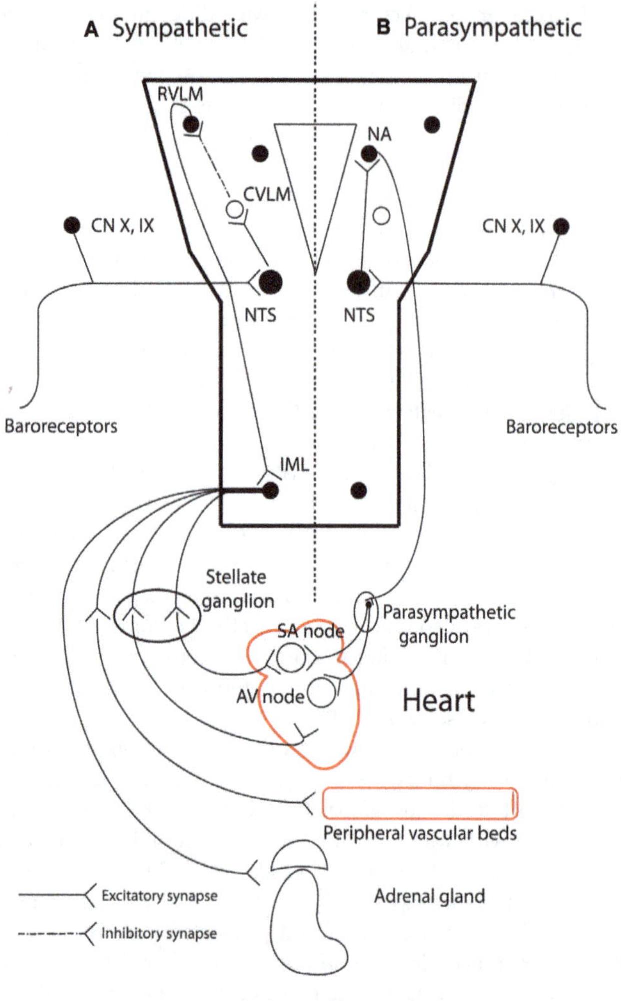

FIGURE 2 | The main peripheral and neural centers involved in autonomic cardiovascular regulation. (A) Sympathetic baroreflex arm: sensory neurons in the periphery transmit baroreceptor information via a glutamatergic synapse to the nucleus tractus solitaries (NTS) in the medulla. NTS neurons project to and excite neurons in the caudal ventrolateral medulla (CVLM). CVLM neurons in turn project and inhibit (via a GABAergic synapse) presympathetic neurons in the rostral ventrolateral medulla (RVLM). Spinally projecting presympathetic RVLM neurons make direct connections with sympathetic preganglionic neurons in the intermediolateral (IML) spinal column, which projects sympathetic outflow to effector organs. **(B)** Parasympathetic control of heart rate: NTS neurons receive baroreceptor and chemoreceptor information and relay via a glutamatergic pathway to the nucleus ambiguous (NA). Cardioinhibitory neurons in NA then project to the heart via the vagus nerve, which mediates its effect via muscarinic receptors in the heart. Adapted from Pilowsky and Goodchild (2002). *GABA*, gamma-Aminobutyric acid; SA, sinoatrial; AV, atrioventricular.

heart is regulated in this manner within the cardio-respiratory system (**Figure 2**). Afferent nerves convey baroreceptor and chemoreceptor inputs to the cardio-respiratory centers within the brainstem and generally opposing reflex responses are mediated by the sympathetic and parasympathetic efferent to the heart, blood vessels, and other effector organs such as the adrenal glands. Both sympathetic and parasympathetic systems are made up of central and peripheral components. The central component consists of cell groups in the brain and spinal cord, and myelinated preganglionic neurons. It is responsible for maintenance of autonomic tone, and integration of afferent inputs to generate appropriate autonomic reflexes. Much of the basic structure involved in the reflex control of the cardiovascular system is contained within the medulla. Integrated and behaviorally appropriate responses also require reciprocal connections between the medulla, pons, midbrain, and hypothalamus (Spyer, 1994). The peripheral component consists of ganglia and unmyelinated postganglionic afferent and efferent fibers innervating the heart and associated effector organs (e.g., blood vessels). It is increasingly recognized that the pattern of cardiac innervation peripherally may be important in cardiac arrhythmogenesis (Verrier and Antzelevitch, 2004).

As described above, the murine models used to study (patho)physiology are often global knockouts or knock-ins. It is conceivable (and probably very likely) that there are contributions to the phenotype from the effects on inhibitory G protein signaling in the nervous system. $G\alpha_{i1}$, $G\alpha_{i2}$, and $G\alpha_{i3}$ are ubiquitously expressed but $G\alpha_o$ protein expression is restricted mainly to the central and peripheral nervous systems, endocrine cells, and cardiomyocytes (Wettschureck and Offermanns, 2005). Expression of $G\alpha_o$ is greatest in the brain where it is estimated to constitute around 1% of all membrane proteins (Sternweis and Robishaw, 1984). Mice lacking the α subunit of G_o are smaller and weaker than their littermates, have greatly reduced life expectancy and display numerous neurological abnormalities including hyperalgesia, tremors, seizures, and increased motor activity with an extreme turning behavior (Jiang and Bajpayee, 2009).

GIRK channels are widely distributed in neuronal and endocrine tissues and play key roles in generating late inhibitory postsynaptic potentials and modulating hormone release in addition to their cardiac functions. In the central nervous system, GIRK channels hyperpolarize neurons in response to activation by neurotransmitters including adenosine, somatostatin, 5-HT, and opioids, and is composed of heterotetramers of Kir3.1, Kir3.2, and Kir3.3 and homotetramers of Kir3.2 (Lüscher et al., 1997; Lüscher and Slesinger, 2010). Pharmacological investigations of GIRK channels and studies in animal models suggest that GIRK activity has an important role in physiological responses, including pain perception and memory modulation. Abnormal GIRK function has been implicated in altering neuronal excitability and cell death, which may be important in the pathophysiology of diseases such as epilepsy, Down's syndrome, Parkinson's disease, and drug addiction (Lüscher and Slesinger, 2010). There is limited study of GIRK's role in autonomic traffic. Feldman and colleagues found reduced BP depressor effects of the I_1-imidazoline receptor (I_1R) selective ligands administered intracisternally in rabbits pretreated with TertiapinQ suggesting that the central sympatho-inhibitory effects of I_1R ligands are mediated by GIRK channels (Yoro Sy et al., 2008).

The regulation of neurotransmitter release at presynaptic terminals is an important mechanism underlying the modulation of synaptic transmission in the nervous system. Inhibitory regulation of neurotransmitter release via inhibitory G proteins is mediated by various G protein coupled receptors like α2-adrenoceptors, μ- and δ-opioid receptors, GABA-B receptors, adenosine A1, or endocannabinoid CB1-receptors. A major mechanism by which these G proteins mediate the inhibition of transmitter release is the direct inhibitory modulation of the action potential-evoked Ca^{2+} entry to the presynaptic terminal by the Gβγ subunit, which is required to trigger neurotransmitter release. N- and P/Q-type calcium channels that are concentrated at nerve terminals as well as R-type calcium channels have been shown to be inhibited via $G\alpha_{i/o}$-coupled receptors (Dolphin, 2003).

There is evidence showing selectivity of inhibitory G protein coupling to voltage gated Ca^{2+} channels. Neuropeptide Y (NPY) and bradykinin both inhibit N-type Ca^{2+} channels *in vitro*, and pertussis toxin treatment could completely abolish this inhibition. Addition of purified bovine $G\alpha_o$ subunits effectively restored the NPY modulation of Ca^{2+} currents while purified $G\alpha_{i1}$ or $G\alpha_{i2}$ had little or no effect. Interestingly, the bradykinin inhibitory effects on Ca^{2+} currents in pertussis toxin-treated cells was only partially restored by the addition of either purified $G\alpha_o$ or $G\alpha_{i2}$, even at high concentrations. Complete restoration required a combination of both $G\alpha_o$ and $G\alpha_{i2}$ proteins suggesting that $G\alpha_o$ and $G\alpha_{i2}$ proteins may couple to distinct subpopulations of bradykinin receptors since $G\alpha_o$ nor $G\alpha_{i2}$ protein alone cannot compensate the loss of the other (Ewald et al., 1989). $G\alpha_o$ antibodies in the superior cervical ganglion has also been shown to reduce calcium current inhibition by noradrenaline in superior cervical ganglion neurons (Caulfield et al., 1994). Signaling via $G\alpha_o$ has also been implicated in vesicular glutamate transporter within the central nervous system (Winter et al., 2005) and GAP43 receptor signaling for neuronal pathfinding (Strittmatter et al., 1990).

In vivo experiments manipulating the expression of inhibitory G proteins and its subtypes either directly with knockout models or indirectly by manipulation of their regulatory proteins have shed limited light on their physiological importance and relative contribution to the peripheral and central control of autonomic heart rate regulation. Methodologically, autonomic tone *in vivo* has been quantified by indirect methods such as catecholamine sampling and analysis of HRV. The baroreceptor reflex is the prototypical cardiovascular reflex studied and is commonly quantified by computation of baroreflex set point and gain from ambulatory BP recordings, although more direct methods have been described (Ma et al., 2002; Young and Davisson, 2011).

Interestingly, mice overexpressing RGS insensitive $G\alpha_{i2}$ were tachycardic during the daytime, have an enlarged heart and hyperdynamic echo profile. Along with reduced viability, growth retardation, and multiple neurological deficit, the cardiovascular phenotype observed was attributed to increased central sympathetic tone (Huang et al., 2006). To study the cardiac specific effect of enhanced $G\alpha_{i2}$ signaling, isoproterenol-stimulated beating isolated perfused hearts were studied and showed the expected enhancement of muscarinic mediated bradycardia (Fu et al., 2007).

Mice deficient in RGS2 were found to be hypertensive but with normal HR suggestive of resetting of baroreceptor sensitivity. There was an associated increase in urinary catecholamine secretion and reduction in both LF and HF power of HRV suggesting increased central sympathetic tone (Gross et al., 2005). This along with data on the RGS insensitive $G\alpha_{i2}$ mice described above implies that overactivity of inhibitory G proteins may contribute to increased central sympathetic tone. In our study of global $G\alpha_o$ knockout mice (Zuberi et al., 2008), in addition to the neurological abnormalities previously described, we found the mice to be tachycardic with loss of diurnal rhythm and fairly selective loss of the LF component of HRV with preserved total power. However, carbachol still had a negative chronotropic effect. This is suggestive of increased sympathetic tone, likely to be of central origin.

Significant progress has been made in our understanding of the autonomic nervous system and the effects upon cardiac function. Nonetheless, further study of the chronic alterations in the autonomic nervous system and their cardiac consequences may prove useful in the prevention of cardiac disease and provide valuable treatment modalities (Brodde and Michel, 1999).

CONCLUSION AND FUTURE DIRECTIONS

It is clear that inhibitory G proteins and their associated RGS proteins play a critical role in autonomic signaling at multiple levels. Their role in mediating the parasympathetic tone to the heart is well established. What is unclear is their role in autonomic traffic in the central autonomic circuits. This will need further elucidation to dissect the role of autonomic tone in cardiac pathophysiology. What is also unclear is what role the autonomic nervous system and the specific signaling molecules have in generating cardiac arrhythmia. Mice with global G protein deletion often have reduced viability and are difficult to work with and it can be unclear at which level signaling is contributing to the phenotype. Use of more refined temporal and spatial conditional deletion strategies would circumvent some of the problems and help define the relative role of inhibitory G proteins and its subtypes in the central and peripheral autonomic control of the heart.

REFERENCES

Aistrup, G. L., Villuendas, R., Ng, J., Gilchrist, A., Lynch, T. W., Gor- don, D., Cokic, I., Mottl, S., Zhou,R., Dean, D. A., Wasserstrom, J. A., Goldberger, J. J., Kadish, A. H., and Arora, R. (2009). Targeted G-protein inhibition as a novel approach to decrease vagal atrial fibrillation by selective parasympathetic attenua- tion. *Cardiovasc. Res.* 83, 481–492.

Bauer, A., McDonald, A. D., Nasir, K.,Peller, L., Rade, J. J., Miller, J. M., Heldman, A. W., and Donahue, J. K. (2004). Inhibitory G protein over- expression provides physiologically relevant heart rate control in per- sistent atrial fibrillation. *Circulation* 110, 3115–3120.

Bender, K., Nasrollahzadeh, P., Timpert, M., Liu, B., Pott, L., and Kienitz, M. C. (2008). A role for RGS10 in adrenergic modulation of G- protein-activated K+ (GIRK) chan- nel current in rat atrial myocytes. *J. Physiol. (Lond.)* 586, 2049–2060.

Benjamin, E. J., Wolf, P. A., D'Agostino, R. B., Silbershatz, H., Kannel, W. B., and Levy, D. (1998). Impact of atrial fibrillation on the risk of death: the Framingham Heart Study. *Circula- tion* 98, 946–952.

Bettoni, M., and Zimmermann, M. (2002). Autonomic tone variations before the onset of paroxysmal atrial fibrillation. *Circulation* 105, 2753–2759.

Boknik, P., Grote-Wessels, S., Barteska, G., Jiang, M., Müller, F. U., Schmitz, W., Neumann, J., and Birnbaumer, L. (2009). Genetic disruption of G proteins, G(i2)alpha or G(o)alpha, does not abolish inotropic and chronotropic effects of stimulat- ing muscarinic cholinoceptors in atrium. *Br. J. Pharmacol.* 158, 1557–1564.

Bösche, L. I., Wellner-Kienitz, M.-C., Bender, K., and Pott, L. (2003). G protein-independent inhibition of GIRK current by adenosine in rat atrial myocytes overexpressing A1 receptors after adenovirus-mediated gene transfer. *J. Physiol. (Lond.)* 550, 707–717.

Brack, K. E., Patel, V. H., Coote, J. H., and Ng, G. A. (2007). Nitric oxide mediates the vagal protective effect on ventricular fibrillation via effects on action potential duration restitu- tion in the rabbit heart. *J. Physiol. (Lond.)* 583, 695–704.

Brodde, O. E., and Michel, M. C. (1999). Adrenergic and muscarinic recep- tors in the human heart. *Pharmacol. Rev.* 51, 651–690.

Caulfield, M. P., Jones, S., Vallis, Y., Buckley, N. J., Kim, G. D., Milligan, G., and Brown, D. A. (1994). Mus- carinic M-current inhibition via G alpha q/11 and alpha-adrenoceptor inhibition of Ca2+ current via G alpha o in rat sympathetic neu- rones. *J. Physiol. (Lond.)* 477(Pt 3), 415–422.

Cifelli, C., Rose, R. A., Zhang, H., Voigtlaender-Bolz, J., Bolz, S.-S., Backx, P. H., and Heximer, S. P. (2008). RGS4 regulates parasympa- thetic signaling and heart rate con- trol in the sinoatrial node. *Circ. Res.* 103, 527–535.

Coumel, P., Attuel, P., Lavallee, J., Flam- mang, D., Leclercq, J. F., and Slama, R. (1978). The atrial arrhythmia syn- drome of vagal origin. *Arch. Mal. Coeur. Vaiss.* 71, 645–656.

DeGeorge, B. R. J., Gao, E., Boucher, M., Vinge, L. E., Martini, J. S., Raake, P. W., Chuprun, J. K., Harris, D. M., Kim, G. W., Soltys, S., Eckhart, A. D., and Koch, W. J. (2008). Tar- geted inhibition of cardiomyocyte Gi signaling enhances susceptibility to apoptotic cell death in response to ischemic stress. *Circulation* 117, 1378–1387.

DiFrancesco, D. (2010). The role of the funny current in pacemaker activity. *Circ. Res.* 106, 434–446.

Dizayee, S., Kaestner, S., Kuck, F., Hein, P., Klein, C., Piekorz, R. P., Meszaros, J., Matthes, J., Nurnberg, B., and Herzig, S. (2011). Galphai2- and Galphai3-specific regulation of voltage-dependent L-type calcium channels in cardiomyocytes. *PLoS ONE* 6, e24979. doi:10.1371/jour- nal.pone.0024979

Dobrev, D., Friedrich, A., Voigt, N., Jost, N., Wettwer, E., Christ, T., Knaut, M., and Ravens, U. (2005). The G protein-gated potassium current I(K,ACh) is constitutively active in patients with chronic atrial fibrilla- tion. *Circulation* 112, 3697–3706.

Dolphin, A. C. (2003). G protein modulation of voltage-gated cal- cium channels. *Pharmacol. Rev.* 55, 607–627.

Doupnik, C. A., Xu, T., and Shinaman, J. M. (2001). Profile of RGS expres- sion in single rat atrial myocytes. *Biochim. Biophys. Acta* 1522, 97–107.

Duan, S. Z., Christe, M., Milstone, D. S., and Mortensen, R. M. (2007). Go but not Gi2 or Gi3 is required for muscarinic regulation of heart rate and heart rate variability in mice. *Biochem. Biophys. Res. Com- mun.* 357, 139–143.

El-Sherif, N., Zeiler, R. H., Craelius, W., Gough, W. B., and Henkin, R. (1988). QTU prolongation and polymorphic ventricu- lar tachyarrhythmias due to bradycardia-dependent early afterdepolarizations. Afterde- polarizations and ventricular arrhythmias. *Circ. Res.* 63, 286–305.

Eschenhagen, T., Mende, U., Nose, M., Schmitz, W., Scholz, H., Haverich, A., Hirt, S., Doring, V., Kalmar, P., and Hoppner, W. (1992). Increased mes- senger RNA level of the inhibitory G protein alpha sub- unit Gi alpha-2 in human end-stage heart failure. *Circ. Res.* 70, 688–696.

Ewald, D. A., Pang, I. H., Sternweis, P. C., and Miller, R. J. (1989). Dif- ferential G protein-mediated cou- pling of neurotransmitter receptors to Ca2+ channels in rat dorsal root ganglion neurons in vitro. *Neuron* 2, 1185–1193.

Fischmeister, R., and Hartzell, H. C. (1986). Mechanism of action of acetylcholine on calcium current in single cells from frog ventricle. *J. Physiol. (Lond.)* 376, 183–202.

Foerster, K., Groner, F., Matthes, J., Koch, W. J., Birnbaumer, L., and Herzig, S. (2003). Cardioprotection specific for the G protein Gi2 in chronic adrenergic signaling through beta 2- adrenoceptors. *Proc. Natl. Acad. Sci. U.S.A.* 100, 14475–14480.

Fu, Y., Huang, X., Piao, L., Lopatin, A. N., and Neubig, R. R. (2007). Endogenous RGS proteins modu- late SA and AV nodal functions in isolated heart: implications for sick sinus syndrome and AV block. *Am. J. Physiol. Heart Circ. Physiol.* 292, H2532–H2539.

Fu,Y., Huang, X., Zhong, H., Mortensen, R. M., D'Alecy, L. G., and Neubig, R. R. (2006). Endogenous RGS proteins and G alpha subtypes differentially control muscarinic and adenosine- mediated chronotropic effects. *Circ. Res.* 98, 659–666.

Gehrmann, J., Meister, M., Maguire, C. T., Martins, D. C., Hammer, P. E., Neer, E. J., Berul, C. I., and Mende, U. (2002). Impaired parasympathetic heart rate control in mice with a reduction of functional G protein betagamma-subunits. *Am. J. Physiol. Heart Circ. Physiol.* 282, H445–56.

Gross, V., Tank, J., Obst, M., Plehm, R., Blumer, K. J., Diedrich, A., Jor- dan, J., and Luft, F. C. (2005). Autonomic nervous system and blood pressure regulation in RGS2- deficient mice. *Am. J. Physiol. Regul. Integr. Comp. Physiol.* 288, R1134–R1142.

Haissaguerre, M., Jais, P., Shah, D. C., Takahashi, A., Hocini, M., Quiniou, G., Garrigue, S., Le Mouroux, A., Le Metayer, P., and Clementy, J. (1998). Spontaneous initiation of atrial fib- rillation by ectopic beats originating in the pulmonary veins. *N. Engl. J. Med.* 339, 659–666.

Hirayama, Y., and Hartzell, H. C. (1997). Effects of protein phosphatase and kinase inhibitors on Ca2+ and Cl– currents in guinea pig ventricu- lar myocytes. *Mol. Pharmacol.* 52, 725–734.

Ho, K. K., Pinsky, J. L., Kannel, W. B., and Levy, D. (1993). The epidemi- ology of heart failure: the Framing- ham Study. *J. Am. Coll. Cardiol.* 22, 6A–13A.

Hollinger, S., and Hepler, J. R. (2002). Cellular regulation of RGS proteins: modulators and integrators of G protein signaling. *Pharmacol. Rev.* 54, 527–559.

Huang, X., Fu, Y., Charbeneau, R. A., Saunders, T. L., Taylor, D. K., Hankenson, K. D., Russell, M. W., D'Alecy, L. G., and Neubig, R. R. (2006). Pleiotropic phenotype of a genomic knock-in of an RGS- insensitive G184S Gnai2 allele. *Mol. Cell. Biol.* 26, 6870–6879.

Jalife, J. (2003). Rotors and spiral waves in atrial fibrillation. *J. Cardiovasc. Electrophysiol.* 14, 776–780.

Jiang, M., and Bajpayee, N. S. (2009). Molecular mechanisms of go signal- ing. *Neurosignals* 17, 23–41.

Kardestuncer, T., Wu, H., Lim, A. L., and Neer, E. J. (1998). Cardiac myocytes express mRNA for ten RGS proteins: changes in RGS mRNA expression in ventricular myocytes and cultured atria. *FEBS Lett.* 438, 285–288.

Karschin, C., Schreibmayer, W., Das- cal, N., Lester, H., Davidson, N., and Karschin, A. (1994). Distri- bution and localization of a G- protein-coupled inwardly rectifying K+ channel in the rat. *FEBS Lett.* 348, 139–144.

Kasanuki, H., Ohnishi, S., Ohtuka, M., Matsuda, N., Nirei, T., Iso- gai, R., Shoda, M., Toyoshima, Y., and Hosoda, S. (1997). Idiopathic ventricular fibrillation induced with vagal activity in patients without obvious heart disease. *Circulation* 95, 2277–2285.

Kolman, B. S., Verrier, R. L., and Lown, B. (1975). The effect of vagus nerve stimulation upon vulnerabil- ity of the canine ventricle: role of sympathetic-parasympathetic inter- actions. *Circulation* 52, 578–585.

Kovoor, P., Wickman, K., Maguire, C. T., Pu, W., Gehrmann, J., Berul, C. I., and Clapham, D. E. (2001). Evalua- tion of the role of I(KACh) in atrial fibrillation using a mouse knock- out model. *J. Am. Coll. Cardiol.* 37, 2136–2143.

Krapivinsky, G., Gordon, E. A., Wick- man, K., Velimirovic, B., Krapivin- sky, L., and Clapham, D. E. (1995). The G-protein-gated atrial K+ channel IKACh is a hetero- multimer of two inwardly rectifying K(+)-channel proteins. *Nature* 374, 135–141.

Lakatta, E. G., and DiFrancesco, D. (2009). What keeps us ticking: a funny current, a calcium clock, or both? *J. Mol. Cell. Cardiol.* 47, 157–170.

Leaney, J. L., and Tinker, A. (2000). The role of members of the pertus- sis toxin-sensitive family of G pro- teins in coupling receptors to the activation of the G protein-gated inwardly rectifying potassium chan- nel. *Proc. Natl. Acad. Sci. U.S.A.* 97, 5651–5656.

Leenhardt, A., Glaser, E., Burguera, M., Nürnberg, M., Maison-Blanche, P., and Coumel, P. (1994). Short- coupled variant of torsade de pointes. A new electrocardiographic entity in the spectrum of idiopathic ventricular tachyarrhythmias. *Circu- lation* 89, 206–215.

Lei, M., Brown, H. F., and Terrar, D. A. (2000). Modulation of delayed recti- fier potassium current, iK, by isopre- naline in rabbit isolated pacemaker cells. *Exp. Physiol.* 85, 27–35.

Logothetis, D. E., Kurachi, Y., Galper, J., Neer, E. J., and Clapham, D. E. (1987). The beta gamma subunits of GTP-binding proteins activate the muscarinic K+ channel in heart. *Nature* 325, 321–326.

Lüscher, C., Jan, L. Y., Stoffel, M., Malenka, R. C., and Nicoll, R. A. (1997). G protein-coupled inwardly rectifying K+ channels (GIRKs) mediate postsynaptic but not presy- naptic transmitter actions in hip- pocampal neurons. *Neuron* 19, 687–695.

Lüscher, C., and Slesinger, P. A. (2010). Emerging roles for G protein- gated inwardly rectifying potassium (GIRK) channels in health and dis- ease. *Nat. Rev. Neurosci.* 11, 301–315.

Ma, X., Abboud, F. M., and Chapleau, M. W. (2002). Analysis of afferent, cen- tral, and efferent components of the baroreceptor reflex in mice. *Am. J. Physiol. Regul. Integr. Comp. Physiol.* 283, R1033–R1040.

Maltsev, V. A., and Lakatta, E. G. (2008). Dynamic interactions of an intracel- lular Ca2+ clock and membrane ion channel clock underlie robust initia- tion and regulation of cardiac pace- maker function. *Cardiovasc. Res.* 77, 274–284.

McCleskey, E. W., Fox, A. P., Feldman, D., and Tsien, R. W. (1986). Differ- ent types of calcium channels. *J. Exp. Biol.* 124, 177–190.

Moss, A. J., and Kass, R. S. (2005). Long QT syndrome: from channels to car- diac arrhythmias. *J. Clin. Invest.* 115, 2018–2024.

Nagata, K., Ye, C., Jain, M., Milstone, D. S., Liao, R., and Mortensen, R. M. (2000). Galpha(i2) but not Galpha(i3) is required for muscarinic inhibition of contractility and calcium currents in adult cardiomyocytes. *Circ. Res.* 87, 903–909.

Nattel, S. (2002). New ideas about atrial fibrillation 50 years on. *Nature* 415, 219–226.

Nattel, S., Burstein, B., and Dobrev, D. (2008). Atrial remodeling and atrial fibrillation: mechanisms and impli- cations. *Circ. Arrhythm. Electrophys- iol.* 1, 62–73.

Noseworthy, P. A., and Newton-Cheh, C. (2008). Genetic determinants of sudden cardiac death. *Circulation* 118, 1854–1863.

Ochi, R., Momose, Y., Oyama, K., and Giles, W. R. (2006). Sphingosine- 1-phosphate effects on guinea pig atrial myocytes: alterations in action potentials and K+ currents. *Cardio- vasc. Res.* 70, 88–96.

Ono, K., Masumiya, H., Sakamoto, A., Christé, G., Shijuku, T., Tanaka, H., Shigenobu, K., and Ozaki, Y. (2001). Electrophysiological analysis of the negative chronotropic effect of endothelin-1 in rabbit sinoatrial node cells. *J. Physiol. (Lond.)* 537, 467–488.

Ono, K., Tsujimoto, G., Sakamoto, A., Eto, K., Masaki, T., Ozaki, Y., and Satake, M. (1994). Endothelin-A receptor mediates cardiac inhibition by regulating calcium and potassium currents. *Nature* 370, 301–304.

Owen, V. J., Burton, P. B., Mullen, A. J., Birks, E. J., Barton, P., and Yacoub, M. H. (2001). Expression of RGS3, RGS4 and Gi alpha 2 in acutely failing donor hearts and end- stage heart failure. *Eur. Heart J.* 22, 1015–1020.

Pappone, C., Santinelli, V., Manguso, F., Vicedomini, G., Gugliotta, F., Augello, G., Mazzone, P., Torto- riello, V., Landoni, G., Zangrillo, A., Lang, C., Tomita, T., Mesas, C., Mas- tella, E., and Alfieri, O. (2004). Pul- monary vein denervation enhances long-term benefit after circum- ferential ablation for paroxysmal atrial fibrillation. *Circulation* 109, 327–334.

Pilowsky, P. M., and Goodchild, A. K. (2002). Baroreceptor reflex pathways and neurotransmitters: 10 years on. *J. Hypertens.* 20, 1675–1688.

Poole-Wilson, P. A., Swedberg, K., Cle- land, J. G., Di Lenarda, A., Han- rath, P., Komajda, M., Lubsen, J., Lutiger, B., Metra, M., Remme, W. J., Torp-Pedersen, C., Scherhag, A., and Skene, A. (2003). Com- parison of carvedilol and meto- prolol on clinical outcomes in patients with chronic heart fail- ure in the Carvedilol Or Metopro- lol European Trial (COMET): ran- domised controlled trial. *Lancet* 362, 7–13.

Posokhova, E., Wydeven, N., Allen, K. L., Wickman, K., and Martemyanov, K. A. (2010). RGS6/Gss5 complex accelerates IKACh gating kinetics in atrial myocytes and modulates parasympathetic regulation of heart rate. *Circ. Res.* 107, 1350–1354.

Pruvot, E., Thonet, G., Vesin, J. M., van- Melle, G., Seidl, K., Schmidinger, H., Brachmann, J., Jung, W., Hoffmann, E., Tavernier, R., Block, M., Pod- czeck, A., and Fromer, M. (2000). Heart rate dynamics at the onset of ventricular tachyarrhythmias as retrieved from implantable cardioverter-defibrillators in patients with coronary artery disease. *Circulation* 101, 2398–2404.

Rudolph, U., Spicher, K., and Birn- baumer, L. (1996). Adenylyl cyclase inhibition and altered G pro- tein subunit expression and ADP- ribosylation patterns in tissues and cells from Gi2 alpha-/-mice. *Proc. Natl. Acad. Sci. U.S.A.* 93, 3209–3214.

Sharifov, O. F., Fedorov, V. V., Beloshapko, G. G., Glukhov, A. V., Yushmanova, A. V., and Rosen- shtraukh, L. V. (2004). Roles of adrenergic and cholinergic stim- ulation in spontaneous atrial fibrillation in dogs. *J. Am. Coll. Cardiol.* 43, 483–490.

Spyer, K. M. (1994). Annual review prize lecture. Central nervous mech- anisms contributing to cardiovascu- lar control. *J. Physiol. (Lond.)* 474, 1–19.

Stauss, H. M. (2003). Heart rate vari- ability. *Am. J. Physiol. Regul. Integr. Comp. Physiol.* 285, R927–R931.

Sternweis, P. C., and Robishaw, J. D. (1984). Isolation of two pro- teins with high affinity for gua- nine nucleotides from membranes of bovine brain. *J. Biol. Chem.* 259, 13806–13813.

Strittmatter, S. M., Valenzuela, D., Kennedy, T. E., Neer, E. J., and Fish- man, M. C. (1990). G0 is a major growth cone protein subject to reg- ulation by GAP-43. *Nature* 344, 836–841.

Swedberg, K., Komajda, M., Böhm, M., Borer, J. S., Ford, I., Dubost- Brama, A., Lerebours, G., Tavazzi, L., and SHIFT Investigators. (2010). Ivabradine and outcomes in chronic heart failure (SHIFT): a randomised placebo-controlled study. *Lancet* 376, 875–885.

Thireau, J., Zhang, B. L., Poisson, D., and Babuty, D. (2007). Heart rate variability in mice: a theoretical and practical guide. *Exp. Physiol.* 93, 83–94.

Tuomi, J. M., Chidiac, P., and Jones, D. L. (2010). Evidence for enhanced M3 muscarinic receptor function and sensitivity to atrial arrhythmia in the RGS2-deficient mouse. *Am. J. Physiol. Heart Circ. Physiol.* 298, H554–H561.

Valenzuela, D., Han, X., Mende, U., Fankhauser, C., Mashimo, H., Huang, P., Pfeffer, J., Neer, E. J., and Fishman, M. C. (1997). G alpha(o) is necessary for muscarinic regulation of Ca2+ channels in mouse heart. *Proc. Natl. Acad. Sci. U.S.A.* 94, 1727–1732.

Verrier, R. L., and Antzelevitch, C. (2004). Autonomic aspects of arrhythmogenesis: the enduring and the new. *Curr. Opin. Cardiol.* 19, 2–11.

Voigt, N., Maguy, A., Yeh, Y. H., Qi, X., Ravens, U., Dobrev, D., and Nattel, S. (2008). Changes in I K, ACh single- channel activity with atrial tachy- cardia remodelling in canine atrial cardiomyocytes. *Cardiovasc. Res.* 77, 35–43.

Wakili, R., Voigt, N., Kaab, S., Dobrev, D., and Nattel, S. (2011). Recent advances in the molecular patho- physiology of atrial fibrillation. *J. Clin. Invest.* 121, 2955–2968.

Waxman, M. B., and Wald, R. W. (1977). Termination of ventricu- lar tachycardia by an increase in cardiac vagal drive. *Circulation* 56, 385–391.

Welzig, C. M., Shin, D. G., Park, H. J., Kim, Y. J., Saul, J. P., and Galper, J. B. (2003). Lipid lowering by pravastatin increases parasym- pathetic modulation of heart rate. *Circulation* 108, 2743–2746.

Wettschureck, N., and Offermanns, S. (2005). Mammalian G proteins and their cell type specific functions. *Physiol. Rev.* 85, 1159–1204.

Wickman, K., Nemec, J., Gendler, S. J., and Clapham, D. E. (1998). Abnormal heart rate regulation in GIRK4 knockout mice. *Neuron* 20, 103–114.

Wieland, T., and Mittmann, C. (2003). Regulators of G-protein signalling: multifunctional proteins with impact on signalling in the cardio- vascular system. *Pharmacol. Ther.* 97, 95–115.

Wijffels, M. C., Kirchhof, C. J., Dor- land, R., and Allessie, M. A. (1995). Atrial fibrillation begets atrial fibril- lation. A study in awake chronically instrumented goats. *Circulation* 92, 1954–1968.

Winter, S., Brunk, I., Walther, D. J., Höltje, M., Jiang, M., Peter, J.-U., Takamori, S., Jahn, R., Birnbaumer, L., and Ahnert-Hilger, G. (2005). Galphao2 regulates vesicular gluta- mate transporter activity by chang- ing its chloride dependence. *J. Neu- rosci.* 25, 4672–4680.

Wong, Y. H., Federman, A., Pace, A. M., Zachary, I., Evans, T., Pouysségur, J., and Bourne, H. R. (1991). Mutant alpha subunits of Gi2 inhibit cyclic AMP accumulation. *Nature* 351, 63–65.

Yang, J., Huang, J., Maity, B., Gao, Z., Lorca, R. A., Gudmundsson, H., Li, J., Stewart, A., Swaminathan, P. D., Ibeawuchi, S. R., Shepherd, A., Chen, C. K., Kutschke, W., Mohler, P. J., Mohapatra, D. P., Anderson, M. E., and Fisher, R. A. (2010). RGS6, a modulator of parasympa- thetic activation in heart. *Circ. Res.* 107, 1345–1349.

Yoro Sy, G., Urosevic, D., Fellmann, L., Greney, H., Bousquet, P., and Feld- man, J. (2008). G-protein inwardly rectifying potassium channels are involved in the hypotensive effect of I1-imidazoline receptor selec- tive ligands. *J. Hypertens.* 26, 1025–1032.

Young, C. N., and Davisson, R. L. (2011). In vivo assessment of neurocardio-vascular regulation in the mouse: principles, progress, and prospects. *Am. J. Physiol. Heart Circ. Physiol.* 301, H654–H662.

Zheng, M., Zhu, W., Han, Q., and Xiao, R. P. (2005). Emerging con- cepts and therapeutic implications of beta-adrenergic receptor sub- type signaling. *Pharmacol. Ther.* 108, 257–268.

Zuberi, Z., Birnbaumer, L., and Tinker,

A. (2008). The role of inhibitory het- erotrimeric G proteins in the control of in vivo heart rate dynamics. *Am. J. Physiol. Regul. Integr. Comp. Physiol.* 295, R1822–R1830.

Zuberi, Z., Nobles, M., Sebastian, S., Dyson, A., Lim, S. Y., Breckenridge, R., Birnbaumer, L., and Tinker, A. (2010). Absence of the inhibitory G-protein Galphai2 predisposes to ventricular cardiac arrhythmia. *Circ. Arrhythm. Electrophysiol.* 3, 391–400.

13

Mouse models of *SCN5A*-related cardiac arrhythmias

Mickael Derangeon[1,2,3], Jérôme Montnach[1,2,3], Isabelle Baró[1,2,3] and Flavien Charpentier[1,2,3] *

[1] INSERM, UMR 1087, l'Institut du Thorax, Nantes, France
[2] CNRS, UMR 6291, l'Institut du Thorax, Nantes, France
[3] Université de Nantes, Nantes, France

***Correspondence:**
Flavien Charpentier, INSERM, UMR1087, CNRS UMR6291, l'Institut du Thorax, IRT-UN, 8 quai Moncousu, BP 70721, 44007 Nantes Cedex 1, France.
e-mail: flavien.charpentier@inserm.fr

Mutations of *SCN5A* gene, which encodes the α-subunit of the voltage-gated Na^+ channel $Na_V1.5$, underlie hereditary cardiac arrhythmic syndromes such as the type 3 long QT syndrome, cardiac conduction diseases, the Brugada syndrome, the sick sinus syndrome, a trial standstill, and numerous overlap syndromes. Patch-clamp studies in heterologous expression systems have provided important information to understand the genotype-phenotype relationships of these diseases. However, they could not clarify how *SCN5A* mutations can be responsible for such a large spectrum of diseases, for the late age of onset or the progressiveness of some of these diseases and for the overlapping syndromes. Genetically modified mice rapidly appeared as promising tools for understanding the pathophysiological mechanisms of cardiac *SCN5A*-related arrhythmic syndromes and several mouse models have been established. This review presents the results obtained on these models that, for most of them, recapitulate the clinical phenotypes of the patients. This includes two models knocked out for Nav1.5 β1 and β3 auxiliary subunits that are also discussed. Despite their own limitations that we point out, the mouse models still appear as powerful tools to elucidate the pathophysiological mechanisms of *SCN5A*-related diseases and offer the opportunity to investigate the secondary cellular consequences of *SCN5A* mutations such as the expression remodeling of other genes. This points out the potential role of these genes in the overall human phenotype. Finally, they constitute useful tools for addressing the role of genetic and environmental modifiers on cardiac electrical activity.

Keywords: $Na_V1.5$, arrhythmia, conduction disease, long QT syndrome, Brugada syndrome, sinus node dysfunction

Mutations in the *SCN5A* gene, which encodes the α-subunit of the cardiac voltage-gated Na^+ channel $Na_V1.5$, underlie hereditary arrhythmic syndromes (so-called cardiac channelopathies). On one hand, gain-of-function mutations, that increase the late component of the Na^+ current (I_{Na}) and thus prolong the ventricular action potential, are responsible for the type 3 long QT syndrome (LQT3; Moss and Kass, 2005). On the other hand, loss-of-function mutations decrease I_{Na} and are responsible for cardiac conduction diseases (Schott et al., 1999; Tan et al., 2001; Probst et al., 2003), Brugada syndrome (Gussak et al., 1999), sick sinus syndrome (Benson et al., 2003), and atrial standstill (Groenewegen et al., 2003). To complicate matters further, some *SCN5A* mutations can lead to more complex diseases associating different phenotypic traits such as, for instance, bradycardia, conduction disease, LQT3, and Brugada syndrome (so-called overlap syndromes; Bezzina et al., 1999; Kyndt et al., 2001; Grant et al., 2002; Rossenbacker et al., 2004; Smits et al., 2005; for review, see Remme et al., 2008). Finally, there is also an association between *SCN5A* genetic defects and susceptibility to dilated cardiomyopathy (DCM; McNair et al., 2004) and atrial fibrillation (Laitinen-Forsblom et al., 2006; Ellinor et al., 2008).

Although patch-clamp studies in heterologous expression systems have provided a great deal of information to understand the genotype-phenotype relationships of these diseases, these models could not clarify how loss-of-function-mutations can be responsible for such a large spectrum of diseases and the late age of onset or the progressiveness of some of them. They are even less adapted to overlap syndromes.

Genetically modified mice thus appeared as promising tools for understanding the pathophysiological sequence of cardiac *SCN5A*-related channelopathies and several mouse models have been established (**Table 1**). Fortunately, whereas some genetically modified mice related to K^+ channel dysfunction did not reach investigators' expectations because of major electrophysiological differences between mice and men (Nerbonne et al., 2001; Charpentier et al., 2004), mouse models of inherited *SCN5A* channelopathies, on the contrary, appeared to be informative.

MODELS FOR THE LQT3 SYNDROME

SCN5A-related long QT syndrome (LQT3; Wang et al., 1995) is less frequent but often more lethal than LQT1 and LQT2 (Priori et al., 2003). Like in other LQT syndromes, the abnormal prolongation of ventricular repolarization is associated with a susceptibility to a specific polymorphic ventricular tachycardia called *torsades de pointes* and ventricular fibrillation, leading to syncope and sudden death. Clinically, LQT3 is characterized by an increased duration of the ST segment with a late appearance of the T-wave (Moss, 2002). Bradycardia and pauses occurring at rest, and more particularly during sleep, are often at the origin of the arrhythmias. However, fatal tachycardia-induced arrhythmias have also been reported for a third of the patients (Schwartz et al., 2001). Two thirds of the *SCN5A* mutations found in LQT3 alter the fast inactivation process

Table 1 | Mouse models of *SCN5A*-related cardiac genetic diseases.

Mouse	Genetic modification	Human disease	ECG phenotype	Arrhythmias	Effect on I_{Na}	Original publication
Scn5a$^{\Delta/+}$	KI/heterozygote/ 150-5KPQ-1507 del	LQT3	QT prolongation	VT EADs *in vitro*	Increased late current	Nuyens et al. (2001), Head et al. (2005)
h*SCN5A*-N1325S	Tg/point mutation	LQT3	QT prolongation	VT EADs *in vitro*	Delayed inactivation increased late current	Tian et al. (2004)
Scn5a$^{\pm}$	KO/heterozygote	Brugada, PCCD	P wave, PR and QRS prolongation	Triggered VT (spontaneous in old)	≈50% decrease in peak current	Papadatos et al. (2002)
Scn5a$^{1798insD/+}$	KI/heterozygote/ insertion	Overlap syndrome (LQT3 – Brugada – CCD)	PR, QRS and QT prolongation	Sinus pauses EADs *in vitro*	≈40% decrease in peak current, increased late current	Remme et al. (2006)
SCN5A-D1275N	RMCE/hetero- and homozygote/ point mutation	Arrhythmogenic DCM	Bradycardia, P wave, PR and QRS prolongation	AT/AF, VT and sinus node dysfunction in homozygote	≈50% decrease in peak current (heterozygote)	Watanabe et al. (2011)
Scn1b$^{-/-}$	KO/hetero- and homozygote	LQT3	Bradycardia and QT prolongation (homozygote)	Not investigated	≈60% increase in peak and late current (homzygote)	Lopez-Santiago et al. (2007)
Scn3b$^{-/-}$	KO/homozygote	Brugada, CCD	Bradycardia, P wave and PR prolongation	Triggered VT spontaneous and triggered AT	≈50% decrease in peak current, negative shift of steady-state inactivation	Hakim et al. (2008)

AT, atrial tachycardia; AF, atrial fibrillation; DCM, dilated cardiomyopathy; del, deletion; EAD, early afterdepolarization; KI, knock-in; KO, knockout; LQT3, type 3 long QT syndrome; PCCD, progressive cardiac conduction defects; RMCE, recombinase mediated cassette exchange; VT, ventricular tachycardia; Tg, transgenic.

of the channel (Zimmer and Surber, 2008). For example, the first identified mutation, which leads to the deletion of three amino acids (1505-KPQ-1507) in the inactivation domain of $Na_V1.5$, results in a persistent inward Na^+ current (Wang et al., 1996) and prolongation of the action potential plateau phase (Moss and Kass, 2005).

SCN5A$^{\Delta 1505\text{-}1507KPQ/+}$ KNOCK-IN MOUSE

Nuyens et al. (2001) generated a knock-in mouse model lacking the same KPQ residues. Mice heterozygous for this mutation (*Scn5a*$^{\Delta/+}$) showed typical features of the LQT3 syndrome and spontaneously developed ventricular arrhythmias. Compared with wild-type mice, transmembrane action potentials recorded in ventricular preparations were markedly prolonged in *Scn5a*$^{\Delta/+}$ mice and showed a steeper "heart rate" versus "action potential duration" relationship (Nuyens et al., 2001). Action potential amplitude and upstroke velocity were not altered. Whole-cell patch-clamp recordings performed on cardiomyocytes confirmed the increase in late inward Na^+ current previously observed in heterologous expression system, which explains the action potential prolongation (Wang et al., 1996). Surprisingly, there was also a two-fold increase in the peak Na^+ current density, which could not be explained by an over-expression of $Na_V1.5$ or changes in the steady-state activation and inactivation of the current. However, this finding was not confirmed in a more recent study on the same model (Fredj et al., 2006) and the reason for this discrepancy remains to be clarified. Nuyens et al.'s (2001) study also revealed an acceleration of the recovery from inactivation, a property that might favor re-entrant arrhythmias. Indeed, intracardiac pacing with extra stimuli, short-long-short pacing sequences and abrupt accelerations of heart rate reproducibly induced polymorphic ventricular arrhythmias in *Scn5a*$^{\Delta/+}$ mice but not in wild-type mice. The *Scn5a*$^{\Delta/+}$ mice were also characterized by a paradoxical transient action potential prolongation upon abrupt acceleration of pacing rate that favored the occurrence of early after depolarizations. This prolongation was blocked by the Na^+ channel blocker mexiletine and the adrenergic agonist isoproterenol. It can be explained by the increase of both fast and slow components of the Na^+ current which causes a sudden increase of Na^+ load, and secondarily of Ca^{2+} load. As a consequence, during each action potential, the increased Ca^{2+} release from the sarcoplasmic reticulum activates a larger Na/Ca exchanger current which generates early after depolarizations. The autonomic modulation of cardiac electrical activity and arrhythmias of *Scn5a*$^{\Delta/+}$ mice has been recently investigated in more details both *in vivo* in freely moving mice and *ex vivo* (Fabritz et al., 2010). As expected from clinical investigations, cholinergic stimulation was shown to favor arrhythmias by inducing bradycardia. In contrast, β-adrenergic stimulation suppressed arrhythmias by shortening repolarization and increasing cardiac rate, while β-blockers had no effect on their own.

A second *Scn5a*$^{\Delta/+}$ mouse line, exhibiting the same phenotype as the previous line, was created (Head et al., 2005) and submitted to an extended pharmacological analysis. Electrophysiological studies performed on Langendorff-perfused whole hearts confirmed the anti-arrhythmic properties of mexiletine (Fabritz et al., 2003; Head et al., 2005) and showed that another Na^+ channel inhibitor, flecainide, could also prevent arrhythmias by preferentially inhibiting the late Na^+ current (Fredj et al., 2006), whereas β-blockers were inefficient (Head et al., 2005; Stokoe et al., 2007b;

Sabir et al., 2008). These results have been confirmed in freely moving mice (Fabritz et al., 2010). More recently, it was shown that a specific inhibition of the L-type Ca^{2+} channels with nifedipine was also efficient in preventing arrhythmias through the suppression of early after depolarizations (Thomas et al., 2007). Finally, nicorandil, an activator of the ATP-sensitive K^+ channel, also reduces arrhythmogenicity in *Scn5a*$^{\Delta/+}$ mice (Hothi et al., 2008), confirming previous results obtained with the canine wedge preparation pharmacological model of LQT3 (Shimizu and Antzelevitch, 2000). In contrast, quinidine was proarrhythmic (Sabir et al., 2008). *Ex vivo* studies also confirmed the key role played by bradycardia and increased dispersion of repolarization on the occurrence of spontaneous ventricular arrhythmias (Fabritz et al., 2003). Sudden rate accelerations initially and transiently increased the dispersion of repolarization due to early after depolarizations and action potential alternans (Fabritz et al., 2003; Hothi et al., 2008), as previously observed *in vivo* (Nuyens et al., 2001), and then secondarily suppressed and prevented ventricular tachycardia by decreasing dispersion of repolarization and suppressing early after depolarizations. Arrhythmogenesis, as assessed by programmed electrical stimulation on Langendorff-perfused hearts, has also been associated with abnormal patterns of myocardial activation and abnormally reduced transmural gradients of repolarization resulting from a larger increase in action potential duration in subepicardium than in subendocardium (Stokoe et al., 2007b). In addition, *Scn5a*$^{\Delta/+}$ mice exhibit larger differences between action potential duration and refractory period, so-called local critical interval (APD-ERP), in subepicardial regions than in wild-type mice. Those anomalies may support re-entrant events following premature excitation. More recently, Sabir et al. (2008) proposed that the increases of the slopes of restitution curves (plotting action potential duration versus the preceding diastolic interval; Gilmour, 2003) to values greater than one, rather than increased dispersion of repolarization, was associated with arrhythmogenicity. All these anomalies, including action potential alternans are corrected by nicorandil (Hothi et al., 2008).

Altogether, *Scn5a*$^{\Delta/+}$ mice recapitulate most of the LQT3 associated clinical symptoms. They confirmed previous studies suggesting that arrhythmias in LQT3 syndrome may result from reentries provoked by early after depolarizations and enabled to unveil the mechanisms of tachycardia-induced arrhythmias. Studies of *Scn5a*$^{\Delta/+}$ mice have also provided a rationale for the use of Na^+ channel blockers and pacing to prevent cardiac arrhythmias and sudden death in the context of LQT3, for which β-blockers have shown low efficacy. Finally, they suggest that Ca^{2+} channels inhibitors and ATP-sensitive K^+ channel activators might be interesting pharmacological approaches to prevent arrhythmias in this context.

In addition to early after depolarizations, the occurrence of delayed after depolarizations, resulting from the transient inward current (I_{ti}), was also clearly demonstrated in myocytes of *Scn5a*$^{\Delta/+}$ mice (Fredj et al., 2006). Most recently, Lindegger et al. (2009) showed that I_{ti} induction occurs under conditions of elevated sarcoplasmic reticulum Ca^{2+} content that is most probably related to the mutation-induced increase in late Na^+ current. Indeed, both I_{ti} and its underlying Ca^{2+} wave were suppressed by ranolazine, an antianginal agent well known to block the late Na^+ current (Hale et al., 2008). Whether delayed after depolarizations participate to spontaneous arrhythmic events in *Scn5a*$^{\Delta/+}$ mice, and of course in LQT3 patients, remains to be determined. Investigating the potential anti-arrhythmic effects of ranolazine in this model also remains to be performed.

Patients with LQT syndrome (El Yaman et al., 2008; Johnson et al., 2008; Zellerhoff et al., 2009), including LQT3 (Benito et al., 2008), may be at increased risk for atrial fibrillation. Therefore, the atrial phenotype of *Scn5a*$^{\Delta/+}$ mice was characterized. Using Langendorff-perfused hearts, Blana et al. (2010) showed that atrial action potential duration and effective refractory period were prolonged in *Scn5a*$^{\Delta/+}$ mice. Short runs of rapid pacing-induced a larger increase in post-pacing spontaneous atrial cycle length and action potential duration in *Scn5a*$^{\Delta/+}$ mice than in wild-type mice, leading to the occurrence of atrial tachycardia in *Scn5a*$^{\Delta/+}$ mice but not in wild-type mice. Extra stimuli triggered arrhythmias similarly in wild-type and *Scn5a*$^{\Delta/+}$ mice (in 30–40% of the mice). Contrasting results had been previously observed with the second mouse line suggesting that *Scn5a*$^{\Delta/+}$ mice are protected against pacing-induced atrial tachyarrhythmias when young (3 months; Dautova et al., 2009), whereas they exhibit an increased atrial arrhythmogenicity when old (1 year; Guzadhur et al., 2010). Without excluding the influence of variable experimental conditions, those discrepancies might also rely on the fact that the two lines have different genetic backgrounds, as we will discuss later for the *Scn5a*$^{1798insD/+}$ knock-in mouse. Both mouse lines, however, exhibit decreased heart rate and atrioventricular conduction (prolonged PR interval) versus wild-type mice.

Sinus node dysfunction has been reported in patients with *SCN5A*-related long QT syndrome whether these mutations only lead to an increased late Na^+ current (Moss et al., 1995; Wei et al., 1999) or lead to more complex biophysical alterations of the channel (Bezzina et al., 1999; van den Berg et al., 2001; Grant et al., 2002). Because QT prolongation is more pronounced at lower heart rates, bradycardia represents an important indirect factor in predisposition to lethal arrhythmias in LQT3 families (Schwartz et al., 1995). The mechanisms for LQT3-related bradycardia were investigated for the 1795insD mutation of $Na_V1.5$ (Veldkamp et al., 2003), a mutation inducing an overlap syndrome with bradycardia, conduction disease, LQT3 and Brugada syndrome (Bezzina et al., 1999). This mutation induces both a decrease in Na^+ peak current and the occurrence of a late Na^+ current (see dedicated section below for details). By combining current clamp studies and computational modeling, Veldkamp et al. (2003) suggested that both the decreased availability of Na^+ channels and the increase of late current accounted for bradycardia. However, the effect of action potential prolongation secondary to the increased late current appeared more prominent. The contribution of the late Na^+ current to sinus node dysfunction has been further confirmed on *Scn5a*$^{\Delta/+}$ mice (Wu et al., 2012). *Scn5a*$^{\Delta/+}$ mice exhibit sinus node dysfunction with episodes of bradycardia, sinus pauses, and longer sinus node recovery times. Sino-atrial preparations from *Scn5a*$^{\Delta/+}$ mice had lower intrinsic rate from the sinus node to the surrounding atrium than wild-type preparations. Computational studies confirmed that the decrease in sinus rate could be attributed to the increased late current. *Ex vivo* experiments on sino-atrial preparations also showed that conduction through the sinus node to the surrounding atrium was decreased, a result that computer modeling could only explain by a decrease in Na^+ peak current amplitude, which has not been experimentally confirmed.

hSCN5A-N1325S TRANSGENIC MOUSE MODEL

The N1325S mutation of $Na_V1.5$, located in the intracellular region between segments 4 and 5 of domain III, also causes LQT3 syndrome (Wang et al., 1995). This mutation, like many similar mutations, leads to an increased late inward Na^+ current (Dumaine et al., 1996; Wang et al., 1996). A transgenic mouse with cardiac selective expression of human *SCN5A*-N1325S mutation under the control of the mouse α-myosin heavy chain promoter was established (Tian et al., 2004). Transgenic mice showed some of the typical features of the LQT3 syndrome such as prolonged QT interval, ventricular arrhythmias, and a high rate of sudden deaths due to documented polymorphic ventricular tachycardia and ventricular fibrillation. However, transgenic mice were also characterized by increased heart rate and shorter PR intervals that are not observed in LQT3 patients. Some of these features might result from over-expression of the channel rather than from the mutation itself since short PR interval was also observed in the control mouse over-expressing wild-type h*SCN5A* gene (Zhang et al., 2007).

Voltage-clamp experiments on cardiomyocytes isolated from wild-type and h*SCN5A*-N1325S mice confirmed that the N1325S mutation does not modify the peak current but delays the inactivation process and generates a late persistent current (Tian et al., 2004), which decreases with increasing pacing rates (Yong et al., 2007). Action potentials from h*SCN5A*-N1325S ventricular myocytes were longer than wild-type ones and exhibited early after depolarizations. As in $Scn5a^{\Delta/+}$ mice, mexiletine shortened ventricular action potential duration and prevented arrhythmias (Tian et al., 2004). Interestingly, action potential duration of transgenic but not wild-type myocytes paradoxically increased with pacing rate (Tian et al., 2004) and became highly variable with occurrence of repolarization alternans (Yong et al., 2007). Whether this phenomenon was only transient, as in $Scn5a^{\Delta/+}$ mice, or persisted during long periods of increased pacing rate is unclear. The Ca^{2+} channel blocker verapamil reduced these alternans, suggesting an involvement of intracellular Ca^{2+} deregulation in this phenomenon. Previous studies had shown that patients with long QT syndrome can exhibit T-wave alternans during sinus tachycardia (Cruz Filho et al., 2000; Viskin et al., 2004).

Like the $Scn5a^{\Delta/+}$ mouse model, the h*SCN5A*-N1325S mouse provided key information to our understanding of arrhythmias in LQT3 syndrome. For instance, it showed that the N1325S mutant dysfunction can explain both bradycardia- and non-bradycardia-related arrhythmias observed in patients carrying this mutation (Yong et al., 2007). However, the model might be taken with caution because of the limitations linked to the over-expression of the channel. Indeed, there is a clear relationship between the level of h*SCN5A*-N1325S expression and the extent of QT prolongation, i.e., by 23% with 1–2 copies and by 91% with 10 copies. Most recently, this model was shown to exhibit cardiomyocyte apoptosis, cardiac fibrosis, and contractile dysfunction during aging (Zhang et al., 2011). But signs of heart failure were markedly larger in the mouse line with 10 copies. Although heart failure is probably not related to *SCN5A* over-expression *per se*, because old mice over-expressing 10 times the wild-type channel remained normal, one should better consider the model over-expressing the least the mutant channel to extrapolate the results to the patients. In this second line, left ventricular fractional shortening was less decreased and only 30% of the mice showed features of DCM, a result more consistent with the scarcity of heart failure in LQT3 patients (Nguyen et al., 2008; Shi et al., 2008).

A MODEL FOR THE BRUGADA SYNDROME AND CONDUCTION DISORDERS: THE *Scn5a* KNOCKOUT MOUSE

The Brugada syndrome is a genetic disease which associates ST segment elevation in the right precordial leads V1 to V3 of the ECG, often with signs of conduction slowing, with a high risk of sudden cardiac death secondary to ventricular tachycardia or fibrillation (Gussak et al., 1999; Antzelevitch et al., 2005). In 20–30% of the patients, the disease is related to mutations in *SCN5A* leading to a complete or partial loss-of-function of $Na_V1.5$ (Tan et al., 2003). Loss-of-function mutations are also responsible for inherited Progressive Cardiac Conduction Defects (PCCD), also called Lev-Lenègre disease (Schott et al., 1999), or non-progressive conduction defects (Tan et al., 2001). More recently, PCCD has also been linked to gain-of-function mutations in *TRPM4* gene (Transient Receptor Potential cation channel, subfamily M, member 4), which encodes a Ca^{2+}-activated non-selective channel (Kruse et al., 2009; Liu et al., 2010). PCCD is a slowly evolving disease which progressively affects cardiac conduction leading ultimately to pacemaker implantation to prevent the risk of complete atrioventricular block and Stokes–Adams syncope. Inherited PCCD associates haploinsufficiency of *SCN5A* together with an additional yet unknown mechanism related to aging (Probst et al., 2003). Despite their major clinical differences, Brugada syndrome, and inherited conduction diseases share common features. First, both diseases can be caused by *SCN5A* haploinsufficiency. Second, Brugada patients with *SCN5A* mutations exhibit altered conduction whereas Brugada patients without *SCN5A* mutations do not (Smits et al., 2002). Finally, both Brugada syndrome and PCCD can be found in the same pedigree (Kyndt et al., 2001). In other families, patients carrying loss-of-function mutations can exhibit symptoms of Brugada syndrome, conduction disease, and sick sinus syndrome, either combined or not (Smits et al., 2005). Severe forms of sick sinus syndrome have also been found in patients with double inheritance of *SCN5A* loss-of-function mutations (Benson et al., 2003).

A mouse model with targeted disruption of *Scn5a* gene has been established (Papadatos et al., 2002). Homozygous knockout mouse embryos die during mid-gestation due to severe defects in ventricular morphogenesis whereas heterozygous ($Scn5a^{\pm}$) mice show normal survival. However, 8- to 10-week-old $Scn5a^{\pm}$ mice have several cardiac electrical defects such as decreased atrial and atrioventricular conduction and increased susceptibility to pacing-induced ventricular arrhythmias (Papadatos et al., 2002). Following this initial report, the model was further analyzed to investigate the potential pathophysiological mechanisms involved in the progressive evolution of *SCN5A*-related PCCD (Royer et al., 2005; van Veen et al., 2005). It was found that in addition to atrial and atrioventricular conduction, ventricular conduction was also decreased. Moreover, ECG studies performed on mice ranging from 4 to 71 weeks of age showed that the ventricular phenotype of *Scn5a*$^{\pm}$ mice worsened with age. This feature was confirmed by activation mapping studies performed on Langendorff-perfused hearts. In young *Scn5a*$^{\pm}$ mice, conduction velocity was only affected in the right ventricle. In old mice, right ventricular conduction defect worsened and was in addition associated with conduction velocity defect in the left ventricle. This age-dependent deterioration of ventricular conduction was associated with the occurrence of fibrosis in ventricular myocardium. In some aspects, this phenotype resembles PCCD, although in the later fibrosis was found to be limited to the conduction system area (Lenègre and Moreau, 1963; Lev, 1964). However, it is worth noting that fibrosis has also been observed in patients with the Brugada syndrome (Coronel et al., 2005; Frustaci et al., 2005). More recently, it was shown that *Scn5a*$^{\pm}$ mice display variable degrees of conduction defects when young (10 weeks old): some mice have only mild prolongation of the QRS interval while others have more severe QRS prolongation associated with RR′ or SS′ patterns (Leoni et al., 2010). The extent of fibrotic remodeling was dependent on the severity of the initial conduction disorders: mice with larger QRS prolongation when young have the most severe fibrotic remodeling when they get older, suggesting that the ventricular activation pattern is a key element for triggering remodeling. Whatever their triggering mechanism, fibrosis, and redistribution of connexin 43 expression most likely contribute to the age-dependent degradation of ventricular conduction in the mouse model. Whether *SCN5A*-related inherited PCCD in human also results from a primary decrease in Na^+ current and a secondary progressive fibrosis with aging remains to be clarified. In this context, *Scn5a*$^{\pm}$ mice could be used for testing preventive therapies as an alternative to pacemaker implantation.

In their initial report on the *Scn5a*$^{\pm}$ mouse model, Papadatos et al. (2002) showed that programmed ventricular electrical pacing of Langendorff-perfused hearts induced ventricular tachyarrhythmias in two thirds of *Scn5a*$^{\pm}$ mice but not in wild-type mice and proposed that the model could be used for elucidating the mechanisms of arrhythmias in the context of *SCN5A*-related Brugada syndrome. Pathophysiological findings have implicated the right ventricular outflow tract as the primary location for electrical disorders in Brugada syndrome. Two hypotheses have been proposed to explain both ST segment elevation and occurrence of arrhythmias (Wilde et al., 2010). The first one, mainly based on experimental data obtained in arterially perfused canine right ventricular wedges, implicates alterations in transmural and regional repolarization gradients leading to localized losses of the subepicardial action potential dome and phase 2 reentries as the arrhythmogenic mechanism. The second one, mainly based on clinical studies, implicates abnormal conduction. To elucidate the arrhythmogenic mechanisms in *Scn5a*$^{\pm}$ mice programmed electrical stimulation, monophasic action potential (MAP) recording, and bipolar electrogram recording was performed on Langendorff-perfused hearts. These experiments showed that *Scn5a*$^{\pm}$ mice were characterized by increased electrogram duration with shortening extrasystoles intervals, especially in the right ventricular outflow tract, and increased transmural and regional heterogeneity of MAP duration and refractory periods in the right ventricle with the shortest in the right ventricular outflow tract (Stokoe et al., 2007a; Martin et al., 2010, 2011a,b). *Scn5a*$^{\pm}$ mice also exhibited increased incidence of MAP alternans. As a consequence, ventricular tachycardia occurred earlier in the right ventricular outflow tract (Martin et al., 2011b). All these mechanisms were potentiated by flecainide, a Na^+ channel inhibitor which is well described to favor ST segment elevation and arrhythmias in patients with the Brugada syndrome. Ventricular tachycardia also occurred spontaneously both *in vivo* (Leoni et al., 2010; Martin et al., 2011c) and *ex vivo* (Martin et al., 2011d), but with a much higher incidence under flecainide treatment (Martin et al., 2011c,d). Multielectrode array studies showed that the initiation of spontaneous arrhythmias resulted from a combination of conduction slowing and repolarization heterogeneities leading to lines of conduction blocks and unidirectional conduction (Martin et al., 2011d). Altogether these results seem to contradict the hypothesis that arrhythmias in the Brugada syndrome result from phase 2 re-entrant mechanisms. However, the main limitation of the mouse model is that the ventricular action potential lacks a plateau phase, and for the subepicardial action potential, a spike, and dome morphology, present in larger mammals and prerequisite for phase 2 reentries.

In addition, *Scn5a*$^{\pm}$ mice turned out to be useful for understanding the role of $Na_V1.5$ in sinus node normal function and the pathophysiology of sinus node dysfunction associated to *SCN5A* loss-of-function mutations (Benson et al., 2003; Smits et al., 2005). Indeed, *Scn5a*$^{\pm}$ mice also display moderate bradycardia that can be associated with occasional sino-atrial blocks in older animals (Lei et al., 2005). Lei et al. showed that small central sino-atrial node cells, which do not express $Na_V1.5$, exhibited normal intrinsic pacemaker rate. In contrast, larger peripheral sino-atrial node cells, which normally express $Na_V1.5$, exhibited reduced intrinsic pacemaker rate associated to reduced expression of $Na_V1.5$. These data were consistent with the slower sino-atrial conduction and frequent sino-atrial conduction blocks observed in *Scn5a*$^{\pm}$ sino-atrial node preparations compared to wild-type although they exhibited normal activation patterns. A computer model successfully reproduced these findings and implicated I_{Na} in action potential propagation through the sino-atrial node, from sino-atrial node to atria, and in modifying heart rate through a coupling of sino-atrial node and atrial cells. More recently, this same team has shown that both aging and *Scn5a* disruption affect sino-atrial node function through electrical remodeling and TGF-β_1-mediated fibrosis, with the most severe phenotype observed in old *Scn5a*$^{\pm}$ mice (Hao et al., 2011). Interestingly, this *in vivo* sino-atrial node dysfunction appears less severe than expected from *ex vivo* experiments and computer simulations seems to be due to an increase in sympathetic regulation of sino-atrial node with age, partly explained by an over-expression of β_1-adrenoceptors (Hao et al., 2011).

AN OVERLAP SYNDROME MODEL: THE *Scn5a*$^{1798INSD/+}$ KNOCK-IN MOUSE

In 1999, a *SCN5A* mutation (1795insD) associated with an overlap syndrome of cardiac Na^+ channelopathies was described in a large Dutch family. The patients' ECG presented features of bradycardia, conduction disease, LQT3, and Brugada syndrome (Bezzina et al., 1999). The analysis of the 1795insD mutation biophysical properties led to contrasting results depending on the heterologous expression system used. In *Xenopus oocytes*, the mutation reduced the Na^+ current through a negative shift in voltage-dependence of steady-state inactivation but did not produce the persistent current commonly observed in LQT3 (Bezzina et al., 1999). In contrast, in HEK293 cells, 1795insD mutation disrupted fast inactivation leading to sustained inward Na^+ current that could prolong repolarization at slow heart rates and, at the same time, increased slow inactivation, delaying recovery of Na^+ channel availability between stimuli and reducing the Na^+ current under conditions mimicking fast heart rates (Veldkamp et al., 2000). Computer modeling showed that this dual mechanism could indeed explain the overlap syndrome, depending on the heart rate (Clancy and Rudy, 2002). Because of these discrepancies and because the co-inheritance of other genetic variants besides the 1795insD mutation as a cause of the phenotype complexity in the family could not be ruled out, Remme et al. (2006) generated a knock-in mouse carrying the mouse equivalent (1798insD) of the human *SCN5A*-1795insD mutation. Homozygous mice are not viable. Heterozygous *Scn5a*$^{1798insD/+}$ mice recapitulate many of the pathological features of the patients including sinus node dysfunction, conduction slowing, and QT prolongation at slow rates. Patch-clamp experiments performed on ventricular *Scn5a*$^{1798insD/+}$ cardiomyocytes have shown that action potential duration was longer than in wild-type cardiomyocytes and that this prolongation was more pronounced at slow pacing rates. Also, at fast pacing rates, action potential upstroke velocity, which reflects Na^+ channel availability, was reduced in *Scn5a*$^{1798insD/+}$ mice compared to wild-type. However, the potential biophysical mechanisms thought to explain decreased availability of Na^+ channels in heterologous expression systems were not confirmed in *Scn5a*$^{1798insD/+}$ mice. Indeed, rather than changes in the voltage-dependence of activation and inactivation or slow inactivation properties, dysfunctional mutant channels at the membrane or ineffective trafficking of mutant channels to the membrane more likely explained the marked decrease of Na^+ current in *Scn5a*$^{1798insD/+}$ mice. In addition, a small persistent inward Na^+ current was found in *Scn5a*$^{1798insD/+}$ cardiomyocytes, explaining the prolongation of action potential duration and QT interval. These studies constitute another example of the limitations of heterologous expression systems and illustrate the benefits of genetically engineered mouse models. In summary, the phenotypic characterization of this mouse model has demonstrated that a single *SCN5A* mutation is sufficient to cause an overlap syndrome of cardiac Na^+ channel diseases.

This unique model also represented a useful tool to investigate the impact of genetic and environmental modifiers on cardiac conduction and repolarization. Indeed, also genetic background has often been proposed to affect the phenotypic consequences of ion channel mutations, the identification of genetic modifiers of disease severity in genetically inherited arrhythmias is rare (Scicluna et al., 2008). In order to identify genetic modifiers of conduction disease, Remme et al. (2009) studied the effect of the *Scn5a*-1798insD mutation in mice of two distinct inbred genetic backgrounds. They showed that the phenotype severity of mice carrying the *Scn5a*$^{1798insD/+}$ mutation varies depending on the genetic background. This variability is associated with differential expression of a large number of genes including some encoding ion channels. In particular, ventricular expression levels of $Na_V1.5$ regulatory β4-subunit (encoded by *Scn4b* gene) were markedly reduced in the mouse strain with the most severe conduction defects, leading to a shift of $Na_V1.5$ channel activation curve toward more positive voltages and consequently to a further decrease of I_{Na}. Most recently, these authors went a step further and applied linkage analysis to a F2 cross resulting from the two strains carrying the *Scn5a*-1798insD mutation to identify quantitative trait loci (QTL) for heart rate, ECG parameters, and susceptibility to arrhythmias (Scicluna et al., 2011). This first genetic mapping analysis for cardiac electrical traits in mice identified 3 QTL linked with heart rate (chromosome 4), PR interval (chromosome 3), and QRS interval (chromosome 7) at baseline. Additional significant linkage to chromosome 4 locus was observed for post-flecainide heart rate and ventricular arrhythmias. Unexpectedly, numerous sex-specific QTLs were also identified. Finally, QTL for ECG parameters and arrhythmias coincided at five chromosomal locations suggesting pleiotropic effects at these loci. Interestingly, identified QTLs coincided with chromosomal locations of genes found differentially expressed between the two parental strains in the prior study (Remme et al., 2009). This considerably reduces the number of candidate genes responsible for these QTLs. Nevertheless, additional experiments are still needed to reduce linkage intervals and identify the causal genes. In spite of their success, genome-wide association studies (GWAS) performed in large human populations identified only a very small fraction of heritability of ECG traits and often failed to identify the causal genes. In this context, QTL analysis studies performed in mice could provide independent information pointing to the right genes (Dina, 2011).

A MODEL FOR *SCN5A*-RELATED DILATED CARDIOMYOPATHY: THE *Scn5a*-D1275N MOUSE

The D1275N *SCN5A* mutation has been related to different cardiac diseases. It was first reported in a family affected by atrial standstill, mild conduction disease, and atrial enlargement. However, all affected members also carried a variant in the connexin 40 promoter (Groenewegen et al., 2003). Subsequently, D1275N mutation was reported in a family affected by DCM, sinus node dysfunction, atrial and ventricular tachyarrhythmias and conduction disorders (McNair et al., 2004; Olson et al., 2005; Ge et al., 2008). More recently, it was also reported in a family with atrial tachyarrhythmias, conduction disease, and ventricular enlargement, but without impaired contractility, as opposed to the previous family (Laitinen-Forsblom et al., 2006). Finally, this mutation was also identified in a patient with atrial flutter, atrial standstill, conduction disease, and sinus node dysfunction (Watanabe et al., 2011). Despite these phenotypic differences, patch-clamp studies that have compared wild-type and D1275N channels in heterologous expression systems have not shown major differences in the biophysical properties of the mutant channel (Groenewegen et al., 2003; Gui et al., 2010; Watanabe et al., 2011).

To address this discrepancy, Watanabe et al. (2011) used recombinase mediated cassette exchange to engineer a mouse model expressing the human D1275N mutant channel and compare it to the mouse model expressing the human wild-type channel

(Watanabe et al., 2011). The D1275 allele was associated with slow heart rate and prolonged atrial, atrioventricular and ventricular conduction in a gene-dose-dependent manner, i.e., D1275N homozygous mice had a more severe phenotype. Interestingly, conduction disease increased with age. In addition, sinus node dysfunction, second degree atrioventricular block, atrial tachycardia/fibrillation, and polymorphic ventricular tachycardia occurred in homozygous D1275N mice. Patch-clamp studies of isolated cardiomyocytes demonstrated that D1275N mutation causes a severe decrease in peak I_{Na} by 54% in heterozygous mice and 78% in homozygous mice in relation to a decreased sarcolemmal expression of $Na_V1.5$. Moreover, homozygous D1275N mice exhibited an increased late Na^+ current, leading to prolonged action potential duration. Finally, the mutant was also associated with a gene-dose-dependent reduction of contractile function and DCM. These results are in line with the clinical findings described in the mutation carriers.

Scn1b KNOCKOUT MOUSE

The cardiac Na^+ channel is a heterotrimer composed of $Na_v1.5$, the pore-forming α-subunit, and two auxiliary β-subunits (Meadows and Isom, 2005): a non-covalently linked β1-subunit ($Na_V\beta1$ or β3) and a disulfide-linked subunit ($Na_V\beta2$ or β4). In a genetic screening of 282 probands with Brugada syndrome and 44 with conduction disease, none of whom had mutations in *SCN5A* gene, three mutations in the gene encoding $Na_V\beta1$ (*SCN1B*) were identified in three kindred (Watanabe et al., 2008). Two mutations were located in a newly described alternately spliced transcript, $Na_V\beta1B$ (Qin et al., 2003). Both transcripts are expressed in human heart and to a greater extent in Purkinje fibers than in ventricular myocardium (Watanabe et al., 2008). The E87Q mutation, located in the extracellular immunoglobulin loop of both β1- and β1B-subunits, was identified in a family affected by conduction disease. The two other mutations, which resulted in a β1B-subunit truncated after the amino-acid tryptophan-179, were identified in a family affected with both Brugada syndrome and conduction disease and in a kindred affected with conduction disease. Electrophysiological studies showed that peak I_{Na} amplitude was lower when $Na_v1.5$ was co-expressed with mutant $Na_V\beta1$- and $Na_V\beta1B$-subunits versus wild-type subunits. This result was consistent with the patients' phenotypes.

The cardiac electrophysiological phenotype of a mouse model invalidated for *Scn1b* markedly differed from the phenotype of the patients presented above (Lopez-Santiago et al., 2007). Compared to wild-type mice, *Scn1b* knockout mice exhibited lower heart rates and prolonged QT intervals, without any signs of conduction disease. Surprisingly, loss of $Na_V\beta1$ expression resulted in an increase in both peak and persistent Na^+ current while channel gating and kinetics were unaffected. This increase in current was most likely due to the increased expression of $Na_v1.5$ observed in these mice. Immunostaining studies revealed no alterations in the localization of Na^+ channel α- or β-subunits. Action potentials were prolonged, supporting the increased QT interval. These results are consistent with the observation that the D1790G mutation of *SCN5A*, which affects the interaction of $Na_V1.5$ with $Na_V\beta1$, also leads to a long QT phenotype (Benhorin et al., 1998; An et al., 1998). Once again, studies performed in heterologous expression systems led to contrasting results. Indeed, the D1790G mutation was first found to shift negatively steady-state inactivation of the Na^+ current without increasing its late component (An et al., 1998). The action potential prolongation was attributed to alterations of calcium-sensitive exchange and ion channel currents (Wehrens et al., 2000). By contrast, a second study showed that the mutation-induced a marked prolongation of the late Na^+ current, a result more consistent with the long QT phenotype (Baroudi and Chahine, 2000). Interestingly, the phenotype of *Scn1b* knockout mice resembles that found in a family of patients carrying a mutation on *SCN4B*, the gene encoding the β4-subunit. These patients exhibit a markedly prolonged QT interval (LQT10; Medeiros-Domingo et al., 2007) due to a large increase of the late Na^+ current amplitude, as in LQT3 patients.

Scn3b KNOCKOUT MOUSE

In order to understand better the role of $Na_V\beta3$ subunit on $Na_V1.5$ function, Hakim and co-workers generated a mouse model lacking the *Scn3b* gene (*Scn3b*$^{-/-}$ mouse; Hakim et al., 2008). They showed that the lack of $Na_V\beta3$ induced a ≈30% decrease in cardiac Na^+ peak current amplitude associated with a shift of the steady-state inactivation curve toward negative potentials while other I_{Na} biophysical parameters were not altered, thus confirming previous studies in mammalian heterologous expression system (Ko et al., 2005). As a consequence, *Scn3b*$^{|}$ mice exhibited decreased ventricular conduction, shortened ventricular action potential duration, and refractory period and increased incidence of arrhythmias under programmed electrical stimulation in *ex vivo* Langendorff-perfused hearts (Hakim et al., 2008). Arrhythmogenic incidence was reduced by flecainide and quinidine (Hakim et al., 2010b), in contrast to what had been observed previously for flecainide in *Scn5a*$^{\pm}$ mice (Martin et al., 2011c,d). Like *Scn5a*$^{\pm}$ mice, *Scn3b*$^{-/-}$ mice also exhibited sinus node dysfunction and decreased atrial and atrioventricular conduction, sometimes leading to atrioventricular block (Hakim et al., 2010a). Finally, *Scn3b*$^{-/-}$ mice were more prone than wild-type mice to develop atrial tachycardia and fibrillation upon burst pacing in *ex vivo* Langendorff-perfused hearts. Altogether, these studies suggested that *Scn3b* gene could also be involved in cardiac channelopathies in human.

This hypothesis has been confirmed. Indeed, *SCN3B* mutations have been identified in patients with either Brugada syndrome (Hu et al., 2009), idiopathic ventricular fibrillation (Valdivia et al., 2010) or lone atrial fibrillation (Olesen et al., 2011). All the mutations lead to a loss-of-function of $Na_V\beta3$ and consequently a decrease in cardiac Na^+ current.

CONCLUSION

Most mouse models of *SCN5A*-related cardiac channelopathies recapitulate most of the diverse clinical phenotypes observed in patients. However mouse models also have their own limitation as a phenotype observed in mice may not be encountered in patients. For example, the *Scn1b* knockout mouse shows prolonged ventricular repolarization, a feature that is not seen in patients with *SCN1B* loss-of-function mutations. These discrepancies relate to either species differences or differences between a heterozygous point mutation and complete invalidation of a gene on one allele.

Mouse models also turned out to be powerful tools to elucidate the pathophysiological mechanisms of *SCN5A*-related diseases. For instance, the *Scn5a*$^{1798insD/+}$ mouse clearly demonstrated that a single *SCN5A* mutation is sufficient to cause an overlap syndrome. This mouse also illustrated the limitations of heterologous expression systems in the elucidation of the biophysical consequences of the mutation on the channel function.

Finally, mouse models of Na$_V$1.5 (or Na$_V$1.5-associated proteins) dysfunction offer the unique opportunity to investigate the secondary cellular consequences of *SCN5A* mutations such as the expression remodeling of other genes, which is hardly accessible in the hearts of patients, but that might participate to the overall phenotype and explain some of the differences among patients. The most exiting benefit of mouse models is that they raise new working hypotheses such as the putative link between Na$_V$1.5 loss-of-function and occurrence of fibrosis in the context of PCCD, thereby providing new potential therapeutic approaches. One limitation, though, is that remodeling might be partly species dependent. They also constitute useful tools for future studies addressing as yet unanswered questions, such as the role of genetic and environmental modifiers on cardiac conduction and repolarization.

ACKNOWLEDGMENTS

The authors wish to thank the seventh framework program of the European Union (*EUTrigTreat* collaborative project; grant agreement #241526) for financial support.

REFERENCES

An, R. H., Wang, X. L., Kerem, B., Ben- horin, J., Medina, A., Goldmit, M., and Kass, R. S. (1998). Novel LQT-3 mutation affects Na+ channel activ- ity through interactions between alpha-and beta1-subunits. *Circ. Res.* 83, 141–146.

Antzelevitch, C., Brugada, P., Borggrefe, M., Brugada, J., Brugada, R., Cor- rado, D., Gussak, I., Le Marec, H., Nademanee, K., Perez Riera, A. R., Shimizu, W., Schulze-Bahr, E., Tan, H., and Wilde, A. (2005). Brugada syndrome: report of the second con- sensus conference: endorsed by the Heart Rhythm Society and the Euro- pean Heart Rhythm Association. *Circulation* 111, 659–670.

Baroudi, G., and Chahine, M. (2000). Biophysical phenotypes of SCN5A mutations causing long QT and Bru- gada syndromes. *FEBS Lett.* 487, 224–228.

Benhorin, J., Goldmit, M., MacCluer, J. W., Blangero, J., Goffen, R., Leibovitch, A., Rahat, A., Wang, Q., Medina, A., Towbin, J., and Kerem, B. (1998). Identification of a new SCN5A mutation associated with the long QT syndrome. *Hum. Mutat.* 12, 72–74.

Benito, B., Brugada, R., Perich, R. M., Lizotte, E., Cinca, J., Mont, ., Berruezo, A., Tolosana, J. M., Freixa, X., Brugada, P., and Bru- gada, J. (2008). A mutation in the sodium channel is responsible for the association of long QT syndrome and familial atrial fibrillation. *Heart Rhythm* 5, 1434–1440.

Benson, D. W., Wang, D. W., Dyment, ., Knilans, T. K., Fish, F. A., Strieper, M. J., Rhodes, T. H., and George, A. Jr. (2003). Congenital sick sinus syndrome caused by recessive muta- tions in the cardiac sodium channel gene (SCN5A). *J. Clin. Invest.* 112, 1019–1028.

Bezzina, C., Veldkamp, M. W., van den Berg, M. P., Postma, A. V., Rook, M. B., Viersma, J. W., van Langen, I. M., Tan-Sindhunata, G., Bink-Boelkens, T., van Der Hout, A. H., Mannens, M. M., and Wilde, A. A. (1999). A single Na$^+$ channel mutation caus- ing both long-QT and Brugada syn- dromes. *Circ. Res.* 85, 1206–1213.

Blana, A., Kaese, S., Fortmüller, L., Laak- mann, S., Damke, D., van Bragt, K., Eckstein, J., Piccini, I., Kirchhefer, U., Nattel, S., Breithardt, G., Carmeliet, P., Carmeliet, E., Schotten, U., Ver- heule, S., Kirchhof, P., and Fabritz, L. (2010). Knock-in gain-of-function sodium channel mutation prolongs atrial action potentials and alters atrial vulnerability. *Heart Rhythm* 7, 1862–1869.

Charpentier, F., Demolombe, S., and Escande, D. (2004). Cardiac channelopathies: from men to mice. *Ann. Med.* 36(Suppl. 1), 28–34.

Clancy, C. E., and Rudy, Y. (2002). Na$^+$ channel mutation that causes both Brugada and long-QT syn- drome phenotypes: a simulation study of mechanism. *Circulation* 105, 1208–1213.

Coronel, R., Casini, S., Koopmann, T. T., Wilms-Schopman, F. J., Verkerk, A. O., de Groot, J. R., Bhuiyan, Z., Bezzina, C. R., Veldkamp, M. W., Linnenbank, A. C., van der Wal, A. C., Tan, H. L., Brugada, P., Wilde, A. A., and de Bakker, J. M. (2005). Right ventricular fibrosis and conduction delay in a patient with clinical signs of Brugada syndrome: a com- bined electrophysiological, genetic, histopathologic, and computational study. *Circulation* 112, 2769–2777.

Cruz Filho, F. E., Maia, I. G., Fagun- des, M. L., Barbosa, R. C., Alves, P. A., Sá, R. M., Boghossian, S. H., and Ribeiro, J. C. (2000). Electrical behavior of T-wave polarity alter- nans in patients with congenital long QT syndrome. *J. Am. Coll. Cardiol.* 36, 167–173.

Dautova, Y., Zhang, Y., Sabir, I., Grace, A. A., and Huang, C. L. (2009). Atrial arrhythmogenesis in wild-type and Scn5a+/delta murine hearts modelling LQT3 syndrome. *Pflugers Arch.* 458, 443–457.

Dina, C. (2011). Of 508 mice and 40,000 humans. *J. Mol. Cell. Cardiol.* 50, 377–379.

Dumaine, R., Wang, Q., Keating, M. T., Hartmann, H. A., Schwartz, P. J., Brown, A. M., and Kirsch, E. (1996). Multiple mechanisms of Na$^+$ channel-linked long-QT syn- drome. *Circ. Res.* 78, 916–924.

El Yaman, M., Perry, J., Makielski, J. C., and Ackerman, M. J. (2008). Suppression of atrial fibrillation with mexiletine pharmacotherapy in a young woman with type 1 long QT syndrome. *Heart Rhythm* 5, 472–474.

Ellinor, P. T., Nam, E. G., Shea, M. A., Milan, D. J., Ruskin, J. N., and MacRae, C. A. (2008). Cardiac sodium channel mutation in atrial fibrillation. *Heart Rhythm* 5, 99–105. Fabritz, L., Damke, D., Emmerich, M., Kaufmann, S. G., Theis, K., Blana, A., Fortmüller, L., Laakmann, S., Her- mann, S., Aleynichenko, E., Stein- furt, J., Volkery, D., Riemann, B., Kirchhefer, U., Franz, M. R., Brei- thardt, G., Carmeliet, E., Schäfers, M., Maier, S. K., Carmeliet, P., and Kirchhof, P. (2010). Auto- nomic modulation and antiarrhyth- mic therapy in a model of long QT syndrome type 3. *Cardiovasc. Res.* 87, 60–72.

Fabritz, L., Kirchhof, P., Franz, M. R., Nuyens, D., Rossenbacker, T., Ottenhof, A., Haverkamp, W., Bre- ithardt, G., Carmeliet, E., and Carmeliet, P. (2003). Effect of pacing and mexiletine on disper- sion of repolarisation and arrhyth- mias in DeltaKPQ SCN5A (long QT3) mice. *Cardiovasc. Res.* 57, 1085–1093.

Fredj, S., Lindegger, N., Sampson, K. J., Carmeliet, P., and Kass, R. S. (2006). Altered Na$^+$ channels promote pause-induced spontaneous diastolic activity in long QT syn- drome type 3 myocytes. *Circ. Res.* 99, 1225–1232.

Frustaci, A., Priori, S. G., Pieroni, M., Chimenti, C., Napolitano, C., Rivolta, I., Sanna, T., Bellocci, F., and Russo, M. A. (2005). Car- diac histological substrate in patients with clinical phenotype of Bru- gada syndrome. *Circulation* 112, 3680–3687.

Gussak, I., Antzelevitch, C., Bjerregaard, P., Towbin, J. A., and Chaitman, B. R. (1999). The Brugada syn- drome: clinical, electrophysiologic and genetic aspects. *J. Am. Coll. Cardiol.* 33, 5–15.

Ge, J., Sun, A., Paajanen, V., Wang, S., Su, C., Yang, Z., Li, Y., Wang, S., Jia, J., Wang, K., Zou, Y., Gao, L., Wang, K., and Fan, Z. (2008).

Molecular and clinical characteri- zation of a novel SCN5A muta- tion associated with atrioventricu- lar block and dilated cardiomyopa- thy. *Circ. Arrhythm. Electrophysiol.* 1, 83–92.

Gilmour, R. F. Jr. (2003). A novel approach to identifying antiarrhyth- mic drug targets. *Drug Discov. Today* 8, 162–167.

Grant, A. O., Carboni, M. P., Neplioueva, V., Starmer, C. F., Memmi, M., Napolitano, C., and Priori, S. (2002). Long QT syndrome, Brugada syn- drome, and conduction system dis- ease are linked to a single sodium channel mutation. *J. Clin. Invest.* 110, 1201–1209.

Groenewegen, W. A., Firouzi, M., Bezzina, C. R., Vliex, S., van Lan- gen, I. M., Sandkuijl, L., Smits, J. P., Hulsbeek, M., Rook, M. B., Jongsma, H. J., and Wilde, A. A. (2003). A cardiac sodium chan- nel mutation cosegregates with a rare connexin40 genotype in famil- ial atrial standstill. *Circ. Res.* 92, 14–22.

Gui, J., Wang, T., Jones, R. P., Trump, D., Zimmer, T., and Lei, M. (2010). Multiple loss-of-function mechanisms contribute to SCN5A- related familial sick sinus syn- drome. *PLoS ONE* 5, e10985. doi:10.1371/journal.pone.0010985

Guzadhur, L., Pearcey, S. M., Duehmke, R. M., Jeevaratnam, K., Hohmann, A. F., Zhang, Y., Grace, A. A., Lei, M., and Huang, C. L. (2010). Atrial arrhythmogenicity in aged *Scn5a*+/DeltaKPQ mice modeling long QT type 3 syndrome and its relationship to Na+ channel expression and cardiac conduction. *Pflugers Arch.* 460, 593–601.

Hakim, P., Brice, N., Thresher, R., Lawrence, J., Zhang, Y., Jackson, A. P., Grace, A. A., and Huang, C. L. (2010a). Scn3b knockout mice exhibit abnormal sino-atrial and cardiac conduction properties. *Acta Physiol. (Oxf.)* 198, 47–59.

Hakim, P., Thresher, R., Grace, A. A., and Huang, C. L. (2010b). Effects of flecainide and quinidine on action potential and ventricular arrhyth- mogenic properties in Scn3b knock- out mice. *Clin. Exp. Pharmacol. Physiol.* 37, 782–789.

Hakim, P., Gurung, I. S., Pedersen, T. H., Thresher, R., Brice, N., Lawrence, J., Grace, A. A., and Huang, C. L. (2008). Scn3b knockout mice exhibit abnormal ventricular electrophysi- ological properties. *Prog. Biophys. Mol. Biol.* 98, 251–266.

Hale, S. L., Shryock, J. C., Belardinelli, L., Sweeney, M., and Kloner, R. A. (2008). Late sodium current inhi- bition as a new cardioprotective approach. *J. Mol. Cell. Cardiol.* 44, 954–967.

Hao, X., Zhang, Y., Zhang, X., Nirmalan, M., Davies, L., Konstantinou, D., Yin, F., Dobrzynski, H., Wang, X., Grace, A. A., Zhang, H., Boyett, M., Huang, C. L., and Lei, M. (2011). TGF-β1- mediated fibrosis and ion channel remodeling are key mechanisms in producing the sinus node dysfunc- tion associated with SCN5A defi- ciency and aging. *Circ. Arrhythm. Electrophysiol.* 4, 397–406.

Head, C. E., Balasubramaniam, R., Thomas, G., Goddard, C. A., Lei, M., Colledge, W. H., Grace, A. A., and Huang, C. L. (2005). Paced electrogram fractionation analysis of arrhythmogenic tendency in DeltaKPQ Scn5a mice. *J. Cardiovasc. Electrophysiol.* 16, 1329–1340.

Hothi, S. S., Booth, S. W., Sabir, I. N., Killeen, M. J., Simpson, F., Zhang, Y., Grace, A. A., and Huang, C. L. (2008). Arrhythmogenic substrate and its modification by nicorandil in a murine model of long QT type 3 syndrome. *Prog. Biophys. Mol. Biol.* 98, 267–280.

Hu, D., Barajas-Martinez, H., Burash- nikov, E., Springer, M., Wu, Y., Varro, A., Pfeiffer, R., Koopmann, T. T., Cordeiro, J. M., Guerchicoff, A., Pollevick, G. D., and Antzelevitch, C. (2009). A mutation in the beta 3 sub- unit of the cardiac sodium channel associated with Brugada ECG phe- notype. *Circ. Cardiovasc. Genet.* 2, 270–278.

Johnson, J. N., Tester, D. J., Perry, J., Salisbury, B. A., Reed, C. R., and Ackerman, M. J. (2008). Prevalence of early-onset atrial fibrillation in congenital long QT syndrome. *Heart Rhythm* 5, 704–709.

Ko, S. H., Lenkowski, P. W., Lee, H. C., Mounsey, J. P., and Patel, M. K. (2005). Modulation of Na(v)1.5 by beta1 - and beta3-subunit co- expression in mammalian cells. *Pflugers Arch.* 449, 403–412.

Kruse, M., Schulze-Bahr, E., Corfield, V., Beckmann, A., Stallmeyer, B., Kurt- bay, G., Ohmert, I., Schulze-Bahr, E., Brink, P., and Pongs, O. (2009). Impaired endocytosis of the ion channel TRPM4 is associated with human progressive familial heart block type I. *J. Clin. Invest.* 119, 2737–2744.

Kyndt, F., Probst, V., Potet, F., Demolombe, S., Chevallier, J. C., Baró, I., Moisan, J. P., Boisseau, P., Schott, J. J., Escande, D., and Le Marec, H. (2001). Novel SCN5A mutation leading either to isolated cardiac conduction defect or Bru- gada syndrome in a large French family. *Circulation* 104, 3081–3086.

Laitinen-Forsblom, P. J., Mäkynen, P., Mäkynen, H., Yli-Mäyry, S., Vir- tanen, V., Kontula, K., and Aalto- Setälä, K. (2006). SCN5A mutation associated with cardiac conduction defect and atrial arrhythmias. *J. Car- diovasc. Electrophysiol.* 17, 480–485. Lei, M., Goddard, C., Liu, J., Leoni, AL.,

Royer, A., Fung, S. S., Xiao, G., Ma, A., Zhang, H., Charpentier, F., Van- denberg, J. I., Colledge, W. H., Grace, A. A., and Huang, C. L. (2005). Sinus node dysfunction following targeted disruption of the murine cardiac sodium channel gene Scn5a. *J. Physiol. (Lond.)* 567, 387–400.

Lenègre, J., and Moreau, P. (1963). Le bloc auriculo-ventriculaire chronique. Etude anatomique, clinique et histologique. *Arch. Mal. Coeur. Vaiss.* 56, 867–888.

Leoni, A. L., Gavillet, B., Rougier, J. S., Marionneau, C., Probst, V., Le Scouarnec, S., Schott, J. J., Demolombe, S., Bruneval, P., Huang, C. L., Colledge, W. H., Grace, A. A., Le Marec, H., Wilde, A. A., Mohler, P. J., Escande, D., Abriel, H., and Charpentier, F. (2010). Vari- able Na(v)1.5 protein expression from the wild-type allele correlates with the penetrance of cardiac con- duction disease in the Scn5a(±) mouse model. *PLoS ONE* 5, e9298. doi:10.1371/journal.pone.0009298

Lev, M. (1964). Anatomic basis for atri- oventricular block. *Am. J. Med.* 37, 742–748.

Lindegger, N., Hagen, B. M., Marks, A. R., Lederer, W. J., and Kass, R. S. (2009). Diastolic transient inward current in long QT syndrome type 3 is caused by Ca2+ overload and inhibited by ranolazine. *J. Mol. Cell. Cardiol.* 47, 326–334.

Liu, H., El Zein, L., Kruse, M., Guina- mard, R., Beckmann, A., Bozio, A., Kurtbay, G., Mégarbané, A., Ohmert, I., Blaysat, G., Villain, E., Pongs, O., and Bouvagnet, P. (2010). Gain-of- function mutations in TRPM4 cause autosomal dominant isolated car- diac conduction disease. *Circ. Cardiovasc. Genet.* 3, 374–385.

Lopez-Santiago, L. F., Meadows, L. S., Ernst, S. J., Chen, C., Malhotra, J. D., McEwen, D. P., Speelman, A., Noebels, J. L., Maier, S. K., Lopatin, A. N., and Isom, L. L. (2007). Sodium channel Scn1b null mice exhibit pro- longed QT and RR intervals. *J. Mol. Cell. Cardiol.* 43, 636–647.

Martin, C. A., Grace, A. A., and Huang, C. L. (2011a). Refractory disper- sion promotes conduction distur- bance and arrhythmias in a Scn5a (±) mouse model. *Pflugers Arch.* 462, 495–504.

Martin, C. A., Grace, A. A., and Huang, C. L. (2011b). Spatial and temporal heterogeneities are localized to the right ventricular outflow tract in a heterozygotic Scn5a mouse model. *Am. J. Physiol. Heart Circ. Physiol.* 300, H605–H616.

Martin, C. A., Zhang, Y., Grace, A. A., and Huang, C. L. (2011c). In vivo studies of Scn5a± mice model- ing Brugada syndrome demonstrate both conduction and repolarization abnormalities. *J. Electrocardiol.* 43, 433–439.

Martin, C. A., Guzadhur, L., Grace, A. A., Lei, M., and Huang, C. L. (2011d). Mapping of re-entrant spontaneous polymorphic ventricular tachycar- dia in a Scn5a± mouse model. *Am. J. Physiol. Heart Circ. Physiol.* 300, H1853–H1862.

Martin, C. A., Zhang, Y., Grace, A. A., and Huang, C. L. (2010). Increased right ventricular repolarization gra- dients promote arrhythmogenesis in a murine model of Brugada syn- drome. *J. Cardiovasc. Electrophysiol.* 21, 1153–1159.

McNair, W. P., Ku, L., Taylor, M. R., Fain, P. R., Dao, D., Wolfel, E., and Mestroni, L., and Familial Cardiomyopathy Registry Research Group. (2004). SCN5A mutation associated with dilated cardiomy- opathy, conduction disorder, and arrhythmia. *Circulation* 110, 2163–2167.

Meadows, L. S., and Isom, L. L. (2005). Sodium channels as macro- molecular complexes: implications for inherited arrhythmia syndromes. *Cardiovasc. Res.* 67, 448–458.

Medeiros-Domingo, A., Kaku, T., Tester, D. J., Iturralde-Torres, P., Itty, A., Ye, B., Valdivia, C., Ueda, K., Canizales- Quinteros, S., Tusié-Luna, M. T., Makielski, J. C., and Ackerman, M. J. (2007). SCN4B-encoded sodium channel beta4 subunit in congenital long-QT syndrome. *Circulation* 116, 134–142.

Moss, A. J. (2002). T-wave patterns asso- ciated with the hereditary long QT syndrome. *Card. Electrophysiol. Rev.* 6, 311–315.

Moss, A. J., and Kass, R. S. (2005). Long QT syndrome: from channels to car- diac arrhythmias. *J. Clin. Invest.* 115, 2018–2024.

Moss, A. J., Zareba, W., Benhorin, J., Locati, E. H., Hall, W. J., Robin- son, J. L., Schwartz, P. J., Towbin, J. A., Vincent, G. M., Lehmann, M. H., Keating, M. T., MacCluer, J. W., and Timothy, K. W. (1995). ECG T-wave patterns in geneti- cally distinct forms of the hereditary long QT syndrome. *Circulation* 92, 2929–2934.

Nerbonne, J. M., Nichols, C. G., Schwarz, T. L., and Escande, D. (2001). Genetic manipulation of cardiac K^+ channel function in mice: what have we learned, and where do we go from here? *Circ. Res.* 89, 944–956.

Nguyen, T. P., Wang, D. W., Rhodes, T. H., and George, A. L. Jr. (2008). Divergent biophysical defects caused by mutant sodium channels in dilated cardiomyopathy with arrhythmia. *Circ. Res.* 102, 364–371.

Nuyens, D., Stengl, M., Dugarmaa, S., Rossenbacker, T., Compernolle, V., Rudy, Y., Smits, J. F., Flameng, W., Clancy, C. E., Moons, L., Vos, M. A., Dewerchin, M., Benndorf, K., Collen, D., Carmeliet, E., and Carmeliet, P. (2001). Abrupt rate accelerations or premature beats cause life-threatening arrhythmias in mice with long-QT3 syndrome. *Nat. Med.* 7, 1021–1027.

Olesen, M. S., Jespersen, T., Nielsen, J. B., Liang, B., Møller, D. V., Hedley, P., Christiansen, M., Varró, A., Olesen, S. P., Haunsø, S., Schmitt, N., and Svendsen, J. H. (2011). Mutations in sodium channel β-subunit SCN3B are associated with early-onset lone atrial fibrillation. *Cardiovasc. Res.* 89, 786–793.

Olson, T. M., Michels, V. V., Ballew, J. D., Reyna, S. P., Karst, M. L., Her- ron, K. J., Horton, S. C., Rodehef- fer, R. J., and Anderson, J. L. (2005). Sodium channel mutations and sus- ceptibility to heart failure and atrial fibrillation. *JAMA* 293, 447–454.

Papadatos, G. A., Wallerstein, P. M., Head, C. E., Ratcliff, R., Brady, P. A., Benndorf, K., Saumarez, R. C., Trezise, A. E., Huang, C. L., Vanden- berg, J. I., Colledge, W. H., and Grace, A. A. (2002). Slowed conduction and ventricular tachycardia after targeted disruption of the cardiac sodium channel gene Scn5a. *Proc. Natl. Acad. Sci. U.S.A.* 99, 6210–6215.

Priori, S. G., Schwartz, P. J., Napolitano, C., Bloise, R., Ronchetti, E., Grillo, M., Vicentini, A., Spazzolini, C., Nas- toli, J., Bottelli, G., Folli, R., and Cap- pelletti, D. (2003). Risk stratification in the long-QT syndrome. *N. Engl. J. Med.* 348, 1866–1874.

Probst, V., Kyndt, F., Potet, F., Trochu, J. N., Mialet, G., Demolombe, S., Schott, J. J., Baró, I., Escande, D., and Le Marec, H. (2003). Hap- loinsufficiency in combination with aging causes SCN5A-linked hered- itary Lenègre disease. *J. Am. Coll. Cardiol.* 41, 643–652.

Qin, N., D'Andrea, M. R., Lubin, M. L., Shafaee, N., Codd, E. E., and Cor- rea, A.

M. (2003). Molecular cloning and functional expression of the human sodium channel beta1B sub- unit, a novel splicing variant of the beta1 subunit. *Eur. J. Biochem.* 270,4762–4770.

Remme, C. A., Scicluna, B. P., Verk- erk, A. O., Amin, A. S., van Brun- schot, S., Beekman, L., Deneer, V. H., Chevalier, C., Oyama, F., Miyazaki, H., Nukina, N., Wilders, R., Escande, D., Houlgatte, R., Wilde, A. A., Tan, H. L., Veldkamp, M. W., de Bakker, J. M., and Bezzina, C. R. (2009). Genetically determined dif-ferences in sodium current charac-teristics modulate conduction dis-ease severity in mice with cardiacsodium channelopathy. *Circ. Res.* 104, 1283–1292.

Remme, C. A., Verkerk, A. O., Nuyens, D., van Ginneken, A. C., van Brun- schot, S., Belterman, C. N., Wilders, R., van Roon, M. A., Tan, H. L., Wilde, A. A., Carmeliet, P., de Bakker, J. M., Veldkamp, M. W., and Bezzina, C. R. (2006). Over- lap syndrome of cardiac sodium channel disease in mice carrying the equivalent mutation of human SCN5A-1795insD. *Circulation* 114, 2584–2594.

Remme, C. A., Wilde, A. A., and Bezzina, C. R. (2008). Cardiac sodium chan- nel overlap syndromes: different faces of SCN5A mutations. Trends *Cardiovasc.* Med. 18, 78–87.

Rossenbacker, T., Carroll, S. J., Liu, H., Kuipéri, C., de Ravel, T. J. L., Devriendt, K., Carmeliet, P., Kass, R. S., and Heidbüchel, H. (2004). Novel pore mutation in SCN5A manifests as a spectrum of phenotypes rang- ing from atrial flutter, conduction disease, and Brugada syndrome to sudden cardiac death. *Heart Rhythm* 1, 610–615.

Royer, A., van Veen, T. A., Le Bouter, S., Marionneau, C., Griol-Charhbili, V., Leoni, A. L., Steenman, M., van Rijen, H. V., Demolombe, S., God- dard, C. A., Richer, C., Escoubet, B., Jarry-Guichard, T., Colledge, W. H., Gros, D., de Bakker, J. M., Grace, A. A., Escande, D., and Charpentier, F. (2005). Mouse model of SCN5A- linked hereditary Lenegre's disease: age-related conduction slowing and myocardial fibrosis. *Circulation* 111, 1738–1746.

Sabir, I. N., Li, L. M., Jones, V. J., Goddard, C. A., Grace, A. A., and Huang, C. L. (2008). Criteria for arrhythmogenicity in genetically-modified Langendorff-perfused murine hearts modelling the congenital long QT syndrome type 3 and the Brugada syndrome. *Pflugers Arch.* 455, 637–651.

Schott, J. J., Alshinawi, C., Kyndt, F., Probst, V., Hoorntje, T. M., Huls-beek, M., Wilde, A. A., Escande, D.,Mannens, M. M., and Le Marec, H. (1999). Cardiac conduction defectsas sociate with mutations in SCN5A. *Nat. Genet.* 23, 20–21.

Schwartz, P. J., Priori, S. G., Locati, E. H., Napolitano, C., Cantu, F., Tow- bin, J. A., Keating, M. T., Ham-moude, H., Brown, A. M., Chen, L. K., and Colatsky, T. J. (1995).

Long-QT syndrome patients with mutations of the SCN5A and HERG genes have differential responses to Na+ channel blockade and to increases in heart rate: implications for gene-specific therapy. *Circulation* 92, 3381–3386.

Schwartz, P. J., Priori, S. G., Spazzolini, C., Moss, A. J., Vincent, G. M., Napolitano, C., Denjoy, I., Guich- eney, P., Breithardt, G., Keating, M. T., Towbin, J. A., Beggs, A. H., Brink, P., Wilde, A. A., Toivonen, L., Zareba, W., Robinson, J. L., Timothy, K. W., Corfield, V., Wat- tanasirichaigoon, D., Corbett, C., Haverkamp, W., Schulze-Bahr, E., Lehmann, M. H., Schwartz, K., Coumel, P., and Bloise, R. (2001). Genotype-phenotype correlation in the long-QT syndrome: gene-specific triggers for life-threatening arrhythmias. *Circulation* 103, 89–95.

Scicluna, B. P., Tanck, M. W., Remme, C. A., Beekman, L., Coronel, R., Wilde, A. A., and Bezzina, C. R. (2011). Quantitative trait loci for electrocar- diographic parameters and arrhyth- mia in the mouse. J. Mol. *Cell. Car- diol.* 50, 380–389.

Scicluna, B. P., Wilde, A. A., and Bezzina, C. R. (2008). The primary arrhyth- mia syndromes: same mutation, dif- ferent manifestations. Are we start- ing to understand why? *J. Cardio- vasc. Electrophysiol.* 19, 445–452.

Shi, R., Zhang, Y., Yang, C., Huang, C., Zhou, X., Qiang, H., Grace, A. A., Huang, C. L., and Ma, A. (2008). The cardiac sodium channel muta- tion delQKP 1507-1509 is associ- ated with the expanding phenotypic spectrum of LQT3, conduction dis- order, dilated cardiomyopathy, and high incidence of youth sudden death. *Europace* 10, 1329–1335.

Shimizu, W., and Antzelevitch, C. (2000). Effects of a K(+) channel opener to reduce transmural dis- persion of repolarization and pre- vent torsade de pointes in LQT1, LQT2, and LQT3 models of the long-QT syndrome. *Circulation* 102, 706–712.

Smits, J. P., Eckardt, L., Probst, V., Bezzina, C. R., Schott, J. J., Remme, C. A., Haverkamp, W., Breithardt, G., Escande, D., Schulze-Bahr, E., LeMarec, H., and Wilde, A. A. (2002). Genotype- phenotype relationship in Brugada syndrome: electrocardiographic fea- tures differentiate SCN5A-related patients from non-SCN5A-related patients. *J. Am. Coll. Cardiol.* 40,350–356.

Smits, J. P., Koopmann, T. T., Wilders, R., Veldkamp, M. W., Opthof, T., Bhuiyan, Z. A., Mannens, M. M., Balser, J. R., Tan, H. L., Bezzina, C. R., and Wilde, A. A. (2005). A mutation in the human cardiac sodium chan- nel (E161K) contributes to sick sinus syndrome, conduction disease and Brugada syndrome in two families. *J. Mol. Cell. Cardiol.* 38, 969–981.

Stokoe, K. S., Balasubramaniam, R., Goddard, C. A., Colledge, W. H., Grace, A. A., and Huang, C. L.(2007a). Effects of flecainide and quinidine on arrhythmogenic prop- erties of Scn5a± murine hearts modelling the Brugada syndrome. J. *Physiol. (Lond.)* 581, 255–275.

Stokoe, K. S., Thomas, G., Goddard, C. A., Colledge, W. H., Grace, A. A., and Huang, C. L. (2007b). Effects of flecainide and quinidine on arrhyth- mogenic properties of Scn5a+/Delta murine hearts modelling long QT syndrome 3. *J. Physiol. (Lond.)* 578, 69–84.

Tan, H. L., Bezzina, C. R., Smits, J. P., Verkerk, A. O., and Wilde, A. A. (2003). Genetic control of sodium channel function. *Cardiovasc. Res.* 57, 961–973.

Tan, H. L., Bink-Boelkens, M. T., Bezzina, C. R., Viswanathan, P. C., Beaufort-Krol, G. C., van Tintelen, P. J., van den Berg, M. P., Wilde, A. A., and Balser, J. R. (2001). A sodium- channel mutation causes isolated cardiac conduction disease. *Nature* 409, 1043–1047.

Thomas, G., Gurung, I. S., Killeen, M. J., Hakim, P., Goddard, C. A., Mahaut-Smith, M. P., Colledge, W. H., Grace, A. A., and Huang, C. L. (2007). Effects of L-type Ca2+ channel antagonism on ventricular arrhythmogenesis in murine hearts containing a modification in the Scn5a gene modelling human long QT syndrome 3. *J. Physiol. (Lond.)* 578, 85–97.

Tian, X. L., Yong, S. L., Wan, X., Wu, L., Chung, M. K., Tchou, P. J., Rosenbaum, D. S., Van Wag- oner, D. R., Kirsch, G. E., and Wang, Q. (2004). Mechanisms by which SCN5A mutation N1325S causes cardiac arrhythmias and sud-den death in vivo. *Cardiovasc. Res.* 61, 256–267.

Valdivia, C. R., Medeiros-Domingo, A., Ye, B., Shen, W. K., Algiers, T. J., Ackerman, M. J., and Makielski, J. C. (2010). Loss-of-function muta- tion of the SCN3B-encoded sodium channel {beta}3 subunit associated with a case of idiopathic ventricu- lar fibrillation. *Cardiovasc. Res.* 86, 392–400.

van den Berg, M. P., Wilde, A. A. M., Viersma, J. W., Brouwer, J., Haaksma, J., van der Hout, A. H., Stolte- Dijkstra, I., Bezzina, C. R., van Lan- gen, I. M., Beaufort-Krol, G. C. M., Cornel, J. H., and Crijns, H. J. G. M. (2001). Possible bradycardic mode of death and successful pace-maker treatment in a large family with features of long QT syndrome type 3 and Brugada syndrome. *J. Cardiovasc. Electrophysiol.* 12, 630–636.

Valdivia, C. R., Medeiros-Domingo, A., Ye, B., Shen, W. K., Algiers, T. J., Ackerman, M. J., and Makielski, J. C. (2010). Loss-of-function muta- tion of the SCN3B-encoded sodium channel {beta}3 subunit associated with a case of idiopathic ventricu-lar fibrillation. *Cardiovasc. Res.* 86, 392–400.

van den Berg, M. P., Wilde, A. A. M., Viersma, J. W., Brouwer, J., Haaksma, J., van der Hout, A. H., Stolte- Dijkstra, I., Bezzina, C. R., van Lan- gen, I. M., Beaufort-Krol, G. C. M., Cornel, J. H., and Crijns, H. J. G. M. (2001). Possible bradycardic mode of death and successful pace- maker treatment in a large family with features of long QT syndrome type 3 and Brugada syndrome. *J. Cardiovasc. Electrophysiol.* 12, 630–636.

van Veen, T. A., Stein, M., Royer, A., Le Quang, K., Charpentier, F., Colledge, W. H., Huang, C. L., Wilders, R., Grace, A. A., Escande, D., de Bakker, J. M., and van Rijen, H. V. (2005). Impaired impulse propagation in Scn5a- knockout mice: combined contribu- tion of excitability, connexin expres- sion, and tissue architecture in relation to aging. *Circulation* 112, 1927–1235.

Veldkamp, M. W., Viswanathan, P. C., Bezzina, C., Baartscheer, A., Wilde, A. A., and Balser, J. R. (2000). Two distinct congenital arrhyth- mias evoked by a multidysfunc- tional Na^+ channel. Circ. Res. 86, E91–E97.

Veldkamp, M. W., Wilders, R., Baartscheer, A., Zegers, J. G., Bezzina, C. R., and Wilde, A. A. (2003). Contribution of sodium channel mutations to bradycar- dia and sinus node dysfunction in LQT3 families. *Circ. Res.* 92, 976–983.

Viskin, S., Rosso, R., Rogowski, O., Bel- hassen, B., Levitas, A., Wagshal, A., Katz, A., Fourey, D., Zeltser, D., Oliva, A., Pollevick, G. D., Antzelevitch, C., and Rozovski, U. (2004). Provoca- tion of sudden heart rate oscilla- tion with adenosine exposes abnor- mal QT responses in patients with long QT syndrome: a bedside test for diagnosing long QT syndrome. *Eur. Heart J.* 27, 469–475.

Wang, D. W., Yazawa, K., George, A. L. Jr., and Bennett, P. B. (1996). Characterization of human car- diac Na^+ channel mutations in the congenital long QT syndrome. *Proc. Natl. Acad. Sci. U.S.A.* 93, 13200–13205.

Wang, Q., Shen, J., Li, Z., Timothy, K., Vincent, G. M., Priori, S. G., Schwartz, P. J., and Keating, M. T. (1995). Cardiac sodium channel mutations in patients with long QT syndrome, an inherited cardiac arrhythmia. *Hum. Mol. Genet.* 4, 1603–1607.

Watanabe, H., Koopmann, T. T., Le Scouarnec, S.,Yang, T., Ingram, C. R., Schott, J. J., Demolombe, S., Probst, V., Anselme, F., Escande, D., Wies- feld, A. C., Pfeufer, A., Kääb, S., Wich- mann, H. E., Hasdemir, C., Aizawa, Y., Wilde, A. A., Roden, D. M., and Bezzina, C. R. (2008). Sodium channel beta1 subunit mutations associated with Brugada syndrome and cardiac conduction disease in humans. *J. Clin. Invest.* 118, 2260–2268.

Watanabe, H., Yang, T., Stroud, D. M., Lowe, J. S., Harris, L., Atack, T. C., Wang, D. W., Hipkens, S. B., Leake, B., Hall, L., Kupershmidt, S., Chopra, N., Magnuson, M. A., Tan- abe, N., Knollmann, B. C., George, A. L. Jr., and Roden, D. M. (2011). Striking In vivo phenotype of a disease-associated human SCN5A mutation producing minimal changes in vitro. *Circulation* 124, 1001–1011.

Wehrens, X. H., Abriel, H., Cabo, C., Benhorin, J., and Kass, R. S. (2000).

Arrhythmogenic mechanism of an LQT-3 mutation of the human heart Na(+) channel alpha-subunit: a computational analysis. *Circulation* 102, 584–590.

Wei, J., Wang, D. W., Alings, M., Fish, F., Wathen, M., Roden, D. M., and George, A. L. (1999). Congenital long-QT syndrome caused by a novel mutation in a conserved acidic domain of the cardiac Na+ channel. Circulation 99, 3165–3171.

Wilde, A. A., Postema, P. G., Di Diego, J. M., Viskin, S., Morita, H., Fish, J. M., and Antzelevitch, C. (2010). The pathophysiologi- cal mechanism underlying Brugada syndrome: depolarization ver- sus repolarization. *J. Mol. Cell. Car- diol.* 49, 543–553.

Wu, J., Zhang, Y., Zhang, X., Cheng, L., Lammers, W. J., Grace, A. A., Fraser, J.A., Zhang, H., Huang, C. L., and Lei, M. (2012). Altered sino atrial node function and intra-atrial con- duction in murine gain-of-function Scn5a+/{Delta}KPQ hearts suggest an overlap syndrome. Am. J. Phys- iol. *Heart Circ. Physiol.* 302, H1510– H1523.

Yong, S. L, Ni, Y., Zhang, T., Tester, D. J., Ackerman, M. J., and Wang, Q. K. (2007). Characterization of the cardiac sodium channel SCN5A mutation, N1325S, in single murine ventricular myocytes. Biochem. *Biophys. Res. Commun.* 352, 378–383.

Zellerhoff, S., Pistulli, R., Mönnig, G., Hinterseer, M., Beckmann, B. M., Köbe, J., Steinbeck, G., Kääb, S., Haverkamp, W., Fabritz, L., Gradaus, R., Breithardt, G., Schulze-Bahr, E., Böcker, D., and Kirchhof, P. (2009). Atrial Arrhythmias in long- QT syndrome under daily life con- ditions: a nested case control study. J. *Cardiovasc. Electrophysiol.* 20, 401–407.

Zhang, T., Yong, S. L., Drinko, J. K., Popovic, Z. B., Shryock, J. C., Belar- dinelli, L., and Wang, Q. K. (2011). LQTS mutation N1325S in car- diac sodium channel gene SCN5A causes cardiomyocyte apoptosis, car- diac fibrosis and contractile dysfunc- tion in mice. *Int. J. Cardiol.* 147, 239–245.

Zhang, T., Yong, S. L., Tian, X. L., and Wang, Q. K. (2007). Cardiac- specific overexpression of SCN5A gene leads to shorter P wave dura- tion and PR interval in transgenic mice. *Biochem. Biophys. Res. Com- mun.* 355, 444–450.

Zimmer, T., and Surber, R. (2008). SCN5A channelopathies – an update on mutations and mecha- nisms. *Prog. Biophys. Mol. Biol.* 98, 120–136.

14

Genetics and epigenetics of arrhythmia and heart failure

Burcu Duygu, Ella M. Poels and Paula A. da Costa Martins*

Department of Cardiology, CARIM School for Cardiovascular Diseases, Maastricht University, Maastricht, Netherlands

Correspondence:
Paula A. da Costa Martins, Department of Cardiology, CARIM School for Cardiovascular Diseases, Maastricht University, Maastricht, ER 6229, Netherlands
e-mail: p.dacostamartins@maastrichtuniversity.nl

Heart failure (HF) is the end stage of several pathological cardiac conditions including myocardial infarction, cardiac hypertrophy and hypertension. Various molecular and cellular mechanisms are involved in the development of HF. At the molecular level, the onset of HF is associated with reprogramming of gene expression, including downregulation of the alpha-myosin heavy chain (α-MHC) gene and sarcoplasmic reticulum Ca^{2+} ATPase genes and reactivation of specific fetal cardiac genes such as atrial natriuretic factor and brain natriuretic peptide. These deviations in gene expression result in structural and electrophysiological changes, which eventually progress to HF. Cardiac arrhythmia is caused by altered conduction properties of the heart, which may arise in response to ischemia, inflammation, fibrosis, aging or from genetic factors. Because changes in the gene transcription program may have crucial consequences as deteriorated cardiac function, understanding the molecular mechanisms involved in the process has become a priority in the field. In this context, various studies besides having identified different DNA methylation patterns in HF patients, have also focused on specific disease processes and their underlying mechanisms, also introducing new concepts such as epigenomics. This review highlights specific genetic mutations associated with the onset and progression of HF, also providing an introduction to epigenetic mechanisms such as histone modifications, DNA methylation and RNA-based modification, and highlights the relation between epigenetics, arrhythmogenesis and HF.

Keywords: arrhythmias, heart failure, genetic predisposition to disease, epigenetic regulation, microRNAs, pharmacoepigenomics

INTRODUCTION

Genetic mutations can contribute to the diverse pathologies of heart failure (HF) by altering structure and therefore, the function of proteins responsible for various cellular activities (Creemers et al., 2011). While several studies have been devoted to the evaluation of genetic factors related to heart disease and genetic complications, much less is known about the relevance of epigenetics. The term "epigenetics" is defined as changes in gene expression that cannot be explained by changes in DNA sequence (Egger et al., 2004) but rather result from alterations related to packaging and/or translation of genetic information (Bird, 2007). Epigenetic mechanisms can be acquired or heritable and constitute a mean by which interactions between genes and environment can occur. Epigenetic regulation occurs by three key mechanisms: (i) methylation of CpG islands, mediated by DNA methyltransferases (DNMTs), (ii) modification of histone proteins and (iii) microRNAs (miRNAs). Such modifications will lead to differential expression of similar information depending on the surrounding conditions, resulting in gene activation or silencing. Although epigenetic variability of genetic information is part of normal development and differentiation, it also depends on exogenous stimuli (e.g., smoking, drug abuse) and can, therefore, reflect the influence of those factors on the development of disease (Feinberg, 2007). The role of epigenetics has been mainly evaluated in cancer but recent studies have begun to address the involvement of epigenetics in the development and progression of cardiovascular diseases (CVD).

Heart failure is the end stage of several pathological cardiac conditions including myocardial infarction (MI), cardiac hypertrophy and hypertension. Various molecular and cellular mechanisms are involved in the development of HF. At the molecular level, the onset of HF is associated with reprogramming of gene expression, including downregulation of the alpha-myosin heavy chain (α-MHC) gene and sarcoplasmic reticulum Ca^{2+} ATPase genes and reactivation of specific fetal cardiac genes such as atrial natriuretic factor (ANF) and brain natriuretic peptide (BNP; Herron and McDonald, 2002; Olson et al., 2006). These deviations in gene expression result in structural and electrophysiological changes, which eventually progress to HF. Cardiac arrhythmia is caused by altered conduction properties of the heart, which may arise in response to ischemia, inflammation, fibrosis, aging or from genetic factors. Because changes in the gene transcription program may have crucial consequences such as deteriorated cardiac function, understanding the molecular mechanisms involved in the process has become a priority in the field. In this context, various studies besides having identified different DNA methylation patterns in HF patients (Movassagh et al., 2011a,b), have also focused on specific disease processes (Yan et al., 2010; Kim et al., 2011) and their underlying mechanisms (Baccarelli and Bollati, 2009; Handy et al., 2011; Shirodkar and Marsden, 2011), also introducing new concepts such as epigenomics. This review highlights specific genetic mutations associated to the onset and progression of HF, also providing an introduction to epigenetic mechanisms such as histone modifications, DNA methylation and RNA-based modification, and highlights the relation between epigenetics, arrhythmogenesis and HF.

GENETICS OF HEART FAILURE

Genetic forms of HF are mainly known as familial dilated cardiomyopathy (FDCM). There are, however, two other familial forms of cardiomyopathy: hypertrophic cardiomyopathy (FHCM) and arrhythmogenic right ventricular cardiomyopathy (ARVC). In fact, FHCM is the most common form of inherited HF with a prevalence of 1 in every 500 individuals (Rodriguez et al., 2009). FHCM is mainly defined as unexplained left ventricular hypertrophy with increased heart mass (Elliott and McKenna, 2004). The majority of patients with FHCM (approximately 60%) exhibit autosomal dominant mutations in genes encoding for sarcomere proteins such as β-myosin heavy chain (MYH7), cardiac myosin binding protein C (MYBPC3), cardiac troponin T (TNNT2), troponin I (TNNI3), alpha-tropomyosin (TPM1), myosin light chains (MYL2 and MYL3) and cardiac actin (ACTCI; Morita et al., 2008, 2010; Lopes and Elliott, 2013).

Familial dilated cardiomyopathy is characterized as idiopathic DCM with a prevalence of 20–50% determined by epidemiological studies using family history and clinical, electrocardiographic and echocardiographic screening of first-degree relatives (Michels et al., 1992; Grunig et al., 1998). FDCM is mainly inherited in an autosomal dominant manner (approximately 90%) however, X-linked (5–10%) and much less commonly autosomal recessive (AR) or mitochondrial inheritance have also been reported (Hershberger et al., 2009). A genetic cause of FDCM was identified in 30–35% cases and mainly mutant variants of Laminin A/C (LMNA) have been reported as the most common cause of FDCM (in 7.3% of patients with DCM; Hershberger et al., 2009; Hershberger and Siegfried, 2011). In a recent study, Titin (TTN) truncating mutations were attributed as the cause of FDCM in 27% of a total of 312 DCM patients (Herman et al., 2012). Furthermore, GATA zinc finger domain containing protein 1 (GATAD1) has been identified as a disease-causing gene for AR DCM by genome-wide mapping and exome sequencing in a unique family (Theis et al., 2011).

EPIGENETIC MECHANISMS

There are several epigenetic mechanisms in eukaryotes and many have already been linked to cardiac development, CVD and/or HF. The main alterations encompassing epigenetics in CVD are described below and include ATP-dependent chromatin remodeling, DNA methylation, histone modification and RNA-based mechanisms.

CHROMATIN REMODELING THROUGH ATP-DEPENDENT ENZYMES

The ATP-dependent chromatin-remodeling complexes do not perform covalent modifications of the DNA or histones but rather use energy derived from ATP hydrolysis to move, destabilize, eject or restructure nucleosomes. There are four different families of ATP-dependent chromatin remodeling complexes: switching defective/sucrose non-fermenting complexes (SWI/SNF); imitation switch complexes (ISWI); chromodomain, helicase, DNA binding complexes (CHD) and inositol-requiring 80 complexes (INO80; Li, 2002; Yang and Seto, 2008; Clapier and Cairns, 2009; Ho and Crabtree, 2010). Although all members of each family have distinct flanking domains, they all share an evolutionarily conserved SWI-like ATPase catalytic domain that serves as vehicle to adjust histone-DNA contacts for DNA movement and chromatin restructuring. In turn, the other domains act in the recognition of covalently modified histones, modulation of ATPase activity and/or interaction with other chromatin and transcription factors. Consequently, these unique domains and their associated proteins determine the genomic targeting specificity and biological functions of each family of chromatin remodelers. In fact, chromatin modification through ATP-dependent enzymes is associated with regulation of expression of distinct gene programs in organ development and adaptation (Ho and Crabtree, 2010).

DNA METHYLATION

DNA methylation is the most common epigenetic modification in the mammalian genome. This long-term stable epigenetic modulation involves the addition of a methyl group to the 5′ carbon of a cytosine by DNMT enzymes (**Figure 1**) and mostly occurs at the CpG (cytosine preceding guanosine) dinucleotide sequences, also known as CpG islands, in the mammalian genome (Feinberg, 2008). CpG islands, in contrast to the remainder genome, are cytosine-guanosine-rich sequences (CpG-rich), generally not methylated (Deaton and Bird, 2011), and mostly acting as sites of transcription initiation once they are associated with promoter regions of genes (~70% of gene promoters; Li et al., 1993; Saxonov et al., 2006). DNA methylation is known to be catalyzed by three different DNMTs: DNMT1, DNMT3a and DNMT3b (Broadbent et al., 2008), where DNMT1 is the core enzyme in mammals. Methylation of DNA is considered a maintenance function of DNMTs as it results in post-replicative restoration of hemi-methylated sites to full methylation (Laird, 2003). Reduction of DNMT1 activity may result in demethylation and recent studies even showed that this is an active process (Bhutani et al., 2011). However this has not been shown yet for the cardiovascular system.

DNA methylation is, generally, attributed to gene silencing by hampering the accessibility of *cis*-DNA binding elements present in the promoter regions of genes of the transcriptional machinery (Suzuki and Bird, 2008) and plays a crucial role in the regulation of chromatin structure including X chromosome inactivation, genomic imprinting, silencing of repetitive DNA elements and transposon transcription (Li et al., 1993; Panning and Jaenisch, 1996; Li, 2002). Moreover, DNA methylation has been linked to biological processes underlying various diseases from cancer (Feinberg and Tycko, 2004) to CVD, such as hypertension (Millis, 2011), diabetes (Ling and Groop, 2009; MacFarlane et al., 2009), atherosclerosis and inflammation (Wierda et al., 2010).

HISTONE MODIFICATIONS

The eukaryotic DNA is tightly compact and organized in chromatin. The nucleosome is the central unit of chromatin and is composed of an octomer center of two copies of each histone protein (H2A, H2B, H3, and H4; Jenuwein and Allis, 2001) around which a DNA segment of 14–150 base pairs is looped.

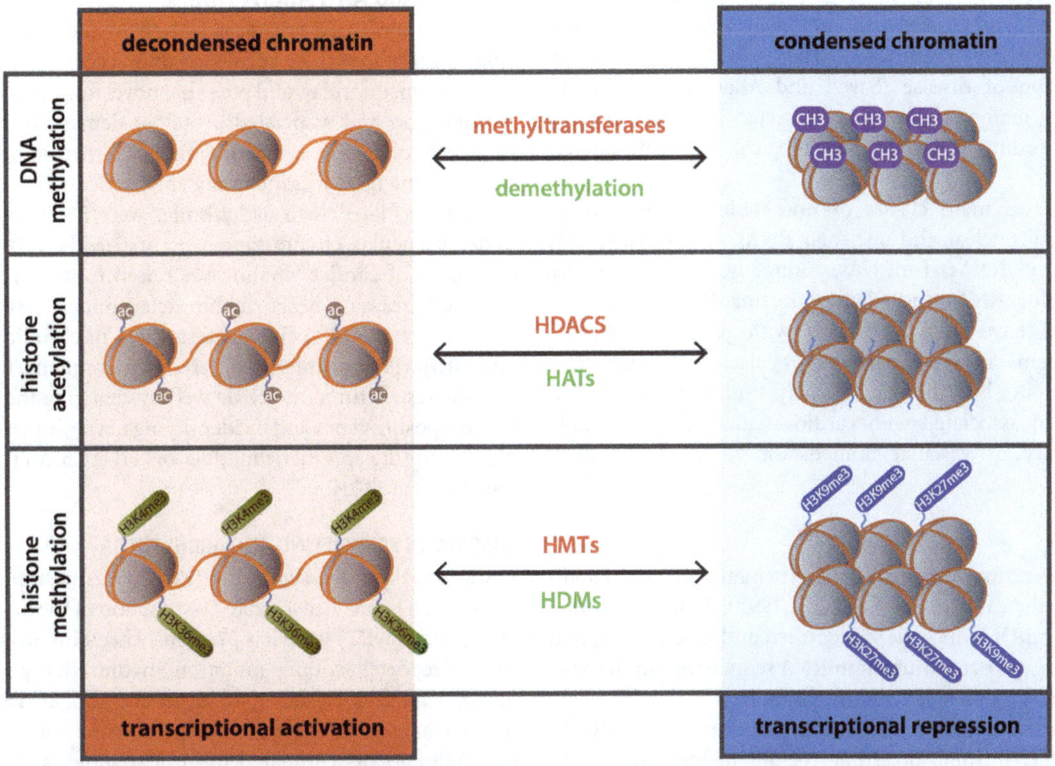

FIGURE 1 | Schematic representation of the role of DNA methylation and histone modifications in transcriptional gene regulation.

Each histone has an amino-terminal tail that protrudes from the surface of the nucleosome and which can be subjected to various posttranscriptional modifications such as phosphorylation, sumoylation, ubiquitination, methylation, ADP-ribosylation, proline isomerization, deimination and acetylation (Handy et al., 2011). These modifications lead to conformational changes in the chromatin resulting in altered gene expression (Margueron and Reinberg, 2010) depending on whether DNA becomes accessible (euchromatin) or inaccessible (heterochromatin) for transcription (**Figure 1**).

HISTONE ACETYLATION

Histone acetylation occurs at the lysine residues of the histone tails resulting in de-condensation of the chromatin structure and serving as a binding site for bromodomain proteins and transcriptional activators, and eventually leading to transcriptional activation (Elliott and McKenna, 2004; Rodriguez et al., 2009). Conversely, histone deacetylation induces chromatin condensation and therefore transcriptional repression (Clayton et al., 2006; Shahbazian and Grunstein, 2007; **Figure 1**). Acetylation of histones is a dynamic process mediated by two counteracting enzyme families, the histone acetyltransferases (HATs) and histone deacetylases (HDACs). The harmony between the activities of these two sets of enzymes is a crucial element during regulation of gene expression and its deregulation is linked to several pathological conditions varying from cancer to CVD (Ordovas and Smith, 2010; Burgess, 2012).

HISTONE METHYLATION

Other key modulator of posttranslational regulation is histone methylation which can occur on all basic amino acid residues of the histone tail; arginines, lysine and histidines (Cheung and Lau, 2005). In addition, different amino acids can be methylated to a different extent and while lysine can be subjected to mono-, di- and trimethylation, arginine residues can only become mono- or dimethylated (Cheung and Lau, 2005). Methylation of histones is a dynamic process mediated by histone methyltransferases (HMTs) and histone demethylases (HDMs; Teperino et al., 2010) and, unlike acetylation, histone methylation can induce either activation or repression of gene expression depending on the target sites and degree of methylation (Lachner and Jenuwein, 2002; **Figure 1**). In contrast to histone acetylation, histone methylation governed mainly by HMTs SUV39H1 and G9a (Martin and Zhang, 2005; Shi and Whetstine, 2007), has long been considered to be a permanent epigenetic mark (Jenuwein and Allis, 2001). However, the discovery of new players such as HDMs has shifted the paradigm and, in fact, several studies showed that histone methylation is tightly regulated in inflammatory and metabolic disorders (Saccani and Natoli, 2002; Villeneuve et al., 2008; Brasacchio et al., 2009).

RNA-BASED MECHANISMS

It is now proven and accepted that the majority of the genomic DNA is transcribed as non-coding RNAs and that such RNA species play pivotal regulatory roles during development (Sayed and Abdellatif, 2011), in response to environmental adversity (Ferguson, 2011), and at the onset and progression of disease (Sayed and Abdellatif, 2011). In this context, many studies were directed at revealing the role of non-coding RNAs in physiological and pathological processes.

There are two main classes of non-coding RNAs: infrastructural (small nuclear and nucleolar RNAs, ribosomal RNAs) and regulatory RNAs (miRNAs, long non-coding RNAs, small interfering RNAs and Piwi-interacting RNAs). To date, only miRNAs have been associated with epigenetic regulatory mechanisms in HF. Epigenetic regulation through long non-coding RNAs have been extensively studied in cancer but have also been associated with cardiovascular disease, mainly in maintenance of vascular homeostasis (Robb et al., 2004; Li et al., 2010).

MICRORNAs

MicroRNAs were first described in the nematode *Caenorhabditis elegans*, in the early 1990s (Lee et al., 1993). From then on, a multitude of miRNAs have been identified and investigated, and presently there are ~1600 human miRNA sequences annotated at miRBase19 (Kozomara and Griffiths-Jones, 2011).

MiRNAs are transcribed as primary transcripts (pri-miRNA) from intergenic, intronic or exonic regions in the genome, by RNA polymerase II. These pri-miRNAs fold into an hairpin shape with a five prime (5′) capped (mGpppG) and a polyadenylated tail which is subsequently cleaved by an enzyme complex composed of the RNase III endonuclease Drosha and the dsRNA binding protein Pasha (also known as DiGeorge critical region 8; DGCR8; Lee et al., 2003, 2004). The resulting shorter (70–100 nucleotide in length) hairpin-shaped precursor miRNA (pre-miRNA) is transported from the nucleus into the cytoplasm by Ran-GTP and exportin-5 (Kim, 2004). In the cytoplasm, pre-miRNAs are further processed by a RNase III enzyme, Dicer, into a short (20–25 nucleotides in length) transient double stranded RNA molecule. At this stage, the formed mature RNA molecule is included in a protein complex – the so-called RNA-inducing silencing complex (RISC), while the passenger strand is degraded (Winter et al., 2009). The RISC-miRNA complex specifically targets mRNA sequences leading to negative regulation of protein synthesis or mRNA degradation (Winter et al., 2009). One miRNA can regulate a vast number of mRNAs simultaneously (Lewis et al., 2005) by predominantly acting through destabilization of target mRNAs and subsequently leading to reduced protein output (Guo et al., 2010). Therefore, decreased protein production can result from a combination of mRNA destabilization and translational inhibition. MiRNAs have been shown to be involved in different pathological processes such as cancer and CVD (Lujambio and Lowe, 2012; Quiat and Olson, 2013). While in cancer epigenetic mechanisms have been widely associated with silencing of miRNA-encoding genes and thus recognized to greatly influence the expression of genetic information, only recently the importance of such mechanisms have started to be addressed in CVD, and more specifically in HF.

EPIGENETICS AND ARRHYTHMIA

Recent technological advances in DNA sequencing have enabled epigenome mapping and provided unprecedented insight into the distribution, interplay, and potential novel functions of chromatin modification and associated proteins. Remarkably, when using such technologies in evaluating the heart rhythm prominence of selected gene networks including epigenetic modulators, not previously associated with arrhythmia, were identified as relevant under particular circumstances. A first evidence for epigenetic regulation of cardiac rhythm was raised from a study conducting microarrays on heart rhythm determinants (HRD) on tissue from mice exposed to either intermittent or chronic hypoxia and untreated wild type mice. A different environment (hypoxia) profoundly restructured the HRD web by changing the hierarchy of the composing genes and by identifying new role players. This was the case for the epigenetic modulators HDAC5, Mef2b and Mef2c (Iacobas et al., 2010).

CHROMATIN REMODELING AND ARRHYTHMIA

Postural tachycardia syndrome (POTS) has multiple symptoms, one of such being tachycardia. Dysfunction of the norepinephrine transporter (NET) gene has previously been implicated in POTS, with a reported coding mutation in the NET gene (SLC6A2; Bayles et al., 2012). Head-up tilt experiments in POTS patients and showed that the expression of norepinephrine transported is lower in POTS patients compared to healthy subjects. In the absence of altered SLC6A2 gene sequence or promoter methylation, the observed reduced expression of norepinephrine was directly correlated with chromatin modifications. Changes in expression were attributable to increased binding of the repressive methyl CpG-binding protein 2 (MeCP2) regulatory complex, in association with an altered histone modification composition at the promoter region of the SLC6A2 gene (Bayles et al., 2012).

DNA METHYLATION AND ARRHYTHMIA

The KCNQ1 gene is located on chromosome 11 in a region that contains a cluster of 6 genes that are expressed from either only the maternal or the paternal allele. In mice, the KCNQ1 overlapping transcript (KCNQ1ot1) is transcribed from a promoter located in intron 10 of the KCNQ1 gene. This promoter region is a CpG island and undergoes methylation on the maternal chromosome, preventing transcription, and therefore allowing expression of the gene cluster. However, this promoter region is not methylated on the paternal chromosome allowing expression of the regulatory transcript and suppressing the expression of the gene cluster (Mancini-DiNardo et al., 2003). The maternal allele is transcribed in early embryogenesis with the paternal allele being progressively methylated and therefore only activated during late embryogenesis.

Variable imprinting of the KCNQ1 gene provides a possible explanation for the existence of long QT syndrome (LQTS) in the absence of a coding sequence mutation in KCNQ1. Paternal imprinting is probably relieved in cardiac tissue, meaning that during differentiation methylation of the paternal chromosome must occur to block production of the suppressive KCNQot1 transcript. Mutations that disrupt the CpG island could prevent methylation and silence the paternal allele in the heart

(Mancini-DiNardo et al., 2003; Bokil et al., 2010). A more recent study by Fatima et al. (2012) associates epigenetic modifications with regulation of the ATP sensitive potassium channel (KATP). In cardiac myocytes, different isoform combinations of the SURx (SUR1, SUR2) and Kir6.2 (KCNJ11) will be responsible for distinct physiological and pharmacological properties, depending on the isoforms expressed. Promotor CpG methylation appears to be one of the regulators of SURx isoform expression and therefore, regulated or aberrant CpG methylation might play a role in controlling channel structure and function under different conditions (Fatima et al., 2012).

HISTONE MODIFICATIONS IN ARRHYTHMIA

Histone deacetylases-1 and -2 have important functions in regulating cardiac gene expression and cardiomyocyte differentiation. While myocardium-specific deletion of either HDAC-1 or HDAC-2 results in no apparent cardiac phenotype, specific deletion of both in the murine myocardium, results in death within 2 weeks after birth, due to cardiac arrhythmias and dilated cardiomyopathy (Montgomery et al., 2007). This is likely caused by upregulation of genes that encode for fetal calcium channels and skeletal muscle-specific contractile proteins, including hyperpolarization-activated non-selection cation current (If) and T-type Ca^{2+} current (ICa, T), both involved in calcium handling. Such genes are normally transcriptionally repressed by the RE1-silencing transcription factor (REST) through class I and IIa HDACs. Knockout of both HDAC-1 and -2 seems to result in incapacity of REST to repress these fetal genes, resulting in, among other things, arrhythmia (Montgomery et al., 2007; Chang and Bruneau, 2012).

Ablation of PAX-interacting protein 1 (PTIP), a key component of the histone H3 lysine 4 (H3K4me) methyltransferase complex, leads to reduced H3K4me expression levels and is sufficient to alter subsequent gene expression profiles. One of those H3K4me-regulated genes is the Kv channel-interacting protein 2 (Kcnip2), a regulator of cardiac repolarization current that is known to have functions in arrhythmogenesis. Regulation of Kcnip2 by H3K4me leads to decreased sodium current and action potential upstroke velocity and significantly prolonged action potential duration (APD), thereby increasing the risk of lethal ventricular arrhythmias. These results suggest that maintaining H3K4me marks is necessary for the stability of a specific transcriptional program and cellular homeostasis (Stein et al., 2011; Chang and Bruneau, 2012).

In Duchenne muscular dystrophy (DMD) more than 30% of deaths result from a progressive deterioration in cardiac function. Ventricular arrhythmia is a common complication in DMD patients and a risk factor for sudden cardiac death. Colussi et al. (2010) used X-chromosome-linked muscular dystrophy (mdx) mice, a model for DMD, and treated them with the histone deactylase inhibitor suberoylanilide hydroxamic acid (SAHA). In resting state there was no difference between treated and untreated groups, however, upon restraint, an increase was seen in ventricular arrhythmias in untreated mdx animals compared to mdx SAHA- treated animals or wild type control animals. Epicardial recordings revealed prolongation of the QRS complex in mdx-untreated mice in comparison to mdx-SAHA treated mice and WT mice, together with a significant reduction in impulse propagation velocity. Further analysis revealed that SAHA induces connexin 40 (Cx40), Cx37 and Cx32 remodeling but expression of Cx43 and Cx45 remains unaltered. Treatment with SAHA not only reversed Cx43 lateralization, which was observed in mdx- untreated animals, but also re-induced $Na_v1.5$ expression. This indicates that in mdx mice SAHA attenuates arrhythmias by mechanisms in which connexin-remodeling and sodium channel re-expression may play a role (Colussi et al., 2010).

Atrial fibrillation (AF), induced by atrial fibrosis, seems to also be epigenetically regulated and this was suggested in a study sought to determine whether the HDAC inhibitor trichostatin A (TSA) reduces the amount of atrial fibrosis and concomitant AF (Liu et al., 2008). Transgenic mice overexpressing the homeo-domain-only protein (HopX-Tg), which recruits HDAC activity to induce cardiac hypertrophy were either treated or untreated with TSA and compared to control groups. Invasive electrical stimulation induced more atrial arrhythmias in HopX-Tg untreated mice than in HopX-Tg TSA-treated mice. TSA reduced atrial arrhythmia duration and atrial fibrosis in HopX-Tg animals. In the HopX-Tg untreated mice, atrial Cx40 was found to be lower than in WT mice, a phenomenon that was abrogated by introducing TSA in these mice. Myocardial angiotensin II levels were similar between groups, suggesting that HDAC-inhibition reverses atrial fibrosis, Cx40 remodeling and atrial arrhythmia vulnerability, rendering the atrium almost refractory to arrhythmia inducibility, independent of angiotensin II in cardiac hypertrophy (Liu et al., 2008).

NON-CODING RNA IN ARRHYTHMIAS

Several studies have been conducted to look at the association between miRNAs and arrhythmias. MiRNA expression profiles were shown to differ in right atrial disease, with 47 miRNAs being differentially expressed between disease and control states, whereas similar changes in expression could not be found in left atrial disease (Cooley et al., 2012; Kim, 2013). In a different study, miRNAs that were differentially expressed between AF and sinus rhythm in patients with mitral stenosis were showed by microarrays (Xiao et al., 2011; Kim, 2013). These data indicate that miRNAs play a role in regulating cardiac conduction and in the induction of arrhythmias.

Multiple studies have shown that miR-208a plays an important role in action potential conduction. Overexpression of miR-208a leads to arrhythmia, cardiac fibrosis and hypertrophy, and is a strong predictor of cardiac death (Oliveira-Carvalho et al., 2013). Genetic deletion of miR-208a, on the other hand, also leads to an increased risk of AF and other arrhythmias, due to aberrant conduction mainly caused by dysregulation of Cx40 (Callis et al., 2009; Oliveira-Carvalho et al., 2013). Similarly, also miR-328 is upregulated not only in animal models of AF but also in human tissue samples from AF patients. Overexpression of miR-328 in mice increased vulnerability to AF as confirmed by diminished L-type Ca^{2+} current and shortened atrial APD. AF vulnerability could be reversed by concomitant inhibition of the miRNA by an antagomir (Lu et al., 2010; Kim, 2013).

The most well established cardiac conduction-related miRNA is by far, miR-1. This miRNA plays a role in myotonic dystrophy, a disease where degeneration of the conduction system occurs and increased CACNA1C (CAV 1.2) expression, a cardiac L-type Ca^{2+} channel gene, is observed (Kim, 2013). The involvement of miR-1 in electrocardiophysiology was further confirmed by a targeted deletion of miR-1-2 by Zhao et al. (2007), which lead to a high rate of sudden death, caused by conduction blockade due to direct targeting of Irx5, a transcription factor that regulates cardiac repolarization. In rats, induction of MI by occlusion of the left anterior descending artery results in miR-1 upregulation and arrhythmia exacerbation but treating the animals with an antisense inhibitor could abrogate these effects. Furthermore, miR-1 also directly targets KCNJ2, which encodes for the calcium channel subunit Kir 2.1, providing a possible mechanism for increase of arrhythmias in MI (Yang et al., 2007). The role of miR-1 in arrhythmogenesis was further confirmed in humans where atrial cells from AF patients display a 86% decrease in miR-1expression, a subsequent increased Kir 2.1 protein expression and an increase in I_{k1} density (Girmatsion et al., 2009; Kim, 2013). MiR-1 is also involved in cardiac electrical remodeling in viral myocarditis where it is upregulated, resulting in decreased Cx43, which is required for transfer of electric activation, and indicating that miR-1 plays a role in intercellular communication.

Another prominent miRNA in the regulation of cardiac conduction is miR-133. Matkovich et al. (2010) showed that an increase in miR-133a leads to prolonged QT intervals. This miRNA is highly and preferentially expressed in cardiac and skeletal muscle and is known to regulate cardiac ion channels such as Kv4- encoded $I_{to,f}$ (Kcnip2; Matkovich et al., 2010; Kim, 2013). Furthermore, the catalytic and regulatory subunits of protein phosphatase 2A (PP2A) are decreased in cardiomyocytes in chronic HF and were shown to be targets of both miR-1 and miR-133. Because pharmacologic inhibition of PP2A leads to altered diastolic Ca^{2+} waves this indicates a role for these two miRNAs in calcium handling (Belevych et al., 2011; Kim, 2013).

Interestingly, a relation between nicotine abuse and cardiac arrhythmias has been suggested by several studies. Nicotine treatment of canine atrial fibroblasts, resulted in upregulation of transforming growth factor beta-1 (TGF-β1) and TGF- beta receptor type II levels (TGF-βRII), with concomitant decreased levels of miR-133 and miR-590, both directly targeting TGF-β1 and TGF-βRII. This effect was abolished by synthetic downregulation of both miRNAs (Shan et al., 2009; Kim, 2013).

Apart from miR-1 and miR-133, there are several other miRNAs that have been associated with regulation of cardiac conduction to some extent. This is the case for miR-212 that seems to regulate inward rectifier K^{+} current density by targeting Kir 2.1 (Kim, 2013), and for miR-21 which is increased in the left atria of patients with AF and which abrogation leads to repression of atrial fibrosis and AF (Adam et al., 2012; Cardin et al., 2012; Kim, 2013). Furthermore, conditional overexpression of miR-17-92 in cardiac and smooth muscle tissue results in both dilated, HCM as well as in arrhythmias. An increase in atrial and ventricular ectopy, as well as increased susceptibility to arrhythmia was observed in homozygous and heterozygous animals. After programmed electrical stimulation all transgenic animals developed sustained and lethal ventricular tachycardia (VT) or ventricular fibrillation (VF) and these effects were mainly caused by dysregulation of two downstream targets of miR-17-92, the lipid phosphatase and tensin homolog PTEN and Cx43 (Danielson et al., 2013). Likewise, also miR-155 and miR-181 have been associated with cardiac conduction defects. Circulating levels of miR-155 are upregulated in patients with specific angiotensin receptor type 1 (AT1R) polymorphisms that have been shown to be associated with an increased risk of ventricular tachyarrhythmias and sudden death (Blanco et al., 2012). In turn, miR-181a seems to play a role in VT after MI (Li et al., 2009). Altogether, the data available regarding the relation between miRNAs and arrhythmias establish miRNAs as crucial players in regulating cardiac electrophysiology and electric potential conduction through an array of different mechanisms.

EPIGENETIC CONTROL OF HEART FAILURE

Recent genetic and biochemical studies indicate that epigenetic changes play a crucial role in the development of cardiac hypertrophy and HF, with dysregulation in histone acetylation status being directly linked to impaired contraction of cardiac myocytes. In fact, it has been shown that there is a cardiac chamber – specific histone acetylation pattern suggesting that cardiac ventricular chambers are epigenetically distinct (Mathiyalagan et al., 2010).

ATP-DEPENDENT ENZYMES AND CHROMATIN REMODELING IN HF

ATP-dependent chromatin remodeling complexes play crucial roles in vertebrates, mainly in organ development and adaptation. Most of them have been associated with heart development and only a few were implicated in heart disease. The BAF (brahma-associated factor) complex is the vertebrate homolog of the yeast SWI/SNF family of chromatin remodelers. In mammals, this complex contains 12 protein components from which an ATPase subunit encoded by either *Brm* (brahma) or *Brg1* (brahma-related gene 1). These two subunits, although highly homologous, exhibit distinctive functions in vivo. While several studies have demonstrated that individual subunits of the BAF complex are essential during heart development (Lickert et al., 2004; Takeuchi et al., 2007; Takeuchi and Bruneau, 2009) and may be implicated in human congenital diseases (Kitagawa et al., 2003; Bajpai et al., 2010), BRG1 was recently involved in cardiac disease (Hang et al., 2010). In embryos, *Brg1* promotes myocyte proliferation and it preserves fetal cardiac differentiation by interacting with HDACs and poly (ADP ribose) polymerase (PARP) to repress α-MHC to β-MHC shift. *Brg1* (also known as *Smarca4*) is not expressed in the adult heart but it is reactivated by stress conditions such as pressure overload. Once reactivated, Brg1 forms a complex with its embryonic partners (HDAC and PARP), to induce the pathologic α-MHC to β-MHC shift. Adult myocardial gene deletion of Brg1 inhibited cardiac hypertrophic growth and reversed the MHC switch. Accordingly, Brg1 is activated in patients with HCM, correlating with disease severity and MHC changes (Hang et al., 2010). PPAR is a nuclear enzyme known to respond to DNA damage and facilitate repair. Besides DNA repair, PPAR-1 also modulates chromatin to control the transcriptional machinery in response to diverse stimuli. Such stimuli induce PPAR activation and PAR-dependent striping of histones from chromatin, thereby favoring the opening of chromatin to allow transcriptional regulation (Tulin and Spradling, 2003; Kim et al., 2004). PARP is activated in cardiac hypertrophy and its activity is increased in murine and human failing hearts (Pillai et al., 2005b; Xiao et al., 2005). Deletion of PARP-1 in mice or pharmacological inhibition of PARP activity decreases cardiac hypertrophy induced by angiotensin II (Pillai et al., 2006) or pressure overload (Pillai et al., 2005a; Xiao et al., 2005), delays the progression from hypertensive cardiomyopathy to HF (Bartha et al., 2009), decreases cell death and HF after MI (Palfi et al., 2006) and diminishes myocardial ischemia/reperfusion injury (Szabo et al., 2002).

Although very preliminary, there seems to be a link, at the chromatin level, between fetal hearts and adult diseased hearts, and in the future, targeting the regulation of chromatin remodeling processes may become a promising approach to prevent or maybe even reverse pathological cardiac hypertrophic growth and HF.

DNA METHYLATION IN HEART FAILURE

Unlike in other diseases such as cancer, the role of DNA methylation in HF remains elusive. Movassagh et al. (2010) compared genome-wide methylation profiles of left ventricle tissue from HF patients and healthy controls by methylated DNA immunoprecipitation-chip (MeDIP-chip), in which immunoprecipitation of methylated DNA is followed by microarray hybridization and further validated by bisulfite sequencing. As a result, three differentially methylated angiogenesis-related loci have been identified and correlated to differential expression levels of the corresponding gene (Movassagh et al., 2010). Hyper-methylation of the 5′ regulatory region of platelet endothelial cell adhesion molecule 1 (PECAM-1) and hypo-methylation of the angiomotin-like protein 2 (AMOTL2) in failing hearts correlated with reduced expression of those genes, while hyper-methylation within the Rho GTPase activating protein 24 gene (ARHGAP24) is correlated with increased expression of ARHGAP24 in failing hearts (Movassagh et al., 2010). Moreover, a follow up study (Movassagh et al., 2011a) generated a genome-wide DNA methylation map of human hearts and revealed a significant decrease in global promoter methylation of genes with increased expression in failing hearts (Movassagh et al., 2011a). The genome-wide methylation profile of patients with idiopathic dilated cardiomyopathy was recently generated (Haas et al., 2013). In an attempt to validate the methylation profiling of the 20 most differentially methylated genes, MassARRAY and Bisulfite sequencing were used in a large independent cohort (30 patients; Baccarelli and Bollati, 2009). Interestingly, 12 (out of 20) genes showed similar methylation patterns between the two independent studies. Such approach allowed the identification of two novel genes with differential methylation profiles between patient and control subjects, lymphocyte antigen 75 (ly75) and adenosine A2a receptor (adora2a). Curiously, downregulation of those genes in zebrafish by using specific morpholino technology resulted in reduced ventricular contractility and HF (Haas et al., 2013). More recently, DNA methylation was found to be responsible for the hypermutability of distinct cardiac genes. This is the case for the cardiac isoform of the myosin binding protein C gene (Mybpc3) that has a significantly higher level of exonic methylation of CpG sites than the skeletal isoform (Mybpc2; Meurs and Kuan, 2011). This suggests that there are unique aspects of the Mybpc3 gene or its epigenetic environment that are prone to generate genetic mutations.

Very recently, a report in the Journal of the American Heart Association (Bellavia et al., 2013) provided evidence for the effects of ambient particulate-matter (PM) on blood pressure (BP). In humans, exposure to fine and coarse concentrated ambient particles (CAPs) induce blood hypomethylation of *Alu*, a transposable repeated element, and Toll-like receptor 4 (TLR4). Hypomethylation of both factors was found to be associated with increased systolic BP after exposure. This is of great interest since many epidemiological studies (O'Toole et al., 2008; Brook et al., 2010) have reported a correlation between PM exposure, cardiovascular disease and death, and may, therefore, represent a novel mechanism that mediates environmental effects on BP and indirectly cardiovascular disease and HF.

HISTONE MODIFICATION IN HEART FAILURE

Histone acetylation

Cardiac hypertrophy is the initial response to cardiac stress leading to adverse cardiac remodeling and eventually to HF. In order to elucidate the underlying mechanisms behind the development of cardiac hypertrophy, the role of histone acetylation/deacetylation has been extensively studied. Gusterson et al. (2003) and Morita et al. (2010) demonstrated that overexpression of the transcriptional co-activators CREB binding protein (CRB) or p300, individually, could induce hypertrophic growth of cardiomyocytes depending on their histone HAT activity. Consequently, inhibition of these co-activators repressed phenylephrine (PE)-induced hypertrophic cell growth (Gusterson et al., 2003). High expression and induced activity of HAT were observed in animals subjected to pressure overload, compared to sham operated animals, while heterozygous p300 transgenic animals revealed limited cardiac hypertrophy with preserved cardiac function when subjected to pressure overload (Morita et al., 2010). Intriguingly, another study showed that p300 transgenic animals develop HF at baseline, as indicated by high mortality, adverse remodeling and impaired cardiac function (Yanazume et al., 2003). Although these studies indicate that p300 is a crucial modulator of cardiac remodeling they do not specifically address the importance of its HAT activity in vivo. To assess this question, studies with transgenic animals carrying a mutant form of p300, with no HAT activity, were performed revealing a rescue of MI-induced pathological remodeling as well as preserved cardiac function compared to intact p300-carrying transgenic animals (Miyamoto et al., 2006). These responses to p300 modulation in vivo are, most likely, related to the fact that p300 can directly acetylate non-histone proteins such as hypertrophy-responsive transcriptional factors like MEF2 (Wei et al., 2008) and GATA-4 (Yanazume et al., 2003; Miyamoto et al., 2006).

The regulation of gene expression by HDACs seems to be more complex. HDACs are divided into four different classes (class-I, -IIa, -IIb and -IV) based on differences in their structure, enzymatic function, expression patterns and subcellular localization. Class I HDACs (HDAC1, 2, 3 and 8) are expressed ubiquitously and predominantly localized in the nucleus. Class IIa HDACs (HDAC4, 5, 7, and 9) shuttle between the nucleus and the cytoplasm and are strictly expressed in muscle, heart and brain tissues (Haberland et al., 2009). A first demonstration of the relevant role of HDAC activity in cardiomyocytes derived from a study where myocardial differentiation of monkey ES cells was facilitated by TSA, an HDAC inhibitor (Hosseinkhani et al., 2007). Furthermore, differential chromatin scanning (DCS) is a technique used to genome-widely profile HDAC targets enabling the isolation of genomic fragments associated with histones and, therefore, carrying different acetylation marks (Kaneda et al., 2005). Such studies provide a basis for all following studies into the role of epigenetic modifications in cardiac disorders (**Table 1**). Interestingly, the two classes of HDACs show opposite roles in cardiac hypertrophy with class I HDACs being pro-hypertrophic and class IIa HDACs being anti-hypertrophic (Zhang et al., 2002; Antos et al., 2003; Chang et al., 2004). Induced expression of HDAC2 in cardiomyocytes mimics hypertrophic growth in an Akt-dependent manner. In vivo, class I HDAC2 overexpressing transgenic animals develop cardiac hypertrophy whereas HDAC2-null animals are protected from cardiac hypertrophic response after stimulation either by pressure overload or isoproteranol (ISO) administration (Trivedi et al., 2007). Similar to HATs, HDACs also interact with DNA binding proteins regulating their activity. For instance, class IIa HDACs (HDAC4, -5, -7 and -9) can directly interact with MEF2 leading to inhibition of MEF2 activity and subsequent reduced cardiac hypertrophy (Backs and Olson, 2006). On the other hand, when MEF2 is discharged of HDACs, it may become an available target for HATs binding which in turn leads to enhanced activity of MEF2 (Backs and Olson, 2006).

Besides transcriptional factors, HATs and HDACs can also interact with sarcomeric proteins. PCAF, a HAT, class II HDAC4 co-localizes with cardiomyocyte sarcomeres in the Z-disk whereas class I HDAC3 localize mainly in the A-band (Gupta et al., 2008; Samant et al., 2011). In addition, inhibition of HDAC4 results in altered calcium sensitivity and therefore altered contractility. HDAC4 has an unique docking site for the binding of calcium/calmodulin-dependent kinase II (CaMKII), which is absent in other class IIa HDACs. Phosphorylation of HDAC4 by CaMKII promotes nuclear export and derepression of HDAC target genes, which, in cardiomyocytes, will lead to hypertrophic growth (Backs et al., 2006), indicating a central role for CaMKII-HDAC4 signaling pathways in the development of cardiac hypertrophy. From the HDAC class IIb, HDAC6 catalytic activity seems to be consistently increased in stressed myocardium and is activated by different extracellular stimuli in cultured cardiac myocytes (Lemon et al., 2011). Recently, Cao et al. (2011) showed that inhibition of HDAC by TSA (HDAC inhibitor) treatment limits cardiac hypertrophy by suppressing autophagy. Further in vitro experiments, by selective downregulation of HDAC isoforms in cardiomyoctes, indicated HDAC1/2 as responsible for PE-induced autophagy (Cao et al., 2011). Autophagy is a self-degradative process during development and in response to nutrient stress, and can be altered under pathological conditions (Wang et al., 2013). Increasing evidence suggests more distinctive roles for HDACs besides only acting as histone deacetyltransferases.

Histone methylation

The most widely studied histone methylations are lysine methylations: histone H3 lysine 4 (H3K4), H3K9, H3K27, H3K36, H3K79 and H4K20 (Martin and Zhang, 2005). There is limited information about the function of histone methylation in HF. It is known that differential methylation patterns for H3K4 and H3K9 occur in the vicinity of various gene clusters of failing human hearts (Kaneda et al., 2009). Because such sets of genes encode proteins that function in the same signal transduction pathways and H3K9 mark-profile seems to be less sensitive to disease status, this indicates differential H3K4 marking during the development of HF (Kaneda et al., 2009). Furthermore, in a Dahl salt-sensitive rat model of congestive heart failure (CHF), genome-wide histone methylation analysis revealed H3K4me3 and H3K9me3 as the most abundant histone methylation marks (Kaneda et al., 2009). Interestingly, mapping of H3K4me3 and H3K9me3 enriched regions in the genome of human CHF samples compared to controls revealed many HF-associated genes located in these regions (Kaneda et al., 2009). Moreover, histone methylation has been shown to mark not only protein coding genes but also non-coding RNA regions (Movassagh et al., 2011a). The genome wide mapping of H3K36me3 in end-stage failing human hearts allowed to identify 4 novel non-coding RNA regions, which have active transcription and might be involved in HF (Movassagh et al., 2011a). This differential profile of histone methylation marks found in both human and animal samples suggests a potential role for HMTs and HDMs in HF. Accordingly, JMJD2A, a histone trimethyl demetyhlase (Kooistra and Helin, 2012), is found to be upregulated in human HCM patients compared to control (Zhang et al., 2011). Moreover, transgenic mice with cardiac-specific overexpression of JMJD2A develop exaggerated cardiac hypertrophy compared to control mice following transverse aortic constriction (TAC) whereas *jmjd2a*-null animals seem to be protected against TAC-induced cardiac stress (Zhang et al., 2011). All in all, these experiments indicate a potential modulator function for histone modification in HF.

NON-CODING RNA IN HEART FAILURE

Post-transcriptional regulation of gene expression is mainly achieved by non-coding RNA molecules including miRNAs and, based on rather recent findings, long-noncoding RNAs (lncRNAs).

Comparison of miRNA expression profiles in healthy and failing heart samples from humans or animal models revealed differential miRNA expression patterns indicating their potential involvement in the development and progression of HF. In this regard, miRNA microarray analysis of cardiac tissue from mouse models of cardiac hypertrophy and CHF detected five upregulated miRNAs (namely miR-24, miR-125b, miR-195, miR-199a and miR-214), which were further confirmed in idiopathic end stage failing human hearts (van Rooij et al., 2006). Furthermore, mice overexpressing miR-195 developed pathological remodeling, impaired cardiac function and subsequently HF (van Rooij et al., 2006). Besides distinct expression signatures of miRNAs in healthy and failing hearts, the differential miRNA expression profile among failing hearts is dependent on the underlying HF etiology (Ikeda et al., 2007; Sucharov et al., 2008). Ikeda et al. (2007) found 14 aortic stenosis-specific miRNAs while a set of other eight miRNAs were mainly expressed in a cardiomyopathic form of HF. In a similar study, different sets of miRNAs were found for

Table 1 | Role of HDACs in heart disease.

Class	Chromatin modifying factor	Modulation	Phenotype	Mechanism
Class I	HDAC2	Germline deletion	Lethal at birth, Surviving adults are resistant to hypertrophy	Suppression of SRF and GATA4-dependent gene expression; Inhibition of hypertrophic Akt/GSK3β pathway
		Overexpression in myocardium	Cardiac hypertrophy	Activation of hypertrophic Akt/GSK3β pathway
		Deletion in myocardium	No cardiac phenotype	Redundancy with HDAC1
		Deletion of HDAC1 and HDAC2	Lethal at 2 weeks after birth: arrhythmias, dilated cardiomyopathy	Interaction with REST: repression of fetal genes involved in calcium handling and contractility
	HDAC3	Overexpression	Cardiac hyperplasia without hypertrophy	Suppression of Cdk inhibitors: promotion of cardiomyocyte proliferation
		Deletion in myocardium	Lethality at 3-4 months of age: cardiac hypertrophy, fibrosis, defects in fatty acid metabolism and lipid accumulation in the heart	Suppression of PPARα activity on gene promoters involved in metabolic regulation
Class II	HDAC5/HDAC9	Germline deletion	Enhanced hypertrophic response to cardiac stress; female hearts are protected from ischemia injury	Suppression of Mef2 and CAMTA2; suppression of Mef2-ERα-VEGFa pathway
Class III	SIRT1	Overexpression in myocardium	Low-moderate expression of SIRT1 reduces cardiac hypertrophy; High levels induces cardiac hypertrophy and apoptosis	SIRT1 expression is activated by cardiac stress and regulates the response to stress in a dose-dependent manner
	SIRT3	Germline deletion	Cardiac hypertrophy and fibrosis at 2 months of age	Inhibition the proapoptotic activity of Bax
		Overexpression in myocardium	Resistant to stress-induced cardiac hypertrophy	Activation of FOXO3a-dependent pathways; attenuation of the prohypertrophic MAPK/ERK and PI3K/Akt pathways.
	SIRT7	Germline deletion	Cardiac fibrosis, hypertrophy and shortened lifespan	Deacetylation of p53; protection from stress-induced apoptosis

idiopathic dilated and ischemic cardiomyopathy (Sucharov et al., 2008). Furthermore, the expression levels of miRNAs can vary as the disease progresses (Bagnall et al., 2012). This was shown in a double transgenic mouse model, harboring mutations in both the myosin heavy chain gene and the cardiac troponin I gene, resulting in severe HCM and premature mortality by age of 21 days. Global miRNA profiles in those mice, at age of 10 and 16 days, revealed stable downregulation of specific miRNAs such as miR-1 and miR-133, suggesting a functional role for these miRNAs throughout the progression to HF. Counterwise, miR-31 was upregulated at the end-stage of HF which points to a specific function for this miRNA during the final phase of the disease (Bagnall et al., 2012).

Another miRNA microarray profiling study has been carried out in human end-stage CHF with or without left ventricular assist device (LVAD) compared to healthy subjects (Matkovich et al., 2009). Twenty-eight miRNAs were differentially expressed in diseased hearts regardless of LVAD support and, interestingly, the expression levels of 20 of those miRNAs were either normalized or reversed in the CHF group after LVAD support suggesting an eventual value of such miRNAs as prognostic tools for end-stage CHF patients (Matkovich et al., 2009). Recent data also emphasizes the variations between adult and child idiopathic dilated cardiomyopathy patients, regarding their miRNA expression profile (Stauffer et al., 2013). Naga Prasad et al. (2009) performed miRNA microarrays in end stage dilated cardiomyopathic hearts (with >15 ejection fraction) followed by in silico network analysis in order to obtain a global picture of the molecular networks and key proteins regulated by the dysregulated miRNAs. As a result, eight miRNAs displayed different expression levels in DCM subjects compared to controls and two out of these eight miRNAs, namely miR-7 and miR-378, were novel miRNAs, shown for the first time to be downregulated in end stage failing hearts (Naga Prasad et al., 2009). Confirmation of network analysis revealed upregulation of erythroblastic leukemia viral oncogene homolog 2 (ERBB2) and collagen, type I, alpha 1 (Col1A1) which are predicted targets of miR-7 and thus, confirming that the regulatory function of miRNAs results in alterations of global signaling networks during development and progression towards cardiac hypertrophy and HF (Naga Prasad et al., 2009).

A more recent study, besides showing that miRNA expression profiles differ between healthy and failing hearts, in consensus with previous findings, also demonstrated that failing adult hearts and fetal hearts display similar miRNA profiles supporting the paradigm of reactivation of a fetal gene program (Thum et al., 2007; Barry et al., 2008) at onset and/or during the development of HF.

On top of these profiling studies, a myriad of selected miRNAs were associated with cardiac disease-specific roles. miRNAs have also become a research focus on defining novel biomarkers of HF by characterizing miRNA patterns in easy accessible sources such as serum, plasma and even whole blood, and specific miRNA signatures have been identified as biomarkers of MI (Meder et al., 2011).

Interestingly, but not yet studied in the context of CVD, miRNA genes can be subject of DNA methylation with direct impact on the miRNA expression levels. Epigenetic-regulation of miRNA genes was mainly showed, so far, for different types of cancer. miRNAs such as miR-127 and miR-137 are sensitive to DNMT inhibitors and chromatin-modifying drugs. Interestingly, the miR-127 gene is embedded in a CpG island and is subject of epigenetic silencing (Saito et al., 2006). Because miR-127 is physiologically expressed as a member of a miRNA cluster together with miR-136, -431, -432 and -433 not only in normal tissues but also in cultured fibroblasts this could hint for a role of epigenetic regulation of this miR in cardiovascular disease, e.g., fibrosis, but this remains to be clarified (Saito et al., 2006). Similarly, the promoter region of miR-137 is heavily methylated in cancer cell lines and this is reversible after treatment with DNMT inhibitors (Balaguer et al., 2010).

To date, the epigenetic regulation of miRNA expression through methylation of CpG islands or other modifications in the promoter regions that encode for specific miRNAs has not been assessed in the context of CVD. Nevertheless, the above-mentioned studies strongly suggest a crucial role for such mechanisms at the onset of cardiovascular pathologies.

PHARMACOEPIGENETICS IN HEART FAILURE

The existent therapies for HF seem to be insufficient since HF remains the leading cause of death in the developed countries. Therefore there is an increasing necessity for finding novel therapeutic targets. Because the wide variability in an individual's disease predisposition and response to treatment is only partially ascribed to heritable factors, epigenetical modifications diverging from DNA methylation to non-coding RNAs have gained much attention in several diseases, including HF (Feinberg, 2007; Mano, 2008). Therefore, epigenetic changes are currently being considered as therapeutic approaches in synergy with nucleotide variations at the drug response level (Szyf, 2004). This rapidly emerging new discipline, so-called pharmacoepigenomics, assesses the influence of epigenetic factors in the interindividual variation to drugs with the ultimate goal of discovering novel therapeutic targets (Ingelman-Sundberg et al., 2007). To date, the most advances have been made in the oncology field (Ingelman-Sundberg et al., 2007). However, the knowledge obtained from such studies combined with the knowledge on the role of epigenetic modifications is being applied to other complex forms of disease including HF.

In this context, several studies performed in animal models of disease endorse modifiers of epigenetic marks as therapeutic target points. Curcumin, a natural compound found in the spice trumeric, has an HAT inhibitory activity with specificity to p300/CREB-binding protein. It has been shown to rescue pathological cardiac remodeling and preserve cardiac function in two different rat models of HF, namely the salt-sensitive Dahl rats and in rats that were subjected to MI (Morimoto et al., 2008). An analogous study suggests that administration of curcumin in combination with a conventional therapy such as angiotension conversion enzyme inhibitors (ACEi), in MI-induced rats results in a beneficial additive effect on cardiac function (Sunagawa et al., 2011). Additionally, TSA, an HDAC inhibitor, was showed to blunt the hypertrophic response of cardiomyocytes to PE-treatment in a dose dependent manner and excluding the eventual cytotoxic effect of TSA (Antos et al., 2003). Moreover, treatment with TSA and valproic acid (VPA), another HDAC inhibitor, was able to attenuate cardiac hypertrophic growth in transgenic mice with cardiac overexpression of the atypical homeodomain protein Hop, known to be able to inhibit certain cardiac-gene expression by blocking serum response factor (SRP) transcription activity in a HDAC dependent way (Kook et al., 2003). TSA is also able to attenuate pathological cardiac remodeling in other mouse models such as isoprotenol-, angiotensin II- and pressure overload-induced hypertrophy (Kook et al., 2003; Kee et al., 2006).

Considering that epigenetics regulates phenotypic variation in health and disease, it is conceivable to expect that understanding and controlling the epigenome will prime great developments in the prevention and treatment of common diseases, including HF.

CONCLUSION

The dynamic aspects of epigenetics may not only provide more accurate evidences to the role of changing environmental factors in the drug response, associating the environment with the genome, but also offer a way to reactivate silenced genes. While pharmacogenetics has been very valuable in the identification of interindividual variation in drug uptake and metabolism, epigenomics offers yet another layer of information that may help developing more personalized therapy. In the oncology field, epigenetic drugs have already entered the clinical arena and methylation patterns are used as biomarkers to subtype and stage various cancers as a critical and more personalized care (Coppede, 2011; Litzow, 2011).

It is clear that epigenetic modifications such as DNA methylation, histone modifications and RNA-based mechanisms are the molecular targets for disadvantageous environmental stimuli and may lead to the onset of other complex and heterogeneous diseases such as arrhythmia and HF. However, additional research is obviously necessary to further clarify how epigenetic mechanisms impact the onset and development of heart disease, to eventually identify new druggable targets in HF and allowing disease classification or risk stratification.

REFERENCES

Adam, O., Löhfelm, B., Thum, T., Gupta, S. K., Puhl, S. L., Schäfers, H. J., et al. (2012). Role of miR-21 in the pathogenesis of atrial fibro- sis. *Basic Res. Cardiol.* 107, 278. doi: 10.1007/s00395-012-0278-0

Antos, C. L., McKinsey, T. A., Dre- itz, M., Hollingsworth, L. M., Zhang, C. L., Schreiber, K., et al. (2003). Dose-dependent blockade to cardiomyocyte hypertrophy by histone deacetylase inhibitors. *J. Biol. Chem.* 278, 28930–28937. doi: 10.1074/jbc.M303113200

Baccarelli, A., and Bollati, V. (2009). Epigenetics and envi- ronmental chemicals. *Curr. Opin. Pediatr.* 21, 243–251. doi: 10.1097/MOP.0b013e32832925cc

Backs, J., and Olson, E. N. (2006). Control of cardiac growth by histone acetylation/deacetylation. *Circ. Res.* 98, 15–24. doi: 10.1161/01.RES.0000197782.21444.8f

Backs, J., Song, K., Bezprozvannaya, S., Chang, S., and Olson, E. N. (2006). CaM kinase II selectively sig- nals to histone deacetylase 4 dur- ing cardiomyocyte hypertrophy. *J. Clin. Invest.* 116, 1853–1864. doi: 10.1172/JCI27438

Bagnall, R. D., Tsoutsman, T., Shephard, R. E., Ritchie, W., and Semsarian, C. (2012). Global microRNA profiling of the mouse ventricles during development of severe hypertrophic cardiomyopa- thy and heart failure. *PLoS ONE* 7:e44744. doi: 10.1371/journal.pone. 0044744

Bajpai, R., Chen, D. A., Rada-Iglesias, A., Zhang, J., Xiong, Y., Helms, J., et al. (2010). CHD7 cooperates with PBAF to control multipotent neural crest formation. *Nature* 463, 958–962. doi: 10.1038/nature08733

Balaguer, F., Link, A., Lozano, J. J., Cua- trecasas, M., Nagasaka, T., Boland, C. R., et al. (2010). Epigenetic silenc- ing of miR-137 is an early event in colorectal carcinogenesis. *Cancer Res.* 70, 6609–6618. doi: 10.1158/0008- 5472.CAN-10-0622

Barry, S. P., Davidson, S. M., and Townsend, P. A. (2008). Molecular regulation of cardiac hypertrophy. *Int. J. Biochem. Cell Biol.* 40, 2023–2039. doi: 10.1016/j.biocel.2008.02.020

Bartha, E., Solti, I., Kereskai, L., Lan- tos, J., Plozer, E., Magyar, K., et al. (2009). PARP inhibition delays tran- sition of hypertensive cardiopathy to heart failure in spontaneously hyper- tensive rats. *Cardiovasc. Res.* 83, 501–510. doi: 10.1093/cvr/cvp144

Bayles, R., Harikrishnan, K. N., Lam- bert, E., Baker, E. K., Agrotis, A., Guo, L., et al. (2012). Epigenetic modification of the norepinephrine transporter gene in postural tachycar- dia syndrome. *Arterioscler. Thromb. Vasc. Biol.* 32, 1910–1916. doi: 10.1161/ATVBAHA.111.244343

Belevych, A. E., Sansom, S. E., Ter- entyeva, R., Ho, H. T., Nishi-jima, Y., Martin, M. M., et al. (2011). MicroRNA-1 and -133 increase arrhythmogenesis in heart failure by dissociating phosphatase activity from RyR2 complex. *PLoS ONE* 6:e28324. doi: 10.1371/jour- nal.pone.0028324

Bellavia, A., Urch, B., Speck, M., Brook, R. D., Scott, J. A., Albetti, B., et al. (2013). DNA hypomethyla- tion, ambient particulate matter, and increased blood pressure: findings from controlled human exposure experiments. *J. Am. Heart Assoc.* 2, e000212.

Bhutani, N., Burns, D. M., and Blau, H. M. (2011). DNA demethylation dynamics. *Cell* 146, 866–872. doi: 10.1016/j.cell.2011.08.042

Bird, A. (2007). Perceptions of epi- genetics. *Nature* 447, 396–398. doi: 10.1038/nature05913

Blanco, R. R., Austin, H., Vest, R. N. III, Valadri, R., Li, W., Lassegue, B., et al. (2012). Angiotensin recep- tor type 1 single nucleotide poly- morphism 1166A/C is associated with malignant arrhythmias and altered circulating miR-155 levels in patients with chronic heart failure. *J. Card. Fail.* 18, 717–723. doi: 10.1016/j.cardfail.2012.06.531

Bokil, N. J., Baisden, J. M., Radford, D. J., and Summers, K. M. (2010). Molecular genetics of long QT syn- drome. *Mol. Genet. Metab.* 101, 1–8. doi: 10.1016/j.ymgme.2010.05.011

Brasacchio, D., Okabe, J., Tikel- lis, C., Balcerczyk, A., George, P., Baker, E. K., et al. (2009). Hyper- glycemia induces a dynamic coop- erativity of histone methylase and demethylase enzymes associated with gene-activating epigenetic marks that coexist on the lysine tail. *Diabetes* 58, 1229–1236. doi: 10.2337/db08-1666

Broadbent, H. M., Peden, J. F., Lorkowski, S., Goel, A., Ongen, H., Green, F., et al. (2008). Susceptibility to coronary artery dis- ease and diabetes is encoded by dis- tinct, tightly linked SNPs in the ANRIL locus on chromosome 9p. *Hum. Mol. Genet.* 17, 806–814. doi: 10.1093/hmg/ddm352

Brook, R. D., Rajagopalan, S., Pope, C. A. III, Brook, J. R., Bhatna- gar, A., Diez-Roux, A. V., et al. (2010). Particulate matter air pollu- tion and cardiovascular disease: an update to the scientific statement from the American Heart Association. *Circulation* 121, 2331–2378. doi: 10.1161/CIR.0b013e3181dbece1

Burgess, D. J. (2012). Cancer genomics: histone modification at the gene level. *Nat. Rev. Genet.* 13, 148–149.

Callis, T. E., Pandya, K., Seok, H. Y., Tang, R. H., Tatsuguchi, M., Huang, Z. P., et al. (2009). MicroRNA-208a is a regulator of cardiac hypertro- phy and conduction in mice. *J. Clin. Invest.* 119, 2772–2786. doi: 10.1172/JCI36154

Cao, D. J., Wang, Z. V., Battiprolu, P. K., Jiang, N., Morales, C. R., Kong, Y., et al. (2011). Histone deacetylase (HDAC) inhibitors atten- uate cardiac hypertrophy by sup- pressing autophagy. *Proc. Natl. Acad. Sci. U.S.A.* 108, 4123–4128. doi: 10.1073/pnas.1015081108

Cardin, S., Guasch, E., Luo, X., Naud, P., Le Quang, K., Shi, Y., et al. (2012). Role for MicroRNA-21 in atrial profibrillatory fibrotic remodeling associated with exper- imental postinfarction heart fail- ure. *Circ. Arrhythm. Electrophysiol.* 5, 1027–1035. doi: 10.1161/CIR- CEP.112.973214

Chang, C. P., and Bruneau, B. G. (2012). Epigenetics and cardiovascu- lar development. *Annu. Rev. Physiol.* 74, 41–68. doi: 10.1146/annurev-physiol-020911-153242

Chang, S., McKinsey, T. A., Zhang, L., Richardson, J. A., Hill, J. A., and Olson, E. N. (2004). His- tone deacetylases 5 and 9 govern responsiveness of the heart to a sub- set of stress signals and play redun- dant roles in heart development. *Mol. Cell. Biol.* 24, 8467–8476. doi: 10.1128/MCB.24.19.8467-8476.2004

Cheung, P., and Lau, P. (2005). Epigenetic regulation by histone methylation and histone variants. *Mol. Endocrinol.* 19, 563–573. doi: 10.1210/me.2004-0496

Clapier, C. R., and Cairns, B. R. (2009). The biology of chromatin remodeling complexes. *Annu. Rev. Biochem.* 78, 273–304. doi: 10.1146/ annurev. biochem.77.062706.153223

Clayton, A. L., Hazzalin, C. A., and Mahadevan, L. C. (2006). Enhanced histone acetylation and transcription: a dynamic perspec- tive. *Mol. Cell* 23, 289–296. doi: 10.1016/j.molcel.2006.06.017

Colussi, C., Berni, R., Rosati, J., Straino, S., Vitale, S., Spallotta, F., et al. (2010). The histone deacetylase inhibitor suberoylanilide hydroxamic acid reduces cardiac arrhythmias in dystrophic mice. *Cardiovasc. Res.* 87, 73–82. doi: 10.1093/cvr/ cvq035

Cooley, N., Cowley, M. J., Lin, R. C., Marasco, S., Wong, C., Kaye, M., et al. (2012). Influence of atrial fibrillation on microRNA expression profiles in left and right atria from patients with valvular heart disease. *Physiol. Genomics* 44, 211–219. doi: 10.1152/physiolge- nomics.00111.2011

Coppede, F. (2011). Epigenetic biomarkers of colorectal can- cer: focus on DNA methylation. *Cancer Lett.* doi: 10.1016/j.canlet. 2011.12.030 [Epub ahead of print].

Creemers, E. E., Wilde, A. A., and Pinto, Y. M. (2011). Heart failure: advances through genomics. *Nat. Rev. Genet.* 12, 357–362. doi: 10.1038/nrg2983

Danielson, L. S., Park, D. S., Rotllan, N., Chamorro-Jorganes, A., Guijarro, M. V., Fernandez-Hernando, C., et al. (2013). Cardiovascular dysregulation of miR-17-92 causes a lethal hyper- trophic cardiomyopathy and arrhyth- mogenesis. *FASEB J.* 27, 1460–1467. doi: 10.1096/fj.12-221994

Deaton, A. M., and Bird, A. (2011). CpG islands and the regulation of tran- scription. *Genes Dev.* 25, 1010–1022. doi: 10.1101/gad.2037511

Egger, G., Liang, G., Aparicio, A., and Jones, P. A. (2004). Epigenetics in human disease and prospects for epi- genetic therapy. *Nature* 429, 457–463. doi: 10.1038/nature02625

Elliott, P., and McKenna, W. J. (2004). Hypertrophic cardiomyopa- thy. *Lancet* 363, 1881–1891. doi: 10.1016/S0140-6736(04)16358-7

Fatima, N., Schooley, J. F. Jr., Clay- comb, W. C., and Flagg, T. P. (2012). Promoter DNA methyla- tion regulates murine SUR1 (Abcc8) and SUR2 (Abcc9) expression in HL-1 cardiomyocytes. *PLoS ONE* 7:e41533. doi: 10.1371/journal. pone. 0041533

Feinberg, A. P. (2007). Phenotypic plas- ticity and the epigenetics of human disease. *Nature* 447, 433–440. doi: 10.1038/nature05919

Feinberg, A. P. (2008). Epigenet- ics at the epicenter of modern medicine. *JAMA* 299, 1345–1350. doi: 10.1001/jama.299.11.1345

Feinberg, A. P., and Tycko, B. (2004). The history of cancer epigenetics. *Nat. Rev. Cancer* 4, 143–153. doi: 10.1038/nrc1279

Ferguson, L. R. (2011). RNA silenc- ing: mechanism, biology and responses to environmental stress. *Mutat. Res.* 714, 93–94. doi: 10.1016/j. mrfmmm.2011.07.007

Girmatsion, Z., Biliczki, P., Bonauer, A., Wimmer-Greinecker, G., Scherer, M., Moritz, A., et al. (2009). Changes in microRNA-1 expression and IK1 up-regulation in human atrial fibril- lation. *Heart Rhythm* 6, 1802–1809. doi: 10.1016/j.hrthm.2009.08.035

Grunig, E., Tasman, J. A., Kücherer, H., Franz, W., Kübler, W., and Katus, H. A. (1998). Frequency and phenotypes of familial dilated cardiomyopathy. *J. Am. Coll. Cardiol.* 31, 186–194. doi: 10.1016/S0735-1097(97)00434-8

Guo, H., Ingolia, N. T., Weissman, J. S., and Bartel, D. P. (2010). Mammalian microRNAs predomi- nantly act to decrease target mRNA levels. *Nature* 466, 835–840. doi: 10.1038/nature09267

Gupta, M. P., Samant, S. A., Smith, S. H., and Shroff, S. G. (2008). HDAC4 and PCAF bind to cardiac sarcom- eres and play a role in regulating myofilament contractile activity. *J. Biol. Chem.* 283, 10135–10146. doi: 10.1074/jbc. M710277200

Gusterson, R. J., Jazrawi, E., Adcock, I. M., and Latchman, D. S. (2003). The transcriptional co-activators CREB- binding protein (CBP) and p300 play a critical role in cardiac hyper- trophy that is dependent on their histone acetyltransferase activity. *J. Biol. Chem.* 278, 6838–6847. doi: 10.1074/jbc. M211762200

Haas, J., Frese, K. S., Park, Y. J., Keller, A., Vogel, B., Lin- droth, A. M., et al. (2013). Alter- ations in cardiac DNA methylation in human dilated cardiomyopathy. *EMBO Mol. Med.* 5, 413–429. doi: 10.1002/emmm.201201553

Haberland, M., Montgomery, R. L., and Olson, E. N. (2009). The many roles of histone deacetylases in development and physiology: impli- cations for disease and therapy. *Nat. Rev. Genet.* 10, 32–42. doi: 10.1038/nrg2485

Handy, D. E., Castro, R., and Loscalzo, J. (2011). Epigenetic modifications: basic mechanisms and role in car- diovascular disease. *Circulation* 123, 2145–2156. doi: 10.1161/CIRCULA- TIONAHA.110.956839

Hang, C. T., Yang, J., Han, P., Cheng, H. L., Shang, C., Ashley, E., et al. (2010). Chromatin regulation by Brgl under- lies heart muscle development and disease. *Nature* 466, 62–67. doi: 10.1038/nature09130

Herman, D. S., Lam, L., Taylor, M. R., Wang, L., Teekakirikul, P., Christodoulou, D., et al. (2012). Truncations of titin causing dilated cardiomyopathy. *N. Engl. J. Med.* 366, 619–628. doi: 10.1056/NEJ- Moa1110186

Herron, T. J., and McDonald, K. S. (2002). Small amounts of alpha-myosin heavy chain iso- form expression significantly increase power output of rat car- diac myocyte fragments. *Circ. Res.* 90, 1150–1152. doi: 10.1161/01.RES. 0000022879.57270.11

Hershberger, R. E., Lindenfeld, J., Mestroni, L., Seidman, C. E., Tay- lor, M. R., Towbin, J. A., et al. (2009). Genetic evaluation of car- diomyopathy – a Heart Failure Soci- ety of America practice guideline. *J. Card. Fail.* 15, 83–97. doi: 10.1016/j.cardfail.2009.01.006

Hershberger, R. E., and Siegfried, J. D. (2011). Update 2011: clin- ical and genetic issues in famil- ial dilated cardiomyopathy. *J. Am. Coll. Cardiol.* 57, 1641–1649. doi: 10.1016/j.jacc.2011.01.015

Ho, L., and Crabtree, G. R. (2010). Chromatin remodelling during development. *Nature* 463, 474–484. doi: 10.1038/nature08911

Hosseinkhani, M., Hasegawa, K., Ono, K., Kawamura, T., Takaya, T., Mori- moto, T., et al. (2007). Trichostatin A induces myocardial differentiation of monkey ES cells. *Biochem. Bio- phys. Res. Commun.* 356, 386–391. doi: 10.1016/j. bbrc.2007.02.151

Iacobas, D. A., Iacobas, S., and Haddad,G. G. (2010). Heart rhythm genomic fabric in hypoxia. *Biochem. Biophys. Res. Commun.* 391, 1769–1774. doi: 10.1016/j. bbrc.2009.12.151

Ikeda, S., Kong, S. W., Lu, J., Bisp- ing, E., Zhang, H., Allen, P. D., et al. (2007). Altered microRNA expression in human heart dis- ease. *Physiol. Genomics* 31, 367–373. doi: 10.1152/physiolge- nomics.00144.2007

Ingelman-Sundberg, M., Sim, S. C., Gomez, A., and Rodriguez-Antona, C. (2007). Influence of cytochrome P450 polymorphisms on drug ther- apies: pharmacogenetic, pharma- coepigenetic and clinical aspects. *Pharmacol. Ther.* 116, 496–526. doi: 10.1016/j.pharmthera.2007.09.004

Jenuwein, T., and Allis, C. D. (2001). Translating the histone code. *Science* 293, 1074–1080. doi: 10.1126/sci-ence.1063127

Kaneda, R., Takada, S., Yamashita, Y., Choi, Y. L., Nonaka-Sarukawa, M., Soda, M., et al. (2009). Genome-wide histone methylation profile for heart failure. *Genes Cells* 14, 69–77. doi: 10.1111/j.1365-2443.2008.01252.x

Kaneda, R., Ueno, S., Yamashita, Y., Choi, Y. L., Koinuma, K., Takada, S., et al. (2005). Genome-wide screen- ing for target regions of histone deacetylases in cardiomyocytes. *Circ. Res.* 97, 210–218. doi: 10.1161/01. RES.0000176028.18423.07

Kee, H. J., Sohn, I. S., Nam, K. I., Park, J. E., Qian, Y. R., Yin, Z., et al. (2006). Inhibition of histone deacetylation blocks cardiac hyper- trophy induced by angiotensin II infusion and aortic banding. *Circu- lation* 113, 51–59. doi: 10.1161/CIR- CULATIONAHA.105.559724

Kim, G. H. (2013). MicroRNA reg- ulation of cardiac conduction and arrhythmias. *Transl. Res.* 161, 381– 392. doi: 10.1016/j.trsl.2012.12.004

Kim, G. H., Ryan, J. J., Marsboom, G., and Archer, S. L. (2011). Epigenetic mechanisms of pulmonary hyperten- sion. *Pulm. Circ.* 1, 347–356. doi: 10.4103/2045-8932.87300

Kim, M. Y., Mauro, S., Gévry, N.,Lis, J. T., and Kraus, W. L. (2004). NAD+-dependent modulation of chromatin structure and transcrip- tion by nucleosome binding proper- ties of PARP-1. *Cell* 119, 803–814. doi: 10.1016/j.cell.2004.11.002

Kim, V. N. (2004). MicroRNA pre- cursors in motion: exportin-5 medi- ates their nuclear export. *Trends Cell Biol.* 14, 156–159. doi: 10.1016/j.tcb.2004.02.006

Kitagawa, H., Fujiki, R., Yoshimura, K., Mezaki, Y., Uematsu, Y., Matsui, D., et al. (2003). The chromatin- remodeling complex WINAC targets a nuclear receptor to promoters and is impaired in Williams syndrome. *Cell* 113, 905–917. doi: 10.1016/S0092-8674(03)00436-7

Kooistra, S. M., and Helin, K. (2012). Molecular mechanisms and potential functions of histone demethylases. *Nat. Rev. Mol. Cell Biol.* 13, 297–311. Kook, H., Lepore, J. J., Gitler, A. D., Lu,

M. M., Wing-Man Yung, W., Mackay, J., et al. (2003). Cardiac hypertrophy and histone deacetylase-dependent transcriptional repression mediated by the atypical homeodomain pro- tein Hop. *J. Clin. Invest.* 112, 863–871. Kozomara, A., and Griffiths-Jones, S. (2011). miRBase: integrat- ing microRNA annotation and deep-sequencing data. *Nucleic Acids Res.* 39, D152–D157. doi: 10.1093/nar/ gkq1027

Lachner, M., and Jenuwein, T. (2002). The many faces of histone lysine methylation. *Curr. Opin. Cell Biol.* 14, 286–298. doi: 10.1016/S0955- 0674(02)00335-6

Laird, P. W. (2003). The power and the promise of DNA methylation mark- ers. *Nat. Rev. Cancer* 3, 253–266. doi: 10.1038/nrc1045

Lee, R. C., Feinbaum, R. L., and Ambros, V. (1993). The C. elegans hete- rochronic gene lin-4 encodes small RNAs with antisense complementar- ity to lin-14. *Cell* 75, 843–854. doi: 10.1016/0092-8674(93)90529-Y

Lee, Y., Ahn, C., Han, J., Choi, H., Kim, J., Yim, J., et al. (2003). The nuclear RNase III Drosha initiates microRNA processing. *Nature* 425, 415–419. doi: 10.1038/nature01957

Lee, Y., Kim, M., Han, J., Yeom, K. H., Lee, S., Baek, S. H., et al. (2004). MicroRNA genes are transcribed by RNA polymerase II. *EMBO J.* 23, 4051–4060. doi: 10.1038/sj.emboj.7600385

Lemon, D. D., Horn, T. R., Cavasin, M. A., Jeong, M. Y., Haubold, K. W., Long, C. S., et al. (2011). Cardiac HDAC6 catalytic activity is induced in response to chronic hypertension. *J. Mol. Cell. Cardiol.* 51, 41–50. doi: 10.1016/j.yjmcc.2011.04.005

Lewis, B. P., Burge, C. B., and Bartel, D. P. (2005). Conserved seed pairing, often flanked by adenosines, indicates that thousands of human genes are microRNA targets. *Cell* 120, 15–20. doi: 10.1016/j.cell.2004.12.035

Li, E. (2002). Chromatin modifi- cation and epigenetic reprogram- ming in mammalian development. *Nat. Rev. Genet.* 3, 662–673. doi: 10.1038/nrg887

Li, E. (2002). Chromatin modifi- cation and epigenetic reprogram- ming in mammalian development. *Nat. Rev. Genet.* 3, 662–673. doi: 10.1038/nrg887

Li, E., Beard, C., and Jaenisch, R. (1993). Role for DNA methylation in genomic imprinting. *Nature* 366, 362–365. doi: 10.1038/366362a0

Li, K., Blum, Y., Verma, A., Liu, Z., Pramanik, K., Leigh, N. R., et al. (2010). A noncoding antisense RNA in tie-1 locus regulates tie-1 func- tion in vivo. *Blood* 115, 133–139. doi: 10.1182/blood-2009-09-242180

Li, Y. G., Zhang, P. P., Jiao, K. L., and Zou, Y. Z. (2009). Knock- down of microRNA-181 by lentivirus mediated siRNA expression vector decreases the arrhythmogenic effect of skeletal myoblast transplantation in rat with myocardial infarction. *Microvasc. Res.* 78, 393–404. doi: 10.1016/j.mvr.2009.06.011

Lickert, H., Takeuchi, J. K., Von Both, I., Walls, J. R., McAuliffe, F., Adamson, S. L., et al. (2004). Baf60c is essential for function of BAF chromatin remod- elling complexes in heart develop- ment. *Nature* 432, 107–112. doi: 10.1038/nature03071

Ling, C., and Groop, L. (2009). Epi- genetics: a molecular link between environmental factors and type 2 dia- betes. *Diabetes* 58, 2718–2725. doi: 10.2337/db09-1003

Litzow, M. R. (2011). Novel thera- peutic approaches for acute lym- phoblastic leukemia. *Hematol. Oncol. Clin. North Am.* 25, 1303–1317. doi: 10.1016/j.hoc.2011.09.019

Liu, F., Levin, M. D., Petrenko, N. B., Lu, M. M., Wang, T., Yuan, L. J., et al. (2008). Histone- deacetylase inhibition reverses atrial arrhythmia inducibility and fibrosis in cardiac hypertrophy inde- pendent of angiotensin. *J. Mol. Cell. Cardiol.* 45, 715–723. doi: 10.1016/j.yjmcc.2008.08.015

Lopes, L. R., and Elliott, P. M. (2013). Genetics of heart fail- ure. *Biochim. Biophys. Acta* doi: 10.1016/j.bbadis.2012.12.012 [Epub ahead of print].

Lu, Y., Zhang, Y., Wang, N., Pan, Z., Gao, X., Zhang, F., et al. (2010). MicroRNA-328 contributes to adverse electrical remodeling in atrial fibrillation. *Circulation* 122, 2378–2387. doi: 10.1161/CIRCULA- TIONAHA.110.958967

Lujambio, A., and Lowe, S. W. (2012). The microcosmos of can- cer. *Nature* 482, 347–355. doi: 10.1038/nature10888

MacFarlane, A. J., Strom, A., and Scott, F. W. (2009). Epigenetics: decipher- ing how environmental factors may modify autoimmune type 1 diabetes. *Mamm. Genome* 20, 624–632. doi: 10.1007/s00335-009-9213-6

Mancini-DiNardo, D., Steele, S. J., Ingram, R. S., and Tilghman, S. M. (2003). A differentially methy- lated region within the gene Kcnq1 functions as an imprinted promoter and silencer. *Hum. Mol. Genet.* 12, 283–294. doi: 10.1093/hmg/ ddg024

Mano, H. (2008). Epigenetic abnormal- ities in cardiac hypertrophy and heart failure. *Environ. Health Prev. Med.*13, 25–29. doi: 10.1007/s12199-007-0007-8

Margueron, R., and Reinberg, D. (2010). Chromatin structure and the inheritance of epigenetic informa- tion. *Nat. Rev. Genet.* 11, 285–296. doi: 10.1038/nrg2752

Martin, C., and Zhang, Y. (2005). The diverse functions of histone lysine methylation. *Nat. Rev. Mol. Cell Biol.* 6, 838–849. doi: 10.1038/nrm1761

Mathiyalagan, P., Chang, L., Du, X. J., and El-Osta, A. (2010). Cardiac ventricular chambers are epigenet- ically distinguishable. *Cell Cycle* 9, 612–617. doi: 10.4161/cc.9.3.10612

Matkovich, S. J., Van Booven, D. J., Youker, K. A., Torre-Amionem, G., Diwan, A., Eschenbacher, W. H., et al. (2009). Reciprocal regulation of myocardial microRNAs and messen- ger RNA in human cardiomyopathy and reversal of the microRNA sig- nature by biomechanical support. *Circulation* 119, 1263–1271. doi: 10.1161/CIRCULATIONAHA.108.813576

Matkovich, S. J., Wang, W., Tu, Y., Eschenbacher, W. H., Dorn, L. E., Condorelli, G., et al. (2010). MicroRNA-133a protects against myocardial fibrosis and mod- ulates electrical repolarization without affecting hypertrophy in pressure-overloaded adult hearts. *Circ. Res.* 106, 166–175. doi: 10.1161/CIRCRESAHA.109.202176

Meder, B., Keller, A., Vogel, B., Haas, J., Sedaghat-Hamedani, F., Kayvan- pour, E., et al. (2011). MicroRNA signatures in total peripheral blood as novel biomarkers for acute myocar- dial infarction. *Basic Res. Cardiol.* 106, 13–23. doi: 10.1007/s00395-010-0123-2

Meurs, K. M., and Kuan, M. (2011). Differential methylation of CpG sites in two isoforms of myosin binding protein C, an important hyper- trophic cardiomyopathy gene. *Envi- ron. Mol. Mutagen* 52, 161–164. doi: 10.1002/em.20596

Michels, V. V., Moll, P. P., Miller, F. A., Tajik, A. J., Chu, J. S., Driscoll, D. J., et al. (1992). The frequency of familial dilated cardiomyopathy in a series of patients with idio- pathic dilated cardiomyopathy. *N. Engl. J. Med.* 326, 77–82. doi: 10.1056/NEJM199201093260201

Millis, R. M. (2011). Epigenetics and hypertension. *Curr. Hypertens. Rep.* 13, 21–28. doi: 10.1007/s11906-010-0173-8 Miyamoto, S., Kawamura, T., Mori- moto, T., Ono, K., Wada, H., Kawase, Y., et al. (2006). Histone acetyltrans- ferase activity of p300 is required for the promotion of left ventric- ular remodeling after myocardial infarction in adult mice in vivo. *Circulation* 113, 679–690. doi: 10.1161/CIRCULATIONAHA.105.585182

Montgomery, R. L., Davis, C. A., Pot- thoff, M. J., Haberland, M., Fielitz, J., Qi, X., et al. (2007). Histone deacety- lases 1 and 2 redundantly regulate cardiac morphogenesis, growth, and contractility. *Genes Dev.* 21, 1790–1802. doi: 10.1101/gad.1563807

Morimoto, T., Sunagawa, Y., Kawamura, T., Takaya, T., Wada, H., Naga- sawa, A., et al. (2008). The dietary compound curcumin inhibits p300 histone acetyltransferase activity and prevents heart failure in rats. *J. Clin. Invest.* 118, 868–878.

Morita, H., Nagai, R., Seidman, J. G., and Seidman, C. E. (2010). Sarcomere gene mutations in hyper- trophy and heart failure. *J. Cardio- vasc. Transl. Res.* 3, 297–303. doi: 10.1007/s12265-010-9188-4

Morita, H., Rehm, H. L., Menesses, A., McDonough, B., Roberts, A. E., Kucherlapati, R., et al. (2008). Shared genetic causes of cardiac hypertrophy in children and adults. *N. Engl. J. Med.* 358, 1899–1908. doi: 10.1056/NEJMoa075463

Movassagh, M., Choy, M. K., God- dard, M., Bennett, M. R., Down, T. A., and Foo, R. S. (2010). Differen- tial DNA methylation correlates with differential expression of angiogenic factors in human heart failure. *PLoS ONE* 5:e8564. doi: 10.1371/jour- nal.pone.0008564

Movassagh, M., Choy, M. K., Knowles, D. A., Cordeddu, L., Haider, S., Down, T., et al. (2011a). Distinct epigenomic features in end-stage fail- ing human hearts. *Circulation* 124, 2411–2422.

Movassagh, M., Vujic, A., and Foo, R. (2011b). Genome-wide DNA methy- lation in human heart failure. *Epige- nomics* 3, 103–109.

Naga Prasad, S. V., Duan, Z. H., Gupta, M. K., Surampudi, V. S., Volinia, S., Calin, G. A., et al. (2009). Unique microRNA profile in end-stage heart failure indicates alterations in specific cardiovascular signaling networks. *J. Biol. Chem.* 284, 27487–27499. doi: 10.1074/jbc.M109.036541

Oliveira-Carvalho, V., Carvalho, V. O., and Bocchi, E. A. (2013). The emerging role of miR-208a in the heart. *DNA Cell Biol.* 32, 8–12. doi: 10.1089/dna.2012.1787

Olson, E. N., Backs, J., and McKin- sey, T. A. (2006). Control of car- diac hypertrophy and heart failure by histone acetylation/deacetylation. *Novartis Found. Sym.* 274, 3–12. doi: 10.1002/0470029331.ch2

Ordovas, J. M., and Smith, C. E. (2010). Epigenetics and cardiovas- cular disease. *Nat. Rev. Cardiol.* 7, 510–519. doi: 10.1038/nrcardio.2010.104

O'Toole, T. E., Conklin, D. J., and Bhatnagar, A. (2008). Environmen- tal risk factors for heart disease. *Rev. Environ. Health* 23, 167–202. doi: 10.1515/REVEH.2008.23.3.167

Palfi, A., Toth, A., Hanto, K., Deres, P., Szabados, E., Szereday, Z., et al. (2006). PARP inhibition prevents postinfarction myocardial remodeling and heart failure via the protein kinase C/glycogen syn- thase kinase-3beta pathway. *J. Mol. Cell. Cardiol.* 41, 149–159. doi: 10.1016/j.yjmcc.2006.03.427

Panning, B., and Jaenisch, R. (1996). DNA hypomethylation can activate Xist expression and silence X-linked genes. *Genes Dev.* 10, 1991–2002. doi: 10.1101/gad.10.16.1991

Pillai, J. B., Gupta, M., Rajamohan, S. B., Lang, R., Raman, J., and Gupta, M. P. (2006). Poly(ADP- ribose) polymerase-1-deficient mice are protected from angiotensin II- induced cardiac hypertrophy. *Am. J. Physiol. Heart Circ. Physiol.* 291, H1545–H1553.

Pillai, J. B., Isbatan, A., Imai, S., and Gupta, M. P. (2005a). Poly(ADP- ribose) polymerase-1-dependent car- diac myocyte cell death during heart failure is mediated by NAD+ deple- tion and reduced Sir2alpha deacety- lase activity. *J. Biol. Chem.* 280, 43121–43130.

Pillai, J. B., Russell, H. M., Raman, J., Jeevanandam, V., and Gupta, M. P. (2005b). Increased expression of poly(ADP-ribose) polymerase-1 contributes to caspase-independent myocyte cell death during heart fail- ure. *Am. J. Physiol. Heart Circ. Phys- iol.* 288, H486–H496.

Quiat, D., and Olson, E. N. (2013). MicroRNAs in cardiovascular dis- ease: from pathogenesis to prevention and treatment. *J. Clin. Invest.* 123, 11–18. doi: 10.1172/JCI62876 Robb, G. B., Carson, A. R., Tai, S.

C., Fish, J. E., Singh, S., Yamada, T., et al. (2004). Post-transcriptional regulation of endothelial nitric-oxide synthase by an overlapping anti- sense mRNA transcript. *J. Biol. Chem.* 279, 37982–37996. doi: 10.1074/jbc.M400271200

Rodriguez, J. E., McCudden, C. R., and Willis, M. S. (2009). Familial hypertrophic cardiomyopathy: basic concepts and future molecular diag- nostics. *Clin. Biochem.* 42, 755–765. doi: 10.1016/j.clinbiochem.2009.01. 020

Saccani, S., and Natoli, G. (2002). Dynamic changes in histone H3 Lys 9 methylation occurring at tightly reg- ulated inducible inflammatory genes. *Genes Dev.* 16, 2219–2224. doi: 10.1101/gad.232502

Saito, Y., Liang, G., Egger, G., Friedman, J. M., Chuang, J. C., Coetzee, G. A., et al. (2006). Specific activation of microRNA- 127 with downregulation of the proto-oncogene BCL6 by chromatin- modifying drugs in human cancer cells. *Cancer Cell* 9, 435–443. doi: 10.1016/j.ccr.2006.04.020

Samant, S. A., Courson, D. S., Sundare- san, N. R., Pillai, V. B., Tan, M., Zhao, Y., et al. (2011). HDAC3-dependent reversible lysine acetylation of cardiac myosin heavy chain isoforms modu- lates their enzymatic and motor activ- ity. *J. Biol. Chem.* 286, 5567–5577. doi: 10.1074/jbc.M110.163865

Saxonov, S., Berg, P., and Brutlag, D. L. (2006). A genome-wide analysis of CpG dinucleotides in the human genome distinguishes two distinct classes of promoters. *Proc. Natl. Acad. Sci. U.S.A.* 103, 1412–1417. doi: 10.1073/pnas.0510310103

Sayed, D., and Abdellatif, M. (2011). MicroRNAs in development and dis- ease. *Physiol. Rev.* 91, 827–887. doi: 10.1152/physrev.00006.2010

Shahbazian, M. D., and Grunstein, M. (2007). Functions of site-specific his- tone acetylation and deacetylation. *Annu. Rev. Biochem.* 76, 75–100. doi: 10.1146/annurev.biochem.76.052705. 162114

Shan, H., Zhang, Y., Lu, Y., Zhang, Y., Pan, Z., Cai, B., et al. (2009). Down- regulation of miR-133 and miR- 590 contributes to nicotine-induced atrial remodelling in canines. *Car- diovasc. Res.* 83, 465–472. doi: 10.1093/cvr/cvp130

Shi, Y., and Whetstine, J. R. (2007). Dynamic regulation of his- tone lysine methylation by demethy- lases. *Mol. Cell* 25, 1–14. doi: 10.1016/j.molcel.2006.12.010

Shirodkar, A. V., and Marsden, P. A. (2011). Epigenetics in cardiovascular disease. *Curr. Opin. Cardiol.* 26, 209–215. doi: 10.1097/HCO.0b013e328345986e

Stauffer, B. L., Russell, G., Nunley, K., Miyamoto, S. D., and Sucharov, C. C. (2013). miRNA expression in pediatric failing human heart. *J. Mol. Cell. Cardiol.* 57, 43–46. doi: 10.1016/j.yjmcc.2013.01.005

Stein, A. B., Jones, T. A., Herron, T. J., Patel, S. R., Day, S. M., Nou- jaim, S. F., et al. (2011). Loss of H3K4 methylation destabilizes gene expression patterns and physiologi- cal functions in adult murine car- diomyocytes. *J. Clin. Invest.* 121, 2641–2650. doi: 10.1172/JCI44641

Sucharov, C., Bristow, M. R., and Port, J. D. (2008). miRNA expres- sion in the failing human heart: functional correlates. *J. Mol. Cell. Cardiol.* 45, 185–192. doi: 10.1016/j.yjmcc.2008.04.014

Sunagawa, Y., Morimoto, T., Wada, H., Takaya, T., Katanasaka, Y., Kawamura, T., et al. (2011). A natural p300-specific histone acetyl- transferase inhibitor, curcumin, in addition to angiotensin-converting enzyme inhibitor, exerts beneficial effects on left ventricular systolic function after myocardial infarction in rats. *Circ. J.* 75, 2151–2159. doi: 10.1253/circj.CJ-10-1072

Suzuki, M. M., and Bird, A. (2008). DNA methylation land- scapes: provocative insights from epigenomics. *Nat. Rev. Genet.* 9, 465–476. doi: 10.1038/nrg2341

Szabo, G., Bährle, S., Stumpf, N., Son- nenberg, K., Szabó, E. E., Pacher, P., et al. (2002). Poly(ADP-Ribose) polymerase inhibition reduces reper- fusion injury after heart transplan- tation. *Circ. Res.* 90, 100–106. doi: 10.1161/hh0102.102657

Szyf, M. (2004). Toward a discip- ine of pharmacoepigenomics. *Curr. Pharmacogenomics* 2, 357–377. doi: 10.2174/1570160043377358

Takeuchi, J. K., and Bruneau, B. G. (2009). Directed transdifferentiation of mouse mesoderm to heart tissue by defined factors. *Nature* 459, 708–711. doi: 10.1038/nature08039

Takeuchi, J. K., Lickert, H., Bisgrove, B. W., Sun, X., Yamamoto, M., Chawengsaksophak, K., et al. (2007). Baf60c is a nuclear Notch signaling component required for the estab- lishment of left-right asymmetry. *Proc. Natl. Acad. Sci. U.S.A.* 104, 846– 851. doi: 10.1073/pnas.0608118104

Teperino, R., Schoonjans, K., and Auw- erx, J. (2010). Histone methyl trans- ferases and demethylases; can they link metabolism and transcription? *Cell Metab.* 12, 321–327.

Theis, J. L., Sharpe, K. M., Mat- sumoto, M. E., Chai, H. S., Nair, A. A., Theis, J. D., et al. (2011). Homozygosity mapping and exome sequencing reveal GATAD1 muta- tion in autosomal recessive dilated cardiomyopathy. *Circ. Cardiovasc. Genet.* 4, 585–594. doi: 10.1161/CIR- CGENETICS.111.961052

Thum, T., Galuppo, P., Wolf, C., Fiedler, J., Kneitz, S., van Laake, L. W., et al. (2007). MicroRNAs in the human heart: a clue to fetal gene reprogram- ming in heart failure. *Circulation* 116, 258–267. doi: 10.1161/CIRCU- LATIONAHA.107.687947

Trivedi, C. M., Luo, Y., Yin, Z., Zhang, M., Zhu, W., Wang, T., et al. (2007). Hdac2 regulates the cardiac hyper- trophic response by modulating Gsk3 beta activity. *Nat. Med.* 13, 324–331. doi: 10.1038/nm1552

Tulin, A., and Spradling, A. (2003). Chromatin loosening by poly(ADP)-ribosepolymerase (PARP) at *Drosophila* puff loci. *Science* 299, 560–562. doi: 10.1126/science.1078764

van Rooij, E., Sutherland, L. B., Liu, N., Williams, A. H., McAnally, J., Gerard, R. D., et al. (2006). A signature pat- tern of stress-responsive microRNAs that can evoke cardiac hypertrophy and heart failure. *Proc. Natl. Acad. Sci. U.S.A.* 103, 18255–18260. doi: 10.1073/pnas.0608791103

Villeneuve, L. M., Reddy, M. A., Lant- ing, L. L., Wang, M., Meng, L., and Natarajan, R. (2008). Epigenetic histone H3 lysine 9 methylation in metabolic memory and inflamma- tory phenotype of vascular smooth muscle cells in diabetes. *Proc. Natl. Acad. Sci. U.S.A.* 105, 9047–9052. doi: 10.1073/pnas.0803623105

Wang, Z. V., Ferdous, A., and Hill, J. A. (2013). Cardiomyocyte autophagy: metabolic profit and loss. *Heart Fail. Rev.* 18, 585–594. doi: 10.1007/s10741-012-9350-y Wei, J. Q., Shehadeh, L. A., Mitrani, J. M., Pessanha, M., Slepak, T. I., Webster, K. A., et al. (2008). Quantitative control of adaptive car- diac hypertrophy by acetyltrans- ferase p300. *Circulation* 118, 934– 946. doi: 10.1161/CIRCULATION- AHA.107.760488

Wierda, R. J., Geutskens, S. B., Jukema, J. W., Quax, P. H., and van den Elsen, P. J. (2010). Epigenetics in atherosclerosis and inflammation. *J. Cell. Mol. Med.* 14, 1225–1240. doi: 10.1111/j.1582-4934.2010.01022.x

Winter, J., Jung, S., Keller, S., Gre- gory, R. I., and Diederichs, S. (2009). Many roads to maturity: microRNA biogenesis pathways and their regula- tion. *Nat. Cell Biol.* 11, 228–234. doi: 10.1038/ncb0309-228

Xiao, C. Y., Chen, M., Zsengellér, Z., Li, H., Kiss, L., Kollai, M., et al. (2005). Poly(ADP-Ribose) poly- merase promotes cardiac remodel- ing, contractile failure, and transloca- tion of apoptosis-inducing factor in a murine experimental model of aortic banding and heart failure. *J. Phar- macol. Exp. Ther.* 312, 891–898. doi: 10.1124/jpet.104.077164

Xiao, J., Liang, D., Zhang, Y., Liu, Y., Zhang, H., Liu, Y., et al. (2011). MicroRNA expression sig- nature in atrial fibrillation with mitral stenosis. *Physiol. Genomics* 43, 655–664. doi: 10.1152/physiolge- nomics.00139.2010

Yan, M. S., Matouk, C. C., and Mars- den, P. A. (2010). Epigenetics of the vascular endothelium. *J. Appl. Phys- iol.* 109, 916–926. doi: 10.1152/jap-plphysiol.00131.2010

Yanazume, T., Hasegawa, K., Mori- moto, T., Kawamura, T., Wada, H., Matsumori, A., et al. (2003). Car- diac p300 is involved in myocyte growth with decompensated heart failure. *Mol. Cell. Biol.* 23, 3593–3606. doi: 10.1128/MCB.23.10.3593-3606. 2003

Yang, B., Lin, H., Xiao, J., Lu, Y., Luo, X., Li, B., et al. (2007). The muscle-specific microRNA miR- 1 regulates cardiac arrhythmogenic potential by targeting GJA1 and KCNJ2. *Nat. Med.* 13, 486–491. doi: 10.1038/nm1569

Yang, X. J., and Seto, E. (2008). The Rpd3/Hda1 family of lysine deacety- lases: from bacteria and yeast to mice and men. *Nat. Rev. Mol. Cell Biol.* 9, 206–218. doi: 10.1038/nrm 2346

Zhang, C. L., McKinsey, T. A., Chang, S., Antos, C. L., Hill, J. A., and Olson, E. N. (2002). Class II histone deacety- lases act as signal-responsive repres- sors of cardiac hypertrophy. *Cell* 110, 479–488. doi: 10.1016/S0092- 8674(02)00861-9

Zhang, Q. J., Chen, H. Z., Wang, L., Liu, D. P., Hill, J. A., and Liu, Z. P. (2011). The histone trimethylly- sine demethylase JMJD2A promotes cardiac hypertrophy in response to hypertrophic stimuli in mice. *J. Clin. Invest.* 121, 2447–2456. doi: 10.1172/JCI46277

Zhao, Y., Ransom, J. F., Li, A., Vedan- tham, V., von Drehle, M., Muth, A. N., et al. (2007). Dysregulation of cardiogenesis, cardiac conduc- tion, and cell cycle in mice lacking miRNA-1-2. *Cell* 129, 303–317. doi: 10.1016/j.cell.2007.03.030

15

Transgenic insights linking Pitx2 and atrial arrhythmias

Diego Franco*, Ana Chinchilla and Amelia E. Aránega

Department of Experimental Biology, University of Jaen, Jaen, Spain

Correspondence:
Diego Franco, Department of Experimental Biology, University of Jaen, 23071 Jaen, Spain.
e-mail: dfranco@ujaen.es

Pitx2 is a homeobox transcription factor involved in left–right signaling during embryogenesis. Disruption of left–right signaling in mice within its core nodal/lefty cascade, results in impaired expression of the last effector of the left–right cascade, Pitx2, leading in many cases to absence or bilateral expression of Pitx2 in lateral plate mesoderm (LPM). Loss of Pitx2 expression in LPM results in severe cardiac malformations, including right cardiac isomerism. Pitx2 is firstly expressed asymmetrically in the left but not right LPM, before the cardiac crescent forms, and subsequently, as the heart develops, becomes confined to the left side of the linear heart tube. Expression of Pitx2 is remodeled during cardiac looping, becoming localized to the ventral portion of the developing ventricular chambers, while maintaining a distinct left-sided atrial expression. The importance of Pitx2 during cardiogenesis has been illustrated by the complex and robust cardiac defects observed on systemic deletion of Pitx2 in mice. Lack of Pitx2 expression leads to embryonic lethality at mid-term, and Pitx2-deficient embryos display isomeric hearts with incomplete closure of the body wall. However, whereas the pivotal role of Pitx2 during cardiogenesis is well sustained, its putative role in the fetal and adult heart is largely unexplored. Recent genome-wide association studies have identified several genetic variants highly associated with atrial fibrillation (AF). Among them are genetic variants located on chromosome 4q25 adjacent to PITX2. Since then several transgenic approaches have provided evidences of the role of the homeobox transcription factor PITX2 and atrial arrhythmias. Here, we review new insights into the cellular and molecular links between PITX2 and AF.

Keywords: Pitx2, atrial fibrillation, microRNAs, ion channel, electrophysiology

Cardiac arrhythmia can be defined as a deviation from the normal heart rate and/or rhythm under physiological circumstances which are thus reflected on specific ECG patterns (Bellet, 1971). Atrial arrhythmias may be regular, as in the case of flutter or monomorphic tachycardia, or irregular, as in the case of fibrillation or polymorphic tachycardia (Gussak and Antzelevitch, 2008). We focus herein on atrial fibrillation (AF), the most prevalent type of arrhythmia in humans. AF is characterized by uncoordinated atrial activation with consequent weakening of atrial mechanical function with intact AV conduction (Gussak and Antzelevitch, 2008). AF prevalence ranges from 1% in young adults to >10% of those over 80 years old (Fuster et al., 2001) and is frequently associated with hypertension, coronary disease, valvular diseases, and cardiomyopathies (Kannel et al., 1998), yet in 10–20% of AF patients, no underlying disease is found (Brand et al., 1985), i.e., idiopathic or lone AF. Great insights have been gained concerning the cellular and molecular mechanisms that underlie AF (Schotten et al., 2011; Wakili et al., 2011). Enhanced automaticity in one or several rapidly depolarizing foci leads to AF (Haissaguerre et al., 1998), being frequently located within the superior pulmonary veins, and more rarely within the superior vena cava or coronary sinus (Moe and Abildskov, 1959). Alternatively, multiple wave fronts propagate within the atria, resulting in derived wavelets that self-perpetuate (Arnar et al., 2006). However, the molecular substrates of AF remain obscure.

Although AF is the most prevalent type of arrhythmia, its genetic etiology remains elusive. The first AF genetic locus was reported by Brugada et al. (1997) identifying linkage to chromosome 10q22–q24 and soon thereafter Chen et al. (2003) identify a mutation in KCNQ1. Mutations in KCNQ1 have been subsequently confirmed (Ellinor et al., 2007) as well as in other ion channels including KCNE2, KCNE3, KCNJ2, KCNA5, and SCN5A (Ellinor et al., 2004; Mc Nair et al., 2004; Yang et al., 2004; Xia et al., 2005). Surprisingly, mutations in ion channels would underlie less 1% of AF cases.

The advent of new genetic strategies, in particular genome-wide association studies (GWAS), has shed new light on the genetic bases of arrhythmogenic syndromes and the identification of novel disease-causing genes (Larson et al., 2007). GWAS have identified several genetic variants highly associated with AF, which are located at 9p21, 1q21, 16q22, and 4q25, respectively. On chromosome 9p21, no candidate gene has been linked to AF, and thus its relevance awaits further experimental and functional evidence (Larson et al., 2007). Distinct genetic variants at 1q21 are linked to KCNN3, a potassium channel involved in atrial repolarization (Ellinor et al., 2011) and IL6R, a gene involved in inflammatory response (Schnabel et al., 2011), respectively. Genetic variants at 16q22 are linked to ZFHX3, a zinc finger homeobox transcription factor involved in liver gene expression (Gudbjartsson et al., 2009). However, in both cases 1q21 and 16q22 risk variants, their role in AF remains obscure. Finally, genetic variants on chromosome

4q25 which are strongly associated with lone AF in three distinct populations of European descent (Gudbjartsson et al., 2007) map adjacent to PITX2, which is known to have a critical function in establishing left–right asymmetry (Gage et al., 1999; Lin et al., 1999) and plays a critical role in cardiac development (Campione et al., 1999, 2001; Franco and Campione, 2003) and thus supporting the notion that impaired function of PITX2 might underlie AF (Gudbjartsson et al., 2009).

Pitx2 is a homeobox transcription factor involved in left–right signaling during embryogenesis (Gage et al., 1999; Lin et al., 1999). Disruption of left–right signaling in mice within its core nodal/lefty cascade (Blum et al., 1999; Hamada et al., 2001; Bamforth et al., 2004) results in impaired expression of Pitx2, the last effector of the left–right cascade, being absent or bilateral expressed in lateral plate mesoderm (LPM). Loss of Pitx2 expression in LPM results in severe cardiac malformations, including transposition of the great arteries, double-outlet right ventricle, and right cardiac isomerism (Gage et al., 1999; Lin et al., 1999). However, whereas the pivotal role of Pitx2 during cardiogenesis is well sustained, its putative role in the fetal and adult heart is largely unexplored.

The Pitx2 gene encodes three distinct isoforms, Pitx2a, Pitx2b, and Pitx2c, through alternative splicing and distinct promoter usage (Schweickert et al., 2000). Pitx2c is the most prominent isoform in the developing mouse heart and only weak and transient expression of Pitx2a is observed during early embryonic (E9.5–E12.5) stages, whereas Pitx2b displays progressively decreasing expression in embryonic and fetal stages (D. Franco and A. Aranega, unpublished data). In man, a fourth isoform, PITX2D is also expressed, which acts as a dominant negative isoform (Cox et al., 2002). PITX2 mutations are linked to Axenfeld–Rieger syndrome, which is characterized by abnormal morphogenesis of the anterior segment of the eye, variable degree of maxillary hypoplasia, skeletal abnormalities, and abdominal defects (Hjalt and Semina, 2005). In rodents and avian, Pitx2 displays a highly dynamic expression profile during cardiogenesis. Pitx2 is initially expressed asymmetrically in the left but not right LPM, before the cardiac crescent forms, and subsequently, as the heart develops, becomes confined to the left side of the linear heart tube (Campione et al., 1999, 2001; Franco and Campione, 2003). Pitx2 expression is later remodeled during cardiac looping, becoming confined to the ventral portion of the forming ventricular chambers, while keeping left-sided atrial expression (Campione et al., 2001). With further development, Pitx2 is down-regulated in the ventricular chambers, while high and robust expression of Pitx2 is maintained in the atrial chambers as well as in discrete components of the inflow tract, including the left atrial chamber, left superior caval vein, the pulmonary veins, and the interatrial septum (Franco et al., 2000; Kahr et al., 2011).

The significance of Pitx2 during heart development is illustrated by the complex and robust cardiac defects observed on Pitx2 defective mouse models. Systemic deficiency of Pitx2 leads to embryonic lethality at mid-term, leading to severe cardiovascular defects such as double-outlet right ventricle and right atrial isomerism as well as incomplete closure of the body wall (Gage et al., 1999; Lin et al., 1999; Liu et al., 2001, 2002). Isoform-specific Pitx2 mutants revealed that Pitx2c is the most relevant isoform during cardiogenesis, since lack of Pitx2c expression, but not Pitx2a or Pitx2b, recapitulate the morphogenetic defects similar to systemic Pitx2-deficient mice (Liu et al., 2001). More recently, with the advent of tissue-specific conditional mutants, our understanding of the role of Pitx2 during cardiogenesis has greatly expanded. Ai et al. (2006) revealed that lack of Pitx2 function in the secondary heart field, a subpopulation of cardiovascular progenitor cells emanating from the medio-lateral cardiogenic mesoderm (Kelly et al., 2001), leads to developmental defects reminiscent of systemic Pitx2c null mutants. In addition, further evidence on the role of Pitx2 within the secondary heart field has been reported at the arterial (Nowotschin et al., 2006; Yashiro et al., 2007) and venous (Galli et al., 2008) poles of the heart. Importantly, Pitx2 function is not exclusive related to cardiac precursor cells but is also relevant in differentiated cardiomyocytes as reported by Tessari et al. (2008). Using αMHC-Cre driver mice, these authors demonstrated that functional impairment of Pitx2 in cardiomyocytes leads to cytoarchitectural disarray in ventricular myocytes and to abnormal left–right expression of *Bmp10* in the atria. Unexpectedly, αMHCCrePitx2 mutants do not display atrial isomerism, suggesting that left/right atrial morphological identity is acquired before αMHC-Cre activation. Overall, these data demonstrate a developmental role of Pitx2 with precursor cells as well as in cardiomyocytes, including importantly, morphological structures prone to trigger atrial arrhythmias, yet no evidence of such electrophysiological defects was reported in these studies. Moreover, although it is clearly established that Pitx2 plays a role in pulmonary vein development (Mommersteeg et al., 2007), a frequent AF foci, Pitx2 driven alterations occur in the setting of complex cardiac abnormalities such as atrial isomerism, a condition which is not linked to atrial arrhythmias in men. Therefore, additional evidence is required to fill the gap between Pitx2 function in the embryo and the onset of AF.

Genetic variants at 4q25, close to the Pitx2 locus, are highly associated with AF (Gudbjartsson et al., 2007), providing the conjecture thus that Pitx2 dysfunction might be to AF. Linkage of 4q25 AF risk variants have been consistently reported within distinct cohorts, highlighting thus the reproducibility of these findings (Chinchilla et al., 2011; Henningsen et al., 2011; Kiliszek et al., 2011; Schnabel et al., 2011; Delaney et al., 2012; Liu et al., 2012; Olesen et al., 2012). A twofold question arises from this hypothesis, first is whether the 4q25 genetic variants can modulate Pitx2 expression, a question that remains unanswered, and secondly, whether Pitx2 impairment can lead to AF. Reports in human AF right and left atrial biopsies demonstrated that PITX2 expression is severely diminished in AF patients as compared to patients with no clinical history of AF (Chinchilla et al., 2011), validating thus the hypothesis that PITX2 is impaired in AF patients. In addition to the human data, several independent experimental studies have provided evidences for this second issue, using subtle distinct experimental models. Wang et al. (2010) have demonstrated that Pitx2 haploinsufficiency predisposes to AF in electrically stimulated adult mice with structurally normal hearts. These authors reported a developmental link in that Pitx2 inhibits the sinoatrial node gene program in the embryonic left atrium, by regulating Shox2 and Nkx2.5 expression. When Pitx2 function is partially (heterozygous) or completely (null) impaired in the embryonic

(E12.5) mouse heart, Shox2, as well as several other sinoatrial node markers such as Hcn4 and Tbx3, are ectopically expressed in the forming inflow tract of the heart. These findings are further underscored by the recent study of Ammirabile et al. (2012) using a myocardiac specific conditional Pitx2 mouse model (cardiac troponin T Cre deletor mice). Thus, these observations provide a link between the embryonic function of Pitx2 and AF.

Kirchhof et al. (2011) have recently described impaired gap and tight junction expression in microarray analysis of the left atria of adult Pitx2c heterozygous mutant mice which display no overt structural and/or morphological alterations. These data provide a putative link to AF since mutations in GJA5 (Cx40) are associated with AF (Gollob et al., 2006) and further implicate impaired Pitx2 function at fetal and/or adult stages in predisposition to AF. In line with these findings, recent work in our laboratory using a Pitx2 over-expression model of embryonic stem cell-derived cardiomyocytes (Lozano-Velasco et al., 2011) has shown that Pitx2 does not modify the expression of contractile proteins such as actin and myosin heavy and light-chain isoforms, thus suggesting that Pitx2 does not impair the contractile properties of cardiomyocytes, but importantly, Pitx2 mis-expression impairs connexin-40 expression.

In addition, our recent work using atrial-specific conditional Pitx2 mouse mutants, in which right-sided sinoatrial node formation is intact, also supports a role of Pitx2 impairment on the onset of left-sided electrophysiological defects (Chinchilla et al., 2011) which are prone substrates for AF. Voltage-gated sodium and inward rectifying K+ (Kir2.1, Kir2.2, and Kir2.3) ion channels are abnormally expressed in the atrial myocardium both in fetal and adult stages of atrial-specific conditional Pitx2 mouse mutants, while cardiac morphogenesis is not compromised. Importantly, inward rectifying K+ channel de-regulation, but not sodium, is mediated by impaired miR-1 expression in atrial-specific conditional Pitx2 mutant mice. As a consequence, in these mice, the action potential amplitude is decreased, while the resting membrane potential is more depolarized. Further evidence on the deregulation of ion channels by Pitx2 impairment has been recently reported also by Kirchhof et al. (2011) using mRNA microarray analyses in Pitx2c heterozygous adult mutant mice. Thus, these data reveal a role for Pitx2 controlling ion channel expression, and thus a link to atrial arrhythmogenesis, as summarized in **Figure 1**.

CONCLUDING REMARKS AND PERSPECTIVE

We have highlighted herein our current knowledge on the role of Pitx2 in the developing and adult heart as well as on the state-of-the-art link between PITX2 and AF. Several studies have shown that Pitx2 is essential for pulmonary vein development (Mommersteeg et al., 2007), a highly recurrent pro-arrhythmogenic region in humans. Experimental evidence has shown that Pitx2 is important for transcriptional regulation in the secondary heart field (Ai et al., 2006), derivatives of which will form the venous pole of the heart. Similarly, additional evidence has revealed a role of Pitx2 in the regulation of cell-to-cell communication proteins and essential ion channels, which modulate critical aspects of the cardiac action potential, as well as a role repressing the sinoatrial node gene program (Wang et al., 2010; Chinchilla et al., 2011; Kirchhof et al., 2011). Overall, these data strongly implicate Pitx2 as an upstream regulator of pro-arrhythmogenic events. However, there are several missing links. The first one is how the identified genetic variants alter Pitx2 expression and to date, this point

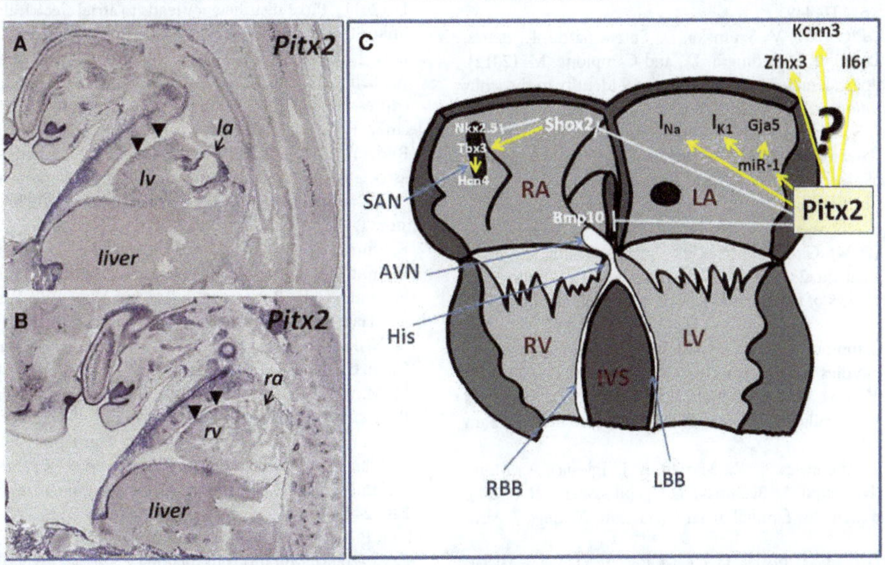

FIGURE 1 | (A,B) Illustrations of Pitx2 expression in the developing fetal embryo (E14.5) in longitudinal histological sections. **(A)** Illustrate the expression of Pitx2 at the level of the left ventricle (lv) and left atria (la), showing the robust expression of Pitx2 in the developing left atrial chamber, whereas **(B)** illustrates the expression of Pitx2 at the level of the right ventricle (rv) and right atrium (ra). Observe the marked contrast of expression between the right atrium (low) and the left atrium (high) as revealed by the arrows. Note also the dorso-ventral difference of Pitx2 expression at the ventricular level [arrowheads, **(A,B)**]. **(C)** Schematic representation of the current state-of-the-art role of Pitx2 in the developing and adult atrial chambers linked to atrial arrhythmogenesis. Pitx2 controls miR-1 expression in the left atrial chamber, providing thus a regulatory mechanism for I_{K1} and Gja1 function. In addition Pitx2 regulates I_{Na} while inhibits the expression right atrial (Bmp10) and sinoatrial (Shox2) markers in the left atrium, which in turn play key regulatory roles on cardiomyocyte cell cycle and pacemaker activity, providing additional links to atrial arrhythmias.

remains unanswered. Secondly, it remains elusive how altered Pitx2 expression would modify conductive elements leading to the onset of AF (although new insights have progressively being gained; **Figure 1**), in particular whether the impaired conductive elements might be deregulated already from embryonic stages, as suggested by Wang et al. (2010) and Ammirabile et al. (2012) or exclusively in the fetal/adult heart as reported by Kirchhof et al. (2011) and Chinchilla et al. (2011). On the basis of the developmental role of Pitx2, it might be postulated that impaired Pitx2 in the developing heart might be a predisposing factor for AF. However, an early defect in Pitx2 function would be expected to have severe consequences for cardiac embryogenesis, and thus it is more likely that fetal or adult dysfunction might underlie Pitx2 predisposition to AF. In addition, it is unclear if Pitx2 deficiency might also lead to impaired formation and/or function of other components of the ventricular cardiac conduction system such as the AV node and the left and right AV bundle branches. Morphological analysis of the ventricular conduction system in the left–right mutant mouse model *iv/iv* suggests that left/right cues can influence AV node formation (Franco and Icardo, 2001). Nonetheless, further studies are required to demonstrate a putative role of Pitx2 in ventricular conduction system deployment.

Interestingly, in addition to reports linking 4q25 risk variants to AF, new GWAS have identified several other genetic variants highly associated with AF, which are located at 9p21, 1q21, and 16q22, respectively. On chromosome 9p21, no candidate gene has been linked to AF, and thus its relevance awaits further experimental and functional evidence (Larson et al., 2007). However, genetic variants at 1q21 are linked to KCNN3 (Ellinor et al., 2011) and IL6R (Schnabel et al., 2011), respectively whereas risk genetic variants at 16q22 are linked to ZFHX3 (Gudbjartsson et al., 2009). To date it remains elusive the putative involvement of these genes in the pathophysiology of AF. A putative scenario might be that PITX2 might modulate these genes. Thus, further insights are required to explore both the links between all GWAS associated genes as well as the cellular and molecular mechanisms that might underlie a functional role between KCNN3, IL6R and ZFHX3, and AF, yet this aspect remains to be elucidated. Thus, new exciting dates are ahead right now.

ACKNOWLEDGMENTS

This work is partially supported by the VI EU Integrated Project "Heart Failure and Cardiac Repair" LSHM-CT-2005-018630 to Diego Franco, a grant from the Junta de Andalucía Regional Council to Diego Franco (CTS-1614), a grant from the Junta de Andalucía Regional Council to Amelia E. Aránega (CTS-03878), and grants from the Ministry of Science and Innovation of the Spanish Government to Diego Franco (MICINN BFU2009-11566) and to Amelia E. Aránega (MICINN BFU-2008-01217). This work is partially supported by a translational CNIC grant (2009-08) to Diego Franco.

REFERENCES

Ai, D., Liu, W., Ma, L., Dong, F., Lu, M. F., Wang, D., Verzi, M. P., Cai, C., Gage, P. J., Evans, S., Black, B. L., Brown, N. A., and Martin, J. F. (2006). Pitx2 regulates cardiac left-right asymme-try by patterning second cardiac lineage-derived myocardium. *Dev. Biol.* 296, 437–449.

Ammirabile, G., Tessari, A., Pignataro, V., Szumska, D., Sutera Sardo, F., Benes, J. Jr., Balistreri, M., Bhattacharya, S., Sedmera, D., and Campione, M. (2012). Pitx2 confers left morphological, molecular, and functional identity to the sinus venosus myocardium. *Cardiovasc.* Res. 93, 291–301.

Arnar, D. O., Thorvaldsson, S., Manolio, T. A., Thorgeirsson, G., Kristjansson, K., Hakonarson, H., and Stefansson, K. (2006). Familial aggregation of atrial fabrillation in Iceland. *Eur. Heart* J. 27, 708–712.

Bamforth, S. D., Bragança, J., Farthing, C. R., Schneider, J. E., Broadbent, C., Michell, A. C., Clarke, K., Neubauer, S., Norris, D., Brown, N. A., Anderson, R. H., and Bhattacharya, S. (2004). Cited2 controls left-right patterning and heart developmentthrough a Nodal-Pitx2c pathway. *Nat. Genet.* 36, 1189–1196.

Bellet, S. (1971). *Clinical Disorders of the Heart Beat,* 3rd Edn. Philadelphia: Lea& Febiger.

Blum, M., Steinbeisser, H., Campione, M., and Schweickert, A. (1999). Vertebrate left-right asymmetry: old studies and new insights. *Cell. Mol. Biol.* 45, 505–516.

Brand, F. N., Abbott, R. D., Kannel, W. B., and Wolf, P. A. (1985). Characteristics and prognosis of lone atrial fibrillation. 30-year follow-up in the Framingham Study. *JAMA* 254, 3449–3453.

Brugada, R., Tapscott, T., Czernuszewicz, G. Z., Marian, A. J., Iglesias, A., Mont, L., Brugada, J., Girona, J., Domingo, A., Bachinski, L. L., and Roberts, R. (1997). Identification of a genetic locus for familial atrial fibrillation. *N. Engl. J. Med.* 336, 905–911.

Campione, M., Ros, M. A., Icardo, J. M., Piedra, E., Christoffels, V. M., Schweickert, A., Blum, M., Franco, D., and Moorman, A. F. (2001). Pitx2 expression defines a left cardiac lineage of cells: evidence for atrial and ventricular molecular isomerism in the iv/iv mice. *Dev. Biol.* 231, 252–264.

Campione, M., Steinbeisser, H., Schweickert, A., Deissler, K., van Bebber, F., Lowe, L. A., Nowotschin, S.,Viebahn, C., Haffter, P., Kuehn, M. R., and Blum, M. (1999). The homeobox gene Pitx2: mediator of asymmetric left-right signaling in vertebrate heart and gut looping. *Development* 126, 1225–1234.

Chen, Y. H., Xu, S. J., Bendahhou, S., Wang, X. L., Wang, Y., Xu, W. Y., Jin, H.-W., Sun, H., Su1, X.-Y., Zhuang, Q. N., Yang, Y.-Q., Li, Y. B., Liu, Y., Xu, H. J., Li, X. F., Ma, N., Mou, C. P., Chen, Z., Barhanin, J., and Huang, W. (2003). KCNQ1 gain-of-function mutation in familial atrial fibrillation. *Science* 299, 251–254.

Chinchilla, A., Daimi, H., Lozano Velasco, E., Dominguez, J. N., Caballero, R., Delpon, E., Tamargo, J., Cinca, J., Hove-Madsen, L., Aranega, A. E., and Franco, D. (2011). Pitx2 insufficiency leads to atrial electrical and structural remodelling linked to arrhythmogenesis. *Circ. Cardiovasc. Genet.* 4, 269–279.

Cox, C. J., Espinoza, H. M., McWilliams, B., Chappell, K., Morton, L., Hjalt, T. A., Semina, E. V., and Amendt, B. A. (2002). Differential regulation of gene expression by PITX2 isoforms. *J. Biol. Chem.* 277, 25001–25010.

Delaney, J. T., Jeff, J. M., Brown, N. J., Pretorius, M., Okafor, H. E., Darbar, D., Roden, D. M., and Crawford, D. C. (2012). Characterization of genome-wide associationidentified variants for atrial fibrillation in African Americans. *PLoS ONE* 7, e32338. doi:10.1371/journal.pone.0032338

Ellinor, P. T., Lunetta, K. L., Glazer, N. L., Pfeufer, A., Alonso, A., Chung, M. K.,Sinner, M. F., de Bakker, P. I., Mueller, M., Lubitz, S. A., Fox, E., Darbar, D.,Smith, N. L., Smith, J. D., Schnabel, R. B., Soliman, E. Z., Rice, K. M., Van Wagoner, D. R., Beckmann, B. M., van Noord, C., Wang, K., Ehret, G. B., Rotter, J. I., Hazen, S. L., Steinbeck, G., Smith, A. V., Launer, L. J., Harris, T. B., Makino, S., Nelis, M., Milan, D. J., Perz, S., Esko, T., Köttgen, A., Moebus, S., Newton-Cheh, C., Li, M., Möhlenkamp, S., Wang, T. J., Kao, W. H., Vasan, R. S., Nöthen, M. M., MacRae, C. A., Stricker, B. H., Hofman, A., Uitterlinden, A. G., Levy, D., Boerwinkle, E., Metspalu, A., Topol, E. J., Chakravarti, A., Gudnason, V., Psaty, B. M., Roden, D. M., Meitinger, T., Wichmann, H. E., Witteman, J. C., Barnard, J., Arking, D. E., Benjamin, E. J., Heckbert, S. R., and Kääb, S. (2011). Common variants in KCNN3 are associated with lone atrial fibrillation. *Nat. Genet.* 42, 240–244.

Ellinor, P. T., Moore, R. K., Patton, K. K., Ruskin, J. N., Pollak, M. R., and Macrae, C. A. (2004). Mutations in the long QT gene, KCNQ1, are an uncommon cause of atrial fibrillation. *Heart* 90, 1487–1488.

Ellinor, P. T., Nam, E. G., Shea, M. A., Milan, D. J., Ruskin, J. N., and MacRae, C. A. (2007). Car- diac sodium channel mutation in atrial fibrillation. *Heart Rhythm* 5, 99–105.

Franco, D., and Campione, M. (2003). The role of Pitx2 during cardiac development. Linking left-right sig- naling and congenital heart dis- eases. *Trends Cardiovasc. Med.* 13, 157–163.

Franco, D., Campione, M., Kelly, R., Zammit, P. S., Buckingham, M., Lamers, W. H., and Moorman, A. F. (2000). Multiple transcriptional domains, with distinct left and right components, in the atrial chambers of the developing heart. *Circ. Res.* 87, 984–991.

Franco, D., and Icardo, J. M. (2001). Molecular characterization of the ventricular conduction sys- tem in the developing mouse heart: topographical correlation in normal and congenitally mal- formed hearts. *Cardiovasc. Res.* 49, 417–429.

Fuster, V., Rydean, L. E., Asinger, R. W., Cannom, D. S., Crijns, H. J., Frye, R. L., Halperin, J. L., Kay, G. N., Klein, W. W., Lévy, S., McNamara, R. L., Prystowsky, E. N., Wann, L. S., Wyse, D. G., and Gibbons, R. J. (2001). ACC/AHA/ESC guidelines for the management of patients with atrial fibrillation. *Circulation* 104, 2118–2150.

Gage, P. J., Suh, H., and Camper, S. A. (1999). Dosage requirement of Pitx2 for development of multiple organs. *Development* 126, 4643–4465.

Galli, D., Domínguez, J. N., Zaffran, S., Munk, A., Brown, N. A., and Buckingham, M. E. (2008). Atrial myocardium derives from the pos- terior region of the second heart field, which acquires left-right iden- tity as Pitx2c is expressed. *Develop- ment* 135, 1157–1167.

Gollob, M. H., Jones, D. L., Krahn, A. D., Danis, L., Gong, X. Q., Shao, Q., Liu, X., Veinot, J. P., Tang, A. S., Stewart, A. F., Tesson, F., Klein, G. J., Yee, R., Skanes, A. C., Guiraudon, G. M., Ebihara, L., and Bai, D. (2006). Somatic mutations in the connexin 40 gene (GJA5) in atrial fibrillation. *N. Engl. J. Med.* 354, 2677–2688.

Gudbjartsson, D. F., Arnar, D. O., Hel- gadottir, A., Gretarsdottir, S., Holm, H., Sigurdsson, A., Jonasdottir, A., Baker, A., Thorleifsson, G., Krist- jansson, K., Palsson, A., Blondal, T., Sulem, P., Backman, V. M., Hardar- son, G. A., Palsdottir, E., Helga- son, A., Sigurjonsdottir, R., Sverris- son, J. T., Kostulas, K., Ng, M. C., Baum, L., So, W. Y., Wong, K. S., Chan, J. C., Furie, K. L., Greenberg, S. M., Sale, M., Kelly, P., MacRae, C. A., Smith, E. E., Rosand, J., Hillert, J., Ma, R. C., Ellinor, P. T., Thorgeirsson, G., Gulcher, J. R., Kong, A., Thorsteinsdottir, U., and Stefansson, K. (2007). Variants conferring risk of atrial fibrillation on chromosome 4q25. *Nature* 448, 353–357.

Gudbjartsson, D. F., Holm, H., Gretarsdottir, S., Thorleifsson, G., Wal- ters, G. B., Thorgeirsson, G., Walters, G. B., Thorgeirsson, G., Gulcher, J., Mathiesen, E. B., Njølstad, I., Nyrnes, A., Wilsgaard, T., Hald, E. M., Hveem, K., Stoltenberg, C., Kucera, G., Stubblefield, T., Carter, S., Roden, D., Ng, M. C., Baum, L., So, W. Y., Wong, K. S., Chan, J. C., Gieger, C., Wichmann, H. E., Gschwendtner, A., Dichgans, M., Kuhlenbäumer, G., Berger, K., Ringelstein, E. B., Bevan, S., Markus, H. S., Kostu- las, K., Hillert, J., Sveinbjörnsdót- tir, S., Valdimarsson, E. M., Løchen, M. L., Ma, R. C., Darbar, D., Kong, A., Arnar, D. O., Thorsteinsdot- tir, U., and Stefansson, K. (2009). A sequence variant in ZFHX3 on 16q22 associates with atrial fibrilla- tion and ischemic stroke. *Nat. Genet.* 41, 876–878.

Gussak, I., and Antzelevitch, C. (2008). Electrical Diseases of the Heart: Genetics, *mechanisms, Treatment, Prevention*. London: Springer-Verlag.

Haissaguerre, M., Jais, P., Shah, D. C., Takahashi, A., Hocini, M., Quin- iou, G., Garrigue, S., Le Mouroux, A., Le Métayer, P., and Clé- menty, J. (1998). Spontaneous ini- tiation of atrial fibrillation by ectopic beats originating in the pul- monary veins. *N. Engl. J. Med.* 339, 659–666.

Hamada, H., Meno, C., Saijoh, Y., Adachi, H., Yashiro, K., Sakuma, R., and Shiratori, H. (2001). Role of asymmetric signals in left-right pat- terning in the mouse. *Am. J. Med. Genet.* 101, 324–327.

Henningsen, K. M., Olesen, M. S., Haunsoe, S., and Svendsen, J. H. (2011). Association of rs2200733 at 4q25 with early onset of lone atrial fibrillation in young patients. *Scand. Cardiovasc. J.* 45, 324–326.

Hjalt, T. A., and Semina, E. V. (2005). Current molecular understanding of Axenfeld-Rieger syndrome. *Expert Rev. Mol. Med.* 7, 1–17.

Kahr, P. C., Piccini, I., Fabritz, L., Greber, B., Schöler, H., Scheld, H. H., Hoffmeier, A., Brown, N. A., and Kirchhof, P. (2011). System- atic analysis of gene expression differences between left and right atria in different mouse strains and in human atrial tissue. *PLoS ONE* 6, e26389. doi:10.1371/jour- nal.pone.0026389

Kannel, W. B., Wolf, P. A., Benjamin, E. J., and Levy, D. (1998). Prevalence, incidence, prognosis, and predisposing conditions for atrial fibrillation: population-based estimates. *Am. J. Cardiol.* 82, 2N–9N.

Kelly, R. G., Brown, N. A., and Buck- ingham, M. E. (2001). The arter- ial pole of the mouse heart forms from Fgf10-expressing cells in pha- ryngeal mesoderm. *Dev. Cell* 1, 435–440.

Kiliszek, M., Franaszczyk, M., Kozluk, E., Lodzinski, P., Piatkowska, A., Broda, G., Ploski, R., and Opolski, G. (2011). Association between vari- ants on chromosome 4q25, 16q22 and 1q21 and atrial fibrillation in the Polish population. *PLoS ONE* 6, e21790. doi:10.1371/jour- nal.pone.0021790

Kirchhof, P., Kahr, P. C., Kaese, S., Piccini, I., Vokshi, I., Scheld, H. H., Rotering, H., Fortmueller, L., Laakmann, S., Verheule, S., Schot- ten, U., Fabritz, L., and Brown, N. A. (2011). PITX2c is expressed in the adult left atrium, and reduc- ing Pitx2c expression promotes atrial fibrillation inducibility and complex changes in gene expres- sion. *Circ. Cardiovasc. Genet.* 4, 123–133.

Larson, M. G., Atwood, L. D., Benjamin, E. J., Cupples, L. A., D'Agostino, R. B. Sr., Fox, C. S., Govindaraju, D. R., Guo, C. Y., Heard-Costa, N. L., Hwang, S. J., Murabito, J. M., Newton-Cheh, C., O'Donnell, C. J., Seshadri, S., Vasan, R. S., Wang, T. J., Wolf, P. A., and Levy, D. (2007). Framingham Heart Study 100K project: genome-wide associations for cardiovascular disease outcomes. *BMC Med. Genet.* 8(Suppl. 1), S5. doi:10.1186/1471-2350-8-S1-S5

Lin, C. R., Kioussi, C., O'Connell, S., Briata, P., Szeto, D., Liu, F., Izpisúa- Belmonte, J. C., and Rosenfeld, M. G. (1999). Pitx2 regulates lung asymmetry, cardiac positioning and pituitary and tooth morphogenesis. *Nature* 401, 279–282.

Liu, C., Liu, W., Lu, M. F., Brown, N. A., and Martin, J. F. (2001). Regulation of left-right asymmetry by thresh- olds of Pitx2c activity. *Development* 128, 2039–2048.

Liu, C., Liu, W., Palie, J., Lu, M. F., Brown, N. A., and Martin, J. F. (2002). Pitx2c patterns anterior myocardium and aortic arch vessels and is required for local cell move- ment into atrioventricular cushions. *Development* 129, 5081–5091.

Liu, X., Wang, F., Knight, A. C., Zhao, J., and Xiao, J. (2012). Com- mon variants for atrial fibrillation: results from genome-wide associ- ation studies. *Hum. Genet.* 131, 33–39.

Lozano-Velasco, E., Chinchilla, A., Martinez-Fernandez, S., Hernandez- Torres, F., Navarro, F., Lyons, G., Franco, D., and Aránega, A. E. (2011). Pitx2c modulates cardiac specific transcription factor net- works in differentiating cardiomy- ocytes from murine embryonic stem cells. *Cells Tissues Organs(Print)* 194, 349–362.

Mc Nair, W. P., Ku, L., Taylor, M. R., Fain, P. R., Dao, D., Wolfel, E., Mestroni, L., and The Familial Cardiomyopa- thy Registry Research Group. (2004). SCN5A mutation associated with dilated car-diomyopathy, conduc- tion disorder, and arrhythmia. *Cir- culation* 110, 2163–2167.

Moe, G. K., and Abildskov, J. A. (1959). Atrial fibrillation as a self sus- taining arrhythmia independent of focal discharge. *Am. Heart J.* 58, 59–70.

Mommersteeg, M. T., Brown, N. A., Prall, O. W., de Gier-de Vries, C., Harvey, R. P., Moorman, A. F., and Christoffels, V. M. (2007). Pitx2c and Nkx2-5 are required for the formation and identity of the pul- monary myocardium. *Circ. Res.* 101, 902–909.

Nowotschin, S., Liao, J., Gage, P. J., Epstein, J. A., Campione, M., and Morrow, B. E. (2006). Tbx1 affects asymmetric cardiac morphogene- sis by regulating Pitx2 in the sec- ondary heart field. *Development* 133, 1565–1573.

Olesen, M. S., Holst, A. G., Jabbari, J., Nielsen, J. B., Christophersen, I. E., Sajadieh, A., Haunsø, S., and Svendsen, J. H. (2012). Genetic loci on chromosomes 4q25, 7p31, and 12p12 are associated with onset of lone atrial fibrillation before the age of 40 years. *Can. J. Cardiol.* 28, 191–195.

Schnabel, R. B., Kerr, K. F., Lubitz, S. A., Alkylbekova, E. L., Marcus, G. M., Sinner, M. F., Magnani, J. W., Wolf, P. A., Deo, R., Lloyd-Jones, D. M., Lunetta, K. L., Mehra, R., Levy, D., Fox, E. R., Arking, D. E., Mosley, T. H., Müller-Nurasyid, M., Young, T. R., Wichmann, H. E., Seshadri, S., Farlow, D. N., Rot- ter, J. I., Soliman, E. Z., Glazer, N. L., Wilson, J. G., Breteler, M. M., Sotoodehnia, N., Newton-Cheh, C., Kääb, S., Ellinor, P. T., Alonso, A., Benjamin, E. J., Heckbert, S. R., and Candidate Gene Associa- tion Resource (CARe) Atrial Fib- rillation/ Electrocardiography Work- ing Group. (2011). Large-scale can- didate gene analysis in whites and African Americans identifies IL6R polymorphism in relation to atrial fibrillation: the National Heart, Lung, and Blood Institute's Can- didate Gene Association Resource (CARe) project. *Circ. Cardiovasc. Genet.* 4, 557–564.

Schotten, U., Verheule, S., Kirchhof, P., and Goette, A. (2011). Pathophys- iological mechanisms of atrial fib- rillation: a translational appraisal. *Physiol. Rev.* 91, 265–325.

Schweickert, A., Campione, M., Steinbeisser, H., and Blum, M. (2000). Pitx2 isoforms:involvement of Pitx2c but not Pitx2a or Pitx2b in vertebrate left-right asymmetry. *Mech. Dev.* 90, 41–51.

Tessari, A., Pietrobon, M., Notte, A., Cifelli, G., Gage, P. J., Schneider, M. D., Lembo, G., and Campione, M. (2008). Myocardial Pitx2 dif- ferentially regulates the left atrial identity and ventricular asymmetric remodeling programs. *Circ. Res.* 102, 813–822.

Wakili, R., Voigt, N., Kääb, S., Dobrev, D., and Nattel, S. (2011). Recent advances in the molecular patho- physiology of atrial fibrillation. *J. Clin. Invest.* 121, 2955–2968.

Wang, J., Klysik, E., Sood, S., Johnson, R. L., Wehrens, X. H., and Martin, J. F. (2010). Pitx2 prevents susceptibil- ity to atrial arrhythmias by inhibit- ing left-sided pacemaker specifica- tion. *Proc. Natl. Acad. Sci. U.S.A.* 107, 9753–9758.

Xia, M., Jin, Q., Bendahhou, S., He, Y., Larroque, M. M., Chen, Y., Zhou, Q., Yang, Y., Liu, Y., Liu, B., Zhu, Q., Zhou, Y., Lin, J., Liang, B., Li, L., Dong, X., Pan,

Z., Wang, R., Wan, H., Qiu, W., Xu, W., Eurlings, P., Barhanin, J., and Chen, Y. (2005). A Kir2.1 gain-of-function mutation underlies familial atrial fibrillation. *Biochem. Biophys. Res. Commun.* 332, 1012–1019.

Yang, Y., Xia, M., Jin, Q., Bendahhou, S., Shi, J., Chen, Y., Liang, B., Lin, J., Liu, Y., Liu, B., Zhou, Q., Zhang, D., Wang, R., Ma, N., Su, X., Niu, K., Pei, Y., Xu, W., Chen, Z., Wan, H., Cui, J., Barhanin, J., and Chen, Y. (2004). Identification of a KCNE2 gain-of- function mutation in patients with familial atrial fibrillation. *Am. J. Hum. Genet.* 75, 899–905.

Yashiro, K., Shiratori, H., and Hamada, H. (2007). Haemodynamics deter- mined by a genetic programme govern asymmetric development of the aortic arch. *Nature* 450, 285–258.

16

Fibrosis in atrial fibrillation – Role of reactive species and MPO

Kai Friedrichs*[1]*, Stephan Baldus*[2] *and Anna Klinke*[2]**

[1] *Department of Electrophysiology, Cardiovascular Research Center, University Heart Center Hamburg, Hamburg, Germany*
[2] *Department of General and Interventional Cardiology, Cardiovascular Research Center, University Heart Center Hamburg, Hamburg, Germany*

***Correspondence:**
Anna Klinke, Department of Cardiology and Cardiovascular Research Center, University Medical Center Hamburg Eppendorf, University Heart Center Hamburg, Martinistrasse 52, 20246 Hamburg, Germany.
e-mail: aklinke@uke.uni-hamburg.de

Atrial fibrosis with enhanced turnover and deposition of matrix proteins leads to inhomogeneous atrial electrical conduction and gives rise to electrical reentry circuits resulting in atrial fibrillation. The multifactorial pathogenesis of atrial fibrosis involves resident cardiac cells as well as infiltrating leukocytes, both generating and sequestering matrix metalloproteinases (MMPs), a key enzyme family involved in fibrosis. A growing body of evidence points toward an important role of reactive oxygen species (ROS) in the release and activation of pro-MMPs and the stimulation of pro-fibrotic cascades. Myeloperoxidase (MPO), a bactericidal enzyme released from activated polymorphonuclear neutrophils (PMN) is not only associated with a variety of cardiovascular diseases, but has also been shown to be mechanistically linked to atrial fibrosis and fibrillation. MPO catalyzes the generation of reactive species like hypochlorous acid, which affect intracellular signaling cascades in various cells and advance activation of pro-MMPs and deposition of atrial collagen resulting in atrial arrhythmias. Thus, inflammatory mechanisms effectively promote atrial structural remodeling and importantly contribute to the initiation and perpetuation of atrial fibrillation.

Keywords: atrial fibrillation, fibrosis, reactive oxygen species, myeloperoxidase

INTRODUCTION

Atrial fibrillation (AF) remains the most prevalent rhythm disorder affecting 1–1.5% of the population in western industrialized countries and its prevalence is supposed to double within the next 50 years (Go et al., 2001; Savelieva and Camm, 2008). With thromboembolic events as one of the most hazardous complications of this disease, AF emerges as a substantial contributor to morbidity and mortality (Kannel et al., 1982; Tsang et al., 2003; Wang et al., 2003).

AF may be triggered by spontaneous premature depolarizations of myocytes originating, e.g., from the pulmonary veins, alternatively by rapid electrical activity in the form of pulmonary vein tachycardia. Once apparent, AF causes alterations of electrical properties of the atria such as reduction of refractory period, which further propagate the perpetuation of AF (Haïssaguerre et al., 1998).

Consequently, electrical isolation of the pulmonary veins is often an important and effective therapeutic strategy especially in patients with paroxysmal AF or in patients without cardiovascular comorbidities ("lone atrial fibrillation"). But a significant number of patients particularly with persistent or chronic AF remains refractory to this approach, pointing toward involvement of atrial tissue as a substrate in those types of AF (Allessie, 1998; Calkins et al., 2012). In particular cardiovascular diseases such as arterial hypertension, heart failure, coronary artery disease, valvular, or inflammatory disease are independent risk factors to AF. In fact, these disorders are believed to be mechanistically involved, since they participate in electrical, contractile, and structural remodeling of atrial tissue (Kannel et al., 1982).

Still, intercellular and subcellular mechanisms underlying AF remain incompletely understood: besides electrical abnormalities mainly based on ion channel dysfunction and contractile remodeling yielding atrial hypocontractility and atrial dilatation, structural remodeling owing to atrial fibrosis has emerged as one of the key aspects in the pathophysiology of AF (Goette et al., 1996; Iwasaki et al., 2011).

Accumulating evidence now advocates for a critical mechanistic role of inflammatory processes in the pathogenesis of atrial fibrosis. This review intends to summarize the role of reactive species in the development of atrial fibrosis and to elucidate the impact of the leukocyte-derived enzyme myeloperoxidase (MPO) herein.

FIBROSIS IN ATRIAL FIBRILLATION

FIBROSIS – A SUBSTRATE FOR ATRIAL FIBRILLATION

Apart from electrical remodeling and contractile dysfunction, alterations in atrial tissue structure, namely atrial fibrosis, have been shown to increase the susceptibility to AF and may serve as a critical substrate in the formation of the arrhythmia. Additionally, atrial fibrosis is hard to reverse and has therefore been considered as a major contributor in the progression from paroxysmal to persistent or permanent AF (Xu et al., 2004). However, those structural abnormalities must not solely be related to AF but may also be present in patients with underlying or coexisting cardiovascular disease without necessarily increasing the vulnerability to AF.

Fibrosis has been observed in atrial tissue of patients with AF (Kostin et al., 2002; Boldt et al., 2004; Saito et al., 2007). Additionally, a correlation of the degree of atrial fibrosis with the persistence of AF in patients was demonstrated. Furthermore, in patients undergoing cardiovascular surgery, the degree of atrial fibrosis correlated with the risk for postoperative AF (Xu et al., 2004).

Of note, experimental and clinical investigations revealed, that prevention of atrial fibrosis attenuates AF stability, as anti-fibrotic therapeutic strategies (statins, ACE inhibitors, and AT1-receptor blocker) effectively limit AF substrate formation (Li et al., 2001; Kumagai et al., 2004; Sakabe et al., 2004; Milliez et al., 2005; Lee et al., 2006).

Mechanistically, experimental studies have demonstrated fibrosis to account for decreased velocity and increased heterogeneity of electrical conduction (Li et al., 1999; Ausma et al., 2003; Verheule et al., 2003, 2004; Lee et al., 2006; Rudolph et al., 2010).

Fibrosis-driven AF implies the disturbance of electrical conductance due to disruptions of intercellular communication of atrial myocytes. Collagen fibers represent electrical barriers, which can cause asynchronous propagation of electrical activation (de Jong et al., 2011b). The electrical barriers establish adjacent regions of diverging refractory periods (Spach and Boineau, 1997; Lin and Pan, 2008; Goudis et al., 2012). This morphological atrial compartmentalization facilitates the formation of micro- and macro-reentry circuits resulting in a higher susceptibility to AF.

Furthermore, the uncoupling of cardiomyocytes by collagen facilitates ectopic activity to arise in atrial tissue. Physiologic impulse conduction depends on a balance of energy for current conduction between a depolarized region ("source" of the current) and an adjacent repolarized region ("sink"; Nattel et al., 2008). A mismatch of this so called "source-to-sink" effect, which occurs by virtue of impaired myocyte coupling, enables the propagation of early or delayed after depolarizations (EADs or DADs). This is due to the fact that in well-coupled myocardium surrounding myocytes minimize voltage differences of neighboring cells and thereby suppress EAD or DAD propagation, whereas a decrease of the source-to-sink effect impairs this compensation (Nattel et al., 2008; Xie et al., 2010).

Interestingly, apart from matrix deposition also direct fibroblast-myocyte interactions contribute to electrophysiological alterations. Activated fibroblasts modify conduction velocities in cultured cardiomyocyte monolayers, and it was proven that a direct heterocellular electrotonic communication between cells can induce depolarization of the myocytes (Miragoli et al., 2007; Vasquez et al., 2010).

These electrical and structural characteristics of fibrotic remodeling give rise to a strong arrhythmogenic potential of this process.

EXTRACELLULAR MATRIX, MMPs, AND FIBROBLASTS

The myocardial extracellular matrix (ECM) consists of matrix proteins such as collagens and fibronectin, proteoglycans, and basement membrane proteins like laminins (Hagiwara, 2010). It further comprises various proteases and signaling molecules (Spinale, 2007). The predominant matrix proteins in myocardial ECM are the collagens type I and III, which are deposited in the myocardial interstitium in a fibrillar architecture to ensure myocardial stability and organization (Spinale, 2007). These proteins are arranged in a physiological balance of synthesis and degradation – with a disturbed balance associating with cardiac disease (Swynghedauw, 1999; de Jong et al., 2011a). Enhanced synthesis and deposition of ECM proteins can occur either as *replacement* fibrosis related to cell death or as *reactive* fibrosis. In particular interstitial reactive fibrosis has been identified to be highly pro-arrhythmic in the atrial myocardium (de Jong et al., 2011b). Whereas the myocardial production of ECM proteins is mainly carried out by fibroblasts and to a lesser extent by cardiomyocytes and smooth muscle cells, their degradation occurs primarily via matrix metalloproteinases (MMPs). MMPs comprise a family of proteolytic enzymes with a variety of different substrates. They are produced as inactive pro-enzymes mostly by fibroblasts, but also by cardiomyocytes and leukocytes, and can be activated by cleavage of their pro-peptide. In turn, inhibition of MMPs is due to tissue-inhibitors of MMPs (TIMPs). The interrelation of fibrotic remodeling and MMPs is complex and still not yet fully elucidated. Although active MMPs degrade matrix proteins, pro-fibrotic states are mostly accompanied by increased instead of decreased MMP-activity (Li et al., 2000; Nattel et al., 2005). Whether increased MMP expression and activity during states of myocardial remodeling reflects cause or consequence still remains to be fully determined. Pro-fibrotic molecules like TGF-β1 and the plasmin system are known to activate MMPs (Jugdutt, 2003; de Jong et al., 2011a). Thus, MMP-activity might be merely an epiphenomenon of the fibrotic process. However, accumulating evidence supports the notion of a causal role of MMPs in fibrosis and their activity is regarded to result in enhanced instead of reduced ECM deposition, which is particularly valid for the gelatinases MMP-2 and -9 (de Jong et al., 2011a). This assumption is supported by observations, that long-term inhibition of MMPs suppresses fibrosis (Nattel et al., 2005; Moe et al., 2008). This pro-fibrotic effect of MMPs might be due to the concomitant release of matrix-embedded bioactive molecules like cytokines as TNF-α and IL-1β (Flesch et al., 2003; Diwan et al., 2004), growth factors like TGF-β1 and angiotensin II (ATII), and endothelin-1 (Dell'Italia et al., 1997; Wei et al., 1999; Ergul et al., 2000; Multani et al., 2005), which further spur the fibrotic cascade. Furthermore, fragments of matrix proteins themselves form bioactive molecules, so called *matrikines*, which serve as ligands of leukocyte integrins and other cell activating receptors and effectively stimulate connective tissue formation (Li et al., 2000; Mott and Werb, 2004). Importantly, protein composition, organization, and cross-links rather than just the extent of deposition is considered relevant for the matrix pro-arrhythmic potential (Li et al., 2000; Pellman et al., 2010). It is known that MMP-degraded physiological collagens are replaced by fibrous interstitial deposits of various unorganized ECM proteins.

Collectively, enhanced matrix turnover affects signaling cascades of cardiomyocytes, fibroblasts, endothelial cells, and leukocytes creating an inflammatory milieu, which results in increased fibrotic remodeling (**Figure 1**).

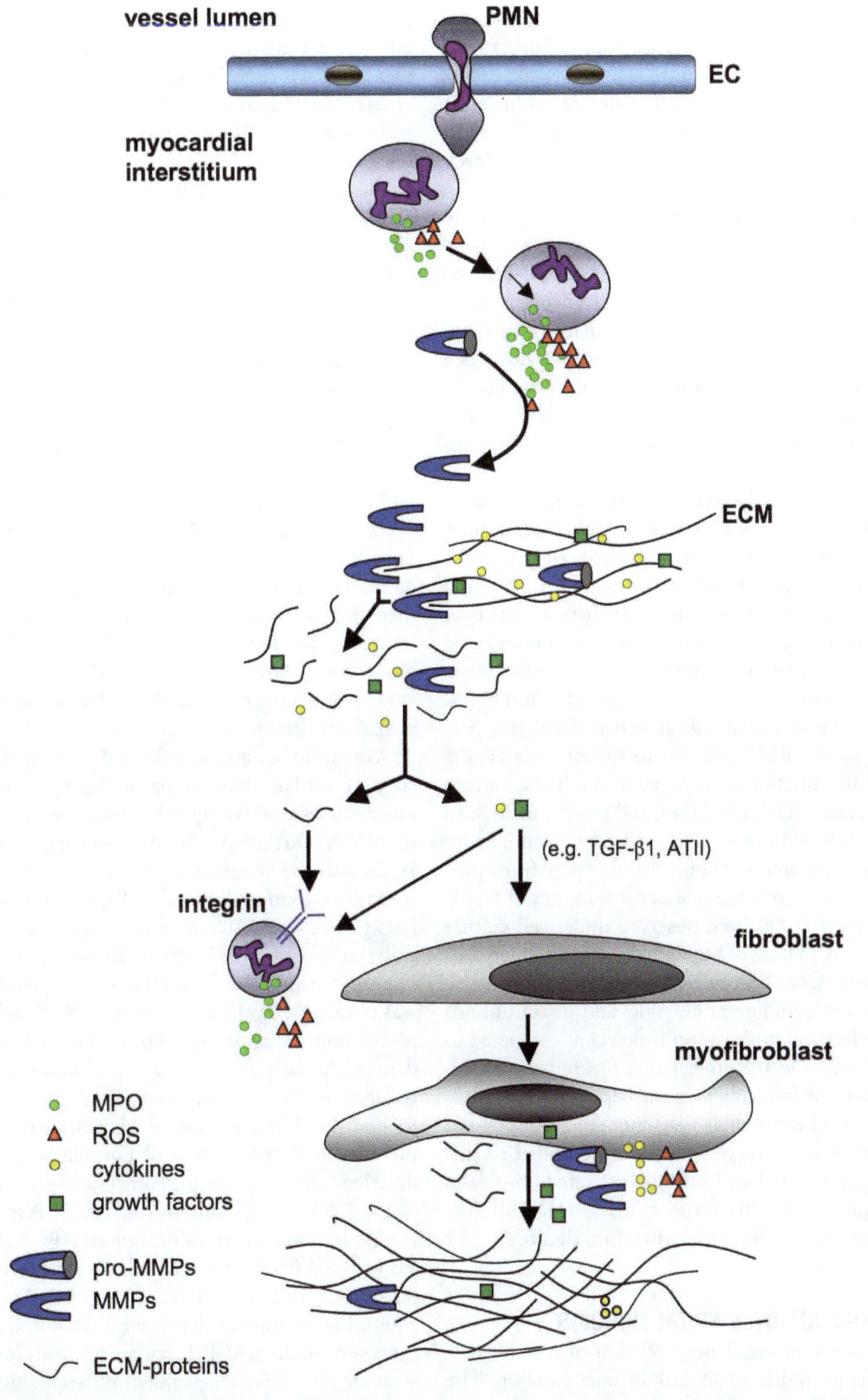

FIGURE 1 | Schematic overview of fibrotic remodeling triggered by reactive species. Neutrophils infiltrating the myocardial interstitium release MPO and ROS, which induce the activation of further neutrophils with sequestration of MPO, ROS, and pro-MMPs. Resident and leukocyte-derived pro-MMPs are converted by MPO and ROS to active MMPs, which degrade the ECM resulting in a release of ECM-protein fragments and embedded cytokines, growth factors, and MMPs. These molecules stimulate leukocytes to secrete further ROS and MPO as well as fibroblasts to differentiate into myofibroblasts. The latter produce cytokines, growth factors, pro-MMPs, and ECM proteins building up a fibrotic matrix. Abbreviations: EC, endothelial cell; ECM, extracellular matrix; MMP, matrix metalloproteinase; MPO, myeloperoxidase; PMN, polymorphonuclear neutrophil; ROS, reactive oxygen species.

The significance of ECM-turnover and MMPs for AF has clearly been pointed out in a number of experimental and clinical studies illustrating that MMP levels are associated with AF in patients with cardiovascular disease (Xu et al., 2004; Gai et al., 2009), demonstrating that MMP inhibition attenuates AF inducibility and maintenance (Moe et al., 2008) and showing that AF recurrence after ablation therapy is associated with MMP serum levels (Kato et al., 2009; Okumura et al., 2011).

Interestingly, the atrial myocardium is especially prone to fibrotic remodeling. Verheule et al. (2003) for example demonstrated that mice with cardiac overexpression of TGF-β1 developed solely atrial but not ventricular fibrosis. Healthy atrial myocardium not only contains more fibroblasts than ventricular myocardium (Hinescu et al., 2006; Burstein et al., 2008), but also displays a more pronounced response to pro-fibrotic stimuli. Atrial fibroblasts exhibit a markedly different gene expression profile and a profoundly increased disposition to proliferate and differentiate in culture and *in vivo* as compared to ventricular fibroblasts (Burstein et al., 2008). Upon differentiation the active fibroblast phenotype is referred to as *myofibroblast*. Myofibroblasts differ significantly from fibroblasts and are the principal cell type in the myocardium to produce growth factors, cytokines, MMPs, and ECM proteins (Yue et al., 2011). Moreover, they have a more pronounced disposition to migrate and to proliferate (Vasquez et al., 2011). Thus, the differentiation of fibroblasts to myofibroblasts is a central and important pro-fibrotic event. Besides fibroblasts, cardiac epithelial, and endothelial cells as well as circulating precursors can undergo the differentiation to myofibroblasts (Kis et al., 2011). The differentiation is provoked by mechanical stress, reactive oxygen species (ROS), cytokines, and growth factors. In particular TGF-β1, but also PDGF, ATII, and catecholamines are known to stimulate this process (Rohr, 2009). Apart from promoting the fibrotic cascade myofibroblasts *per se* may exert highly arrhythmogenic effects. It has been observed under cell-culture conditions and *in vivo*, that myofibroblasts have distinct electrophysiological properties. On the one hand, they can act as passive electrical conduits, but promote rather slow and discontinuous conduction, since electrical propagation is slower as compared to myocytes (Rohr, 2009). On the other hand, myofibroblasts can lead to ectopic activity by inducing myocyte depolarization. Electrotonic interaction via heterocellular gap-junctional coupling of myofibroblasts with cardiomyocytes has been described to differ significantly from that derived from non-activated fibroblasts (Rohr, 2009; Vasquez et al., 2011; Yue et al., 2011). This further underscores the potentially pro-arrhythmic significance of myofibroblasts.

OXIDATIVE STRESS PROMOTES ATRIAL FIBROSIS

Oxidative stress denotes an unbalanced relation of reactive oxidants and antioxidants and is a hallmark of inflammation. The major sources of reactive species in cardiac cells are mitochondria, xanthine oxidase, uncoupled NO-synthase and in particular NADPH-oxidases (Murdoch et al., 2006). Apart from resident cardiac cells, infiltrated leukocytes account for a large portion of ROS and reactive nitrogen species (RNS) in myocardial tissue via production of superoxide and release of pro-oxidant enzyme systems like MPO.

IMPACT OF REACTIVE SPECIES ON MMPs AND CARDIAC CELLS

Reactive oxygen and nitrogen species exert direct effects on MMPs both on a transcriptional and posttranslational level. The former implies primarily activation of mitogen-activated protein kinases (MAPK) and the Jak/Stat kinase pathway in cardiac cells, which leads to activation of transcription factors inducing MMP release (Siwik and Colucci, 2004; Spinale, 2007). Several *in vitro* studies demonstrate that hydrogen peroxide (H_2O_2) induces an increase in MMP release from endothelial cells or cardiac fibroblasts (Belkhiri et al., 1997; Siwik et al., 2001). Moreover, cytokine-induced superoxide production in cardiomyocytes or macrophages increased MMP transcription via MAPK activation (Gurjar et al., 2001; Yoo et al., 2002; Spallarossa et al., 2006). Apart from that, the impact of ROS and RNS on MMP transcription, in particular on MMP-2 and -9, has been proven *in vivo* and *ex vivo* in ischemia and reperfusion models or isolated perfused hearts (Wang et al., 2002, 2005; Scholz et al., 2004; Wainwright, 2004).

Many studies have documented posttranslational effects of ROS and RNS on MMPs (Rajagopalan et al., 1996; Fu et al., 2001; Gu et al., 2002; Wang et al., 2002; Yoon et al., 2002; Zhang et al., 2002; Spinale, 2007). Not only *in vitro* and in cell-culture, but also *in vivo* and *ex vivo* the cleavage of the pro-peptide is known to be directly mediated by reactive species. Activation of pro-MMP-2 and -9 has been observed in the presence of H_2O_2 (Rajagopalan et al., 1996; Siwik et al., 2001; Yoon et al., 2002), peroxynitrite (Rajagopalan et al., 1996; Wang et al., 2002), and hypochlorous acid (HOCl; Fu et al., 2001, 2003).

As mentioned above, ROS and RNS modulate the activation state of cardiac cells, in particular by activating MAPKs and other redox-sensitive signaling pathways. Apart from the release of MMPs, further pro-fibrotic pathways are induced thereby: H_2O_2 and the superoxide-generating system xanthine/xanthine oxidase led to modulation of collagen synthesis in cardiac fibroblasts (Siwik et al., 2001). Interestingly, a reduced production of collagen was observed herein. However, *in vivo* studies proved increased deposition of collagen in dependence on ROS, as it was observed in rat hearts following ATII-dependent superoxide production (Zhao et al., 2008). Here, treatment with antioxidants simultaneously to ATII-application reduced the myocardial collagen volume and prevented in part the expression of TGF-β1 and the differentiation of fibroblasts to myofibroblasts. The pro-fibrotic differentiation of fibroblasts to myofibroblasts – as described above – is amongst others also provoked by ROS (Hecker et al., 2009; Barnes and Gorin, 2011). Peroxynitrite for example induced nuclear translocation of NFκ-B in fibroblasts, which led to the differentiation to myofibroblasts with enhanced production of TGF-β, fibronectin, and collagen I (Ichikawa et al., 2008). Furthermore, it has been disclosed, that TGF-β1-induced expression of the NADPH-oxidase isoform Nox4 is mainly responsible for the TGF-β1-dependent differentiation of fibroblasts. In fact, the released superoxide led to activation of the well-known downstream target of TGF-β1, i.e., Smad 2/3 (Cucoranu et al., 2005). Likewise, Nox2 was identified in different animal models to mediate pro-fibrotic effects (Murdoch et al., 2006). Interstitial fibrosis induced by ATII- or aldosterone-administration or transaortic banding has been described to be markedly reduced in Nox2-deficient mice, which was related to changes in expression of collagen and growth factors and activation of NF-κB (Bendall et al., 2002; Sun et al., 2002; Grieve et al., 2006; Johar et al., 2006). Moreover, the involvement of NADPH-oxidases in the activation of pro-fibrotic cascades in cardiac cells has been observed in mice with cardiac deficiency or overexpression of the NADPH-oxidase subunit Rac-1 (Li et al., 2010; Reil et al., 2010; Adam et al., 2011). Interestingly, ROS are described to provoke the formation of an inflammasome – a cytosolic multiprotein complex, which leads to the expression of IL-1β in cardiac fibroblasts with subsequent enhancement of fibrosis (Kawaguchi et al., 2011).

LEUKOCYTES IN ATRIAL FIBRILLATION

Leukocytes account for the major source of ROS at inflammatory sites with polymorphonuclear neutrophils (PMN) being the first cell type to infiltrate affected tissue.

Whereas the impact of signaling cascades and ROS-formation within cardiac cells was solidified, the role of leukocytes for the development of AF remained undefined. Recent observations however now provide evidence for a causal role of these cells in AF. Elevated atrial leukocyte infiltration is not only found in patients with AF with an underlying structural heart disease (Yamashita, 2007; Chen et al., 2008) as well as in patients with lone AF (Frustaci et al., 1997), but also independently predicts post-surgery AF (Lamm et al., 2006; Ramlawi et al., 2007). Moreover, leukocyte adhesion molecules like VCAM-1 are elevated in animal models and in patients with AF (Goette et al., 2008). So far, it remains unclear whether this is cause or consequence of the atrial arrhythmia. However, the leukocytes' armament of cytokines like IL-6 and TNF-α, proteases like MMP-8 and -9 and peroxidases like MPO, all of which have been shown to be involved in atrial remodeling (Han et al., 2001; Saba et al., 2005; Spinale, 2007; Rudolph et al., 2010), advocates for an important role of leukocytes in AF.

ROLE OF MYELOPEROXIDASE

MPO AND REACTIVE SPECIES

As stated above, cardiovascular disorders like hypertension, coronary artery disease, and heart failure are important risk factors for AF. Myeloperoxidase (MPO) is not only secreted in a variety of these diseases and in AF itself, but has also been identified to be mechanistically linked to these disorders (Nicholls and Hazen, 2005; Lau and Baldus, 2006), which calls for a deeper understanding of MPO's contribution.

MPO is a heme peroxidase expressed in myeloid cells – in particular in neutrophils MPO makes up to 5% of the protein dry weight. It is stored in azurophilic granules, which secrete the enzyme into the phagosome or extracellular environment upon activation of the PMN. H_2O_2 is the essential substrate necessary to convert MPO to an oxidized form (compound I). This in turn reacts with various oxidizable molecules resulting in the generation of ROS and RNS. Primarily (pseudo)halides serve as substrates, with chloride being the most abundant one in physiological environments leading to the formation of HOCl, which is the strongest bactericidal oxidant produced by PMN (**Figure 2**). However, deficiency of MPO in mice and humans is unexpectedly hardly related to increased susceptibility for infections (Klebanoff, 1970, 2005). Importantly, besides bacterial proteins, HOCl affects various biological targets within the host, including intracellular signaling proteins (Midwinter et al., 2001; Lane et al., 2010), heme proteins, glycoproteins, and lipids (Rees et al., 2010; Szuchman-Sapir et al., 2010; Maitra et al., 2011). In particular the chlorination of tyrosine residues leading to the formation of 3- or 3-,5-(di)chlorotyrosine is considered a marker of MPO's activity. In addition, these posttranslational modifications also influence structure and function of the affected molecules. For example, MPO-derived oxidants were proven to alter MAPK signaling pathways in macrophages by oxidation of protein thiol residues (Lane et al., 2010). Furthermore, thiol group oxidation by MPO inhibited sarco/endoplasmic reticulum Ca^{2+}-ATPase (SERCA) activity and perturbed Ca^{2+} homeostasis in endothelial cells (Cook et al., 2012).

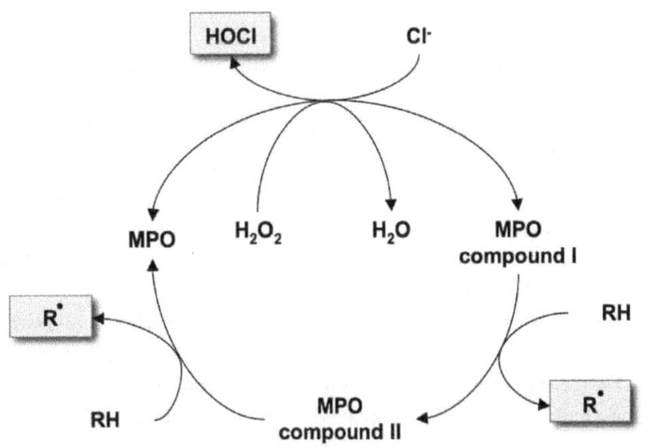

FIGURE 2 | Halogenation and peroxidase cycle of MPO. MPO reacts with H_2O_2 to form compound I, which oxidizes chloride to build the reactive oxidant hypochlorous acid (HOCl). Alternatively, compound I reacts with oxidizable molecules (RH) like ascorbate or tyrosine to form radical intermediates (Rbullet) via compound II.

Apart from the oxidation of halides MPO compound I also reacts via compound II with various organic and inorganic substrates like aromatic amino acids or ascorbate producing radical intermediates (Eiserich et al., 2002; **Figure 2**). An important finding in the field of cardiovascular disease is the prevalent reaction of these radical intermediates with nitric oxide (NO; Eiserich et al., 2002). This not only leads to the reduction of NO-bioavailability, but also forms the reactive nitrating agent nitric dioxide. In cardiomyocytes, MPO-dependent protein nitration was shown to effectively promote apoptosis (Yan et al., 2010). As a further consequence of NO-oxidation, impaired endothelial function became obvious in experimental *ex vivo* (Eiserich et al., 2002) and *in vivo* studies and in human subjects (Rudolph et al., 2007, 2011).

Thus, chlorination, nitration, and other MPO-induced oxidative modifications of host tissue disturb the physiological function of endothelial and myocardial components. Apart from MPO's potency to generate reactive species, also its high affinity to biological structures, which is due to its cationic charge, reinforces the pathophysiological significance of the enzyme.

MPO PROMOTES FIBROSIS

As described above, ROS and RNS mediate fibrotic remodeling via activation of MMPs and various intracellular signaling cascades in cardiac cells. Of note, both of these mechanisms also apply to MPO. Fu et al. (2001) described the activation of MMP-7 by HOCl via oxidation of a cysteine residue in the active site leading to autolytic cleavage of the pro-peptide. MPO's regulatory effect on MMP expression and activation might furthermore be related to the consumption of NO, as a decrease in myocardial NO-bioavailability has been shown to induce MMP-2 release (Wang et al., 2005). In addition, oxidation of a critical cysteine residue induced the inactivation of TIMP-1 (Wang et al., 2007; **Figure 3**). *In vivo*, wild-type (WT) mice treated with ATII displayed enhanced activity of MMP-2 and MMP-9 and elevated MMP-9 protein amount in atrial tissue as compared to MPO-deficient (*Mpo*$^{-/-}$) mice (Rudolph et al., 2010). This was accompanied by a significant increase in atrial fibrosis in ATII-treated WT mice, which was blunted in *Mpo*$^{-/-}$.

In contrast, in a model of acute myocardial infarction the level of pro-MMP-9 and MMP-2 in myocardial tissue was decreased in WT as compared to *Mpo*$^{-/-}$ mice on day 3 after ligation of the left descending coronary artery (Askari et al., 2003). The authors interpreted these unexpected findings by MPO-dependent consumption of H_2O_2: increased bioavailability of H_2O_2 in *Mpo*$^{-/-}$ mice was assumed to lead to MMP expression and activation. However, collagen deposition was markedly delayed in *Mpo*$^{-/-}$ as compared to WT mice upon AMI in this study. This observation underlines the complexity of the interrelation of ECM deposition and MMP-activity – in particular in the setting of myocardial infarction (Jugdutt, 2003). The differences between WT and *Mpo*$^{-/-}$ mice in myocardial remodeling in this model were related to MPO-dependent inhibition of the plasmin activator-inhibitor-1 (PAI-1), which resulted in elevated plasmin activity in WT myocardium. As the fibrinolytic enzyme plasmin has been shown to activate TGF-β1 as well as MMPs (Loskutoff and Quigley, 2000; Zheng and Harris, 2004), and as PAI-1$^{-/-}$ mice display enhanced fibrotic remodeling as compared to WT (Xu et al., 2010), MPO was noted for affecting myocardial remodeling via PAI-1-inhibition (**Figure 3**). Whether this mechanism is also of significance in atrial myocardium remains to be investigated.

Apart from MPO's impact on proteolytic enzyme systems, additional mechanisms are initiated by MPO, which may account for its pro-fibrotic properties: given that leukocytes with their high potency to generate reactive species and to secrete cytokines and MMPs are strongly suggested to contribute to fibrosis formation, MPO's ability to enhance the recruitment of leukocytes (Klinke et al., 2011) might be a pro-fibrotic event. Moreover, MPO not only leads to infiltration of leukocyte but also directly activates MAPK and NADPH-oxidase of PMN via interaction with their integrins CD11b/CD18 (Lau et al., 2005). In addition, activation of macrophages with enhanced production of cytokines is also mediated by MPO (Lefkowitz et al., 1992). Recent data now suggest that MPO-derived HOCl also activates MAPK in cardiomyocytes and endothelial cells (unpublished; **Figure 4**).

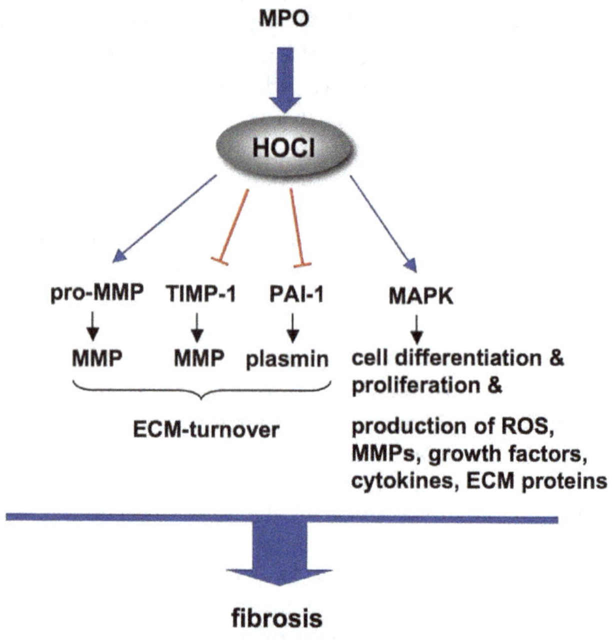

FIGURE 3 | Molecular targets of HOCl mediating fibrosis. MPO-derived HOCl leads to conversion of inactive pro-MMP to active MMP, inactivates TIMP-1 and PAI-1, which results in enhanced ECM-turnover. Activation of MAPKs in various cells initiates pro-fibrotic cascades. Abbreviations: ECM, extracellular matrix; HOCl, hypochlorous acid; MAPK, mitogen-activated protein kinase; MMP, matrix metalloproteinase; PAI-1, plasmin activator-inhibitor-1; ROS, reactive oxygen species; TIMP-1, tissue-inhibitor of MMPs.

Whether MPO-derived reactive species affect fibroblast differentiation, collagen expression, and other processes as described for ROS remains elusive so far.

MPO IN ATRIAL FIBRILLATION

MPO's potency to generate ROS and RNS, its impact on fibrotic remodeling, and its high abundance in leukocytes, which are found to accumulate in fibrillating atria, suggest the enzyme to critically contribute to the formation and maintenance of AF.

In a canine surgical incision model, MPO deposition in the atria was found to correlate with an inhomogeneity of electrical conduction (Ishii et al., 2005). Likewise, surgical induction of pericarditis in dogs lead to marked epicardial injury with reduced expression of connexin-40 and -43 and pronounced accumulation of MPO-positive leukocytes (Ryu et al., 2007; Goldstein et al., 2008). Prednisone treatment in this model prevented the occurrence of atrial flutter, which was accompanied by profoundly reduced MPO immunostaining in the atrial tissue. Furthermore, in patients following AF-ablation an early recurrence of AF was associated with increased MPO plasma levels (Richter et al., 2012). Likewise, increased plasma levels and enhanced atrial deposition of MPO were detected in patients with paroxysmal AF (Rudolph et al., 2010). Whereas these findings remain descriptive without proving a causal role, a clear mechanistic link between MPO and AF development was disclosed within the latter study (Rudolph et al., 2010). As described above, ATII-treated *Mpo*$^{-/-}$ mice were

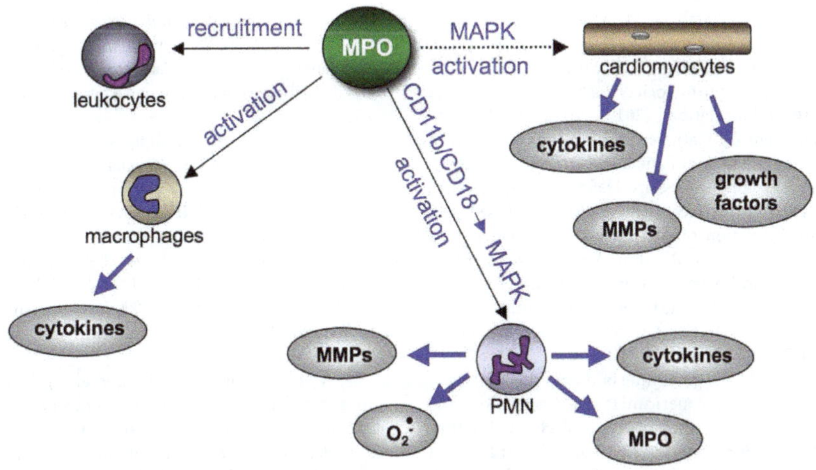

FIGURE 4 | Effect of MPO on cardiac cells and leukocytes contributing to pro-fibrotic remodeling. MPO promotes the recruitment of leukocytes and initiates cytokine secretion from macrophages. Furthermore, MPO activates MAPKs in PMN via CD11b/CD18 integrins, which induces secretion of MMPs, superoxide, cytokines, and MPO. Potentially (dashed line), MPO activates pro-fibrotic pathways in cardiomyocytes via MAPKs. Abbreviations: MAPK, mitogen-activated protein kinase; MMP, matrix metalloproteinase; MPO, myeloperoxidase.

found to be protected of fibrotic atrial remodeling as compared to WT mice. These animals showed markedly attenuated vulnerability to AF upon programmed and burst atrial electrophysiological stimulation as compared to MPO-competent animals. This observation was accompanied by inhomogeneous atrial electrical conduction in ATII-treated WT but not in $Mpo^{-/-}$ mice assessed by an electrophysiological mapping technique. MPO-activity and resultant modifications in atrial tissue following ATII-treatment in WT mice was evidenced by mass-spectromic analysis of chlorotyrosine. Of note, chronic intravenous infusion of MPO led to a profound and dose-dependent increase in AF vulnerability in WT and $Mpo^{-/-}$ mice. These data underscore the importance of MPO for atrial arrhythmias, but also shed light on the function of ATII herein: whereas ATII exerts direct effects on cardiac fibroblasts and myocytes and stimulates the release of MMPs, its ability to activate leukocytes appears to be of great significance. ATII was proven to induce PMN degranulation in the current study (Rudolph et al., 2010) with elevation of MPO concentrations in plasma and atrial tissue of WT mice. The attenuated atrial fibrosis and fibrillation in MPO-naïve animals suggests, that MPO is in part mandatory for ATII-dependent effects.

Taken together, these findings point out that inflammatory processes and in particular MPO-derived reactive species are critically involved in the pathogenesis of AF.

OUTLOOK

Atrial fibrosis is a critical contributor in AF initiation and perpetuation. The pathogenesis of atrial fibrosis is multifactorial and oftentimes related to hypertension, heart failure, or coronary artery disease. So far, the detailed mechanisms, which trigger fibrotic remodeling and account for enhanced deposition of ECM proteins in the atria remain incompletely understood. MPO, with its high potency to generate reactive species and its impact on cellular signaling cascades has evolved as an important mediator in atrial fibrosis and fibrillation. Inhibition of MPO's catalytic activity under conditions of established risk factors for AF might emerge as a potential therapeutic target. However, MPO secretion occurs under a large variety of inflammatory conditions and MPO-derived reactive species exhibit a broad range of biological targets. Thus, further studies are necessary to elucidate MPO's distinct mechanistic implications and therapeutic potentials in AF.

REFERENCES

Adam, O., Theobald, K., Lavall, D., Grube, M., Kroemer, H. K., Ameling, S., Schäfers, H. J., Böhm, M., and Laufs, U. (2011). Increased lysyl oxidase expression and collagen cross-linking during atrial fibrillation. *J. Mol. Cell. Cardiol.* 50, 678–685.

Allessie, M. A. (1998). Atrial electrophysiologic remodeling: another vicious circle? *J. Cardiovasc. Electrophysiol.* 9, 1378–1393.

Askari, A. T., Brennan, M. L., Zhou, X., Drinko, J., Morehead, A., Thomas, J. D., Topol, E. J., Hazen, S. L., and Penn, M. S. (2003). Myeloperoxidase and plasminogen activator inhibitor 1 play a central role in ventricular remodeling after myocardial infarction. *J. Exp. Med.* 197, 615–624.

Ausma, J., van der Velden, H. M., Lenders, M. H., van Ankeren, E. P., Jongsma, H. J., Ramaekers, F. C., Borgers, M., and Allessie, M. A. (2003). Reverse structural and gap-junctional remodeling after prolonged atrial fibrillation in the goat. *Circulation* 107, 2051–2058.

Barnes, J. L., and Gorin, Y. (2011). Myofibroblast differentiation during fibrosis: role of NAD(P)H oxidases. *Kidney Int.* 79, 944–956.

Belkhiri, A., Richards, C., Whaley, M., McQueen, S. A., and Orr, F. W. (1997). Increased expression of activated matrix metalloproteinase-2 by human endothelial cells after sublethal H2 O2 exposure. *Lab. Invest.* 77, 533–539.

Bendall, J. K., Cave, A. C., Heymes, C., Gall, N., and Shah, A. M. (2002). Pivotal role of a gp91(phox)-containing NADPH oxidase in angiotensin II- induced cardiac hypertrophy in mice. *Circulation* 105, 293–296.

Boldt, A., Wetzel, U., Lauschke, J., Weigl, J., Gummert, J., Hindricks, G., Kottkamp, H., and Dhein, S. (2004). Fibrosis in left atrial tissue of patients with atrial fibrillation with and without underlying mitral valve disease. *Heart* 90, 400–405.

Burstein, B., Libby, E., Calderone, A., and Nattel, S. (2008). Differential behaviors of atrial versus ventricular fibroblasts: a potential role for platelet-derived growth factor in atrial-ventricular remodeling differences. *Circulation* 117, 1630–1641.

Calkins, H., Kuck, K. H., Cappato, R., Brugada, J., Camm, A. J., Chen, S. A., Crijns, H. J., Dami-ano, R. J., Davies, D. W., DiMarco, J., Edgerton, J., Ellenbogen, K., Ezekowitz, M. D., Haines, D. E., Haissaguerre, M., Hindricks, G., Iesaka, Y., Jackman, W., Jalife, J., Jais, P., Kalman, J., Keane, D.,

Kim, Y. H., Kirchhof, P., Klein, G., Kot- tkamp, H., Kumagai, K., Lindsay, B. D., Mansour, M., Marchlinski, F. E., McCarthy, P. M., Mont, J. L., Morady, F., Nademanee, K., Nakagawa, H., Natale, A., Nattel, S., Packer, D. L., Pappone, C., Prystowsky, E., Raviele, A., Reddy, V., Ruskin, J. N., Shemin,

R. J., Tsao, H. M., Wilber, D., and Heart Rhythm Society Task Force on Catheter and Surgical Ablation of Atrial Fibrillation. (2012). 2012 HRS/EHRA/ ECAS Expert Consensus Statement on Catheter and Surgical Ablation of Atrial Fibrillation: Recommendations for Patient Selection, Procedural Techniques, Patient Management and Follow-up, Definitions, Endpoints, and Research Trial Design: A report of the Heart Rhythm Society (HRS) Task Force on Catheter and Surgical Ablation of Atrial Fibrillation. Developed in partnership with the European Heart Rhythm Association (EHRA), a registered branch of the European Society of Cardiology (ESC) and the European Cardiac Arrhythmia Society (ECAS); and in collaboration with the American College of Cardiology (ACC), American Heart Association (AHA), the Asia Pacific Heart Rhythm Society (APHRS), and the Society of Thoracic Surgeons (STS). Endorsed by the governing bodies of the American College of Cardiology Foundation, the American Heart Association, the European Cardiac Arrhythmia Society, the European Heart Rhythm Association, the Society of Thoracic Surgeons, the Asia Pacific Heart Rhythm Society, and the Heart Rhythm Society. *Heart Rhythm.* [Epub ahead of print].

Chen, M. C., Chang, J. P., Liu, W. H., Yang, C. H., Chen, Y. L., Tsai, T. H., Wang, Y. H., and Pan, K. L. (2008). Increased inflammatory cell infiltration in the atrial myocardium of patients with atrial fibrillation. *Am. J. Cardiol.* 102, 861–865.

Cook, N. L., Viola, H. M., Sharov, V. S., Hool, L. C., Schöneich, C., and Davies, M. J. (2012). Myeloperoxidase-derived oxidants inhibit sarco/ endoplasmic reticulum Ca^{2+}-ATPase activity and perturb Ca^{2+} homeostasis in human coronary artery endothelial cells. *Free Radic. Biol. Med.* 52, 951–961.

Cucoranu, I., Clempus, R., Dikalova, A., Phelan, P. J., Ariyan, S., Dikalov, S., and Sorescu, D. (2005). NAD(P)H oxidase 4 mediates transforming growth factor-beta1-induced differentiation of cardiac fibroblasts into myofibroblasts. *Circ. Res.* 97, 900–907.

de Jong, S., van Veen, T. A., de Bakker, J. M., Vos, M. A., and van Rijen, H. V. (2011a). Biomarkers of myocardial fibrosis. *J. Cardiovasc. Pharmacol.* 57, 522–535.

de Jong, S., van Veen, T. A., van Rijen, H. V., and de Bakker, J. M. (2011b). Fibrosis and cardiac arrhythmias. *J. Cardiovasc. Pharmacol.* 57, 630–638. Dell'Italia, L. J., Meng, Q. C., Balcells, E., Wei, C. C., Palmer, R., Hageman,

G. R., Durand, J., Hankes, G. H., and Oparil, S. (1997). Compartmentalization of angiotensin II generation in the dog heart. Evidence for independent mechanisms in intravascular and interstitial spaces. *J. Clin. Invest.* 100, 253–258.

Diwan, A., Dibbs, Z., Nemoto, S., DeFreitas, G., Carabello, B. A., Sivasubramanian, N., Wilson, E. M., Spinale, F. G., and Mann, D. L. (2004). Targeted overexpression of noncleavable and secreted forms of tumor necrosis factor provokes disparate cardiac phenotypes. *Circulation* 109, 262–268.

Eiserich, J. P., Baldus, S., Brennan, M. L., Ma, W., Zhang, C., Tousson, A., Castro, L., Lusis, A. J., Nauseef, W. M., White, C. R., and Freeman, B. A. (2002). Myeloperoxidase, a leukocyte-derived vascular NO oxidase. *Science* 296, 2391–2394.

Ergul, A., Walker, C. A., Goldberg, A., Baicu, S. C., Hendrick, J. W., King, M. K., and Spinale, F. G. (2000). ET-1 in the myocardial interstitium: relation to myocyte ECE activity and expression. *Am. J. Physiol. Heart Circ. Physiol.* 278, H2050–H2056.

Flesch, M., Höper, A., Dell'Italia, L., Evans, K., Bond, R., Peshock, R., Diwan, A., Brinsa, T. A., Wei, C. C., Sivasubramanian, N., Spinale, F. G., and Mann, D. L. (2003). Activation and functional significance of the renin-angiotensin system in mice with cardiac restricted overexpression of tumor necrosis factor. *Circulation* 108, 598–604.

Frustaci, A., Chimenti, C., Bellocci, F., Morgante, E., Russo, M. A., and Maseri, A. (1997). Histological substrate of atrial biopsies in patients with lone atrial fibrillation. *Circulation* 96, 1180–1184.

Fu, X., Kassim, S. Y., Parks, W. C., and Heinecke, J. W. (2001). Hypochlorous acid oxygenates the cysteine switch domain of pro-matrilysin (MMP-7). A mechanism for matrix metalloproteinase activation and atherosclerotic plaque rupture by myeloperoxidase. *J. Biol. Chem.* 276, 41279–41287.

Fu, X., Kassim, S. Y., Parks, W. C., and Heinecke, J. W. (2003). Hypochlorous acid generated by myeloperoxidase modifies adjacent tryptophan and glycine residues in the catalytic domain of matrix metalloproteinase-7 (matrilysin): an oxidative mechanism for restraining proteolytic activity during inflammation. *J. Biol. Chem.* 278, 28403–28409.

Gai, X., Lan, X., Luo, Z., Wang, F., Liang, Y., Zhang, H., Zhang, W., Hou, J., and Huang, M. (2009). Association of MMP-9 gene polymorphisms with atrial fibrillation in hypertensive heart disease patients. *Clin. Chim. Acta* 408, 105–109.

Go, A. S., Hylek, E. M., Phillips, K. A., Chang, Y., Henault, L. E., Selby, J. V., and Singer, D. E. (2001). Prevalence of diagnosed atrial fibrillation in adults: national implications for rhythm management and stroke prevention: the AnTicoagulation and Risk Factors in Atrial Fibrillation (ATRIA) Study. *JAMA* 285, 2370–2375.

Goette, A., Bukowska, A., Lendeckel, U., Erxleben, M., Hammwöhner, M., Strugala, D., Pfeiffenberger, J., Röhl, F. W., Huth, C., Ebert, M. P., Klein, H. U., and Röcken, C. (2008). Angiotensin II receptor blockade reduces tachycardia-induced atrial adhesion molecule expression. *Circulation* 117, 732–742.

Goette, A., Honeycutt, C., and Langberg, J. J. (1996). Electrical remodeling in atrial fibrillation. Time course and mechanisms. *Circulation* 94, 2968–2974.

Goldstein, R. N., Ryu, K., Khrestian, C., van Wagoner, D. R., and Waldo, A. L. (2008). Prednisone prevents inducible atrial flutter in the canine sterile pericarditis model. *J. Cardiovasc. Electrophysiol.* 19, 74–81.

Goudis, C. A., Kallergis, E. M., and Vardas, P. E. (2012). Extracellular matrix alterations in the atria: insights into the mechanisms and perpetuation of atrial fibrillation. *Europace* 14, 623–630.

Grieve, D. J., Byrne, J. A., Siva, A., Layland, J., Johar, S., Cave, A. C., and Shah, A. M. (2006). Involvement of the nicotinamide adenosine dinucleotide phosphate oxidase isoform Nox2 in cardiac contractile dysfunction occurring in response to pressure overload. *J. Am. Coll. Cardiol.* 47, 817–826.

Gu, Z., Kaul, M., Yan, B., Kridel, S. J., Cui, J., Strongin, A., Smith, J. W., Liddington, R. C., and Lipton, S.

A. (2002). S-nitrosylation of matrix metalloproteinases: signaling pathway to neuronal cell death. *Science* 297, 1186–1190.

Gurjar, M. V., Deleon, J., Sharma, R. V., and Bhalla, R. C. (2001). Role of reactive oxygen species in IL-1 beta-stimulated sustained ERK activation and MMP-9 induction. *Am. J. Physiol. Heart Circ. Physiol.* 281, H2568–H2574. Hagiwara, N. (2010). Inflammation and atrial fibrillation. *Circ. J.* 74, 246–247.

Haïssaguerre, M., Jaïs, P., Shah, D. C., Takahashi, A., Hocini, M., Quiniou, G., Garrigue, S., Le Mouroux, A., Le Métayer, P., and Clémenty, J. (1998). Spontaneous initiation of atrial fibrillation by ectopic beats originating in the pulmonary veins. *N. Engl. J. Med.* 339, 659–666.

Han, Y. P., Tuan, T. L., Wu, H., Hughes, M., and Garner, W. L. (2001). TNF-alpha stimulates activation of pro-MMP-2 in human skin through NF-(kappa)B mediated induction of MT1-MMP. *J. Cell. Sci.* 114, 131–139.

Hecker, L., Vittal, R., Jones, T., Jagirdar, R., Luckhardt, T. R., Horowitz,

J. C., Pennathur, S., Martinez, F. J., and Thannickal, V. J. (2009). NADPH oxidase-4 mediates myofibroblast activation and fibrogenic responses to lung injury. *Nat. Med.* 15, 1077–1081.

Hinescu, M. E., Gherghiceanu, M., Mandache, E., Ciontea, S. M., and Popescu, L. M. (2006). Interstitial Cajal-like cells (ICLC) in atrial myocardium: ultrastructural and immunohistochemical characterization. *J. Cell. Mol. Med.* 10, 243–257. Ichikawa, T., Sugiura, H., Koarai, A., Yanagisawa, S., Kanda, M., Hayata, A., Furukawa, K., Akamatsu, K., Hirano, T., Nakanishi, M., Matsunaga, K., Minakata, Y., and Ichinose, M. (2008). Peroxynitrite augments fibroblast-mediated tissue remodeling via myofibroblast differentiation. *Am. J. Physiol. Lung Cell Mol. Physiol.* 295, L800–L808.

Ishii, Y., Schuessler, R. B., Gaynor, S. L., Yamada, K., Fu, A. S., Boineau, J. P., and Damiano, R. J. (2005). Inflammation of atrium after cardiac surgery is associated with inhomogeneity of atrial conduction and atrial fibrillation. *Circulation* 111, 2881–2888.

Iwasaki, Y. K., Nishida, K., Kato, T., and Nattel, S. (2011). Atrial fibrillation pathophysiology: implications for management. *Circulation* 124, 2264–2274.

Johar, S., Cave, A. C., Narayanapanicker, A., Grieve, D. J., and Shah, A. M. (2006). Aldosterone mediates angiotensin II-induced interstitial cardiac fibrosis via a Nox2-containing NADPH oxidase. *FASEB J.* 20, 1546–1548.

Jugdutt, B. I. (2003). Ventricular remodeling after infarction and the extracellular collagen matrix: when is enough enough? *Circulation* 108, 1395–1403.

Kannel, W. B., Abbott, R. D., Savage, D. D., and McNamara, P. M. (1982). Epidemiologic features of chronic atrial fibrillation: the Framingham study. *N. Engl. J. Med.* 306, 1018–1022.

Kato, K., Fujimaki, T., Yoshida, T., Oguri, M., Yajima, K., Hibino, T., and Murohara, T. (2009). Impact of matrix metalloproteinase-2 levels on longterm outcome following pharmacological or electrical cardioversion in patients with atrial fibrillation. *Europace* 11, 332–337.

Kawaguchi, M., Takahashi, M., Hata, T., Kashima, Y., Usui, F., Morimoto, H., Izawa, A., Takahashi, Y., Masumoto, J., Koyama, J., Hongo, M., Noda, T., Nakayama, J., Sagara, J., Taniguchi, S., and Ikeda, U. (2011). Inflammasome activation of cardiac fibroblasts is essential for myocardial ischemia/reperfusion injury. *Circulation* 123, 594–604.

Kis, K., Liu, X., and Hagood, J. S. (2011). Myofibroblast differentiation and survival in fibrotic disease. *Expert Rev. Mol. Med.* 13, e27.

Klebanoff, S. J. (1970). Myeloperoxidase: contribution to the microbicidal activity of intact leukocytes. *Science* 169, 1095–1097.

Klebanoff, S. J. (2005). Myeloperoxidase: friend and foe. *J. Leukoc. Biol.* 77, 598–625.

Klinke, A., Nussbaum, C., Kubala, L., Friedrichs, K., Rudolph, T. K., Rudolph, V., Paust, H. J., Schröder, C., Benten, D., Lau, D., Szocs, K., Furtmüller, P. G., Heeringa, P., Sydow, K., Duchstein, H.-J., Ehmke, H., Schumacher, U., Meinertz, T., Sperandio, M., and Baldus, S. (2011). Myeloperoxidase attracts neutrophils by physical forces. *Blood* 117, 1350–1358.

Kostin, S., Klein, G., Szalay, Z., Hein, S., Bauer, E. P., and Schaper, J. (2002). Structural correlate of atrial fibrillation in human patients. *Cardiovasc. Res.* 54, 361–379.

Kumagai, K., Ogawa, M., Noguchi, H., Yasuda, T., Nakashima, H., and Saku, K. (2004). Electrophysiologic properties of pulmonary veins assessed using a multielectrode basket catheter. *J. Am. Coll. Cardiol.* 43, 2281–2289.

Lamm, G., Auer, J., Weber, T., Berent, R., Ng, C., and Eber, B. (2006). Postoperative white blood cell count predicts atrial fibrillation after cardiac surgery. *J. Cardiothorac. Vasc. Anesth.* 20, 51–56.

Lane, A. E., Tan, J. T., Hawkins, C. L., Heather, A. K., and Davies, M. J. (2010). The myeloperoxidase-derived oxidant HOSCN inhibits protein tyrosine phosphatases and modulates cell signalling via the mitogen-activated protein kinase (MAPK) pathway in macrophages. *Biochem. J.* 430, 161–169.

Lau, D., and Baldus, S. (2006). Myeloperoxidase and its contributory role in inflammatory vascular disease. *Pharmacol. Ther.* 111, 16–26. Lau, D., Mollnau, H., Eiserich, J. P., Freeman, B. A., Daiber, A., Gehling, U.

M., Brummer, J., Rudolph, V., Munzel, T., Heitzer, T., Meinertz, T., and Baldus, S. (2005). Myeloperoxidase mediates neutrophil activation by association with CD11b/CD18 integrins. *Proc. Natl. Acad. Sci. U.S.A.* 102, 431–436.

Lee, K. W., Everett, T. H., Rahmutula, D.,

Guerra, J. M., Wilson, E., Ding, C., and Olgin, J. E. (2006). Pirfenidone prevents the development of a vulnerable substrate for atrial fibrillation in a canine model of heart failure. *Circulation* 114, 1703–1712. Lefkowitz, D. L., Mills, K., Morgan, D., and Lefkowitz, S. S. (1992). Macrophage activation and immunomodulation by myeloperoxidase. *Proc. Soc. Exp. Biol. Med.* 199, 204–210.

Li, D., Fareh, S., Leung, T. K., and Nattel, S. (1999). Promotion of atrial fibrillation by heart failure in dogs: atrial remodeling of a different sort. *Circulation* 100, 87–95.

Li, D., Shinagawa, K., Pang, L., Leung, T. K., Cardin, S., Wang, Z., and Nattel, S. (2001). Effects of angiotensin-converting enzyme inhibition on the development of the atrial fibrillation substrate in dogs with ventricular tachypacing-induced congestive heart failure. *Circulation* 104, 2608–2614.

Li, J., Zhu, H., Shen, E., Wan, L., Arnold, J. M., and Peng, T. (2010). Deficiency of rac1 blocks NADPH oxidase activation, inhibits endoplasmic reticulum stress, and reduces myocardial remodeling in a mouse model of type 1 diabetes. *Diabetes* 59, 2033–2042.

Li, Y. Y., McTiernan, C. F., and Feldman, A. M. (2000). Interplay of matrix metalloproteinases, tissue inhibitors of metalloproteinases and their regulators in cardiac matrix remodeling. *Cardiovasc. Res.* 46, 214–224.

Lin, C. S., and Pan, C. H. (2008). Regulatory mechanisms of atrial fibrotic remodeling in atrial fibrillation. *Cell. Mol. Life Sci.* 65, 1489–1508.

Loskutoff, D. J., and Quigley, J. P. (2000). PAI-1, fibrosis, and the elusive provisional fibrin matrix. *J. Clin. Invest.* 106, 1441–1443.

Maitra, D., Banerjee, J., Shaeib, F., Souza, C. E., and Abu-Soud, H. M. (2011). Melatonin can mediate its vascular protective effect by modulating free iron level by inhibiting hypochlorous acid-mediated hemoprotein heme destruction. *Hypertension* 57, e22.

Midwinter, R. G., Vissers, M. C., and Winterbourn, C. C. (2001). Hypochlorous acid stimulation of the mitogen-activated protein kinase pathway enhances cell survival. *Arch. Biochem. Biophys.* 394, 13–20.

Milliez, P., Deangelis, N., Rucker-Martin, C., Leenhardt, A., Vicaut, E., Robidel, E., Beaufils, P., Delcayre, C., and Hatem, S. N. (2005). Spironolactone reduces fibrosis of dilated atria during heart failure in rats with myocardial infarction. *Eur. Heart J.* 26, 2193–2199.

Miragoli, M., Salvarani, N., and Rohr, S. (2007). Myofibroblasts induce ectopic activity in cardiac tissue. *Circ. Res.* 101, 755–758.

Moe, G. W., Laurent, G., Doumanovskaia, L., Konig, A., Hu, X., and Dorian, P. (2008). Matrix metalloproteinase inhibition attenuates atrial remodeling and vulnerability to atrial fibrillation in a canine model of heart failure. *J. Card. Fail.* 14, 768–776.

Mott, J. D., and Werb, Z. (2004). Regulation of matrix biology by matrix metalloproteinases. *Curr. Opin. Cell Biol.* 16, 558–564.

Multani, M. M., Ikonomidis, J. S., Kim, P. Y., Miller, E. A., Payne, K. J., Mukherjee, R., Dorman, B. H., and Spinale, F. G. (2005). Dynamic and differential changes in myocardial and plasma endothelin in patients undergoing cardiopulmonary bypass. *J. Thorac. Cardiovasc. Surg.* 129, 584–590.

Murdoch, C. E., Zhang, M., Cave, A. C., and Shah, A. M. (2006). NADPH oxidase-dependent redox signalling in cardiac hypertrophy, remodelling and failure. *Cardiovasc. Res.* 71, 208–215.

Nattel, S., Burstein, B., and Dobrev, D. (2008). Atrial remodeling and atrial fibrillation: mechanisms and implications. *Circ. Arrhythm. Electrophysiol.* 1, 62–73.

Nattel, S., Shiroshita-Takeshita, A., Cardin, S., and Pelletier, P. (2005). Mechanisms of atrial remodeling and clinical relevance. *Curr. Opin. Cardiol.* 20, 21–25.

Nicholls, S. J., and Hazen, S. L. (2005). Myeloperoxidase and cardiovascular disease. *Arterioscler. Thromb. Vasc. Biol.* 25, 1102–1111.

Okumura, Y., Watanabe, I., Nakai, T., Ohkubo, K., Kofune, T., Kofune, M., Nagashima, K., Mano, H., Sonoda, K., Kasamaki, Y., and Hirayama, A. (2011). Impact of biomarkers of inflammation and extracellular matrix turnover on the outcome of atrial fibrillation ablation: importance of matrix matalloproteinase-2 as a predictor of atrial fibrillation recurrence. *J. Cardiovasc. Electrophysiol.* 22, 987–993.

Pellman, J., Lyon, R. C., and Sheikh, F. (2010). Extracellular matrix remodeling in atrial fibrosis: mechanisms and implications in atrial fibrillation. *J. Mol. Cell. Cardiol.* 48, 461–467.

Rajagopalan, S., Meng, X. P., Ramasamy, S., Harrison, D. G., and Galis, Z. S. (1996). Reactive oxygen species produced by macrophage-derived foam cells regulate the activity of vascular matrix metalloproteinases in vitro. Implications for atherosclerotic plaque stability. *J. Clin. Invest.* 98, 2572–2579.

Ramlawi, B., Otu, H., Mieno, S., Bood-hwani, M., Sodha, N. R., Clements,

R. T., Bianchi, C., and Sellke, F. W. (2007). Oxidative stress and atrial fibrillation after cardiac surgery: a case-control study. *Ann. Thorac. Surg.* 84, 1166–1172; discussion 1172–1173.

Rees, M. D., Whitelock, J. M., Malle, E., Chuang, C. Y., Iozzo, R. V., Nilasaroya, A., and Davies, M. J. (2010). Myeloperoxidase-derived oxidants selectively disrupt the protein core of the heparan sulfate proteoglycan perlecan. *Matrix Biol.* 29, 63–73.

Reil, J. C., Hohl, M., Oberhofer, M., Kazakov, A., Kaestner, L., Mueller, P., Adam, O., Maack, C., Lipp, P., Mewis, C., Allessie, M., Laufs, U., Böhm, M., and Neuberger, H. R. (2010). Cardiac Rac1 overexpression in mice creates a substrate for atrial arrhythmias characterized by structural remodelling. *Cardiovasc. Res.* 87, 485–493.

Richter, B., Gwechenberger, M., Socas, A., Zorn, G., Albinni, S., Marx, M., Bergler-Klein, J., Binder, T., Wojta, J., and Gössinger, H. D. (2012). Markers of oxidative stress after ablation of atrial fibrillation are associated with inflam- mation, delivered radiofrequency energy and early recurrence of atrial fibrillation. *Clin. Res. Cardiol.* 101, 217–225.

Rohr, S. (2009). Myofibroblasts in diseased hearts: new players in cardiac arrhythmias? *Heart Rhythm* 6, 848–856.

Rudolph, T. K., Wipper, S., Reiter, B., Rudolph, V., Coym, A., Detter, C., Lau, D., Klinke, A., Friedrichs, K., Rau, T., Pekarova, M., Russ, D., Knöll, K., Kolk, M., Schroeder, B., Wegscheider, K., Andresen, H., Schwedhelm, E., Boeger, R., Ehmke, H., and Baldus, S. (2011). Myeloperoxidase deficiency preserves vasomotor function in humans. *Eur. Heart J.* doi: 10.1093/eurheartj/ehr193. [Epub ahead of print].

Rudolph, V., Andrié, R. P., Rudolph, T. K., Friedrichs, K., Klinke, A., Hirsch-Hoffmann, B., Schwoerer, A. P., Lau, D., Fu, X., Klingel, K., Sydow, K., Didié, M., Seniuk, A., von Leitner, E. C., Szoecs, K., Schrickel, J. W., Treede, H., Wenzel, U., Lewalter, T., Nickenig, G., Zimmermann, W. H., Meinertz, T., Böger, R. H., Reichen- spurner, H., Freeman, B. A., Eschen- hagen, T., Ehmke, H., Hazen, S. L., Willems, S., and Baldus, S. (2010). Myeloperoxidase acts as a profibrotic mediator of atrial fibrillation. *Nat. Med.* 16, 470–474.

Rudolph, V., Rudolph, T. K., Hennings, J. C., Blankenberg, S., Schnabel, R., Steven, D., Haddad, M., Knittel, K., Wende, S., Wenzel, J., Munzel, T., Heitzer, T., Meinertz, T., Hübner, C., and Baldus, S. (2007). Activation of polymorphonuclear neutrophils in patients with impaired left ventricular function. *Free Radic. Biol. Med.* 43, 1189–1196.

Ryu, K., Li, L., Khrestian, C. M., Matsumoto, N., Sahadevan, J., Ruehr, M. L., Van Wagoner, D. R., Efimov, I. R., and Waldo, A. L. (2007). Effects of sterile pericarditis on connexins 40 and 43 in the atria: correlation with abnormal conduction and atrial arrhythmias. *Am. J. Physiol. Heart Circ. Physiol.* 293, H1231–H1241.

Saba, S., Janczewski, A. M., Baker, L. C., Shusterman, V., Gursoy, E. C., Feldman, A. M., Salama, G., McTiernan, C. F., and London, B. (2005). Atrial contractile dysfunction, fibrosis, and arrhythmias in a mouse model of cardiomyopathy secondary to cardiac-specific overexpression of tumor necrosis factor-α. *Am. J. Physiol. Heart Circ. Physiol.* 289, H1456–H1467.

Saito, T., Tamura, K., Uchida, D., Saito, T., Togashi, M., Nitta, T., and Sugisaki, Y. (2007). Histopathological features of the resected left atrial appendage as predictors of recurrence after surgery for atrial fibrillation in valvular heart disease. *Circ. J.* 71, 70–78.

Sakabe, M., Fujiki, A., Nishida, K., Sugao, M., Nagasawa, H., Tsuneda, T., Mizumaki, K., and Inoue, H. (2004). Enalapril prevents perpetuation of atrial fibrillation by suppressing atrial fibrosis and over-expression of connexin43 in a canine model of atrial pacing-induced left ventricular dysfunction. *J. Cardiovasc. Pharmacol.* 43, 851–859.

Savelieva, I., and Camm, J. (2008). Update on atrial fibrillation: part I. *Clin. Cardiol.* 31, 55–62.

Scholz, H., Aukrust, P., Damås, J. K., Tonstad, S., Sagen, E. L., Kolset, S. O., Hall, C., Yndestad, A., and Halvorsen, B. (2004). 8-Isoprostane increases scavenger receptor A and matrix metalloproteinase activity in THP-1 macrophages, resulting in long-lived foam cells. *Eur. J. Clin. Invest.* 34, 451–458.

Siwik, D. A., and Colucci, W. S. (2004). Regulation of matrix metallopro-teinases by cytokines and reactive oxygen/nitrogen species in the myocardium. *Heart Fail. Rev.* 9, 43–51.

Siwik, D. A., Pagano, P. J., and Colucci, W. S. (2001). Oxidative stress regulates collagen synthesis and matrix metalloproteinase activity in cardiac fibroblasts. *Am. J. Physiol. Cell Physiol.* 280, C53–C60.

Spach, M. S., and Boineau, J. P. (1997). Microfibrosis produces electrical load variations due to loss of side-to-side cell connections: a major mechanism of structural heart disease arrhythmias. *Pacing Clin. Electrophysiol.* 20, 397–413.

Spallarossa, P., Altieri, P., Garibaldi, S., Ghigliotti, G., Barisione, C., Manca, V., Fabbi, P., Ballestrero, A., Brunelli, C., and Barsotti, A. (2006). Matrix metalloproteinase-2 and - 9 are induced differently by doxorubicin in H9c2 cells: the role of MAP kinases and NAD(P)H oxidase. *Cardiovasc. Res.* 69, 736–745.

Spinale, F. G. (2007). Myocardial matrix remodeling and the matrix metalloproteinases: influence on cardiac form and function. *Physiol. Rev.* 87, 1285–1342.

Sun, Y., Zhang, J., Lu, L., Chen, S. S., Quinn, M. T., and Weber, K. T. (2002). Aldosterone-induced inflammation in the rat heart: role of oxidative stress. *Am. J. Pathol.* 161, 1773–1781.

Swynghedauw, B. (1999). Molecular mechanisms of myocardial remodeling. *Physiol. Rev.* 79, 215–262.

Szuchman-Sapir, A. J., Pattison, D. I., Davies, M. J., and Witting, P. K. (2010). Site-specific hypochlorous acid-induced oxidation of recombinant human myoglobin affects specific amino acid residues and the rate of cytochrome b5-mediated heme reduction. *Free Radic. Biol. Med.* 48, 35–46.

Tsang, T. S., Petty, G. W., Barnes, M. E., O'Fallon, W. M., Bailey, K. R., Wiebers, D. O., Sicks, J. D., Christianson, T. J., Seward, J. B., and Gersh, B. J. (2003). The prevalence of atrial fibrillation in incident stroke cases and matched population controls in Rochester, Minnesota: changes over three decades. *J. Am. Coll. Cardiol.* 42, 93–100.

Vasquez, C., Benamer, N., and Morley, G. E. (2011). The cardiac fibroblast: functional and electrophysiological considerations in healthy and diseased hearts. *J. Cardiovasc. Pharmacol.* 57, 380–388.

Vasquez, C., Mohandas, P., Louie, K. L., Benamer, N., Bapat, A. C., and Morley, G. E. (2010). Enhanced fibroblast-myocyte interactions in response to cardiac injury. *Circ. Res.* 107, 1011–1020.

Verheule, S., Sato, T., Everett, T., Engle, S. K., Otten, D., Rubart-von der Lohe, M., Nakajima, H. O., Nakajima, H., Field, L. J., and Olgin, J. E. (2004). Increased vulnerability to atrial fibrillation in transgenic mice with selective atrial fibrosis caused by overexpression of TGF-beta1. *Circ. Res.* 94, 1458–1465.

Verheule, S., Wilson, E., Everett, T., Shanbhag, S., Golden, C., and Olgin, J. (2003). Alterations in atrial electrophysiology and tissue structure in a canine model of chronic atrial dilatation due to mitral regurgitation. *Circulation* 107, 2615–2622.

Wainwright, C. L. (2004). Matrix metalloproteinases, oxidative stress and the acute response to acute myocardial ischaemia and reperfusion. *Curr. Opin. Pharmacol.* 4, 132–138.

Wang, T. J., Massaro, J. M., Levy, D., Vasan, R. S., Wolf, P. A., D'Agostino, R. B., Larson, M. G., Kannel, W. B., and Benjamin, E. J. (2003). A risk score for predicting stroke or death in individuals with new-onset atrial fibrillation in the community: the Framingham Heart Study. *JAMA* 290, 1049–1056.

Wang, W., Sawicki, G., and Schulz, R. (2002). Peroxynitrite-induced myocardial injury is mediated through matrix metalloproteinase-2. *Cardiovasc. Res.* 53, 165–174.

Wang, W., Viappiani, S., Sawicka, J., and Schulz, R. (2005). Inhibition of endogenous nitric oxide in the heart enhances matrix metalloproteinase-2 release. *Br. J. Pharmacol.* 145, 43–49.

Wang, Y., Rosen, H., Madtes, D. K., Shao, B., Martin, T. R., Heinecke, J. W., and Fu, X. (2007). Myeloperoxidase inactivates TIMP-1 by oxidizing its N-terminal cysteine residue: an oxidative mechanism for regulating proteolysis during inflammation. *J. Biol. Chem.* 282, 31826–31834.

Wei, C. C., Meng, Q. C., Palmer, R., Hageman, G. R., Durand, J., Bradley, W. E., Farrell, D. M., Hankes, G. H., Oparil, S., and Dell'Italia, L. J. (1999). Evidence for angiotensin-converting enzyme- and chymase- mediated angiotensin II formation in the interstitial fluid space of the dog heart in vivo. *Circulation* 99, 2583–2589.

Xie, Y., Sato, D., Garfinkel, A., Qu, Z., and Weiss, J. N. (2010). So lit- tle source, so much sink: requirements for after depolarizations to propagate in tissue. *Biophys. J.* 99, 1408–1415.

Xu, J., Cui, G., Esmailian, F., Plunkett, M., Marelli, D., Ardehali, A., Odim, J., Laks, H., and Sen, L. (2004). Atrial extracellular matrix remodeling and the maintenance of atrial fibrillation. *Circulation* 109, 363–368.

Xu, Z., Castellino, F. J., and Ploplis, V. A. (2010). Plasminogen activator inhibitor-1 (PAI-1) is cardioprotective in mice by main-taining microvascular integrity and cardiac architecture. *Blood* 115, 2038–2047.

Yamashita, T. (2007). Molecular basis of thromboembolism in association with atrial fibrillation. *Circ. J.* 71(Suppl. A), A40–A44.

Yan, Z., Liang, F., Guo, L., Wang, J., Wang, X. L., Cheng, X. L., Ma, X. L., and Liu, H. R. (2010). Myeloperoxidase increased cardiomyocyte protein nitration in mice subjected to nonlethal mechanical trauma. *Biochem. Biophys. Res. Commun.* 393, 531–535.

Yoo, H. G., Shin, B. A., Park, J. S., Lee, K. H., Chay, K. O., Yang, S. Y., Ahn, B. W., and Jung, Y. D. (2002). IL-1beta induces MMP-9 via reactive oxygen species and NF- kappaB in murine macrophage RAW264.7 cells. *Biochem. Biophys. Res. Commun.* 298, 251–256.

Yoon, S. O., Park, S. J., Yoon, S. Y., Yun, C. H., and Chung, A. S. (2002). Sustained production of H(2)O(2) activates pro-matrix metalloproteinase-2 through receptor tyrosine kinases/ phosphatidylinositol 3-kinase/NF-kappa B pathway. *J. Biol. Chem.* 277, 30271–30282.

Yue, L., Xie, J., and Nattel, S. (2011). Molecular determinants of cardiac fibroblast electrical function and therapeutic implications for atrial fibrillation. *Cardiovasc. Res.* 89, 744–753.

Zhang, H. J., Zhao, W., Venkatara-man, S., Robbins, M. E., Buettner, G. R., Kregel, K. C., and Oberley, L. W. (2002). Activation of matrix metalloproteinase-2 by over-expression of manganese superoxide dismutase in human breast cancer MCF-7 cells involves reactive oxygen species. *J. Biol. Chem.* 277, 20919–20926.

Zhao, W., Zhao, T., Chen, Y., Ahokas,

R. A., and Sun, Y. (2008). Oxidative stress mediates cardiac fibrosis by enhancing transforming growth factor-beta1 in hypertensive rats. *Mol. Cell. Biochem.* 317, 43–50.

Zheng, G., and Harris, D. C. (2004). Plasmin in renal interstitial fibrosis: innocent or guilty? *Kidney Int.* 66, 455–456.

17

Induced pluripotent stem cell derived cardiomyocytes as models for cardiac arrhythmias

Maaike Hoekstra[1]*, Christine L. Mummery[2], Arthur A. M. Wilde[1], Connie R. Bezzina[1] and Arie O. Verkerk[3]

[1] *Department of Clinical and Experimental Cardiology, Heart Failure Research Center, Academic Medical Center, University of Amsterdam, Amsterdam, Netherlands*

[2] *Department of Anatomy and Embryology, Leiden University Medical Center, Leiden, Netherlands*

[3] *Department of Anatomy, Embryology, and Physiology, Heart Failure Research Center, Academic Medical Center, University of Amsterdam, Amsterdam, Netherlands*

***Correspondence:**
Maaike Hoekstra, Department of Clinical and Experimental Cardiology, Heart Failure Research Center, Academic Medical Center, University of Amsterdam, room K2-113, Meibergdreef 15, PO Box 22700, 1100 DE Amsterdam, Netherlands.
e-mail: m.hoekstra@amc.uva.nl

Cardiac arrhythmias are a major cause of morbidity and mortality. In younger patients, the majority of sudden cardiac deaths have an underlying Mendelian genetic cause. Over the last 15 years, enormous progress has been made in identifying the distinct clinical phenotypes and in studying the basic cellular and genetic mechanisms associated with the primary Mendelian (monogenic) arrhythmia syndromes. Investigation of the electrophysiological consequences of an ion channel mutation is ideally done in the native cardiomyocyte (CM) environment. However, the majority of such studies so far have relied on heterologous expression systems in which single ion channel genes are expressed in non-cardiac cells. In some cases, transgenic mouse models have been generated, but these also have significant shortcomings, primarily related to species differences. The discovery that somatic cells can be reprogrammed to pluripotency as induced pluripotent stem cells (iPSC) has generated much interest since it presents an opportunity to generate patient- and disease-specific cell lines from which normal and diseased human CMs can be obtained These genetically diverse human model systems can be studied *in vitro* and used to decipher mechanisms of disease and identify strategies and reagents for new therapies. Here, we review the present state of the art with respect to cardiac disease models already generated using IPSC technology and which have been (partially) characterized. Human iPSC (hiPSC) models have been described for the cardiac arrhythmia syndromes, including LQT1, LQT2, LQT3-Brugada Syndrome, LQT8/Timothy syndrome and catecholaminergic polymorphic ventricular tachycardia (CPVT). In most cases, the hiPSC-derived cardiomyoctes recapitulate the disease phenotype and have already provided opportunities for novel insight into cardiac pathophysiology. It is expected that the lines will be useful in the development of pharmacological agents for the management of these disorders.

Keywords: induced pluripotent stem cells, cardiac arrhythmia syndromes, electrophysiology, cardiomyocytes, human, iPS, heart

INTRODUCTION

Cardiac arrhythmias can be life threatening and are a major cause of morbidity and mortality in developed nations (Wolf and Berul, 2008). In older patients, most arrhythmic sudden deaths occur in the setting of acute ischemia or coronary artery diseases (Zipes and Wellens, 1998). In younger patients, the great majority of sudden arrhythmic deaths have an underlying genetic cause (Wilde and Bezzina, 2005). These can be broadly subdivided into those associated with structural heart disease (such as hypertrophic cardiomyopathy) and those associated with electrical disease in the structurally normal heart (Wolf and Berul, 2008).

Over the last 15 years, much progress has been made in identifying the clinical phenotypes and cellular and genetic mechanisms underlying the various primary Mendelian arrhythmia syndromes, including the Long QT syndrome (LQTS), Brugada Syndrome (BrS), and catecholaminergic polymorphic ventricular tachycardia (CPVT) (Wilde and Bezzina, 2005). This has provided important insights into these disorders and as a consequence improved the management of affected patients. The availability of genetic tests has added an important diagnostic tool permitting early (presymptomatic) identification of patients at risk and allowing for the timely implementation of preventive strategies (Hofman et al., 2010). Studies into genotype–phenotype relationships have uncovered important gene-specific aspects of disease and indicated that patient management must take the nature of the gene affected into consideration (Priori, 2004). However, there is considerable variation in phenotypic expression of arrhythmia syndromes even within families carrying the same mutation (Scicluna et al., 2008).

Studying the electrophysiological and molecular consequences of a mutation associated with cardiac arrhythmia is ideally done in the native cardiomyocyte (CM) environment. However, obtaining ventricular cardiac biopsies from patients is a highly invasive procedure and not without significant risk. Consequently the majority of functional studies on specific mutations associated with the Mendelian rhythm disorders have relied on heterologous expression systems, primarily *Xenopus oocytes*, human embryonic kidney (HEK) cells, and Chinese Hamster Ovary (CHO) cells (Watanabe et al., 2008), in which the mutated ion channel of interest is expressed. Such cellular models have significant shortcomings since they lack important constituents of cardiac ion channel macromolecular complexes that might be required to reproduce the exact molecular and electrophysiological phenotype of the mutation. For example, the behavior of the Na^+ channel in cell expression systems seems to be different from that in CMs (Remme et al., 2008). One way of overcoming this has been to generate transgenic mice carrying specific mutations (Sabir et al., 2008). However, the generation of such mouse models is costly and time-consuming and not practical for high-throughput screening of rare inherited arrhythmia mutations. Moreover, there remain crucial differences between mouse and human cardiac electrophysiological characteristics, such as the high basal heart rate (>500 bpm), the very negative action potential (AP) plateau phase, and the short AP compared of the mouse compared to human (Watanabe et al., 2011). These differences are amongst others due to the different biophysical properties in the transient outward currents (I_{to}) of human and mouse (for review, see Nerbonne and Kass, 2005).

The discovery of somatic cell reprogramming to generate induced pluripotent stem cells (iPSC) (Takahashi and Yamanaka, 2006) has created much excitement because of the possibility of producing unique patient- and disease-specific human iPSC (hiPSC) lines (Takahashi and Yamanaka, 2006; Takahashi et al., 2007; Yu et al., 2007). With this technique, somatic cells can be turned into embryonic stem cell-like cells which can differentiate into all cells of the human body and be propagated indefinitely in culture. Thus, hiPSC can provide investigators with genetically diverse human model systems to study mechanisms of disease and identify strategies for potential new therapies. Zhang et al. (2009) were the first to show that hiPSC can differentiate to functional CMs, making it possible to generate patient-specific human CMs which are by definition on different genetic backgrounds. hiPSC-derived CMs (hiPSC-CMs) therefore represent a new model system for studying Mendelian arrhythmia syndromes.

Here we provide a short overview of hiPSC generation, culturing, and differentiation methods. Further we will discuss in detail the electrophysiological characteristics of hiPSC-CMs and review hiPSC models for cardiovascular diseases, including LQT1, LQT2, LQT3/BrS, LQT8/Timothy syndrome, and CPVT.

DERIVATION OF hiPSC MODELS

CELL ORIGIN

Although the first hiPSC lines were derived from dermal fibroblasts (Takahashi et al., 2007) hiPSC can now be generated from a wide variety of somatic cells. It is important to consider easily accessible sources, which are efficient to reprogram and give minimal burden to the patient. Easily accessible sources used successfully for reprogramming include keratinocytes from skin or plucked hair (Aasen et al., 2008), peripheral blood (Loh et al., 2009), mesenchymal cells in fat (Sun et al., 2009), dental pulp (Tamaoki et al., 2010), and oral mucosa (Miyoshi et al., 2010).

CELL REPROGRAMMING

Somatic cells can be reprogrammed to a pluripotent state by introducing pluripotency-associated genes. The first iPSC reported were generated by transducing mouse fibroblasts with four retroviral vectors OCT4, SOX2, KLF4, and C-MYC (Takahashi and Yamanaka, 2006). The first hiPSC were generated using the same four retroviral vectors (Takahashi et al., 2007) or OCT4, SOX2, LIN28, and NANOG (Yu et al., 2007). Later studies reported reprogramming with other combinations and numbers of pluripotency factors. The hiPSC thus generated can be kept in culture indefinitely using a variety of undefined fibroblast feeder cells and fetal calf serum-based methods (Takahashi et al., 2007; Yu et al., 2007) or defined mTESr/Matrigel-based protocols. Transplantation of hiPSC into immune-compromised mice leads to the formation of teratomas with derivatives of the three embryonic germ layers, demonstrating the pluripotent potential of these cells (Takahashi et al., 2007; Yu et al., 2007). In addition, differentiation of hiPSC *in vitro* also results in derivatives of the three germ layers. The review by Narsinh et al. (2011) provides a detailed overview of the methods to reprogram somatic cells to iPSC and discusses the advantages and disadvantages of the different techniques.

GENERATION OF iPSC-DERIVED CARDIOMYOCYTES

When iPSC are removed from differentiation suppression conditions and/or when grown in suspension aggregates [called embryoid bodies (EBs)] spontaneous differentiation to cells of the three germ layers occurs. CMs originate from the mesodermal germ layer, so that CM differentiation first requires efficient differentiation toward the mesodermal lineage. Directed differentiation toward the cardiac lineage is mainly achieved by one of the following strategies: (1) The first involves the formation of EBs in the presence of growth factors and repressors known to influence heart development (Kehat et al., 2001); (2) The second relies on the influence of endoderm on cardiac differentiation during embryogenesis (Mummery et al., 2003). Here, co-culture of iPSC with mouse END-2 is used to produce CMs; (3) The third involves monolayer culture at high density of iPSC seeded on Matrigel with sequential treatment with activin A and BMP4 (Laflamme et al., 2007). This method was developed using human embryonic stem cells (hESC) but has been transferred to hiPSC. Beating areas from differentiated EBs usually appear in 7–10 days. These EBs can be microscopically dissected and dissociated in single cells. For electrophysiological and immunofluorescence analysis, the dissociated cells can be seeded onto glass coverslips.

CHARACTERISTICS OF hiPSC-DERIVED CARDIOMYOCYTES

MOLECULAR AND STRUCTURAL CHARACTERISTICS

The first hiPS-CMs were generated by Zhang et al. (2009). In these cells the investigators examined the gene expression of the transcription factor Nkx2.5, the myofilament proteins cardiac troponin T, α-myosin heavy chain, α-actinin, the atrial and ventricular isoforms of myosin light chain 2, atrial natriuretic factor, and phospholamban (PLN). Low levels of cardiac troponin T and the atrial isoform of myosin light chain 2 were found in undifferentiated hiPSC and high expression of all the cardiac genes were found in the hiPSC-CMs, which was comparable to the expression of these genes in adult ventricular myocardium. Immunohistochemistry showed a typically striated pattern for α-actinin and myosin light chain. However, these cells had multiangular morphologies and relatively disorganized sacromeres (Dick et al., 2010). Novak and co-workers demonstrated by transmission electron microscopy analysis that hiPSC-CM had an immature ultra structure without t-tubuli (Novak et al., 2012).

ACTION POTENTIALS

Using the patch clamp technique, Zhang et al. (2009) were the first to measure the APs in spontaneously contracting cells isolated from hiPSC-EBs. The majority of the cells showed ventricular-like APs (70–74% of cells for two distinct hiPSC lines), but atrial-like and nodal-like APs were also observed. The distinction was made on AP phenotype, with a negative diastolic membrane potential, a rapid AP upstroke and a long plateau phase for ventricular-like APs. The absence of a prominent plateau phase was a characteristic of atrial-like APs, resulting in shorter AP duration compared to ventricular-like APs. Nodal-like APs showed a more positive maximum diastolic potential (MDP), a slower AP upstroke and a prominent phase 4 depolarization. Other studies also described ventricular-like, atrial-like, and sometimes nodal-like APs (Moretti et al., 2010; Fatima et al., 2011; Itzhaki et al., 2011a; Ma et al., 2011; Matsa et al., 2011; Jung et al., 2012; Lahti et al., 2012), with the ventricular-like phenotype being the most prominent AP form (76–48%) (Zhang et al., 2009; Moretti et al., 2010; Itzhaki et al., 2011a; Ma et al., 2011; Lahti et al., 2012). Comparison of hiPSC-CMs to hESC-CMs seems valuable, since hESC-CMs are more established. In hESC-CM, ventricular-like APs are also observed more frequently [50–60% (Zhang et al., 2009, 2011)]. Moretti et al. (2010) employed single-cell reverse-transcriptase-PCR in combination with patch-clamp in the same cell to show that the designation as ventricular-like, atrial-like, and nodal-like APs based on cellular electrophysiological features correlated with gene-expression of specific myocyte-lineage markers.

Table 1 summarizes the reported AP characteristics of hiPSC-CMs, hESC-CMs, and native ventricular CMs. The APs measured in hiPSC-CM differ from APs measured in freshly isolated native CMs (**Table 1**). The first remarkable difference is that most of the hiPSC-CMs studied, including the ventricular-like and atrial-like cells, are spontaneously active, with beating rates between 28 and 108 bpm (**Table 1**). Whether, in these studies, the spontaneous activity was used as a tool for CM selection and that non-beating CMs were also present, or whether it is a typical feature of hiPSC-CMs is unknown. We recently (Davis et al., 2012) performed experiments on non-spontaneously beating hiPSC-CM. For this we selected quiescent cells which were able to contract upon field stimulation. In these non-spontaneous beating hiPSC-CM, the resting membrane potential (RMP) was more negative then the MDP in most studies reporting on spontaneously active hiPSC-CMs (**Table 1**). Compared with native human ventricular CMs, where the reported RMP varies from −81.8 to −87 mV (**Table 1**), the MDP of ventricular-like hiPSC-CM APs is less negative with values ranging from −57 to −75 mV (**Table 1**). In spontaneously beating hiPSC-CM, the ventricular-like AP has a maximal upstroke velocity (dV/dt_{max}) ranging from 9 to 40 V/s which is slow compared to those non-spontaneously beating hiPSC-CM with a dV/dt_{max} of 115 V/s, and native ventricular CMs with a dV/dt_{max} of 215–234 V/s (Magyar et al., 2000).

Table 1 | Action potential characteristics in hiPSC-CM and human ventricular cardiomyocytes.

Cell type	BPM	APD_{90} (ms)	dv/dt_{max} (V/s)	APA (mV)	MDP/RMP (mV)	Exp. conditions	References
iPSC-CM V IMR90C4	43.8 ± 2.7	320.1 ± 17	40.5 ± 4.6	87.7 ± 2.6	−63.5 ± 1.7	37°C, me LJP: corr.	Zhang et al., 2009
iPSC-CM V ForeskinC1	44.2 ± 3.5	312.5 ± 11.2	27.2 ± 3.7	87.9 ± 2.4	−63.3 ± 1.5	37°C, me LJP: corr.	Zhang et al., 2009
iPSC-CM V	68.2 ± 2.7	381.3 ± 35.3	9 ± 0.2	107.8 ± 2.1	−63.5 ± 2.1	35°C, wc LJP:nk	Moretti et al., 2010
iPSC-CM V	72 ± 1.2	314.4 ± 17.6	26.8 ± 6.3	113.2 ± 2.4	−63.4 ± 1.3	36°C, pp LJP: nk	Lahti et al., 2012
iPSC-CM V	35.5 ± 2.1	414.7 ± 21.8	27.8 ± 4.8	101.5 ± 2.5	−75.6 ± 1.2	35–37°C pp, LJP: nk	Ma et al., 2011
iPSC-CM V	28 ± 5	495 ± 36	9.5 ± 1.8	109 ± 3	−57 ± 1	32°C, wc LJP: nk	Itzhaki et al., 2011a
iPSC-CM* ns	60	173.5 ± 12.2	115.7 ± 18.4	106 ± 3.2	−72.4 ± 0.9	37°C, pp LJP: corr	Davis et al., 2012
hESC-CM V	47.1 ± 23.3	247.2 ± 66.7	13.2 ± 6.2	85.4 ± 9.3	−53.9 ± 8.6	37°C, me LJP: nk	He et al., 2003
hESC-CM V		285.8 ± 52.6	11.4 ± 2.8	86.8 ± 52.6	−62.3 ± 8.6	rt, wc LJP: nk	Zhang et al., 2011
VM*	50	213 ± 7	215 ± 33	106.7 ± 1.4	−81.8 ± 3.3	37°C, wc LJP: nk	Magyar et al., 2000
VM endo*	60	330 ± 16	234 ± 28	105 ± 2	−87.1 ± 1	37°C, wc LJP: nk	Drouin et al., 1998
VM epi*	60	351 ± 14	228 ± 11	104 ± 2	−86 ± 1	37°C, wc LJP: nk	Drouin et al., 1998

*iPS-CM V, iPS-CM of ventricular-like phenotype; iPS-CM ns, not specified to action potential type; VM, native human ventricular myocyte; endo, endocardial; epi, epicardial; BPM, beats per minute; APD_{90}, action potential duration at 90% of repolarization; dV/dt_{max}, maximal upstroke velocity; APA, action potential amplitude; MDP, maximum diastolic potential; RMP, resting membrane potential; *, non spontaneous beating cells; hESC-CM V, hESC-CM of ventricular-like phenotype; me, micro electrode; wc, whole cell patch-clamp configuration; ljp: corr, corrected for liquid junction potential; ljp:nk, not known if corrected for liquid junction potential; rt, room temperature.*

The duration of ventricular-like hiPSC-CM APs, for example at 90% of repolarization (APD_{90}), is longer in spontaneous active cells (313–495 ms) compared to non-spontaneously active hiPSC-CMs (173 ms) and native freshly isolated CMs (213–351 ms) (**Table 1**). The AP amplitude (APA) for most ventricular-like hiPSC-CM APs (87–113 mV) is comparable to native ventricular CMs (104–106 mV), which due to the depolarized MDP in hiPSC-CM results in a higher overshoot of the hiPSC-CM AP. The direct comparison between the APs is complicated by the differences in experimental techniques used. Most hiPSC-CM studies used a temperature between 35 and 37°C; only in the study of Itzhaki was a temperature of 32°C used. This could be a possible explanation of the depolarized MDP, slow dV/dt_{max} and long APD_{90} in this latter study (Itzhaki et al., 2011a). The majority of the studies used the ruptured whole-cell patch-clamp technique, and three studies (Ma et al., 2011; Davis et al., 2012; Lahti et al., 2012) used the perforated patch-clamp technique. In the latter technique it is possible to perform experiments more close to physiological conditions since cell dialysis is minimal and EGTA, a buffer for Ca^{2+} ions, is absent.

MEMBRANE CURRENTS

The shape of the AP is the result of the various inwardly and outwardly directed ion currents present in the CM. A schematic overview of the different ionic membrane currents underlying the ventricular AP and their course is depicted in **Figure 1**. Because of the clear differences in AP shape between native CMs and hiPSC-CMs, one can assume that differences exist in the content and function of the various cardiac ion channels between the two cell types. Thus, before hiPSC-CMs can be used as a cell model in the study of cardiac arrhythmia syndrome, it is important to carry out a detailed comparison between the cardiac ion currents in hiPSC-CMs with those in native CMs. In the description of the cardiac ion currents below, a comparison between hiPSC-CMs displaying ventricular-like APs and healthy native human ventricular CMs is made, unless stated otherwise.

Sodium current

The cardiac Na^+ current (I_{Na}) is responsible for the AP upstroke in ventricular CMs [see (Berecki et al., 2010), and primary references cited therein]. Mutations in the genes encoding the α- and β-subunits of the cardiac Na^+ channel can alter the kinetics and availability of the cardiac Na^+ current (Remme et al., 2008). As stated before, the upstroke velocity in hiPSC-CM APs is extremely low compared to the AP upstroke of freshly isolated human ventricular CMs. In hiPSC-CM, I_{Na} was studied in detail in two reports (Ma et al., 2011; Davis et al., 2012). Ma et al. (2011) report a half-maximal potential ($V_{1/2}$) of activation and inactivation of –34.1 and –96.1 mV, respectively. Davis et al. (2012) report a $V_{1/2}$ of activation of ~42 mV. The findings of these studies are consistent with values reported for native human ventricular CMs (Sakakibara et al., 1993) (**Table 2**). The low temperature and

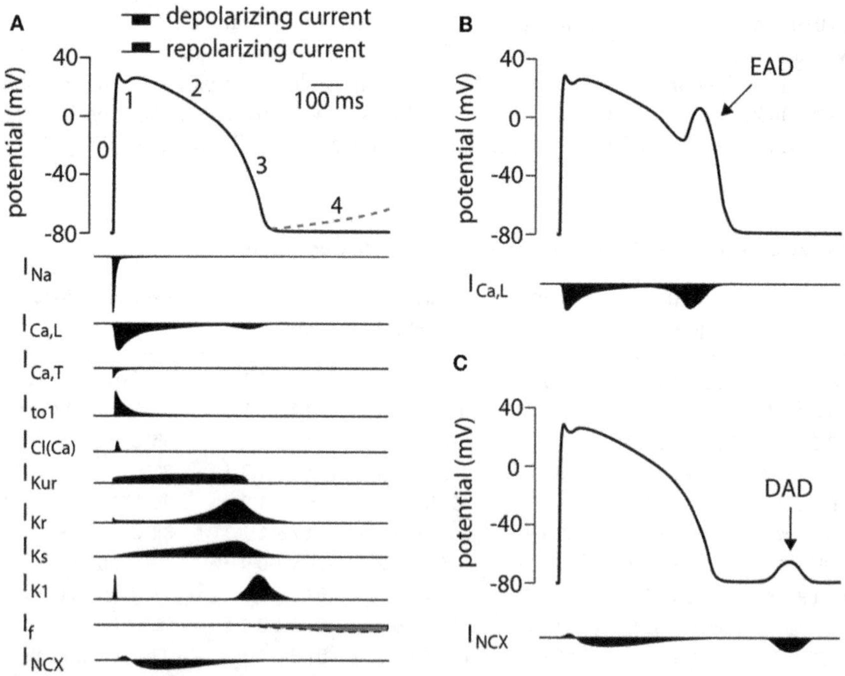

FIGURE 1 | (A) Schematic representation of a human ventricular action potential (top panel). Numbers denote the different phases of the ventricular action potential. The dashed line represents phase 4 depolarization normally present in cells from the conduction system and not in ventricular CMs. Underlying ionic membrane currents and their schematic time course are depicted below. **(B)** Schematic representation of an early afterdepolarization (EAD) and its underlying mechanism. **(C)** Schematic representation of a delayed afterdepolarization (DAD) and its underlying mechanism. I_{Na}, Na^+ current; $I_{Ca,L}$, L-type Ca^{2+} current; $I_{Ca,T}$, T-type Ca^{2+} current; I_{to1}, transient outward current type 1; $I_{Cl(Ca)}$, Ca^{2+} activated Cl^- current, also called I_{to2}; I_{Kur}, ultra rapid component of the delayed rectifier K^+ current, I_{Kr}, rapid component of the delayed rectifier K^+ current; I_{Ks}, slow component of the delayed rectifier K^+ current; I_{K1}, inward rectifier K^+ current; I_f, funny current; I_{NCX}, Na^+/Ca^{2+} exchange current.

Table 2 | Ion channel current and gating properties in hiPS-CM and human cardiomyocytes.

	Cell type	Peak current (pA/pF)	$V_{1/2}$ act (mV)	k act	$V_{1/2}$ inact (mV)	k inact	Exp. conditions	Reference
I_{Na}	iPS-CM	−216.7 ± 18.7	−34.1	5.9	−72.1	−5.7	35–37°C wc, LJP: nk	Ma et al., 2011
	iPS-CM	~280 (Figure 8C)	~ −42 (Figure 8D)				37°C, pp LJP: nc	Davis et al., 2012
	hESC-CM	−72 ± 21	−34	5.7	−78	−4.6	20°C, wc LJP: nk	Jonsson et al., 2012
	VM	−20.2 ± 2.2	−42.4 ± 3.0	6.3 ± 0.5	−100 ± 2.1	−6.3 ± 0.5	17°C, wc LJP: nk	Sakakibara et al., 1993
$I_{Ca,L}$	iPS-CM	−17.1 ± 1.7	−14.9	6.6	−29.1	−4.9	35–37°C wc, LJP: nk	Ma et al., 2011
	iPS-CM	−3.3	~ −45 (Figure 2E)				25°C, wc LJP: nk	Yazawa et al., 2011
	hESC-CM	−4.3 ± 0.6	−12	5.5			37°C, wc LJP: nk	Jonsson et al., 2012
	VM	−10.2 ± 0.6	−4.7 ± 0.7	3.7 ± 0.3	−19.3 ± 1.2	−3.45 ± 0.6	37°C, wc LJP: nk	Magyar et al., 2000
	VM	−3.8 ± 0.5	−4.2 ± 0.8	7 ± 0.3	−23.5 ± 1.4	−5.5 ± 1.4	21–23°C wc, LJP: nk	Mewes and Ravens, 1994
	AM	−2.2 ± 0.3	−12.1 ± 1.3	5.8 ± 0.4	−26.8 ± 1.3	−5.7 ± 0.2	21–23°C wc, LJP: nk	Mewes and Ravens, 1994
I_{to1}	iPS-CM	~2.4 (Figure 6D)					35–37°C wc, LJP: nk	Ma et al., 2011
	iPS-CM	~30 (Suppl. Figure 10A)					35°C, wc LJP: nk	Moretti et al., 2010
	hESC-CM	6.0 ± 0.9					37°C, wc LJP: nk	Sartiani et al., 2007
	VM endo	~5 (Figure 2B)	29.1 ± 1.2	12.9 ± 1.1	−17.6 ± 1.0	−8.9 ± 0.9	35°C, wc LJP: nk	Nabäuer et al., 1996
	VM epi	~16 (Figure 2A)	32.0 ± 1.11	14.9 ± 0.8	−9.5 ± 0.38	−5.1 ± 0.4	35°C, wc LJP: nk	Nabäuer et al., 1996
	VM endo	2.3 ± 0.3	23.1 ± 4.2	12.9 ± 0.8	−25.3 ± 3.0	−4.7 ± 0.8	20–22°C wc, LJP: nk	Wettwer et al., 1994
	VM epi	7.9 ± 0.7	15.4 ± 0.7	9.7 ± 1.6	−31.9 ± 1.5	−4.6 ± 0.2	20–22°C wc, LJP: nk	Wettwer et al., 1994
I_{Kr}	iPS-CM	0.95 ± 0.02	−22.7	4.9			35–37°C wc, LJP: nk	Ma et al., 2011
	iPS-CM	~1.9 (Figure 4A)					35°C, wc LJP: nk	Moretti et al., 2010
	iPS-CM	~1.9 (Figure 5C)					36°C, pp LJP: nk	Lahti et al., 2012
	iPS-CM	~0.55 (Figure 3D)					32°C, wc LJP: nk	Itzhaki et al., 2011a
	hESC-CM	−11.5 ± 1.8					37°C, wc LJP: nk	Jonsson et al., 2012
	VM	~0.25 (Figure 1C)	−5.74	5.63			37°C, wc LJP: nk	Iost et al., 1998
	VM	0.31 ± 0.02					37°C, wc LJP: nk	Magyar et al., 2000
I_{Ks}	iPS-CM	0.31 ± 0.09					35–37°C wc, LJP: nk	Ma et al., 2011
	iPS-CM	~2.5 (Figure 4A)					35°C, wc LJP: nk	Moretti et al., 2010
	hESC-CM	0.65 ± 0.12					37°C, wc LJP: nk	Jonsson et al., 2012
	VM	0.18					37°C, wc LJP: nk	Virag et al., 2001
I_{K1}	iPS-CM	~ −3.8 (Figure 6C)					35–37°C wc, LJP: nk	Ma et al., 2011
	hESC-CM	−2.67 ± 0.3					37°C, wc LJP: nk	Jonsson et al., 2012
	VM	~ −10 (Figure 3B)					37°C, wc LJP: nk	Magyar et al., 2000
I_f	iPS-CM	−4.1 ± 0.3	−84.6	8.8			35–37°C wc, LJP: nk	Ma et al., 2011
	hESC-CM	−10 ± 1.1	−74	4.5			37°C, wc LJP: nk	Jonsson et al., 2012
	VM	−1.18 ± 0.21	−111 ± 0.06				22°C, wc LJP: nk	Hoppe et al., 1998
	SAN	~ −8.0 (Figure 3B)	−96.9 ± 2.7	8.8 ± 0.5			36°C, wc LJP: corr	Verkerk et al., 2007

VM, native human ventricular myocyte; AM, native human atrial myocyte; endo, endocardial; epi, epicardial; SAN; native sinoatrial node myocyte; ~, estimated from figure. I_{Na}, Na^+ current; $I_{Ca,L}$, L-type Ca^{2+} current; I_{to1}, Transient outward current type 1; I_{Kr}, rapid compontent of the delayed rectifier K^+ current; I_{Ks}, slow component of the delayed rectifier K^+ current; I_{K1}, inward rectifier K^+ current; I_f, funny current; $V_{1/2}$ act, potential of half maximal activation; k act, slope factor of activation curve; $V_{1/2}$ inact, potential of half maximal inactivation; k inact, slope factor of inactivation curve hESC-CM; V, hESC-CM of ventricular-like phenotype; wc, whole cell patch-clamp configuration; ljp: corr, corrected for liquid junction potential; ljp: nk, not known if corrected for liquid junction potential, ljp: nc, not corrected for liquid junction potential.

reduced Na^+ concentration used to study the maximal peak I_{Na} in native human ventricular CM (Sakakibara et al., 1993) prevents comparison with the maximal peak I_{Na} measured in hiPSC-CM (Ma et al., 2011; Davis et al., 2012). Other I_{Na} characteristics, such as recovery from inactivation and slow inactivation have not been reported to date. In the presence of the Na^+ channel blocker tetrodotoxin (TTX) the upstroke of the AP in hiPSC-CMs is delayed and the dV/dt_{max} is reduced (Ma et al., 2011). In hESC-derived CMs (hESC-CM) the Na^+ channel blocker lidocaine also reduced the spontaneous beating rate (Kuzmenkin et al., 2009). Whether I_{Na} plays a role in spontaneous activity in hiPSC-CM is unknown. However, hiPSC-CMs have prominent Na^+ currents with characteristics close to that of native human ventricular CMs, despite any information to compare maximal peak I_{Na}, it seems that the low dV/dt_{max} of spontaneously active ventricular-like hiPSC-CM APs seems thus due to lower functional availability of Na^+ channels (related to the relative positive value of the RMP) rather than differences in I_{Na} density.

Calcium current

Two types of Ca^{2+} current exist in the mammalian heart, i.e., the L-type ($I_{Ca,L}$) and T-type ($I_{Ca,T}$) Ca^{2+} current [for review, see (Nerbonne and Kass, 2005)]. Patch clamp studies have demonstrated the presence of the $I_{Ca,L}$ in hiPSC-CM with a $V_{1/2}$ of activation and inactivation of –15 and –29 mV, respectively (Ma et al., 2011). These values are more comparable to those found in native atrial CMs (–12 and –27 mV, for $V_{1/2}$ of activation and inactivation, respectively) (Mewes and Ravens, 1994) than native ventricular myocytes (–4.2 and –4.7 mV and –23.5 and –19.3 mV) (Mewes and Ravens, 1994; Magyar et al., 2000). The maximal peak $I_{Ca,L}$ in hiPSC-CM reported by Ma et al. (2011) is 16.4 pA/pF, which is much higher than the 3.3 pA/pF reported in hiPSC-CM by Yazawa et al. (2011). In native ventricular CMs the amplitudes of the maximal current density varies between 2.2 and 10.2 pA/pF (Mewes and Ravens, 1994; Magyar et al., 2000) The higher maximal peak $I_{Ca,L}$ in the study of Ma et al. (2011) may be explained by the higher extracellular Ca^{2+} and higher temperatures used in their experiments. Blocking of the $I_{Ca,L}$ with nifedipine results in shortening of the AP duration and field potential duration (FDP) with minimal effects on dV/dt_{max} (Itzhaki et al., 2011a; Ma et al., 2011). Long-term application of nifedipine resulted in cessation of beating in some EBs (Itzhaki et al., 2011a).

Functional presence of the $I_{Ca,T}$ has not been reported in hiPSC-CM. Ma et al. (2011) did not find clear evidence for its presence. $I_{Ca,T}$ is present in the human heart conduction system, where it plays a role in facilitation of pacemaker depolarization, but is not functionally present in healthy human native ventricular CMs (Ono and Iijima, 2010). The T-type Ca^{2+} channels are re-expressed in atrial and ventricular CMs under pathological conditions such as cardiac hypertrophy and heart failure (Ono and Iijima, 2010).

Transient outward current

Two transient outward current components are found in native mammalian cardiac cells, one carried by $K^+(I_{to1})$, the other by Cl^- ions (I_{to2}) [for review, see (Nerbonne and Kass, 2005)]. While it is not yet known whether I_{to2} is present in hiPSC-CMs, native human ventricular CMs are known to lack I_{to2} (Verkerk et al., 2001). On the otherhand, I_{to1} has been found in hiPSC-CMs (Moretti et al., 2010; Ma et al., 2011), but data about gating properties are not known. Reported peak current densities of I_{to1} in hiPSC-CM display large variation, namely between 2.4 (Ma et al., 2011) and 30 pA/pF (Moretti et al., 2010), both at 60 mV. Values reported for native ventricular CMs vary between 2.3 and 16 pA/pF (Wettwer et al., 1994; Nabäuer et al., 1996). Although an exact comparison of I_{to1} density between hiPSC-CM and native human CMs is hampered by differences in experimental conditions, I_{to1} current density also depends on the site from which the native ventricular CMs are isolated, with larger current densities reported in human subepicardial ventricular myocytes compared to endocardial ventricular CMs (Beuckelmann et al., 1993; Wettwer et al., 1994).

Studies of I_{to1} block on hiPSC-CM APs have not yet been performed. However, due to the depolarized MDP values in hiPSC-CM, I_{to1} function may be limited because most channels will be inactivated (Varro and Papp, 1992). Further studies are required to address the function of I_{to1} in hiPSC-CM in detail.

The delayed rectifier potassium current

In the mammalian heart, the delayed rectifier K^+ current (I_K) is composed of three different components: the ultrarapid (I_{Kur}), the rapid (I_{Kr}), and the slow (I_{Ks}) components [for review, see (Nerbonne and Kass, 2005)]. To our knowledge, studies to elucidate the presence and function of I_{Kur} in hiPSC-CMs are lacking.

I_{Kr} has been reported in hiPSC-CM with a maximal I_{Kr} density varying between 0.55 and 1.9 pA/pF (Moretti et al., 2010; Itzhaki et al., 2011a; Ma et al., 2011; Lahti et al., 2012), values comparable to those in native human CMs where I_{Kr} densities are between 0.25 and 0.6 pA/pF (Iost et al., 1998; Magyar et al., 2000; Jost et al., 2009). $V_{1/2}$ of activation is –22.7 mV (Ma et al., 2011) in hiPSC-CM and –5.74 mV in native ventricular CMs (Iost et al., 1998) and –14 mV in atrial CMs (Wang et al., 1994). In hiPSC-CMs, blockade of I_{Kr} by E4031 resulted in a significant AP prolongation In addition, E4031 induced early afterdepolarizations (EADs) (Itzhaki et al., 2011a; Ma et al., 2011; Matsa et al., 2011; Lahti et al., 2012), that is afterdepolarization during the AP (**Figure 1B**) due to the reactivation of $I_{Ca,L}$ (Verkerk et al., 2000b). Thus, I_{Kr} plays a prominent role in the repolarization phase of hiPSC-CM APs. Interestingly, in hESC-CM E4031 reduced the beating rate (Kuzmenkin et al., 2009) suggesting that I_{Kr} also plays a role in spontaneous activity.

The presence of I_{Ks} in hiPSC-CMs has been reported in two studies. Ma et al. (2011) found I_{Ks} in 5 out of 16 cells studied, and when present the average I_{Ks} density was 0.31 pA/pF. In contrast, Moretti et al. (2010) measured I_{Ks} in all studied cells and the average density was around 2.5 pA/pF [estimated from Figure 4A (Moretti et al., 2010)]. In native left ventricular human CMs, Virag et al. (2001) identified I_{Ks} in 31 out of 58 cells and the maximal current density was approximately 0.18 pA/pF. In hiPSC-CMs, blockade of I_{Ks} by chromanol 293B results only in minimal prolongation of the AP (Ma et al., 2011). This is consistent with the relative small number of cells exhibiting I_{Ks} and the small I_{Ks} densities found in their study, but contrast with the effects of a loss-of-function I_{Ks} mutation which results in a prominent AP prolongation (see paragraph "LQT1"). A study by Wang et al. (2011) in hESC-CMs suggests altered expression of the β-subunit mink encoded by the *KCNE1* gene, as a mechanism for variable I_{Ks} function in the developing heart and in disease.

Inward rectifier current

In atrial and ventricular CMs, the inward rectifier K^+ current (I_{K1}) is an important contributor to the maintenance of the RMP and contributes to the terminal phase of repolarization (Dhamoon and Jalife, 2005). I_{K1} was found to be present in hiPSC-CM (Ma et al., 2011). I_{K1} density in hiPSC-CM is four times smaller than that reported in native ventricular CMs, 0.9 (Ma et al., 2011) and 3.6 pA/pF (Magyar et al., 2000), respectively. In hESC-CMs I_{K1} is significantly increased in longer cultured hiPSC-CMs, these cells also displayed a flattened diastolic depolarization rate and decreased spontaneous activity (Sartiani et al., 2007).

The small I_{K1} densities in hiPSC-CMs may explain the frequently observed spontaneous activity in these cells. However, whether all hiPSC-CMs have a low I_{K1} density or whether a bias is introduced by the selection of spontaneously active cells for patch-clamp needs to be elucidated.

The acetylcholine-activated K^+ current

The acetylcholine-activated K^+ current ($I_{K,ACh}$) is involved in parasympathetic regulation of heart rate (Tamargo et al., 2004). $I_{K,ACh}$ is to our knowledge not yet studied in hiPSC-CM. Studies addressing the presence of $I_{K,ACh}$ in hiPSC-CM might be particularly important in modeling atrial arrhythmias, as blockers of $I_{K,Ach}$, which leave ventricular repolarization intact, are effective in the treatment of atrial fibrillation (Hashimoto et al., 2006).

The ATP-sensitive K^+ current

The ATP-sensitive K^+ current ($I_{K,ATP}$) has not been studied in detail in hiPSC-CMs. However, the $I_{K,ATP}$ channel openers nicorandil and pinacidil shorten the AP in hiPSC-CMs (Itzhaki et al., 2011a; Matsa et al., 2011), suggesting that $I_{K,ATP}$ channels are present in these cells. Further studies are required to address the presence and function of $I_{K,ATP}$ in hiPSC-CM in detail.

The hyperpolarization-activated "funny" current

The funny current (I_f) is an inward current activating at hyperpolarized membrane potentials [for review, see (Verkerk et al., 2007)]. In human sinoatrial node cells, the current density of I_f at a membrane potential of –130 mV is reported to be 8 pA/pF (Verkerk et al., 2007). I_f is also described in human atrial CMs (El Chemaly et al., 2007) and in human ventricular CMs during heart failure [(Hoppe et al., 1998)]. The current densities reported, however, are much smaller, compared to human sinoatrial node cells. hiPSC-CMs also exhibit I_f (Ma et al., 2011) and the reported current density is 4.1 pA/pF (Ma et al., 2011). The relatively high I_f density in hiPSC-CMs compared to human ventricular CMs might be attributed to the fact that these cells express higher levels of the HCN isoforms (HCN1, 2, 4) as compared to adult human CMs. (Synnergren et al., 2012). In hiPSC-CMs, I_f starts to activate at potentials negative of –60 mV and has a $V_{1/2}$ of activation of –84 mV (Ma et al., 2011) and may therefore have a role in spontaneous activity in these cells. hESC-CMs have comparable characteristics of I_f, and in these cells blockade of I_f with zatebradine resulted in slowing of spontaneous activity due to a reduced diastolic depolarization rate (Sartiani et al., 2007).

Na^+-Ca^{2+} exchange current

The Na^+-Ca^{2+} exchange current (I_{NCX}) is crucial for Ca^{2+} extrusion from the cell and plays a role in the electric activity of mammalian CMs (Sipido et al., 2007). While the functional properties of I_{NCX} have not been studied in hiPSC-CM, the presence of the Na^+-Ca^{2+} exchanger in hiPSC-CM has been demonstrated at the level of the protein (Lee et al., 2011). I_{NCX} is present in hESC-CM and its density increases with maturation (Fu et al., 2010).

In human CMs, Ca^{2+} extrusion by the Na^+/Ca^{2+} exchanger is the major mechanism to balance the Ca^{2+} influx through the $I_{Ca,L}$ (Sipido et al., 2007). In addition, the Na^+/Ca^{2+} exchanger has a function during depolarization where it contributes in its reverse mode (Ca^{2+} influx) to the total amount of Ca^{2+} influx. The amplitude of the I_{NCX} depends on the membrane potential and the intracellular levels of Na^+ ($[Na^+]_i$) and Ca^+ ($[Ca^{2+}]_i$) (Sipido et al., 2007). Altered $[Na^+]_i$ and/or $[Ca^{2+}]_i$ will lead to altered I_{NCX} and can cause cardiac arrhythmias due to spontaneous Ca^{2+} releases from the SR. Studying the I_{NCX} in hiPSC-CM might be of particular interest in cardiac arrhythmia models of CPVT and LQT3. CPVT is associated with mutations in the RyR2 which can lead to increased $[Ca^{2+}]_i$ due to altered gating properties of the RyR2 receptor. In LQT3 syndrome there is an increased persistent I_{Na} (Remme et al., 2006), which might lead to elevated levels of $[Na^+]_i$.

EXCITATION-CONTRACTION COUPLING

hiPSC-CMs display clearly visible contractions. In native adult CMs, a small influx of Ca^{2+} through the L-type Ca^{2+} channels triggers a several-fold multiplied Ca^{2+} release from the sarcoplasmic reticulum (SR) via ryanodine receptors (RyRs). This phenomenon is referred to as "Ca^{2+-}induced Ca^{2+} release" (CICR) (Lee et al., 2011). CICR is the key mechanism underlying excitation-contraction coupling. The key Ca^{2+} handling proteins, RyR2, SR Ca^{2+}-ATPase (SERCA), junctin (Jun), triadin (TRDN), Na^+/Ca^{2+} exchanger (NCX), calsequestrin (CASQ2), L-type Ca^{2+} channel ($Ca_v1.2$), inositol-1,4,5-trisphosphate receptor (IP3R2) and PLN are expressed in hiPSC-CM (Itzhaki et al., 2011b; Lee et al., 2011). Spontaneous rhythmic Ca^{2+} transients are present in hiPSC-CM, and blocking of the $I_{Ca,L}$ by nifedipine, abolishes Ca^{2+} transients (Itzhaki et al., 2011b). The presence of functional SR and RyRs was proven by application of caffeine, which induced a large Ca^{2+} transient (Itzhaki et al., 2011b; Lee et al., 2011), consistent with findings in human ventricular CMs (Piacentino et al., 2003). In addition, ryanodine caused a reduction in the amplitude of the Ca^{2+} transient (Itzhaki et al., 2011b; Lee et al., 2011). The pattern of Ca^{2+} transient in hiPSC-CM was studied by transverse line-scan images and revealed a U-shape Ca^{2+} wavefront (the rise of Ca^{2+} in the periphery is faster than in the center of the cell), which is typical for t-tubule deficient cells (Lee et al., 2011). This suggests that hiPSC-CMs lack t-tubuli, an observation which is in line with that of Novak and co-workers (Novak et al., 2012) who did not find t-tubuli with transmission electron microscopy. This would mean that hiPSC-CMs likely have poor coupling between Ca^{2+} influx through L-type Ca^{2+} channels and Ca^{2+} release from the SR through RyRs.

HUMAN iPSC-CM MODELS FOR INHERITED CARDIAC ARRHYTHMIAS

hiPSC-CM MODELS FOR LQTS

LQT1

Moretti and co-workers (Moretti et al., 2010) were the first to publish on a hiPSC-CM model for a primarily electrical disease, namely LQT1. LQT1 is a repolarization disorder identified by a prolongation of the QT interval on the ECG due to mutations in the *KCNQ1* gene, encoding the α subunit of the K^+ channel responsible of I_{Ks} (Wilde and Bezzina, 2005). They investigators obtained fibroblasts from two, so far, asymptomatic patients, with the *KCNQ*1-G569A mutation and two healthy controls (Moretti et al., 2010). These fibroblasts were infected with retroviruses encoding OCT3/4, SOX2, KLF4, and c-MYC; hiPSC-CMs were differentiated as EBs. In this study AP characteristics and K^+ currents were investigated in spontaneously beating cells. Three different types of AP s were distinguished, that were designated as ventricular-, atrial-, and nodal-like. These investigators also correlated these characteristics with gene-expression analysis of specific myocyte-lineage markers (MLC2v, MLC2a, and HCN4 for ventricular-, atrial- and nodal-like cells, respectively). The delayed rectifier currents were studied in ventricular-like myocytes. In hiPSC-CMs derived from the LQT1 patient (LQT1-iPSC-CM), I_{Ks} peak and tail current densities were reduced by approximately 75%, and I_{Kr} conductance was unaffected. APs of atrial-like and ventricular-like hiPSC-CMs were significantly prolonged in LQT1-iPSC-CMs compared to control (WT-iPSC-CMs). Adaptation of the AP duration to higher pacing frequencies and the response to isoproterenol were impaired in LQT- iPSC-CM. EADs were elicited in response to isoproterenol (a β-adrenergic agonist) in 6 out of 9 LQT1-iPSC-CM and never in WT-iPSC-CM. When propranolol (a non-selective β-blocker) was applied the effect of isoproterenol was blunted. These data are in line with observations in LQT1 patients as these patients suffer from arrhythmias during increased heart rates caused by emotional stress or exercise. The data is also in line with the beneficial effects of β-blockers in suppressing arrythmias in these patients (Ruan et al., 2008). Immunocytochemistry revealed that the *KCNQ*1-G569A mutation leads to impaired trafficking and localization of the mutant channels.

LQT2

Three groups have published on hiPSC-CM models of LQT2 (Itzhaki et al., 2011a,b; Matsa et al., 2011; Lahti et al., 2012). LQT2 is a repolarization disorder caused by mutations in *KCNH2*, encoding I_{Kr} channels (Wilde and Bezzina, 2005).

Itzhaki et al. (2011a) reported on a hiPSC-CMs model generated from dermal fibroblasts obtained from a 28-year-old woman with a diagnosis of familial LQT2 due to the *KCNH2*-A614V mutation. Clinical data of the patient were not shown. Fibroblasts were reprogrammed by retroviral infection with vectors encoding for SOX-2, KLF4, and OCT4. In this study EB formation was used for differentiation of the hiPSC into CMs. In this study APs were measured from spontaneously contracting clusters and the hiPSC-CMs were classified as nodal-, atrial-, and ventricular-like. Prolongation of repolarization and predisposition to the development of EADs was shown in cells with atrial- and ventricular-like APs. For voltage clamp experiments the spontaneously beating clusters were dissociated to single cells. Peak amplitudes of I_{Kr} were found to be significantly smaller in LQT2-iPSC-CM compared to WT-iPSC-CM. FDP corrected for variations in beating frequency were longer in LQT2-iPSC-CM compared to WT-iPSC-CM. When I_{Kr} was blocked by the hERG blocker E4021, the AP prolonged and EADs were seen in 66% of the cells studied. Furthermore, the effects of agents that may have a therapeutic effect in preventing arrhythmias were also studied. These agents include nifedipine, pinacidil, and ryanodine. Because Ca^{2+} influx through L-type Ca^{2+} channels contributes to AP duration and has a role in EAD formation, inhibition of $I_{Ca,L}$ by nifedipine was proposed to be anti-arrhythmic. Another anti-arrhythmic strategy proposed was to augment the repolarization currents, by the $I_{K,ATP}$ channel opener pinacidil. Both interventions resulted in AP shortening and abolished propensity to EADs. This study also demonstrated that ranolazine, a blocker of the persistent I_{Na}, did not shorten the AP duration, but prevented EADs.

Matsa et al. (2011) generated hiPSC-CMs of a symptomatic and an asymptomatic carrier of the G1681A mutation in *KCNH2*. The symptomatic patient, female with a QTc interval of up to 571 ms, experienced 11 episodes of syncope in 12 months. As is typical for LQT2, episodes occurred at arousal from sleep and not during competitive sports. Her mother was the asymptomatic individual studied; although her QTc-interval was prolonged she had not experienced any symptoms. The hiPSC-CMs were derived from punch biopsies of skin, which were reprogrammed by lentiviral delivery of OCT4, SOX2 NANOG, and LIN28; EB formation was used for differentiation of cells into CMs. I_{Kr} current characteristics were not studied. The derived hiPSC-CMs showed APs which were categorized as ventricular-, atrial- and pacemaker-like. Ventricular- and atrial-like APs from the symotomatic patient and her mother showed increased durations compared to APs of the genetically unrelated control; AP duration was less in the maternal hiPSC-CMs compared to those of the patient. Application of isoprenaline resulted in 25% of LQT2-iPSC-CMs in electrophysiological abnormalities, including EADs. Isoprenaline-induced arrhythmias were ameliorated by nadolol or propanolol, non-selective β-blockers. This is in line with the clinical picture in LQT2 as these patients experience arrhythmias due to increased heart rates caused by emotional and similar stress, mainly auditory stimulation and arousal from sleep. As for LQT1, LQT2 patients are often treated with β-blockers for prevention of cardiac events (Ruan et al., 2008). I_{Kr} blockade by E4031 resulted in prolongation of the AP duration and EADs in 30% of the LQT2-iPSC-CMs, but never in control cells. Nicorandil, an $I_{K,ATP}$ channel opener, and PD-118057, an I_{Kr} channel enhancer, shortened the AP in LQT2-iPSC-CM, showing that potassium channel activators can normalize the prolonged repolarization in LQT2.

Lahti et al. (2012) derived hiPSC-CMs from an asymptomatic carrier of the R176W mutation in the *KCNH2*. This mutation is one of the four founder mutations of LQTS cases in Finland, and present in one in 400 Finns (Marjamaa et al., 2009). The QTc intervals of patients carrying the R176W mutation range from 386 to 569 ms, with a mean of 448 ms (Fodstad et al., 2006). In the study of Lahti et al. (2012), fibroblasts were infected with lentivirus followed by retroviruses encoding for OCT4, SOX2, KLF4, and MYC to generate iPSC-CMs. CM differentiation was achieved by co-culturing hiPSC with END-2 cells. APs were divided into two types, atrial- and ventricular-like APs. Only the ventricular-like APs showed significantly increased APD_{90}. The AP frequency had a tendency toward slower frequencies in LQT2-iPSC-CM. EADs were present in 1 of 20 LQT2 iPSC-CMs and were never observed in WT-iPSC-CMs. I_{Kr} step and tail current densities were reduced by 40–46%. The APs of LQT2-iPSC-CMs had a significantly prolonged duration compared to WT AP, especially at low frequencies. The I_{Kr} blocker E4031 provoked EADs in WT-iPSC-CM and LQT2-iPSC-CM, with the effect on LQT2-iPSC-CMs being more pronounced. Sotalol, a non-selective β-blocker elicited EADs only in LQT2-iPSC-CM.

These three studies on LQT2 show that LQT-iPSC-CMs of symptomatic patients show a more severe cellular phenotype than those obtained from asymptomatic patients with the same mutation. However, assessing severity in the hiPSC-CMs system is challenging. For instance, blocking I_{Kr} by E-4031 in WT-iPSC-CMs leads to different findings in different studies. In the study of Matsa et al. (2011) no EADs were provoked by the application of E4031, whereas in the study of Ma et al. (2011) and Lahti et al. (2012) EADs could be provoked in >50% of WT-iPSC-CM. This might reflect diversity of hiPSC-CM lines. However, the differences between the outcomes of these studies might also be caused by the use of different concentrations E-4031. Ma et al. (2011) and Lahti et al. (2012) used a concentration of 100 nmol/l and 500 nmol/l, respectively. The concentration used by Matsa et al. (2011) is not known.

LQT3/Conduction disease/BrS

LQT3 is a repolarization disorder caused by gain-of-function mutations in *SCN5A* encoding the cardiac Na^+ channel. These mutations cause an increased persistent Na^+ current which acts to prolong CM repolarization and increase AP duration (Wilde and Bezzina, 2005). On the otherhand, SCN5A mutations associated with loss of channel function cause conduction disease and Brugada Syndrome (BrS). The latter is an arrhythmia syndrome characterized by ST segment elevation in the right precordial leads of the EGC; SCN5A mutations account for around 20% of BrS cases (Wilde and Bezzina, 2005). Loss of Na^+ channel function leads to a decreased peak I_{Na}, which causes slowing of the upstroke velocity of the AP.

Recently, we have, generated an iPSC-CM model of a patient carrying the *SCN5A*-1795insD mutation (Davis et al., 2012). This mutation gives rise to a phenotype of LQT3 as well as BrS and conduction defects, caused by both gain- and loss-of-function effects on the cardiac Na^+ channel, respectively (Remme et al., 2006, 2009). In this study we generated hiPSC-CMs by transducing fibroblasts with lentiviral vectors encoding OCT4, SOX2, KLF4 and C-MYC (Davis et al., 2012). Cardiac differentiation was induced by co-culture with END-2 cells. In line with the known effects of the mutation in a knock-in mouse model, and in line with the clinical presentation in mutation carriers, we observed a decrease in peak I_{Na} and an increase in persistent I_{Na} in the hiPSC-CMs with *SCN5A*-1795insD compared to genetically unrelated control. APs measured in non-spontaneously active hiPSC-CMs displayed a reduced upstroke velocity and a prolonged duration compared to those derived from a genetically unrelated control.

LQT8/Timothy syndrome

LQT8 and Timothy syndrome are caused by mutation in the *CACNA1C* gene encoding the L-type Ca^{2+} channel. Repolarization disease is only one facet of LQT8 as *CACNA1C* mutations also give rise to other features including syndactyly, heart malformations, and autism spectrum disorders (Yazawa et al., 2011). Yazawa et al. (2011) studied hiPSC-CMs of two patients with LQT8. Fibroblasts were isolated from skin biopsies and were reprogrammed using four retroviruses containing SOX2, OCT3/4, KLF4, and MYC. EBs were used in the generation of hiPSC-CMs. EBs from LQT8/Timothy syndrome hiPSC lines contracted at 30 bpm, whereas control hiPSC-line EBs contracted at a rate of 60 bpm. The LQT8-iPSC-CM showed delay in inactivation of $I_{Ca,L}$ and abnormalities in intracellular Ca^{2+} handling, with larger and prolonged Ca^{2+} transients. Importantly, such aspects of $I_{Ca,L}$ mutations can not be revealed when studying the mutation in a heterologous cell system. The APs of LQT8/Timothy syndrome ventricular-like hiPSC-CMs were three times longer than those of WT hiPSC-CMs. Roscovitine, a compound that increases the voltage-dependent inactivation of the voltage dependent Ca^{2+} channel, reverted the delayed inactivation and restored the irregular Ca^{2+} transients associated with LQT8/Timothy syndrome.

CATECHOLAMINERGIC POLYMORPHIC VENTRICULAR TACHYCARDIA

CPVT is characterized by cateholamine/stress-induced ventricular arrhythmias that can lead to sudden cardiac death in young individuals (Priori and Chen, 2011). CPVT is linked to mutations in the *RYR2* gene, encoding an intracellular Ca^{2+} release channel, and mutations in *CASQ2*, encoding a calcium binding protein in the SR which stores Ca^2. RyR2 and CASQ2 play a role in Ca^{2+} cycling and contractile activity of the CM (Priori and Chen, 2011). To date, three groups have published a CPVT hiPSC model (Fatima et al., 2011; Jung et al., 2012; Novak et al., 2012).

Fatima et al. (2011) studied the F243I mutation in the *RYR2* gene. A skin biopsy of a patient with CPVT carrying the F243I mutation in the *RYR2* gene was taken and fibroblasts derived from this biopsy were infected with retroviruses encoding OCT3/4. SOX2, KLF4, and c-MYC. Cardiac differentiation was achieved by co-culturing with END-2 cells. APs were measured in spontaneously beating single hiPSC-CMs and were categorized as ventricular-, atrial-, and nodal-like APs. Isoproterenol was used to evoke the phenotype. In 22 out of 38 CPVT-iPSC-CMs isoprenaline resulted in a negative chronotropic response and 13 cells exhibited delayed afterdepolarizations (DADs), which are afterdepolarizations after and AP (**Figure 1C**) due to spontaneous SR Ca^{2+} release what activates I_{NCX} (Verkerk et al., 2000a). All control hiPSC-CM showed normal positive chronotropic response. Confocal fluorescence imaging revealed spontaneous local Ca^{2+} release events of higher amplitude and longer duration in CPVT-iPS-CMs. In addition, the CPVT-iPSC-CMs showed a decrease in $I_{Ca,L}$ and Ca^{2+} transients in the presence of forskolin, an adenyl cyclase activator. As the authors state, this is likely due to the large and sustained rise of intracellular Ca^{2+} concentration.

Jung et al. (2012) studied the *RYR2* mutation S406L. Fibroblasts of the patient were transduced with a retroviral vector encoding SOX2, OCT4, KLF4, and c-MYC. To direct the hiPSCs to the cardiac lineage, EB differentiation was used. The CPVT-iPSC-CM showed elevated Ca^{2+} concentrations, a reduced SR Ca^{2+} content, and increased susceptibility to DADs under catecholaminergic stress induced by isoproterenol. Further the authors investigated the ability of dantrolene to rescue the disease phenotype. Dantrolene is a hydrantoin derivative and muscle relaxant, currently used as therapy in cases with malignant hyperthermia, a disorder caused by mutations in the skeletal ryanodine receptor (*RYR1*) (Kobayashi et al., 2009). Dantrolene, restored normal Ca^{2+} spark properties and the arrhythmogenic phenotype.

Novak et al. (2012) studied the effect of the autosomal recessive missense mutation D307H in the *CASQ2* gene. Dermal fibroblasts of two mutation carriers were transduced with a single lentiviral vector containing OCT4, SOX2, KLF4, and c-MYC. Differentiation toward hiPSC-CMs was achieved by EB formation. Spontaneous beating rate of differentiated EBs was significantly lower in CPVT-iPSC-CMs (~26 bpm) compared to control iPSC-CMs (~39 bpm). Isoproterenol induced DADs, oscillatory arrhythmic prepotentials (diastolic voltage oscillation, which appear during the late diastolic depolarization) and increased $[Ca^{2+}]_i$.

CONCLUSIONS AND FUTURE PERSPECTIVES

The hiPSC-CM models described in this review show that it is possible to recapitulate *in vitro* in the hiPSC-CM system the disease phenotype of patients with Mendelian cardiac rhythm disorders. Furthermore, different studies have shown that LQT-iPSC-CMs of symptomatic patients show a more severe cellular phenotype than those obtained from asymptomatic patients with the same mutation (Itzhaki et al., 2011a; Matsa et al., 2011; Lahti et al., 2012). Moreover, hiPSC-CMs can recapitulate a phenotype that cannot be shown in a heterologous expression system (Lahti et al., 2012). For example, Lahti et al. (2012) reported a decrease of ~43% in I_{Kr} density in LQT2- iPSC-CMs with the R176W mutation, which was not revealed in a heterologous expression system. This might reflect, amongst others, differences in cellular environment between the two cell systems or may be due to the effect of high transgene expression as a consequence of the use of a strong promoter in the heterologous expression system. A significant advantage of the hiPSC-CM system is that in this system, in contrast to heterologous expression systems, it also possible to study the effects on the AP and Ca^{2+} cycling.

The responses to some pharmacological agents are studied in hiPSC-CMs. The results are in line with what is seen in patients, healthy human beings, and adult CM. For example β-adrenergic stimulation with isoproterenol leads to a positive chronotropic effect and AP shorterning (Zhang et al., 2009; Moretti et al., 2010) and application of β-blockers blunt the effect of isoproterenol (Moretti et al., 2010). Also the AP shortening effects of $I_{K,ATP}$ openers pinacidil and nicorandil and the I_{Ca} channel blocker nifedipine was captured in hiPSC-CM.

Functional I_{Na} (Ma et al., 2011; Davis et al., 2012), $I_{Ca,L}$(Itzhaki et al., 2011a; Ma et al., 2011; Yazawa et al., 2011), I_{Kr} (Itzhaki et al., 2011a; Ma et al., 2011; Matsa et al., 2011; Lahti et al., 2012) and I_{Ks}(Ma et al., 2011) have been demonstrated in hIPSC-CMs and mutations affecting these channels as well as pharmacological ion channel blockade were shown to impact on the AP. While the functional presence of SR, RyRs and the Ca^{2+} binding protein CASQ2was demonstrated (Itzhaki et al., 2011b; Lee et al., 2011; Novak et al., 2012), studies have shown that the coupling between Ca^{2+} influx through L-type Ca^{2+} channels and Ca^{2+} release from the SR through RyRs is poor as a consequence of the lack of t-tubuli in hiPSC-CMS. Thus, the use of hiPSC-CMs to study certain cardiac arrhythmia syndromes, such as CPVT and LQT8, caused by mutations in one of the Ca^{2+} handling proteins is limited to the study of the biophysical properties of the affected protein. While I_{to1}, I_{K1}, and I_f are present in hiPSC-CMs (Ma et al., 2011), their contribution to electrical activity in these cells has not been proven by pharmacological blockade or through the effect of mutations in the respective genes. Openers of $I_{K,ATP}$ shorten the AP (Itzhaki et al., 2011a; Matsa et al., 2011), so functional presence can be presumed but needs to be studied in more detail. The presence of I_{NCX} is also not studied in detail but its functional presence can also be presumed since intact Ca^{2+} handling has been demonstrated (Itzhaki et al., 2011b; Lee et al., 2011). Up till now there is no evidence for the functional presence or absence of $I_{K,ACh}$.

A difficulty in the use of hiPSC-CM models is their immature electrophysiological phenotype, with depolarized MDP or RMP and slow AP upstroke velocities compared to native CMs. The MDP and upstroke velocity of hiPSC-CMs resemble more those of fetal CMs than adult CMs (Davis et al., 2011). Furthermore, most studies report that hiPSC-CM beat spontaneously, which is also characteristic of fetal CMs (Mummery et al., 2003). Of note, in our study on *quiescent* hiPSC-CMs we recorded a more-negative RMP and a faster AP upstroke velocity (Davis et al., 2012). Considering the importance of I_{K1} for setting the RMP, it is likely that the quiescent hiPSC-CMs have a larger I_{K1} than spontaneously beating hiPSC-CMs. It is not known whether quiescent cells were also present among the hiPSC-CM generated in studies in which spontaneously beating hiPSC-CMs were studied. Possibly, in these studies, the spontaneous activity was used as a tool to recognize CMs. A further consideration is that *cultured* adult CMs show a depolarized MDP and slower AP upstroke velocity compared to freshly isolated adult CMs. The depolarized MDP in cultured CMs is known to be caused by progressive decline in I_{K1} (Mitcheson et al., 1998). Another similarity between cultured ventricular myocytes and hiPSC-CMs is that different AP phenotypes are observed. In many hiPSC-CM studies different AP characteristics are observed and are classified as ventricular-like, atrial-like and nodal-like AP. Similarly, when ventricular CMs are cultured different AP phenotypes are observed after one day in culture, and more pronounced variability is evident after four days in culture (Mitcheson et al., 1998).

Another difficulty is the purity of the population of hiPSC-CMs acquired. With the current techniques it is not possible to acquire a pure population of CMs, the fraction of CMs obtained may vary from 1% to ~50% of the total cells (Dambrot et al., 2011). Moreover, as discussed above, the CMs that are generated are in fact a mixed population of CMs displaying different AP characteristics. One way in which this issue might be addressed is through the use of selectable markers driven by CM lineage-specific promoter elements. However, while this might be useful in selecting CMs as opposed to other cell types, more research is still required for the identification of promoter elements that may be used in selecting for specific CM types (e.g., ventricular versus atrial). Another solution might be found in chemical enhancement of cardiac differentiation. For instance, ascorbic acid enhances cardiac differentiation and minimizes the interline variance and facilitates the structural and functional maturation of hiPSC-CMs (Cao et al., 2012). From hESC-CM research we know that bone morphogenetic protein (BMP) signaling inhibition after mesodermal formation facilitates cardiac development. In this study, also a possibility for ventricular or atrial specific differentiation is shown (Zhang et al., 2011). Inhibition of retinoid (RA) signaling by noggin leads to CM specification into ventricular cells, whereas RA treatment leads to atrial specification (Zhang et al., 2011). Direction of differentiation to nodal like CMs can be achieved by activation of the $Ca2^{+}$ activated potassium channels of small and intermediate conductance (SKCas) by 1-ethyl-2-benzimidazolinone (Kleger et al., 2010). Ventricular specification and electrophysiological maturation of hESC-CMs may also be promoted by microRNAs (miRs). MiR-499 was shown to promote ventricular specification; miR-1 facilitates electrophysiological maturation (Fu et al., 2011).

In summary, iPSC-CM models recapitulate the phenotype of patients with cardiac arrhythmia syndromes. However, the interpretation of electrophysiological data derived from these cells, should be done with caution, since hiPSC-CMs present immature phenotypes and do not recapitulate all the electrical characteristics of an adult CM. Thus, studies addressing the maturity and purity of the hiPSC-CMs acquired are needed, as well as studies to characterize the electrophysiological and pharmacological characteristcs in more detail. Because of this, there are still limitations for the use of this model system in studies on cardiac rhythm disorders, especially if the disease causing mutation is not known. So far, hiPSC-CMs have only been applied as models to the study of disorders for which mutations in particular genes have been identified. Future studies are likely to demonstrate the potential of these cell systems in pointing us to pathophysiological mechanisms for those cases for which no gene mutations are yet known. Another future application of hiPSC-CMs is the use in cardiac safety pharmacology and the development of new drugs. hiPSC-CMs provide researchers with CMs of human origin which are better-suited than CMs of animal origin or heterologous cell systems. Furthermore, hiPSC-CMs provide us with the opportunity to test drugs in disease-specific CMs instead of healthy CMs. Thus, in future studying hiPSC models might lead to novel insights in pathophysiology, improve understanding of genotype-phenotype relationships and could be used in the development and testing of pharmacological agents to treat human cardiac disease.

REFERENCES

Aasen, T., Raya, A., Barrero, M. J., Garreta, E., Consiglio, A., Gonzalez, F., Vassena, R., Bilic, J., Pekarik, V., Tiscornia, G., Edel, M., Boue, S., and Izpisua Belmonte, J. C. (2008). Efficient and rapid generation of induced pluripotent stem cells from human keratinocytes. *Nat. Biotechnol.* 26, 1276–1284.

Berecki, G., Wilders, R., de Jonge, B., van Ginneken, A. C. G., and Verkerk, A. O. (2010). Re-evaluation of the action potential upstroke velocity as a measure of the Na+ current in cardiac myocytes at physiological conditions. *PLoS ONE* 5:e15772. doi: 10.1371/journal.pone.0015772

Beuckelmann, D. J., Nabauer, M., and Erdmann, E. (1993). Alterations of K+ currents in isolated human ventricular myocytes from patients with terminal heart failure. *Circ. Res.* 73, 379–385.

Cao, N., Liu, Z., Chen, Z., Wang, J., Chen, T., Zhao, X., Ma, Y., Qin, L., Kang, J., Wei, B., Wang, L., Jin, Y., and Yang, H. T. (2012). Ascorbic acid enhances the cardiac differentiation of induced pluripotent stem cells through promoting the proliferation of cardiac progenitor cells. *Cell Res.* 22, 219–236.

Dambrot, C., Passier, R., Atsma, D., and Mummery, C. L. (2011). Cardiomyocyte differentiation of pluripotent stem cewlls and their use as cardiac disease models. *Biochem. J.* 434, 25.

Davis, R. P., Casini, S., van den Berg, C. W., Hoekstra, M., Remme, C. A., Dambrot, C., Ward-van Oosterwaard, D., Wilde, A. A. M., Bezzina, C. R., Verkerk, A. O., Freund, C. M. A. H., and Mummery, C. L. (2012). Cardiomyocytes derived from pluripotent stem cells recapitulate electrophysiolgoical characteristics of an overlap syndrome of cardiac sodium channel disease. *Circulation* 125, 3079–3091. Davis, R. P., van den Berg, C. W., Casini, S., Braam, S. R., and Mummery, C. L. (2011). Pluripotent stem cell models of cardiac disease and their implication for drug discovery and development. *Trends Mol. Med.* 17, 475–484.

Dhamoon, A. S., and Jalife, J. (2005). The inward rectifier current (IK1) controls cardiac excitability and is involved in arrhythmogenesis. *Heart Rhythm* 2, 316–324.

Dick, E., Rajamohan, D., Ronksley, J., and Denning, C. (2010). Evaluating the utility of cardiomyocytes from human pluripotent stem cells for drug screening. *Biochem. Soc. Trans.* 38, 1037–1045.

Drouin, E., Lande, G., and Charpentier, F. (1998). Amiodarone reduces transmural heterogeneity of repolarization in the human heart. *J. Am. Coll. Cardiol.* 32, 1063–1067.

El Chemaly, A., Magaud, C., Patri, S., Jayle, C., Guinamard, R., and Bois, P. (2007). The heart rate-lowering agent ivabradine inhibits the pacemaker current If in human atrial myocytes. *J. Cardiovasc. Electrophysiol.* 18, 1190–1196.

Fatima, A., Xu, G., Shao, K., Papadopoulos, S., Lehmann, M., Arnaiz-Cot, J. J., Rosa, A. O., Nguemo, F., Matzkies, M., Dittmann, S., Stone, S. L., Linke, M., Zechner, U., Beyer, V., Hennies, H. C., Rosenkranz, S., Klauke, B., Parwani, A. S., Haverkamp, W., Pfitzer, G., Farr, M., Cleemann, L., Morad, M., Milting, H., Hescheler, J., and Saric, T. (2011). *In vitro* modeling of ryanodine receptor 2 dysfunction using human induced pluripotent stem cells. *Cell. Physiol. Biochem.* 28, 579–592.

Fodstad, H., Bendahhou, S., Rougier, J. S., Laitinen-Forsblom, P. J., Barhanin, J., Abriel, H., Schild, L., Kontula, K., and Swan, H. (2006). Molecular characterization of two founder mutations causing long QT syndrome and identification of compound het- erozygous patients. *Ann. Med.* 38, 294–304.

Fu, J. D., Jiang, P., Liu, J., Chiamvimonvat, N., and Li, R. A. (2010). Na^{+}/Ca^{2+} exchanger is a determinant of excitation contraction coupling in human embryonic stem cell-derived ventricular cardiomyoctes. *Stem Cells Dev.* 19, 773–782.

Fu, J. D., Rushing, S. N., Lieu, D. K., Chan, C. W., Kong, C. W., Geng, L., Wilson, K. D., Chiamvimonvat, N., Boheler, K. R., Wu, J. C., Keller, G.,

Hajjar, R. J., and Li, R. A. (2011). Distinct roles of microRNA-1 and -499 in ventricular specification and functional maturation of human embryonic stem cell-derived cardiomyocytes. *PLoS ONE* 6:e27417. doi: 10.1371/journal.pone.0027417

Hashimoto, N., Yamashita, T., and Tsuruzoe, N. (2006). Tertiapin, a selective IKACh blocker, terminates atrial fibrillation with selective atrial effective refractory period prolongation. *Pharmacol. Res.* 54, 136–141.

He, J. Q., Ma, Y., Lee, Y., Thomson, J. A., and Kamp, T. J. (2003). Human embryonic stem cells develop into multiple types of cardiac myocytes: action potential characterization. *Circ. Res.* 93, 32–39.

Hofman, N., Tan, H. L., Alders, M., van Langen, I. M., and Wilde, A. A. M. (2010). Active cascade screening in primary inherited arrhythmia syndromes; does it lead to prophylactic treatment? *J. Am. Coll. Cardiol.* 55, 2570–2576.

Hoppe, U. C., Jansen, E., Sudkamp, M., and Beuckelmann, D. J. (1998). Hyperpolarization-activated inward current in ventricular myocytes from normal and failing human hearts. *Circulation* 97, 55–65.

Iost, N., Virag, L., Opincariu, M., Szecsi, J., Varro, A., and Papp, J. G. (1998). Delayed rectifier potassium current in undiseased human ventricular myocytes. *Cardiovasc. Res.* 40, 508–515.

Itzhaki, I., Maizels, L., Huber, I., Zwi-Dantsis, L., Caspi, O., Winterstern, A., Feldman, O., Gepstein, A., Arbel, G., Hammerman, H., Boulos, M., and Gepstein, L. (2011a). Modelling the long QT syndrome with induced pluripotent stem cells. *Nature* 471, 225–229.

Itzhaki, I., Rapoport, S., Huber, I., Mizrahi, I., Zwi-Dantsis, L., Arbel, G., Schiller, J., and Gepstein, L. (2011b). Calcium handling in human induced pluripotent stem cell derived cardiomyocytes. *PLoS ONE* 6:e18037. doi: 10.1371/journal.pone.0018037

Jonsson, M. K. B., Vos, M. A., Mirams, G. R., Ducker, G., Sartipy, P., De Boer, T. P., and Van Veen, T. A. B. (2012). Application of human stem cell-derived cardiomyocytes in safety pharmacology requires caution beyond hERG. *J. Mol. Cell. Cardiol.* 52, 998–1008.

Jost, N., Acsai, K., Horvath, B., Banyasz, T., Baczko, I., Bitay, M., Bogats, G., and Nanasi, P. P. (2009). Contribution of I Kr and I K1 to ventricular repolarization in canine and human myocytes: is there any influence of action potential duration? *Basic Res. Cardiol.* 104, 33–41.

Jung, C. B., Moretti, A., Mederos, Y., Schnitzler, M., Iop, L., Storch, U., Bellin, M., Dorn, T., Ruppenthal, S., Pfeiffer, S., Goedel, A., Dirschinger, R. J., Seyfarth, M., Lam, J. T., Sinnecker, D., Gudermann, T., Lipp, P., and Laugwitz, K. L. (2012). Dantrolene rescues arrhythmogenic RYR2 defect in a patient-specific stem cell model of catecholaminergic polymorphic ventricular tachycardia. *EMBO Mol. Med.* 4, 180–191.

Kehat, I., Kenyagin-Karsenti, D., Snir, M., Segev, H., Amit, M., Gepstein, A., Livne, E., Binah, O., Itskovitz-Eldor, J., and Gepstein, L. (2001). Human embryonic stem cells can differentiate into myocytes with structural and functional properties of cardiomyocytes. *J. Clin. Invest.* 108, 407–414.

Kleger, A., Seufferlein, T., Malan, D., Tischerdorf, M., Storch, A., Wolhein, A., Latz, S., Protze, S., Porzner, M., Proepper, C., Brunner, C., Katz, S. F., Varma Pusupati, G., Bullinger, L., Franz, W. M., Koehntop, R., Giehl, K., Spyrantis, A., Wittekindt, O., Lin, Q., Zenke, M., Fleischmann, B. K., Wartenberg, M., Wobus, A. M., Boeckers, T. M., and Liebau, S. (2010). Modulation of calcium-activated potassium channels induces cardiogenesis of pluripotent stem cells and enrichment of pacemaker-like cells. *Circulation* 122, 1823–1836.

Kobayashi, S., Yano, M., Suetomi, T., Ono, M., Tateishi, H., Mochizuki, M., Xu, X., Uchinoumi, H., Okuda, S., Yamamoto, T., Koseki, N., Kyushiki, H., Ikemoto, N., and Matusazaki, M. (2009). Dantrolene, a therapeutic agent for malignant hyperthermia, markedly improves the function of failing cardiomyocytes by stabilizing interdomain interactions within the ryanodine receptor. *J. Am. Coll. Cardiol.* 53, 1993–2005.

Kuzmenkin, A., Liang, H., Xu, G., Pfannkuche, K., Eichhorn, H., Fatima, A., Luo, H., Saric, T., Wernig, M., Jaenisch, R., and Hescheler, J. (2009). Functional characterization of cardiomyocytes derived from murine induced pluripotent stem cells *in vitro*. *FASEB J.* 23, 4168–4180.

Laflamme, M. A., Chen, K. Y., Naumova, A. V., Muskheli, V., Fugate, J. A., Dupras, S. K., Reinecke, H., Xu, C., Hassanipour, M., Police, S., O'Sullivan, C., Collins, L., Chen, Y., Minami, E., Gill, E. A., Ueno, S., Yuan, C., Gold, J., and Murry, C. E. (2007). Cardiomyocytes derived from human embryonic stem cells in pro-survival factors enhance function of infarcted rat hearts. *Nat. Biotechnol.* 25, 1015–1024.

Lahti, A. L., Kujala, V. J., Chapman, H., Koivisto, A. P., Pekkanen-Mattila, M., Kerkela, E., Hyttinen, J., Kontula, K., Swan, H., Conklin, B. R., Yamanaka, S., Silvennoinen, O., and Aalto-Setälä, K. (2012). Model for long QT syndrome type 2 using human iPS cells demonstrates arrhythmogenic characteristics in cell culture. *Dis. Model. Mech.* 5, 220–230.

Lee, Y. K., Ng, K. M., Lai, W. H., Chan, Y. C., Lau, Y. M., Lian, Q., Tse, H. F., and Siu, C. W. (2011). Calcium homeostasis in human induced pluripotent stem cell-derived cardiomyocytes. *Stem Cell. Rev.* 7, 976–986.

Loh, Y. H., Agarwal, S., Park, I. H., Urbach, A., Huo, H., Heffner, G. C., Kim, K., Miller, J. D., Ng, K.,

and Daley, G. Q. (2009). Generation of induced pluripotent stem cells from human blood. *Blood* 113, 5476–5479.

Ma, J., Guo, L., Fiene, S. J., Anson, B. D., Thomson, J. A., Kamp, T. J., Kolaja, K. L., Swanson, B. J., and January, C. T. (2011). High purity human-induced pluripotent stem cell-derived cardiomyocytes: electrophysiological properties of action potentials and ionic currents. *Am. J. Physiol. Heart Circ. Physiol.* 301, H2006–H2017.

Magyar, J., Iost, N., Kortvely, A., Banyasz, T., Virag, L., Szigligeti, P., Varro, A., Opincariu, M., Szecsi, J., Papp, J. G., and Nanasi, P. P. (2000). Effects of endothelin-1 on calcium and potassium currents in undiseased human ventricular myocytes. *Pflugers Arch.* 441, 144–149.

Marjamaa, A., Salomaa, V., Newton-Cheh, C., Porthan, K., Reunanen, A., Karanko, H., Jula, A., Lahermo, P., Väänänen, H., Toivonen, L., Swan, H., Viitasalo, M., Nieminen, M. S., Peltonen, L., Oikarinen, L., Palotie, A., and Kontula, K. (2009). High prevalence of four long QT syndrome founder mutations in the Finnish population. *Ann. Med.* 41, 234–240.

Matsa, E., Rajamohan, D., Dick, E., Young, L., Mellor, I., Staniforth, A., and Denning, C. (2011). Drug evaluation in cardiomyocytes derived from human induced pluripotent stem cells carrying a long QT syndrome type 2 mutation. *Eur. Heart J.* 32, 952–962.

Mewes, T., and Ravens, U. (1994). L-type calcium currents of human myocytes from ventricle of non-failing and failing hearts and from atrium. *J. Mol. Cell. Cardiol.* 26, 1307–1320.

Mitcheson, J. S., Hancox, J. C., and Levi, A. J. (1998). Cultured adult cardiac myocytes: future applications, culture methods, morphological and electrophysiological properties. *Cardiovasc. Res.* 39, 280–300.

Miyoshi, K., Tsuji, D., Kudoh, K., Satomura, K., Muto, T., Itoh, K., and Noma, T. (2010). Generation of human induced pluripotent stem cells from oral mucosa. *J. Biosci. Bioeng.* 110, 345–350.

Moretti, A., Bellin, M., Welling, A., Jung, C. B., Lam, J. T., Bott-Flugel, L., Dorn, T., Goedel, A., Höhnke, C., Hofmann, F., Seyfarth, M., Sinnecker, D., Schömig, A., and Laugwitz, K. L. (2010). Patient-specific induced pluripotent stem-cell models for long-QT syndrome. *N. Engl. J. Med.* 363, 1397–1409.

Mummery, C. L., Ward-van Oostwaard, D., Doevendans, P., Spijker, R., van den Brink, S., Hassink, R., van der Heyden, M., Opthof, T., Pera, M., de la Riviere, A. B., Passier, R., and Tertoolen, L. (2003). Differentiation of human embryonic stem cells to cardiomyocytes: role of coculture with visceral endoderm- like cells. *Circulation* 107, 2733–2740.

Nabäuer, M., Beuckelmann, D. J., Uberfuhr, P., and Steinbeck, G. (1996). Regional differences in current density and rate-dependent properties of the transient outward current in subepicardial and suben- docardial myocytes of human left ventricle. *Circulation* 93, 168–177.

Narsinh, K., Narsinh, K. H., and Wu, J. C. (2011). Derivation of human induced pluripotent stem cells for cardiovascular disease modeling. *Circ. Res.* 108, 1146–1156.

Nerbonne, J. M., and Kass, R. S. (2005). Molecular physiology of cardiac repolarization. *Physiol. Rev.* 85, 1205–1253.

Novak, A., Barad, L., Zeevi-Levin, N., Shick, R., Shtrichman, R., Lorber, A., Itskovitz-Eldor, J., and Binah, O. (2012). Cardiomyocytes generated from CPVTD307H patients are arrhythmogenic in response to beta-adrenergic stimulation. *J. Cell. Mol. Med.* 16, 468–482.

Ono, K., and Iijima, T. (2010). Cardiac T-type Ca^{2+} channels in the heart. *J. Mol. Cell. Cardiol.* 48, 65–70.

Piacentino, V. 3rd., Weber, C. R., Chen, X., Weisser-Thomas, J., Margulies, K. B., Bers, D. M., and Houser, S. R. (2003). Cellular basis of abnormal calcium transients of failing human ventricular myocytes. *Circ. Res.* 92, 651–658.

Priori, S. G. (2004). Inherited arrhyth- mogenic diseases: the complexity beyond monogenic disorders. *Circ. Res.* 94, 140–145.

Priori, S. G., and Chen, S. R. (2011). Inherited dysfunction of sarcoplasmic reticulum Ca^{2+} handling and arrhythmogenesis. *Circ. Res.* 108, 871–883.

Remme, C. A., Scicluna, B. P., Verkerk, A. O., Amin, A. S., van Brunschot, S., Beekman, L., Deneer, V. H. M., Chevalier, C., Oyama, F., Miyazaki, H., Nukina, N., Wilders, R., Escande, D., Houlgatte, R., Wilde, A. A. M., Tan, H. L., Veldkamp, M. W., de Bakker, J. T., and Bezzina, C. R. (2009). Genetically determined differences in sodium current characteristics modulate conduction disease severity in mice with cardiac sodium channelopathy. *Circ. Res.* 104, 1283–1292.

Remme, C. A., Verkerk, A. O., Nuyens, D., van Ginneken, A. C. G., van Brunschot, S., Belterman, C.

A. W., Wilders, R., van Roon, M. A., Tan, H. L., Wilde, A. A. M., Carmeliet, P., de Bakker, J. M. T., Veldkamp, M. W., and Bezzina, C. R. (2006). Overlap syndrome of cardiac sodium channel disease in mice carrying the equivalent mutation of human SCN5A-1795insD. *Circulation* 114, 2584–2594.

Remme, C. A., Wilde, A. A. M., and Bezzina, C. R. (2008). Cardiac sodium channel overlap syndromes: different faces of SCN5A mutations. *Trends Cardiovasc. Med.* 18, 78–87.

Ruan, Y., Liu, N., Napolitano, C., and Priori, S. G. (2008). Therapeutic strategies for long-QT syndrome: does the molecular substrate matter? *Circ. Arrhythm. Electrophysiol.* 1, 290–297.

Sabir, I. N., Killeen, M. J., Grace, A. A., and Huang, C. L. H. (2008). Ventricular arrhythmogenesis: insights from murine models. *Prog. Biophys. Mol. Biol.* 98, 208–218.

Sakakibara, Y., Furukawa, T., Singer, D. H., Jia, H., Backer, C. L., Arentzen, C. E., and Wasserstrom, J. A. (1993). Sodium current in isolated human ventricular myocytes. *Am. J. Physiol.* 265, H1301–H1309.

Sartiani, L., Bettiol, E., Stillitano, F., Mugelli, A., Cerbai, E., and Jaconi, M. E. (2007). Developmental change in cardiomyocytes differentiated from human embryonic stem cells: a molecular and electrophys-iological approach. *Stem Cells* 25, 1136–1144.

Scicluna, B. P., Wilde, A. A. M., and Bezzina, C. R. (2008). The primary arrhythmia syndromes: same mutation, different manifestations. Are we strating to understand why?

J. Cardiovasc. Electrophysiol. 19, 445–452. Sipido, K. R., Bito, V., Antoons, G., Volders, P. G., and Vos, M. A. (2007). Na/Ca exchange and cardiac ventricular arrhythmias. *Ann. N.Y. Acad. Sci.* 1099, 339–348.

Sun, N., Panetta, N. J., Gupta, D. M., Wilson, K. D., Lee, A., Jia, F., Hu, S., Cherry, A. M., Robbins, R. C., Longaker, M. T., and Wu, J. C. (2009). Feeder-free derivation of induced pluripotent stem cells from adult human adipose stem cells. *Proc. Natl. Acad. Sci. U.S.A.* 106, 15720–15725.

Synnergren, J., Améen, C., Jansson, A., and Sartipy, P. (2012). Global transcriptional profilinig reveals similarities and differences between human stem cell-derived cardiomyocyte clusters and heart tissue. *Physiol. Genomics* 44, 245–258.

Takahashi, K., and Yamanaka, S. (2006). Induction of pluripotent stem cells from mouse embryonic and adult fibroblast cultures by defined factors. *Cell* 126, 663–676.

Takahashi, K., Tanabe, K., Ohnuki, M., Narita, M., Ichisaka, T., Tomoda, K., and Yamanaka, S. (2007). Induction of pluripotent stem cells from adult human fibroblasts by defined factors. *Cell* 131, 861–872.

Tamaoki, N., Takahashi, K., Tanaka, T., Ichisaka, T., Aoki, H., Takeda-Kawaguchi, T., Iida, K., Kunisada, T., Shibata, T., Yamanaka, S., and Tezuka, K. (2010). Dental pulp cells for induced pluripotent stem cell banking. *J. Dent. Res.* 89, 773–778.

Tamargo, J., Caballero, R., Gómez, R., Valenzuela, C., and Delpón, E. (2004). Pharmacology of cardiac potassium channels. *Cardiovasc. Res.* 62, 9–33.

Varro, A., and Papp, J. G. (1992). The impact of single cell voltage clamp on the understanding of the cardiac ventricular action potential. *Cardioscience* 3, 131–144.

Verkerk, A. O., Veldkamp, M. W., Baartscheer, A., Schumacher, C. A., Klopping, C., van Ginneken, A. C. G., and Ravesloot, J. H. (2001). Ionic mechanism of delayed afterdepolarizations in ventricular cells isolated from human end-stage failing hearts. *Circulation* 104, 2728–2733.

Verkerk, A. O., Veldkamp, M. W., Bouman, L. N., and van Ginneken, A. C. G. (2000a). Calcium-activated Cl^- current contributes to delayed afterdepolarizations in single Purkinje and ventricular myocytes. *Circulation* 101, 2639–2644.

Verkerk, A. O., Veldkamp, M. W., de Jonge, N., Wilders, R., and van Ginneken, A. C. G. (2000b). Injury current modulates afterde-polarizations in single human ventricular cells. *Cardiovasc. Res.* 47, 124–132.

Verkerk, A. O., Wilders, R., van Borren, M. M. G. J., Peters, R. J. G., Broekhuis, E., Lam, K., Coronel, R., de Bakker, J. M. T., and Tan, H. L. (2007). Pacemaker current (If) in the human sinoatrial node. *Eur. Heart J.* 28, 2472–2478.

Virag, L., Iost, N., Opincariu, M., Szolnoky, J., Szecsi, J., Bogats, G., Szenohradszky, P., Varro, A., and Papp, J. G. (2001). The slow component of the delayed rectifier potassium current in undiseased human ventricular myocytes. *Cardiovasc. Res.* 49, 790–797.

Wang, K., Terrenoir, C., Sampson, K. J., Iyer, V., Osteen, J. D., Lu, J., Keller, G., Kotton, D. N., and Kass, R. S. (2011). Biophysical properties of slow potassium channels in human embryonic stem cell derived cardiomyocytes implicate subunit stoichiometry. *J. Physiol.* 589.24, 6093–6104.

Wang, Z., Fermini, B., and Nattel, S. (1994). Rapid and slow components of delayed rectifier current in human atrial myocytes. *Cardiovasc. Res.* 28, 1540–1546.

Watanabe, H., Yang, T., Stroud, D. M., Lowe, J. S., Harris, L., Atack, T. C., Wang, D. W., Hipkens, S. B., Leake, B., Hall, L., Kupershmidt, S., Chopra, N., Magnuson, M. A., Tanabe, N., Knollmann, B. C., George, A. L. Jr., and Roden, D.

M. (2011). Striking *in vivo* pheno-type of a disease-associated human SCN5A mutation producing minimal changes *in vitro*. *Circulation* 124, 1001–1011.

Watanabe, H., Koopmann, T. T., Le Scouarnec, S., Yang, T., Ingram, C. R., Schott, J. J., Demolombe, S., Probst, V., Anselme, F., Escande, D., Wiesfeld, A. C. P., Pfeufer, A., Kaab, S., Wichmann, H. E., Hasdemir, C., Aizawa, Y., Wilde, A. A. M., Roden, D. M., and Bezzina, C. R. (2008). Sodium channel beta1 subunit mutations associated with Brugada syndrome and cardiac conduction disease in humans. *J. Clin. Invest.* 118, 2260–2268.

Wettwer, E., Amos, G. J., Posival, H., and Ravens, U. (1994). Transient outward current in human ventricular myocytes of subepicardial and subendocardial origin. *Circ. Res.* 75, 473–482.

Wilde, A. A. M., and Bezzina, C. R. (2005). Genetics of cardiac arrhythmias. *Heart* 91, 1352–1358.

Wolf, C. M., and Berul, C. I. (2008). Molecular mechanisms of inherited arrhythmias. *Curr. Genomics.* 9, 160–168.

Yazawa, M., Hsueh, B., Jia, X., Pasca, A. M., Bernstein, J. A., Hallmayer, J., and Dolmetsch, R. E. (2011). Using induced pluripotent stem cells to investigate cardiac phenotypes in Timothy syndrome. *Nature* 471, 230–234.

Yu, J., Vodyanik, M. A., Smuga- Otto, K., Antosiewicz-Bourget, J., Frane, J. L., Tian, S., Nie, J., Jonsdottir, G. A., Ruotti, V., Stewart, R., Slukvin, I. I., and Thomson, J. A. (2007). Induced pluripotent stem cell lines derived from human somatic cells. *Science* 318, 1917–1920.

Zhang, J., Wilson, G. F., Soerens, A. G., Koonce, C. H., Yu, J., Palecek, P., Thomson, J. A., and Kamp, J. (2009). Functional cardiomyocytes derived from human induced pluripotent stem cells. *Circ. Res.* 104, e30–e41.

Zhang, Q., Jiang, J., Han, P., Yuan, Q., Zhang, J., Zhang, X., Xu, Y., Cao, H., Meng, Q., Chen, L., Tian, T., Wang, X., Li, P., Hescheler, J., and Ji, G. (2011). Direct differentiation of atrial and ventricular myocytes from human embryonic stem cells by alternating reinoid signals. *Cell. Res.* 21, 579–587.

Zipes, D. P., and Wellens, H. J. J. (1998). Sudden cardiac death. *Circulation* 98, 2334–2351.

18

Role of cholinergic innervation and RGS2 in atrial arrhythmia

Douglas L. Jones[1,2,3,4]*, Jari M. Tuomi[1†] and Peter Chidiac[1]

[1] Department of Physiology and Pharmacology, The University of Western Ontario, London, ON, Canada
[2] Department of Medicine, The University of Western Ontario, London, ON, Canada
[3] Cardiovascular Group, Lawson Health Research Institute, London Health Sciences Center, London, ON, Canada
[4] Canadian Surgical Technologies and Advance Robotics, Lawson Health Research Institute, London Health Sciences Center, London, ON, Canada

***Correspondence:**
*Douglas L. Jones, Department of Physiology and Pharmacology, University of Western Ontario, London, ON, Canada N6A 5C1.
e-mail: doug.jones@schulich.uwo.ca*

†Present address:
Jari M. Tuomi, Northern Ontario Medical School, Sudbury, ON, Canada.

The heart receives sympathetic and parasympathetic efferent innervation as well as the ability to process information internally via an intrinsic cardiac autonomic nervous system (ICANS). For over a century, the role of the parasympathetics via vagal acetylcholine release was related to controlling primarily heart rate. Although in the late 1800s shown to play a role in atrial arrhythmia, the myocardium took precedence from the mid-1950s until in the last decade a resurgence of interest in the autonomics along with signaling cascades, regulators, and ion channels. Originally ignored as being benign and thus untreated, recent emphasis has focused on atrial arrhythmia as atrial fibrillation (AF) is the most common arrhythmia seen by the general practitioner. It is now recognized to have significant mortality and morbidity due to resultant stroke and heart failure. With the aging population, there will be an unprecedented increased burden on health care resources. Although it has been known for more than half a century that cholinergic stimulation can initiate AF, the classical concept focused on the M2 receptor and its signaling cascade including RGS4, as these had been shown to have predominant effects on nodal function (heart rate and conduction block) as well as contractility. However, recent evidence suggests that the M3 receptor may also playa role in initiation and perpetuation of AF and thus RGS2, a putative regulator of the M3 receptor, may be a target for therapeutic intervention. Mice lacking RGS2 ($RGS2^{-/-}$), were found to have significantly altered electrophysiological atrial responses and were more susceptible to electrically induced AF. Vagally induced or programmed stimulation-induced AF could be blocked by the selective M3R antagonist, darifenacin. These results suggest a potential surgical target (ICANS) and pharmacological targets (M3R, RGS2) for the management of AF.

Keywords: RGS proteins, autonomic nervous system, cholinergic, arrhythmia, atrial fibrillation, intrinsic cardiac autonomic nervous system, heart, M3 muscarinic receptor

INTRODUCTION

This "Special Topic" series explores how regulators of G protein signaling (RGS) proteins share common, yet distinct roles at multiple levels, controlling autonomic regulation of heart function, and what critical questions remain for translational researchers examining the role of these pathways in conditions such as atrial fibrillation (AF), where RGS proteins are currently being assessed as potential druggable targets. Although cholinergic AF has been investigated for decades, exact mechanisms are still controversial (Schotten et al., 2011). AF is highly complex involving multiple mechanisms for its initiation and sustaining the arrhythmia including genetic contributions, structural, ion handling, and autonomic alterations, the complexity of which results in beat-to-beat, second-to-second, and having age-dependent substrate changes. This paper provided some evidence on the role of RGS2 proteins in AF in the mouse. To put this into context, there is a brief introduction of the role of autonomics in AF. For more complete reviews, see a special review issue in Cardiovascular Research 2011 vol. 89 no. 4, and reviews by Dobrev and Nattel (2011), Schotten et al. (2011), Wakili et al. (2011).

HISTORICAL CONCEPTS OF AUTONOMICS IN THE HEART

The heart receives both sympathetic and parasympathetic efferent innervation as well as being able to process information via an intrinsic cardiac autonomic nervous system (ICANS). The ICANS may interact with the efferent nerve supply in a complex fashion to regulate cardiac function and it is thought to act as a "mini-brain on the heart." The neurons of the ICANS are primarily located in five groups of atrial ganglionated plexi (GPs) which have been described by Arora et al. (2003) in the pig. These GPs may represent areas of local control of cardiac muscle (Cardinal et al., 2009). Although close proximity of the neurons to the muscle does not mean exclusive control of the adjacent area, it is an important consideration, and is analogous to the enteric nervous system, which serves as the "local brain" in the intestinal tract (Furness et al., 2004). Subpopulations of intrinsic cardiac neurons express multiple neurotransmitters (Hassall and Burnstock, 1987); however, in Guinea pig posterior ganglia, choline acetyltransferase immunostaining of all neurons indicates major parasympathetic cholinergic input to the myocardium (Mawe et al., 1996).

ATRIAL FIBRILLATION

Atrial fibrillation, the most common clinical arrhythmia (Kannel et al., 1982; Benjamin et al., 1998), is characterized by having abnormal, irregularly irregular, rapid electrical activation. AF is a common health problem in the developed world (Savelieva and Camm, 2001). Its prevalence increases with age, from a prevalence of 0.02% of people of 18–39 years of age to 11.6% of people over 75 years of age (Nixon, 2011). As the population ages, AF will increase the burden on health care resources, both for its therapeutic management, and also due to its serious and costly complications: heart failure and stroke (Dries et al., 1998). Discussion of potential mechanisms for AF, as far back as 1870 (Efimov and Fedorov, 2005), has been separated into two basic themes; those stressing the primary role of the ICANS (referred to as neurogenic AF; Hoffa and Ludwig, 1850; Zipes et al., 1974; Coumel et al., 1978; Liu and Nattel, 1997; Chang et al., 2001; Nattel, 2004), or sometimes called "vagal AF" (Garrey, 1924) and those related exclusively to the role of the atrial muscle itself (referred to as myogenic AF). Both neurogenic (Hoffa and Ludwig, 1850; Zipes et al., 1974; Coumel et al., 1978; Liu and Nattel, 1997; Chang et al., 2001; Nattel, 2004) and myogenic (Vulpain, 1874; MacWilliam, 1887; Garrey, 1914; Moe and Abildskov, 1959; Moe, 1962; Moe et al., 1964; Allessie et al., 1985; Zipes, 1997; Jalife et al., 1998; Skanes et al., 1998; Mandapati et al., 2000) hypotheses have been proposed to account for arrhythmia mechanisms. The separation of AF mechanisms into strictly neurogenic and myogenic types is artificial as they certainly interact and share multiple mechanisms.

Since the studies of Moe and colleagues in the 1950s, AF was shown to be composed of multiple re-entrant wavelets (Nattel, 2002). However, optical mapping studies of AF in isolated sheep atria have found that AF may involve both a high frequency "mother rotor," and fibrillatory conduction of multiple wavelets spawned from the deterministic driver (Kleber, 2000; Jalife, 2003). Remodeling of the atria may also promote the propagation of multiple wavelets as "AF begets AF," indicating that atrial remodeling promotes sustained disorganized activity (Morillo et al., 1995; Shen et al., 2011). AF relies on the interaction of triggers, perpetuators, and a vulnerable substrate for initiation and maintenance of the arrhythmia (Allessie et al., 2001). Triggers combined with dynamic substrates of structural heterogeneities, reduced refractoriness, enhanced spatial dispersion of refractoriness and abnormal impulse conduction initiate and perpetuate the arrhythmia (Nattel et al., 2002). Focal activity originating from the pulmonary veins has been suggested to account for more than 90% of AF triggers (Haissaguerre et al., 2000).

Abnormal impulse initiation and conduction contribute to the mechanism of AT (**Figure 1**), but are also involved in the initiation and maintenance of AF. The rapid rates during AF (Nattel, 2002) promote remodeling of the atria that potentiates AF duration (AF begets AF). There are, however, a number of factors that cause remodeling and "prime" the initial state, promoting rapid triggers (e.g., pulmonary vein ectopy) and susceptibility to fibrillatory conduction necessary for AF. These "clinical risk factors" (Rosiak et al., 2010) for the onset and development of AF are listed in **Figure 2**, for more detail see Dobrev and Nattel (2011). Two factors not mentioned in the Rosiak article are mechanical

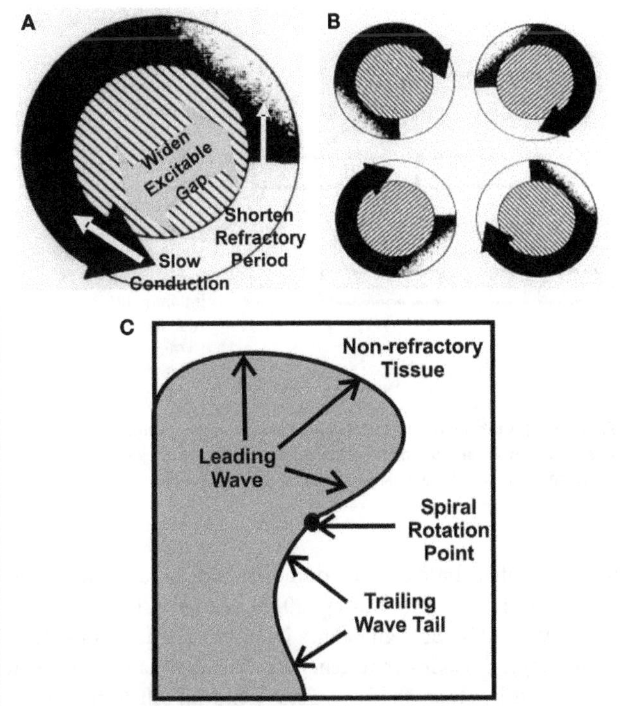

FIGURE 1 | The leading circle, "wave length," of re-entry in atrial fibrillation (AF). The size of a functional re-entry circuit [(**A**), right], depends on the wavelength (WL) which is a product of conduction velocity (CV) and refractory period (RP; WL = CV × RP). Short wavelengths allow multiple circuits [(**B**), left], favoring AF. The wave rotating around a fixed point, rotor [(**C**), lower; Jalife, 2003]. Factors such which slow conduction enhance the potential for multiple smaller waves. Enhanced cholinergics decrease conduction velocity and/or reduce effective refractoriness. Modified connexins also slow conduction. Either, or a combination of both could promote the initiation and sustaining of AF.

stretch and hyperthyroidism (Klein and Ojamaa, 2001; Souza et al., 2012). Although usually associated with other contributing factors such as hypertension or valve disease, stretch and stretch-induced channel conduction can lead to electrical instability. Indeed, interactions between mechanical stretch and cholinergic stimulation has been shown (Yamazaki et al., 2009). Although in embryonic and not the adult atria, there is evidence of interaction between M3 receptors and TREK-2, a stretch activated K^+ channel (Kang et al., 2006). There are also interactions between mechanical stretch and gap junctions (Wang et al., 2000). These interactions can be very complex. For instance, $Cx40^{-/-}$ mice had a lower pacing induced breakdown frequency of 1–1 right atrial impulse conduction than wild type mice but did not present with AF (Bagwe et al., 2005). This indicates that the factors that promote fibrillatory conduction may not necessarily contribute to the mechanism driving AF and may even oppose it. On the other hand, slowed conduction in patients with somatic connexin 40 (Gollob et al., 2006) or connexin 43 mutations (Thibodeau et al., 2010) or mice with mutant connexin 43 (Tuomi et al., 2011) were associated with enhanced arrhythmia susceptibility.

Atrial fibrillation causes remodeling of the atria that promotes long lasting or even permanent AF (Thijssen et al., 2000). AF

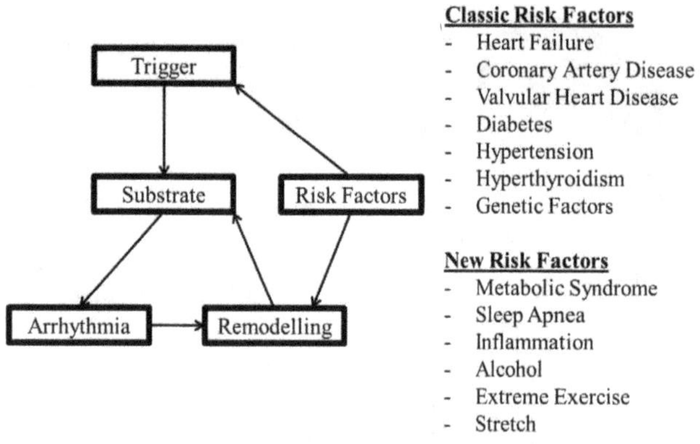

FIGURE 2 | A model of factors involved in arrhythmogenesis and the effect of remodeling with the classical and more recent factors thought to be involved in arrhythmia risk.

can be classified based on its duration and therapeutic history (Nixon, 2011; Yan and Kowey, 2011). Patterns of AF following the ACC/AHA/ESC guidelines include: (1) Paroxysmal (self-terminating), episodes that generally last less than or equal to 7 days (most less than 24 h); (2) Persistent (not self-terminating), usually more than 7 days, and (3) Permanent, cardioversion failed or not attempted. Either paroxysmal or persistent AF may be recurrent (Fuster et al., 2001).

Persistent AF is associated with diffuse macroscopic and histological atrial myocardial changes, i.e., remodeling. Atrial arrhythmia can also cause ventricular remodeling and, if protracted, cardiac failure. This in turn, can feed back on the atria and produce irreversible interstitial atrial fibrosis (Kalifa et al., 2003).

Lone or paroxysmal AF has been shown to be primarily initiated from the pulmonary veins and posterior left atrial regions (Morillo et al., 1995; Haissaguerre et al., 1998), where most of the GP are in contact with the left atrium. Both alterations in vagal responses and a significant increase in AF control (Pappone et al., 2000, 2004; Nademanee et al., 2004; Platt et al., 2004; Nakagawa et al., 2005a,b) were found in patients when the GPs were targeted (Sakamoto et al., 2010) or inadvertently modified during catheter ablation of AF sources in the pulmonary veins. Also, selective ablation of the GPs in pigs abolished the ability to acutely induce AF (Jones et al., 2008b) and reduced the acute inducibility in dogs (Nishida et al., 2011), which persisted in some animals up to 4 weeks following ablation in dogs (Nishida et al., 2011). These observations demonstrate the importance of the ICANS in AF, i.e., neurogenic AF (Hoffa and Ludwig, 1850; Zipes et al., 1974; Coumel et al., 1978; Liu and Nattel, 1997; Chang et al., 2001; Nattel, 2004). Neurogenic or sometimes called "vagal AF" (Garrey, 1924) relies extensively on the action of acetylcholine. The roles of acetylcholine in setting the stage for rotor development and stabilization of the leading sources of AF have been reviewed (Sarmast et al., 2003; Efimov and Fedorov, 2005; Dobrev and Nattel, 2011; Schotten et al., 2011; Wakili et al., 2011). Acetylcholine promotes left to right frequency gradients and enhances the dominant frequency of the AF driver (Mansour et al., 2001). These responses were also dependent on acetylcholine concentration, with higher concentrations resulting in faster dominant frequencies. Previous studies on AF mechanisms commonly focus on dependence on acetylcholine concentration and the expression profiles of receptors and downstream effectors, while ignoring the regulators of the G protein signaling cascades.

ATRIAL MUSCARINIC ACETYLCHOLINE RECEPTORS

Five different subtypes of muscarinic acetylcholine receptors have been cloned. M1, M3, and M5 receptors are $G\alpha q$ coupled receptors, while M2 and M4 receptors are $G\alpha i/o$ coupled. The classical notion is that the cardiac muscarinic acetylcholine receptors are exclusively of the M2 subtype as M2 receptors are the most plentiful. However, there is increasing evidence supporting an important functional role of M3 receptors (Shi et al., 2004; Wang et al., 2004). Of interest, even in the recent review (Schotten et al., 2011), differential effects of cholinergic stimulation, despite its presence in the heart, overlook M3 and are solely related to M2-cholinergic innervation using archival information based on vagal stimulation and atropine blockade "*... heterogeneity in the distribution of... M2-cholinoceptors (4, 343).*" Reference 4 is Alessi et al. (1958). Reference 343 is Liu and Nattel (1997). Both of these references are prior to the description of M3 receptors in the heart. More recently however, novel M2 blockade with NTC-801 was found to block experimental AF, although its effects on M3 receptors were not assessed (Machida et al., 2011). M3 muscarinic receptors were first identified in human atria in Hellgren et al. (2000). Early quantification of M1–M5 muscarinic subtype mRNAs in rat atria utilizing competitive RT-PCR indicated that M2 mRNA represented more than 90% of the total muscarinic mRNA in the atria, while M3 was less than 3% (Krejci and Tucek, 2002). More recently, quantitative PCR showed low level expression of M1, M4, and M5 receptors in the atria, but this may have been due to low level DNA contamination as RNA in most studies was not treated with DNAse (Kitazawa et al., 2009). The functional consequence of co-expression of multiple muscarinic receptor types has been the focus of many studies discussed below, the most compelling of which use M2 and M3 receptor knockout mice.

After 1 week of rapid pacing, Yeh et al. (2007) found approximately a 50% decrease in levels of mRNA encoding M2, M3, and M4 receptor subtypes in both the left atrial appendix and left pulmonary vein region. In contrast, Voigt et al. (2010) found there were differential alterations in samples from atrial appendices of patients with chronic or paroxysmal AF. In paroxysmal AF, basal current was ~2-fold larger in the left versus right atrial appendix, indicating a left-to-right atrial gradient. In both atria, Kir2.1 (I_{K1}) expression was ~2-fold greater in chronic AF but comparable in paroxysmal AF versus patients in sinus rhythm. Kir2.3 levels ($I_{K,ACh}$) were unchanged in chronic AF and the right atrial appendix in paroxysmal AF but were 51% lower in the left atrial appendix in paroxysmal AF. In sinus rhythm carbachol-activated $I_{K,ACh}$ was 70% greater in RA versus LA. This right-to-left atrial gradient was decreased in paroxysmal and chronic AF caused by a selective reduction in $I_{K,ACh}$ in right atrium. Similarly, in sinus rhythm, Kir3.1 and Kir3.4 proteins were greater in right versus left atrium and decreased in the right atrium of paroxysmal and chronic AF. Kir3.1 and Kir3.4 expression was unchanged in the left atrium of paroxysmal and chronic AF (Voigt et al., 2010).

In the heart, M2 receptors inhibit adenylyl cyclase (AC) activity via Gαi and induce activation of the G protein coupled inward rectifier K^+ channel ($GIRK_{3.1/3.4}$ or $I_{K,ACh}$; Kovoor et al., 2001) by Gβγ released from Gαi. Inhibition of adenylyl cyclase production of cAMP reduces the activity of I_f (a cAMP dependent current) and the L-type Ca^{2+} current ($I_{Ca,L}$) through Gαo. $I_{Ca,L}$ is also regulated by Gαi and nitric oxide (Burger et al., 2009a,b). Adenylyl cyclase 5 deficient mice have reduced $I_{Ca,L}$ activity, while Gαi2 knockout mice lack muscarinic regulation of $I_{Ca,L}$ (Chen et al., 2001). M2 receptor inhibition of Gαi decreases cAMP production, which reduces protein kinase A (PKA) activation (Kovoor et al., 2001). PKA, through phosphorylation, increases the activity of $I_{Ca,L}$ and the rapid delayed rectifier potassium channel (I_{Kr}), which promotes repolarization from the plateau phase of cardiac action potential (Tamargo et al., 2004). The inhibition of I_{Kr} prolongs AP duration (Clark et al., 2004).

In the atria, activation of $I_{K,ACh}$ increases membrane K^+ permeability, facilitating an outward current that hyperpolarizes the cell. There is a gradient of $I_{K,ACh}$ current in the mouse atria that, when combined with the heterogeneous distribution of parasympathetic ganglia, may augment the dispersion of atrial refractoriness (Lomax et al., 2003). In mice (Nygren et al., 2004), optically mapped action potential duration was shorter in the left than the right atrium (Nygren et al., 2004) and the cholinergic agonist, carbachol, reduced durations in all areas except the left atrial appendage. GIRK4 knock out ($GIRK4^{-/-}$) mice which lack functional $I_{K,ACh}$ channels have abnormal heart rate regulation and are resistant to carbachol-induced AF (Kovoor et al., 2001). In the SA node, $I_{K,ACh}$ hyperpolarizes the membrane potential, and decreases the pacemaker pre-potential slope, which contributes ~50% to the *in vivo* bradycardic response. In summary, the functions of the M2 receptor include activation of $I_{K,ACh}$ (hyperpolarization), inhibition of I_{Kr} (prolonging repolarization), and inhibition of I_f (negative chronotropy; Hashimoto et al., 2006).

On the other hand, M3 muscarinic receptors couple to Gαq to activate PLC, PKC, and $I_{K,M3}$ (Shi et al., 2004). To date, $I_{K,M3}$ is the only identified K^+ channel activated by Gαq. $I_{K,M3}$ current is highly selective for K^+ and has delayed rectifier properties with a relatively slow activation time constant (~150 ms at +50 mV), which is followed by a partial and slower decay (Wang et al., 2004). The tail current is characterized by an initial rapid rising phase followed by a slow decay with a mean time constant of ~170 ms (Shi et al., 2003). The waveform is similar to that of I_{Kr}; however, it is insensitive to the I_{Kr} blockers dofetilide and E-4031, and to the slow delayed rectifier K^+ current (I_{Ks}) inhibitor, chromanol 293B. $I_{K,M3}$ is blocked by the non-selective muscarinic antagonist, atropine (Wang et al., 2004), and the M3 selective antagonist, darifenacin (Wang et al., 2004, 2007a). M3 content is also altered in patients with chronic AF associated with mitral stenosis (Zhao et al., 2008) and in experimental chronic tachycardia in dogs (Yeh et al., 2007).

Of note, M3 receptor distribution in cardiac tissue was found to be mostly confined to the intercalated disk region (Wang et al., 2004), and thus was also suggested to regulate ventricular gap junction-mediated cell-to-cell conduction (Wang et al., 2007a). Physical and functional interactions between M3 and connexin 43 (Cx43) have been found in rat ventricular myocytes, which were impaired during myocardial ischemia (Yue et al., 2006). Gap junction remodeling is an essential component promoting atrial as well as lethal ventricular tachyarrhythmias (Dupont et al., 2001a,b; Gutstein et al., 2001; Danik et al., 2004; Shiroshita-Takeshita et al., 2007). The functions of the cardiac M3 receptors suggested so far include: (1) depressed inotropy; (2) protection against myocardial ischemia; (3) regulation of cell-to-cell communication, and (4) participation in the generation and maintenance of AF (Wang et al., 2004). Using the M3 receptor antagonist 4-DAMP Wang et al. (2004), concluded that the M3 receptor also mediates, in part, bradycardia elicited by vagal stimulation. However, the pKb of 4-DAMP for M3 is 8.9–9.3, only one order of magnitude greater the pKb for M2 receptors (7.8–8.4). Perhaps the weak inhibition of vagal bradycardia with high dose 4-DAMP used in Wang's study was due to blockade of M2 rather than M3 receptors. On the other hand, vagally induced bradycardia was completely abolished in M2 muscarinic receptor ($M2^{-/-}$) deficient mice but was not affected in M3 muscarinic receptor ($M3^{-/-}$) deficient mice (Fisher et al., 2004), which does not support a role for M3 in bradycardia in the mouse. However, this does not exclude a role for M3-mediated modulation of atrial or AVN function, as analysis of other atrial or AVN functions was not done.

The functional consequence of co-expression of both M2 and M3 receptors in the atria was studied in $M2^{-/-}$, $M3^{-/-}$, and M2/M3 double knockout ($M2^{-/-}/M3^{-/-}$) mice (Kitazawa et al., 2009). In wild type mouse atria, carbachol-induced a negative inotropic response followed by a sustained positive inotropic response. $M3^{-/-}$ mice were devoid of the positive inotropic phase while $M2^{-/-}$ mice had only a positive inotropic response. $M2^{-/-}/M3^{-/-}$ double knockout mice were devoid of any inotropic response (Kitazawa et al., 2009). The susceptibility to arrhythmia was not studied in these mice. However, these results strongly indicate the functional nature of M3 muscarinic receptors present in the atria.

G PROTEIN COUPLED RECEPTORS IN THE HEART

G protein coupled receptors (GPCRs) are seven transmembrane domain cell surface receptors that bind extracellular ligands (hormones, neurotransmitters, and drugs) and transduce signals into the intracellular environment. Most sympathetic and parasympathetic receptors are members of the GPCR superfamily which couple to various downstream signaling cascades including those controlling adenylyl cyclase, Ca^{2+} homeostasis, and ion channels (Wieland et al., 2007). In the heart, GPCRs control the chronotropic (rate of contraction), inotropic (strength of contraction), lusitropic (rate of relaxation), and dromotropic (velocity of conduction) responses to acetylcholine and adrenaline (Wieland et al., 2007). Ligand binding stabilizes or induces a conformational change in its GPCR that activates a coupled intracellular heterotrimeric G protein (Gαβγ). There are four families of mammalian heterotrimeric G proteins including $G_s\alpha$, $G_{i/o}\alpha$, $G_q\alpha$, and $G_{12/13}\alpha$ with various subtypes, effectors, and expression profiles (Milligan and Kostenis, 2006).

RGS2 AND RGS4 IN THE HEART

Regulators of G Protein Signaling proteins were first identified as GTPase activating proteins (GAPs), accelerating the intrinsic

GTPase activity of Gα subunits, as the duration of G protein activation is primarily controlled by GTP hydrolysis. Also, RGS proteins can interfere with G protein binding to effector proteins, separate from their regulation of hydrolysis (Abramow-Newerly et al., 2006). Thus RGS proteins are important limiters of GPCR signaling. Currently, 20 different genes encoding RGS proteins have been identified and divided into four subfamilies, based on their sequence and structural similarities: RZ/A (RGS17, 19, and 20); R4/B (RGS1–5, 8, 13, 16, and 21); R7/C (RGS6, 7, 9, and 11), and R12/D (RGS10, 12, and 14; Bansal et al., 2007). The majority of RGS proteins are GAPs for Gαi/o and many also act on Gαq/11[89]; however, none are GAPs for Gαs but some RGS-like proteins such as p115RhoGEF do have GAP activity on the Gα11/12 subfamily. RGS2, 3, 4, 6, 10, RGSZ2, and GAIP are all found in atrial cardiomyocytes (Doupnik et al., 2001).

The ongoing control of cardiac function by GPCRs is itself modulated by RGS proteins. RGS-insensitive $G\alpha_0$G184S homozygous knock-in (Gαi2GS/GS) embryonic stem cell-derived cardiocytes had enhanced responses to M2 muscarinic but not A1 adenosine receptor stimulation, while analogous GαoGS/GS cardiocytes had enhanced A1 adenosine and M2 receptor mediated responses (Fu et al., 2006). Gαs stimulation of the intrinsic beating rate was almost completely abolished in Gαi2GS/GS cells, likely due to a failure of AC activation resulting from an increase in countervailing inhibitory activity. Gαi2GS/GS insensitive mutant mice also had pronounced (five-fold greater) muscarinic mediated bradycardia and third degree AV nodal block (Fu et al., 2007). These mutant mouse data indicate that in the SA and AV node, M2 receptors primarily couple through Gαi2 to inhibit cAMP production and activation of PKA (Fu et al., 2006, 2007). Adenosine 1 and 3 receptor overexpressing mice have also have prolonged AVN conduction (Kirchhof et al., 2003; Fabritz et al., 2004), which may involve receptor mediated inhibition of adenylyl cyclase 5/6 (AC5/6), primarily coupling through Gαo (Fu et al., 2006, 2007). Susceptibility to atrial arrhythmia has not been examined in these mice. It is currently believed that specific RGS proteins may couple to specific signaling pathways within the cell.

RGS2, a member of the R4/B subfamily, the second most highly expressed RGS protein in the heart (Doupnik et al., 2001), is a selective GAP for Gαq (Zou et al., 2006). This selectivity does not reflect any exceptional affinity for the latter but rather a relatively weak RGS2 affinity for Gαi/o (Ingi et al., 1998; Cladman and Chidiac, 2002) which is due to the substitution of three conserved amino acid residues in its RGS domain that decrease binding affinity to Gαi/o but not Gαq (Heximer et al., 1999). RGS2 also produces a poorly understood inhibitory effect on Gs-activated AC signaling (Sinnarajah et al., 2001; Roy et al., 2006b). The mechanism by which such inhibition occurs does not appear to involve a GAP effect, as RGS2 fails to alter the GTPase activity of either free (Ingi et al., 1998) or receptor-activated Gs (Roy et al., 2003). Some evidence suggests that the inhibitory effect may involve a physical interaction of the N-terminus of RGS2 with the C1 catalytic loop of AC5 (Salim et al., 2003; Beazely and Watts, 2006); however other studies suggest that RGS2 may bind directly to Gαs (Tseng and Zhang, 1998; Ko et al., 2001). In HEK293 cells, GFP-RGS2 tended to localize to the nucleus but was recruited to the plasma membrane by the co-expression of either Gαs or most adenylyl cyclase isoforms, and BRET (bioluminescence resonance energy transfer) interactions between RGS2 and Gαs are not inhibited by adenylyl cyclase (Roy et al., 2006a). RGS2 appears to be important in the desensitization of Gq- and Gs-mediated GPCR receptor signals as it is upregulated by both and moreover it can mediate cross-desensitization between Gαq and Gαs (Sinnarajah et al., 2001; Roy et al., 2006b).

Removal of RGS2's inhibitory effect on Gαq signaling increases Gαq-dependent signaling activity in cardiomyocytes (Zhang et al., 2006). Interestingly, RGS2 has also been shown to be an important target in cardiovascular disease (cardiac hypertrophy and hypertension; Tsang et al., 2010). $RGS2^{-/-}$ mice have a mild to moderate hypertensive phenotype (Heximer et al., 2003; Gross et al., 2005; Tank et al., 2007) that is suggested to be mediated by vascular changes, possibly through angiotensin II, endothelin and/or α-adrenergic receptors, rather than being due to cardiac alterations, although cardiac "contractility," measured by left ventricular *dP/dt*, was not determined (Oliveira-dos-Santos et al., 2000; Heximer et al., 2003). Altered autonomic function and effects mediated via the kidneys may also contribute to elevated blood pressure in these animals (Gu et al., 2009). An increase in mean arterial pressure of ~10 mm Hg was found with Telemetry, while heart rate was unchanged, indicating a resetting of the baroreceptor reflex (Gross et al., 2005). This was confirmed by directly measuring baroreflex sensitivity calculated by cross-spectral analysis of heart rate variability. However, heart rate variability was not different in $RGS2^{-/-}$ compared to $RGS2^{+/+}$ mice (Gross et al., 2005), indicating that the cardiac phenotype was not explained by a baroreflex mediated enhancement of vagal nerve activity. Since RGS2 is a selective regulator of Gαq signaling that can inhibit signaling via M3 receptors in other cell types (Tovey and Willars, 2004; Karakoula et al., 2008), it follows that RGS2 may be an important regulator of M3 muscarinic signaling in the atria. Notably, the scaffolding protein spinophilin, which is present in cardiomyocytes (Bers, 2004), binds to both RGS2 and M3 muscarinic receptors, and thus it may facilitate the inhibition of M3 muscarinic receptor-activated Gq signals, as has been observed with analogous α1-adrenergic signals (Wang et al., 2007b).

RGS4 regulates SA nodal function (Cifelli et al., 2008) via inhibition of parasympathetic signaling and $I_{K,ACh}$ activity. In mice expressing LacZ under the control of the RGS4 promoter, high expression of LacZ-RGS4 was found in the SAN will little expression was observed in the surrounding right atrium. RGS4-null ($RGS4^{-/-}$ mice had lower baseline heart rates and greater increases in heart rate following atropine blockade. High expression of RGS4 (demonstrated by LacZ staining), was also seen in the AV node and $RGS4^{-/-}$ mice were highly susceptible to carbachol-induced AV nodal conduction block when treated with isoproterenol. However, there is limited electrophysiological data describing the location of conduction block, and results were obtained principally in Langendorff hearts (removed from *in vivo* autonomic influences).

As RGS4 was found only in the SA and AV nodal region, the RGS protein regulating parasympathetic signaling and $I_{K,ACh}$ activity in the atrium remained, until recently, unknown. RGS6-deficient ($RGS6^{-/-}$) atrial myocytes exhibited a significant reduction in the time course of $I_{K,ACh}$ activation and deactivation. RGS6$^{-/-}$ mice also displayed bradycardia and AV nodal conduction block indicating that there is at least partial redundancy in RGS protein function *in vivo*.

RGS2 AND ATRIAL ARRHYTHMIA IN THE MOUSE

In both RGS2$^{-/-}$ and C57Bl\6 wild type (WT, control) anesthetized mice (Tuomi et al., 2010) with body temperature maintained within the normal physiological range (36.5–38°C; Connolly and Lynch, 1981) and His bundle recording (**Figure 3**) used to validate correct positioning of the electrode (**Figure 4**), atrial effective refractory periods (AERPs) were heterogeneous, being longer in the high right compared to the mid right atrium. In addition, AERPs were significantly lower in RGS2$^{-/-}$ mice compared to WT mice. M2 receptor and M3 receptor mRNA was not different in RGS2$^{-/-}$ compared to WT mice. Carbachol reduced AERPs in both strains but strain differences persisted. In contrast, the AERPs were increased to similar levels in both strains with atropine. The selective M3 blocker, darifenacin, increased the AERP for the mid atrium of RGS2$^{-/-}$ and WT mice, and eliminated the strain-related differences (Tuomi et al., 2010), supporting a role of RGS2 in atrial function. Of interest, in paroxysmal AF there is a frequency gradient but in chronic AF, the frequency gradient in the left atrium has been shown to be absent (Lazar et al., 2006).

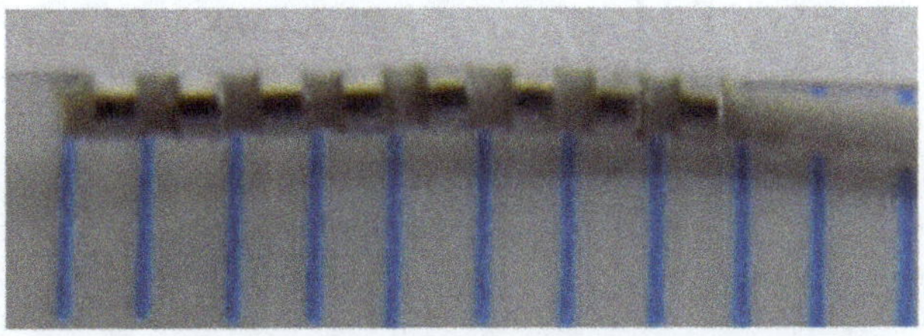

FIGURE 3 | A photograph of an octapolar electrode catheter (CIB'ER Mouse®, NuMED, Inc., Hopkinton, NY, USA) used for recording from the atrium, His bundle region and ventricle of the anesthetized mouse. The small marks on the ruler are 1 mm spacing.

Since vagally induced bradycardia is mediated via M2 but not M3 receptors (Fisher et al., 2004), we compared the effects of cholinergic blockade using darifenacin and atropine on heart rate changes following vagus nerve stimulation. Stimulating the vagus decreased heart rate by 38 ± 6.8% in WT animals. This decrease was abolished by atropine but was unaltered in the presence of darifenacin (Tuomi et al., 2010). This provided evidence that this dose of darifenacin did not affect M2 signaling. Of note, this dose of darifenacin also terminated electrically induced fibrillation in connexin 43 mutant mice (Tuomi et al., 2011).

Both programmed electrical stimulation (Jones et al., 2001) and burst pacing (Jones et al., 2008a) were used to determine susceptibility to atrial arrhythmia induction. A single atrial stimulus induced AF (**Figure 5**). Overall, RGS2$^{-/-}$ mice were more susceptible to electrically induced arrhythmia (**Table 1**; Tuomi et al., 2010).

Atrial fibrillation is very rarely induced by single extrastimuli in large animal and human studies and was thus anticipated to be even less provocable in mice, due to their small size. Thus sensitivity to single extrastimuli in the mouse implies a highly vulnerable myocardial substrate. The duration of induced arrhythmia is also important with "sustained" AF being defined in large animal and human electrophysiological studies as lasting >30 s. Scaling of electrophysiological variables has been related to the BM$^{0.25}$ (Noujaim et al., 2004). Using this relationship, the duration equivalent is in the second range. However as there is no gold standard: indeed not even a convention, we concluded it best to use ranges. Hence, the data were analyzed based on susceptibility to pacing modality and grouped by the duration of the induced arrhythmia, lasting: <10 s; between 10 and 30 s, and >30 s. As expected, WT mice were virtually non-inducible with a single

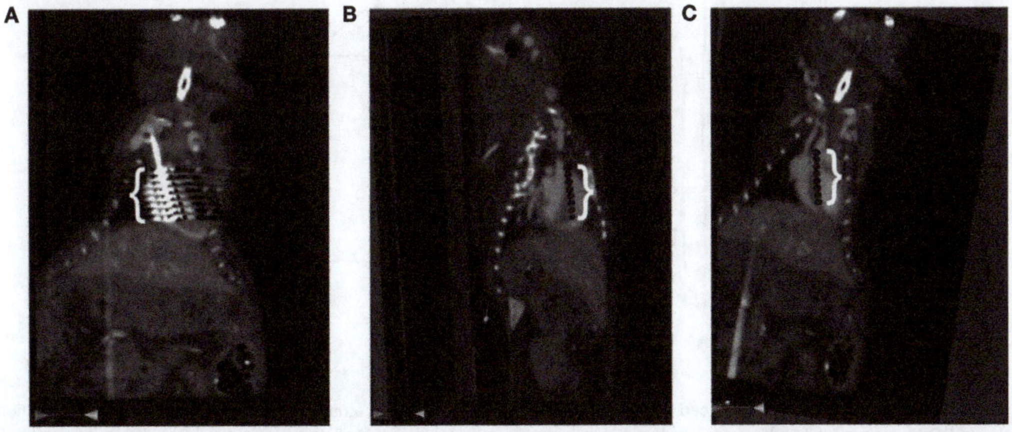

FIGURE 4 | Computed Tomography (CT) of the catheter position in the right heart of the anesthetized mouse. The mouse's head is at the top and tail, off the bottom of each image. **(A)** The white bracket delineates the region of interference from catheter's eight electrodes shown as very bright echoes extending laterally from the catheter. **(B)** A sagittal view of the digitally inserted catheter. The white bracket delineates the position of the catheter's eight electrodes. The bright dots to the left of the torso are from the ribs and those on the left are from the spinal column. **(C)** A coronal view of catheter placement with electrodes three and four across the tricuspid valve. The white bracket delineates the catheter's eight electrodes. The bright dots to the left and right of the torso are from the ribs.

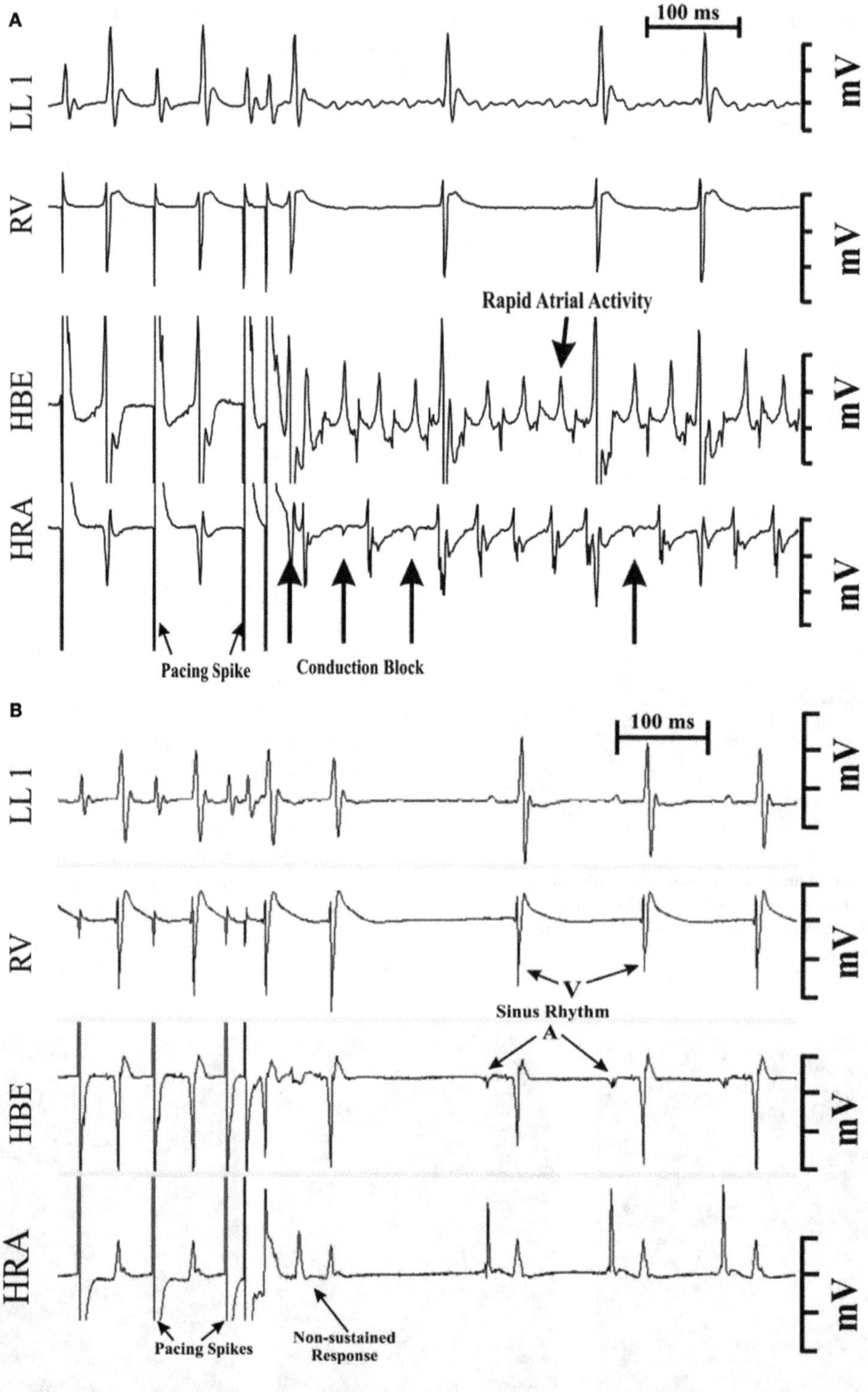

FIGURE 5 | Programmed electrical stimulation-induced atrial fibrillation (AF) in a 1-month-old RGS2−/−mouse (A). Note the conduction block into the high right atrial (HRA) region denoted by the far-field (low amplitude) potential recordings during block. The duration of the arrhythmia was >200 s with an average atrial rate of ~1600 bpm. A similar stimulation protocol failed to induce atrial fibrillation in wild type mice **(B)**. LL1, limb lead 1.RV, right ventricular electrogram. HBE, electrogram from the His bundle region. HRA, recording from the high right atrium.

stimulus (4%, 1/25), compared to burst pacing (40%, 10/25). Carbachol increased the susceptibility to both single extrastimuli (33%, 4/12) and burst pacing (58%, 7/12). Carbachol also prolonged the fibrillation duration with only 2 of 12 untreated mice being sustained, while 5 of the 12 were sustained after carbachol. The atrial stimulation site also affected arrhythmia

Table 1 | Incidence of AT/F induced by PES or burst pacing and maximum duration of induced AT/F with either PES or burst pacing induction.

	Wild type	RGS2$^{-/-}$
INDUCIBILITY		
PES	4% (1/25)	50% (11/22)
Burst (50 Hz, 400 ms pulse)	40% (10/25)	64% (14/22)
DURATION		
No response	60% (15/25)	36% (8/22)
<10 s	20% (5/25)	23% (5/22)
10–30 s	16% (4/25)	18% (4/22)
>30 s	4% (1/25)	23% (5/22)

X^2 analysis of discrete values revealed significant differences in atrial tachycardia/fibrillation (AT/F) susceptibility with programmed electrical stimulation (PES; $P < 0.05$).

susceptibility. Burst pacing more readily induced arrhythmia from the mid right atrium of WT mice (40%, 10/25) compared to those from the high right atrial region (8%, 2/25, $P < 0.05$; Tuomi et al., 2010). This likely reflects the regional AERPs being significantly shorter in the mid-compared to the high right atrium. Electrical heterogeneity may be an important factor in providing a permissive substrate for wave break and re-entry initiation in the atrium.

Rapid focal activity may initiate rotors due to the interaction of a high frequency propagating wave fronts with the refractory tail of the previous wave (Jalife and Pandit, 2005; Vaquero et al., 2008). Immediately after arrhythmia induction, local cycle lengths were often identical in the high right and His bundle regions. However, sometimes at onset, there was regional conduction block into the high right atrium (**Figure 5**), which could be accompanied by heterogeneity in local cycle lengths in RGS2$^{-/-}$ mice, with His bundle electrograms being shorter than those of the high right atrium. Over time, these intervals converged (Tuomi et al., 2010). This pattern is consistent with the concept of a drifting rotor that rapidly became anchored, although it may also indicate a tachycardia with a rapid rate at onset that slowed down as the driving mechanism stabilized. However, rapid onset may combine with the regional refractory heterogeneity to produce functional conduction block/slowing that eventually recovers at slower rates. Of note, the cycle length during arrhythmia was faster than the measured intrinsic AERP in the high right atrial region, suggesting the possibility of electronic interactions from a rotor core causing reduced refractoriness (Vaquero et al., 2008).

In summary, in addition to the previous focus on the role of M2 receptors in atrial arrhythmia, there is evidence that arrhythmia inducibility may be due to parasympathetic M3 receptors and their regulation by RGS2 knockout. RGS2 accelerates the intrinsic GTPase activity of Gαq, thus limiting the lifetime of the activated state, thereby regulating the Gαq coupled M3 receptor and its associated current, $I_{K,M3}$. These data are the first we know that demonstrate a role for RGS proteins in atrial arrhythmia. The RGS2$^{-/-}$ mice were more susceptible to electrically induced AF, and there was a greater percentage of RGS2$^{-/-}$ mice with sustained AF. This strain dependent difference was maintained in the presence of carbachol, while atropine abolished the strain dependent differences. These findings suggest an alteration in muscarinic receptor-gated K^+ flux evidently due to an increase in M3 muscarinic receptor response *per se*.

CONCLUSION

With the aging of the population, there is an increasing drive to identify novel treatments for AF. This will require increased understanding of the signaling pathways and molecular regulators involved in arrhythmia induction, perpetuation, and atrial remodeling. Current medical management of cardiac arrhythmias depends primarily on ion channel blockade, most of which (~70%) are controlled by GPCRs; however, these agents may be proarrhythmic (The Cardiac Arrhythmia Suppression Trial (CAST) Investigators, 1989) and reduce the quality of life of the patients. Thus developing selective agents for cholinergic signaling may provide an effective treatment for AF initiation and perpetuation. Mutations in, or altered expression/function of a variety of RGS proteins could be involved in AF mechanisms in patients, and indeed, changes in RGS2 have been identified in several human cardiovascular phenotypes. Thus, targeting RGS proteins may be important for drug development (Roman et al., 2009). Selective M3R blockade, alone, or in combination with other antiarrhythmic agents, may be useful for patients with AF. However, in mice, oral darifenacin exerted only transient binding to cardiac muscarinic receptors (Yamada et al., 2006), thus its use may be limited.

LIMITATIONS

While these results indicate a role for RGS2 and the M3 muscarinic receptor in promoting AF in the mouse, additional studies will need to directly determine the role of $I_{K,M3}$ activity. Also, it would be beneficial to examine the effects of novel $I_{K,ACh}$ antagonists NTC-801 (Machida et al., 2011) and I_{Kur} antagonist, acacetin (Li et al., 2008). Atrial vulnerability may also be due to a balance of autonomics (Scherlag et al., 2006; Jones et al., 2007). RGS2$^{-/-}$ mice have also been shown to have reduced renal sympathetic nerve activity compared to WT mice (Tank et al., 2007). Although, the lack of a heart rate difference between RGS2$^{-/-}$ and WT mice found in their earlier study (Gross et al., 2005) does not assist in establishing the role of the sympathetic nervous system in atrial susceptibility, the role of the balance between sympathetics and M3 responses remains to be determined. It is also recognized that it may not be possible to directly extrapolate from mouse experiments to the human.

ACKNOWLEDGMENTS

This work was supported in part by the Heart and Stroke Foundation of Ontario (NA6403). Jari Micheal Tuomi was the recipient of an Ontario Graduate Scholarship in Science and Technology and the Canadian Institutes for Health Research CGS Doctoral Research Award. Peter Chidiac holds a Career Investigator Award from the Heart and Stroke Foundation of Ontario. The authors thank Maria Drangova for assistance with the coordinating experiments involving CT Scans and Sarah Detombe for performing the scans.

REFERENCES

Abramow-Newerly, M., Roy, A. A., Nunn, C., and Chidiac, P. (2006). RGS proteins have a signalling com- plex: interactions between RGS pro- teins and GPCRs, effectors, and auxiliary proteins. *Cell. Signal.* 18, 579–591.

Alessi, R., Nusynowitz, M., Abildskov, J. A., and Moe, G. K. (1958). Nonuniform distribution of vagal effects on the atrial refractory period. *Am. J. Physiol.* 194, 406–410.

Allessie, M. A., Boyden, P. A., Camm, A. J., Kleber, A. G., Lab, M. J., Legato, M. J., Rosen, M. R., Schwartz, P. J., Spooner, P. M., Van Wagoner, D. R., and Waldo, A. L. (2001). Pathophys- iology and prevention of atrial fib- rillation. *Circulation* 103, 769–777.

Allessie, M. A., Lammers, W., and Bonke, F. (1985). "Experimental evaluation of Moe's multiple wavelet hypoth- esis of atrial fibrillation," in *Car- diac Electrophysiology and Arrhyth- mias*, eds D. P. Zipes and J. Jarife (New York, NY: Grune & Stratton Inc.), 265–275.

Arora, R. C., Waldmann, M., Hopkins, D. A., and Armour, J. A. (2003). Porcine intrinsic cardiac ganglia. *Anat. Rec.* 271A, 249–258.

Atrial fibrillation is associated with an increased risk for mortality and heart failure progression in patients with asymptomatic and sympto- matic left ventricular systolic dys- function: a retrospective analysis of the SOLVD trials. Studies of left ventricular dysfunction. *J. Am. Coll. Cardiol.* 32, 695–703.

Bagwe, S., Berenfeld, O., Vaidya, D., Morley, G. E., and Jalife, J. (2005). Altered right atrial excita- tion and propagation in connexin 40 knockout mice. *Circulation* 112, 2245–2253.

Bansal, G., Druey, K. M., and Xie, Z. (2007). R4 RGS proteins: regulation of G-protein signaling and beyond. *Pharmacol. Ther.* 116, 473–495.

Beazely, M. A., and Watts, V. J. (2006). Regulatory properties of adenylate cyclases type 5 and 6: a progress report. *Eur. J. Pharmacol.* 535, 1–12. Benjamin, E. J., Wolf, P. A., D'Agostino, R. B., Silbershatz, H., Kannel, W. B., and Levy, D. (1998). Impact of atrial fibrillation on the risk of death: the Framingham Heart Study. *Circula- tion* 98, 946–952.

Bers, D. M. (2004). Macromolecular complexes regulating cardiac ryan- odine receptor function. *J. Mol. Cell. Cardiol.* 37, 417–429.

Burger, D. E., Lu, X., Lei, M., Xiang, F. L., Hammoud, L., Jiang, M., Wang, H., Jones, D. L., Sims, S. M., and Feng, (2009a). Neuronal nitric oxide synthase protects against myocar- dial infarction-induced ventricular arrhythmia and mortality in mice. *Circulation* 120, 1345–1354.

Burger, D. E., Xiang, F. L., Hammoud, L., Jones, D. L., and Feng, Q. (2009b). Erythropoietin protects the heart from ventricular arrhythmia during ischemia and reperfusion via neu- ronal nitric-oxide synthase. *J. Pharmacol. Exp. Ther.* 329, 900–907.

Cardinal, R., Page, P., Vermeulen, M., Ardell, J. L., and Armour, J. A. (2009). Spatially divergent cardiac responses to nicotinic stimulation of ganglionated plexus neurons in the canine heart. *Auton. Neurosci.* 145, 55–62.

Chang, C. M., Wu, T. J., Zhou, S., Doshi, N., Lee, M. H., Ohara, T., Fishbein, M. C., Karagueuzian, H. S., Chen, P. S., and Chen, L. S. (2001). Nerve sprouting and sympathetic hyperin- nervation in a canine model of atrial fibrillation produced by prolonged right atrial pacing. *Circulation* 103, 22–25.

Chen, F., Spicher, K., Jiang, M., Birn- baumer, L., and Wetzel, G. T. (2001). Lack of muscarinic regulation of Ca(2+) channels in G(i2)alpha gene knockout mouse hearts. *Am. J. Phys- iol. Heart Circ. Physiol.* 280, H1989– H1995.

Cifelli, C., Rose, R. A., Zhang, H., Voigtlaender-Bolz, J., Bolz, S. S., Backx, P. H., and Heximer, S. P. (2008). RGS4 Regulates parasympa- thetic signaling and heart rate con- trol in the sinoatrial node. *Circ. Res.* 103, 527–535.

Cladman, W., and Chidiac, P. (2002). Characterization and comparison of RGS2 and RGS4 as GTPase- activating proteins for m2 mus- carinic receptor-stimulated G(i). *Mol. Pharmacol.* 62, 654–659.

Clark, R. B., Mangoni, M. E., Lueger, A., Couette, B., Nargeot, J., and Giles, W. R. (2004). A rapidly activating delayed rectifier K+ current reg- ulates pacemaker activity in adult mouse sinoatrial node cells. *Am. J. Physiol. Heart Circ. Physiol.* 286, H1757–H1766.

Connolly, M. S., and Lynch, C. B. (1981). Circadian variation of strain differences in body temperature and activity in mice. *Physiol. Behav.* 27, 1045–1049.

Coumel, P., Attuel, P., Lavallee, J., Flam- mang, D., Leclercq, J. F., and Slama, R. (1978). The atrial arrhythmia syn- drome of vagal origin. *Arch. Mal. Coeur Vaiss.* 71, 645–656.

Danik, S. B., Liu, F., Zhang, J., Suk, H. J., Morley, G. E., Fishman, G. I., and Gutstein, D. E. (2004). Modulation of cardiac gap junction expression and arrhythmic susceptibility. *Circ. Res.* 95, 1035–1041.

Dobrev, D., and Nattel, S. (2011). New insights into the molecular basis of atrial fibrillation: mechanistic and therapeutic implications. *Car- diovasc. Res.* 89, 689–691.

Doupnik, C. A., Xu, T., and Shinaman, J. M. (2001). Profile of RGS expres- sion in single rat atrial myocytes. *Biochim. Biophys. Acta* 1522, 97–107. Dries, D. L., Exner, D. V., Gersh, B. J., Domanski, M. J., Waclawiw, M. A., and Stevenson, L. W. (1998).

Dupont, E., Ko, Y., Rothery, S., Coppen, S. R., Baghai, M., Haw, M., and Sev- ers, N. J. (2001a). The gap-junctional protein connexin 40 is elevated in patients susceptible to postoperative atrial fibrillation. *Circulation* 103, 842–849.

Dupont, E., Matsushita, T., Kaba, R. A., Vozzi, C., Coppen, S. R., Khan, N., Kaprielian, R., Yacoub, M. H., and Severs, N. J. (2001b). Altered connexin expression in human con- gestive heart failure. *J. Mol. Cell. Cardiol.* 33, 359–371.

Efimov, I. R., and Fedorov, V. V. (2005). Chessboard of atrial fibrillation: reentry or focus? Single or multiple source(s)? Neurogenic or myogenic? *Am. J. Physiol. Heart Circ. Physiol.* 289, H977–H979.

Fabritz, L., Kirchhof, P., Fortmuller, L., Auchampach, J. A., Baba, H. A., Breithardt, G., Neumann, J., Boknik, P., and Schmitz, W. (2004). Gene dose-dependent atrial arrhythmias, heart block, and brady-cardiomyopathy in mice overexpressing A(3) adeno- sine receptors. *Cardiovasc. Res.* 62, 500–508.

Fisher, J. T., Vincent, S. G., Gomeza, J., Yamada, M., and Wess, J. (2004). Loss of vagally mediated bradycardia and bronchoconstriction in mice lacking M2 or M3 muscarinic acetylcholine receptors. *FASEB J.* 18, 711–713.

Fu,Y., Huang, X., Piao, L., Lopatin, A. N., and Neubig, R. R. (2007). Endogenous RGS proteins modulate SA and AV nodal functions in isolated heart: implications for sick sinus syndrome and AV block. *Am. J. Physiol. Heart Circ. Physiol.* 292, H2532–H2539.

Fu,Y., Huang, X., Zhong, H., Mortensen, R. M., D'Alecy, L. G., and Neubig, R. R. (2006). Endogenous RGS proteins and Galpha subtypes differentially control muscarinic and adenosine- mediated chronotropic effects. *Circ. Res.* 98, 659–666.

Furness, J. B., Jones, C., Nurgali, K., and Clerc, N. (2004). Intrinsic primary afferent neurons and nerve circuits within the intestine. *Prog. Neurobiol.* 72, 143–164.

Fuster, V., Ryden, L. E., Asinger, R. W., Cannom, D. S., Crijns, H. J., Frye, R. L., Halperin, J. L., Kay, G. N., Klein, W. W., Levy, S., McNa- mara, R. L., Prystowsky, E. N., Wann, L. S., Wyse, D. G., Gibbons, R. J., Antman, E. M., Alpert, J. S., Faxon, D. P., Fuster, V., Gregoratos, G., Hiratzka, L. F., Jacobs, A. K., Rus- sell, R. O., Smith, S. C. Jr., Klein, W. W., Alonso-Garcia, A., Blomstrom- Lundqvist, C., De, B. G., Flather, M., Hradec, J., Oto, A., Parkhomenko, A., Silber, S., and Torbicki, A. (2001). ACC/AHA/ESC Guidelines for the Management of Patients With Atrial Fibrillation: Executive Summary A Report of the American College of Cardiology/American Heart Associ- ation Task Force on Practice Guide- lines and the European Society of Cardiology Committee for Practice Guidelines and Policy Conferences (Committee to Develop Guidelines for the Management of Patients With Atrial Fibrillation) Developed in Collaboration With the North American Society of Pacing and Electrophysiology. *Circulation* 104, 2118–2150.

Garrey, W. E. (1914). The nature of fib- rillary contraction of the heart. Its relations to tissue mass and form. *Am. J. Physiol.* 33, 397–414.

Garrey, W. E. (1924). Auricular fibrilla- tion. *Physiol. Rev.* 4, 215–250. Gollob, M. H., Jones, D. L., Krahn, A. D., Danis, L., Gong, X. Q., Shao, Q., Liu, X., Veinot, J. P., Tang, A. S., Stewart, A. F., Tesson, F., Klein, G. J., Yee, R., Skanes, A. C., Guiraudon, G. M., Ebi- hara, L. and Bai, D. (2006). Somatic mutations in the connexin 40 gene (GJA5) in atrial fibrillation. *N. Engl. J. Med.* 354, 2677–2688.

Gross, V., Tank, J., Obst, M., Plehm, R., Blumer, K. J., Diedrich, A., Jordan, J., and Luft, F. C. (2005). Autonomic nervous system and blood pressure regulation in RGS2-deficient mice. *Am. J. Physiol. Regul. Integr. Comp. Physiol.* 288, R1134–R1142.

Gu, S., Cifelli, C., Wang, S., and Heximer, S. P. (2009). RGS proteins: identifying new GAPs in the understand- ing of blood pressure regulation and cardiovascular function. *Clin. Sci. (Lond.)* 116, 391–399.

Gutstein, D. E., Morley, G. E., Tamad- don, H., Vaidya, D., Schneider, M. D., Chen, J., Chien, K. R., Stuhlmann, H., and Fishman, G. I. (2001). Conduction slowing and sudden arrhythmic death in mice with cardiac-restricted inactivation of connexin43. *Circ. Res.* 88, 333–339.

Haissaguerre, M., Jais, P., Shah, D. C., Takahashi, A., Hocini, M., Quiniou, G., Garrigue, S., Le Mouroux, A., Le Metayer, P., and Clementy, J. (1998). Spontaneous initiation of atrial fib- rillation by ectopic beats originating in the pulmonary veins. *N. Engl. J. Med.* 339, 659–666.

Haissaguerre, M., Shah, D. C., Jais, P., Hocini, M., Yamane, T., Deisenhofer, I., Garrigue, S., and Clementy, J. (2000). Mapping-guided ablation of pulmonary veins to cure atrial fibril- lation. *Am. J. Cardiol.* 86, 9K–19K.

Hashimoto, N., Yamashita, T., and Tsu- ruzoe, N. (2006). Tertiapin, a selec- tive IKACh blocker, terminates atrial fibrillation with selective atrial effec- tive refractory period prolongation. *Pharmacol. Res.* 54, 136–141.

Hassall, C. J., and Burnstock, G. (1987). Immunocytochemical local- isation of neuropeptide Y and 5- hydroxytryptamine in a subpopu- lation of amine-handling intracar- diac neurones that do not contain dopamine beta-hydroxylase in tissue culture. *Brain Res.* 422, 74–82.

Hellgren, I., Mustafa, A., Riazi, M., Suli- man, I., Sylven, C., and Adem, A. (2000). Muscarinic M3 receptor sub- type gene expression in the human heart. *Cell. Mol. Life Sci.* 57, 175–180.

Heximer, S. P., Knutsen, R. H., Sun, X., Kaltenbronn, K. M., Rhee, M. H., Peng, N., Oliveira-dos-Santos, A., Penninger, J. M., Muslin, A. J., Stein- berg, T. H., Wyss, J. M., Mecham, R. P., and Blumer, K. J. (2003). Hyper- tension and prolonged vasoconstric- tor signaling in RGS2-deficient mice. *J. Clin. Invest.* 111, 445–452.

Heximer, S. P., Srinivasa, S. P., Bern- stein, L. S., Bernard, J. L., Linder, M. E., Hepler, J. R., and Blumer, K. J. (1999). G protein selectivity is a determinant of RGS2 function. *J. Biol. Chem.* 274, 34253–34259.

Hoffa, M., and Ludwig, C. (1850). Einge neueversuche uber herzbewe- gung. *Zeitschrift Rationellen Medizin* 9, 107–144.

Ingi, T., Krumins, A. M., Chidiac, P., Brothers, G. M., Chung, S., Snow, B. E., Barnes, C. A., Lanahan, A. A., Siderovski, D. P., Ross, E. M., Gilman, A. G., and Worley, P. F. (1998). Dynamic regulation of RGS2 suggests a novel mechanism in G- protein signaling and neuronal plas- ticity. *J. Neurosci.* 18, 7178–7188.

Jalife, J. (2003). Rotors and spiral waves in atrial fibrillation. *J. Cardiovasc. Electrophysiol.* 14, 776–780.

Jalife, J., Berenfeld, O., Skanes, A., and Mandapati, R. (1998). Mechanisms of atrial fibrillation: mother rotors or multiple daughter wavelets, or both? *J. Cardiovasc. Electrophysiol.* 9(Suppl. 8), S2–S12.

Jalife, J., and Pandit, S. V. (2005). Ionic mechanisms of wavebreak in fibril- lation. *Heart Rhythm* 2, 660–663.

Jones, D. L., Guiraudon, G. M., Skanes, A. C., and Guiraudon, C. M. (2008a). Anatomical pitfalls during encircling cryoablation of the left atrium for atrial fibrillation therapy in the pig.

J. Interv. Card. Electrophysiol. 21, 187–193. Jones, D. L., Tuomi, J., Ramsay, D., Guiraudon, C. M., Cardinal, R., Page, P., and Guiraudon, G. M. (2008b). Left atrial neuroablation for atrial fibrillation therapy: a fea- sibility study. *J. Interv. Card. Electro Physiol.* 21, 171–172.

Jones, D. L., Petrie, J. P., and, Li, H. G. (2001). Spontaneous, electri- cally, and cesium chloride induced arrhythmia and afterdepolarizations in the rapidly paced dog heart. *Pac- ing Clin. Electrophysiol.* 24(Pt 1), 474–485.

Jones, D. L., Tuomi, J., Ramsay, D., Guiraudon, C. M., Armour, J. A., Cardinal, R., Page, P., and Guiraudon, G. M. (2007). Left atrial neuroablation for atrial fibrillation: a feasibility study. *Can. J. Cardiol.* 23, 225C.

Kalifa, J., Jalife, J., Zaitsev, A. V., Bagwe, S., Warren, M., Moreno, J., Berenfeld, O., and Nattel, S. (2003). Intra-atrial pressure increases rate and organi- zation of waves emanating from the superior pulmonary veins during atrial fibrillation. *Circulation* 108, 668–671.

Kang, D., Han, J., and Kim, D. (2006). Mechanism of inhibition of TREK- 2 (K2P10.1) by the Gq-coupled M3 muscarinic receptor. *Am. J. Physiol. Cell Physiol.* 291, C649–C656.

Kannel, W. B., Abbott, R. D., Sav- age, D. D., and McNamara, P. M. (1982). Epidemiologic features of chronic atrial fibrillation: the Fram- ingham study. *N. Engl. J. Med.* 306, 1018–1022.

Karakoula, A., Tovey, S. C., Brighton, P. J., and Willars, G. B. (2008). Lack of receptor-selective effects of either RGS2, RGS3 or RGS4 on muscarinic M3- and gonadotropin-releasing hormone receptor-mediated sig- nalling through G alpha q/11. *Eur. J. Pharmacol.* 587, 16–24.

Kirchhof, P., Fabritz, L., Fortmuller, L., Matherne, G. P., Lankford, A., Baba, H. A., Schmitz, W., Brei- thardt, G., Neumann, J., and Boknik, P. (2003). Altered sinus nodal and atrioventricular nodal function in freely moving mice overexpressing the A1 adenosine receptor. *Am. J. Physiol. Heart Circ. Physiol.* 285, H145–H153.

Kitazawa, T., Asakawa, K., Nakamura, T., Teraoka, H., Unno, T., Komori, S., Yamada, M., and Wess, J. (2009). M3 muscarinic receptors mediate pos- itive inotropic responses in mouse atria: a study with muscarinic recep- tor knockout mice. *J. Pharmacol. Exp. Ther.* 330, 487–493.

Kleber, A. G. (2000). The fibrillating atrial myocardium. What can the detection of wave breaks tell us? *Cardiovasc. Res.* 48, 181–184.

Klein, I., and Ojamaa, K. (2001). Thy- roid hormone and the cardiovas- cular system. *N. Engl. J. Med.* 344, 501–509.

Ko, J. K., Choi, K. H., Kim, I. S., Jung, E. K., and Park, D. H. (2001). Inducible RGS2 is a cross-talk regulator for parathyroid hormone signaling in rat osteoblast-like UMR106 cells. *Biochem. Biophys. Res. Commun.* 287, 1025–1033.

Kovoor, P., Wickman, K., Maguire, C. T., Pu, W., Gehrmann, J., Berul, C. I., and Clapham, D. E. (2001). Evalua- tion of the role of I(KACh) in atrial fibrillation using a mouse knock- out model. *J. Am. Coll. Cardiol.* 37, 2136–2143.

Krejci, A., and Tucek, S. (2002). Quan- titation of mRNAs for M(1) to M(5) subtypes of muscarinic receptors in rat heart and brain cortex. *Mol. Pharmacol.* 61, 1267–1272.

Lazar, S., Dixit, S., Callans, D. J., Lin, D., Marchlinski, F. E., and Gerstenfeld, E. P. (2006). Effect of pulmonary vein isolation on the left-to-right atrial dominant frequency gradient in human atrial fibrillation. *Heart Rhythm* 3, 889–895.

Li, G. R., Wang, H. B., Qin, G. W., Jin, M. W., Tang, Q., Sun, H. Y., Du, X. L., Deng, X. L., Zhang, X. H., Chen, J. B., Chen, L., Xu, X. H., Cheng, L. C., Chiu, S. W., Tse, H. F., Vanhoutte, P. M., and Lau, C. P. (2008). Acacetin, a natural flavone, selectively inhibits human atrial repolarization potas- sium currents and prevents atrial fibrillation in dogs. *Circulation* 117, 2449–2457.

Liu, L., and Nattel, S. (1997). Differ- ing sympathetic and vagal effects on atrial fibrillation in dogs: role of refractoriness heterogeneity. *Am. J. Physiol.* 273(Pt 2), H805–H816.

Lomax, A. E., Rose, R. A., and Giles, W. R. (2003). Electrophysiological evi- dence for a gradient of G protein- gated K+ current in adult mouse atria. *Br. J. Pharmacol.* 140, 576–584.

Machida, T., Hashimoto, N., Kuwa- hara, I., Ogino, Y., Matsuura, J., Yamamoto, W., Itano, Y., Zamma, A., Matsumoto, R., Kamon, J., Kobayashi, T., Ishiwata, N., Yamashita, T., Ogura, T., and Nakaya, H. (2011). Effects of a highly selective acetylcholine- activated K+ channel blocker on experimental atrial fibrillation. *Circ. Arrhythm. Electrophysiol.* 4, 94–102.

MacWilliam, J. A. (1887). Fibrillar con- traction of the heart. *J. Physiol. (Lond.)* 8: 296.

Mandapati, R., Skanes, A., Chen, J., Berenfeld, O., and Jalife, J. (2000). Stable microreentrant sources as a mechanism of atrial fibrillation in the isolated sheep heart. *Circulation* 101, 194–199.

Mansour, M., Mandapati, R., Beren- feld, O., Chen, J., Samie, F. H., and Jalife, J. (2001). Left-to-right gra- dient of atrial frequencies during acute atrial fibrillation in the iso- lated sheep heart. *Circulation* 103, 2631–2636.

Mawe, G. M., Talmage, E. K., Lee, K. P., and Parsons, R. L. (1996). Expression of choline acetyltrans- ferase immunoreactivity in guinea pig cardiac ganglia. *Cell Tissue Res.* 285, 281–286.

Milligan, G., and Kostenis, E. (2006). Heterotrimeric G-proteins: a short history. *Br. J. Pharmacol.* 147(Suppl. 1), S46–S55.

Moe, G. K. (1962). On the multiple wavelet hypothesis of atrial fibrilla- tion. *Arch. Int. Pharmacodyn. Ther.* 40, 183–189.

Moe, G. K., and Abildskov, J. A. (1959). Atrial fibrillation as a self-sustaining arrhythmia independent of focal discharge. *Am. Heart J.* 58, 59–70.

Moe, G. K., Rheinboldt, W. C., and Abildskov, J. A. (1964). A com- puter model of atrial fibrillation. *Am. Heart J.* 67, 200–220.

Morillo, C. A., Klein, G. J., Jones, D. L., and Guiraudon, C. M. (1995). Chronic rapid atrial pacing. Struc- tural, functional, and electrophys- iological characteristics of a new model of sustained atrial fibrillation. *Circulation* 91, 1588–1595.

Nademanee, K., McKenzie, J., Kosar, E., Schwab, M., Sunsaneewitayakul, B., Vasavakul, T., Khunnawat, C., and Ngarmukos, T. (2004). A new approach for catheter abla- tion of atrial fibrillation: map- ping of the electrophysiologic sub- strate. *J. Am. Coll. Cardiol.* 43, 2044–2053.

Nakagawa, H., Sherlag, B. J., Lockwood, D., Wolf, R. K., Peyton, M., Wu, R., Yokoyama, K., Po, S. S., Her- ring, L., Lazzara, R., Jackmann, W. K., and Armour, J. A. (2005a). Local- ization of left atrial gamglionated plexuses using endocardial and epi- cardial high frequency stimulation in patients with atrial fibrillation. *Heart Rhythm* 2, S10–S11.

Nakagawa, H., Sherlag, B. J., Wu, A. W., Lockwood, D., Yokoyama, K., Her- ring, L., Lazzara, R., and Jackman, W. M. (2005b). Addition of selec- tive ablation of autonomic ganglia to pulmonary vein antrum ablation for treatment of paroxysmal and per- sistent atrial fibrillation. *Circulation* 110, III-543.

Nattel, S. (2002). New ideas about atrial fibrillation 50 years on. *Nature* 415, 219–226.

Nattel, S. (2004). Age, gender, and supraventricular arrhythmias: roles of ion channels, connexins, and tis- sue architecture? *Heart Rhythm* 1, 397–398.

Nattel, S., Allessie, M., and Haissa- guerre, M. (2002). Spotlight on atrial fibrillation-the "complete arrhyth- mia." *Cardiovasc. Res.* 54, 197–203.

Nishida, K., Maguy, A., Sakabe, M., Comtois, P., Inoue, H., and Nattel, S. (2011). The role of pulmonary veins vs. autonomic ganglia in different experimental substrates of canine atrial fibrillation. *Cardiovasc. Res.* 89, 825–833.

Nixon, J. V. (2011). *The AHA Clin- ical Cardiac Consult.* Philadelphia: Lippincott Williams & Wilkins.

Noujaim, S. F., Lucca, E., Munoz, V., Per- saud, D., Berenfeld, O., Meijler, F. L., and Jalife, J. (2004). From mouse to whale: a universal scaling relation for the PR interval of the electrocardio- gram of mammals. *Circulation* 110, 2802–2808.

Nygren, A., Lomax, A. E., and Giles, W. R. (2004). Heterogeneity of action potential durations in isolated mouse left and right atria recorded using voltage-sensitive dye mapping. *Am. J. Physiol. Heart Circ. Physiol.* 287, H2634–H2643.

Oliveira-dos-Santos, A. J., Matsumoto, G., Snow, B. E., Bai, D., Houston, F. P., Whishaw, I. Q., Mariathasan, S., Sasaki, T., Wakeham, A., Ohashi, P. S., Roder, J. C., Barnes, C. A., Siderovski, D. P., and Penninger, J. M. (2000). Regulation of T cell acti- vation, anxiety, and male aggression by RGS2. *Proc. Natl. Acad. Sci. U.S.A.* 97, 12272–12277.

Pappone, C., Rosanio, S., Oreto, G., Toc- chi, M., Gugliotta, F., Vicedomini, G., Salvati, A., Dicandia, C., Mazzone, P., Santinelli, V., Gulletta, S., and Chierchia, S. (2000). Circumferen- tial radiofrequency ablation of pul- monary vein ostia: a new anatomic approach for curing atrial fibrilla- tion. *Circulation* 102, 2619–2628.

Pappone, C., Santinelli, V., Manguso, F., Vicedomini, G., Gugliotta, F., Augello, G., Mazzone, P., Tortoriello, V., Landoni, G., Zangrillo, A., Lang, C., Tomita, T., Mesas, C., Mastella, E., and Alfieri, O. (2004). Pulmonary vein denervation enhances long- term benefit after circumferential ablation for paroxysmal atrial fibril- lation. *Circulation* 109, 327–334.

Platt, M., Mandapati, R., Sherlag, B. J., Yamanashi, W. S., Nagakawa, H., Lazzara, R., and Jackman, W. M. (2004). Limiting the number and extend of radiofrequency applica- tions to terminate atrial fibrilla- tion and subsequently prevent its inducibility. *Heart Rhythm.* 1, S11.

Roman, D. L., Ota, S., and Neubig, R. R. (2009). Polyplexed flow cytome- try protein interaction assay: a novel high-throughput screening para- digm for RGS protein inhibitors. *J. Biomol. Screen.* 14, 610–619.

Rosiak, M., Dziuba, M., Chudzik, M., Cygankiewicz, I., Bartczak, K., Drozdz, J., and Wranicz, J. K. (2010). Risk factors for atrial fibrillation: not always severe heart disease, not always so "lonely." *Cardiol. J.* 17, 437–442.

Roy, A. A., Baragli, A., Bernstein, L. S., Hepler, J. R., Hebert, T. E., and Chidiac, P. (2006a). RGS2 interacts with Gs and adenylyl cyclase in living cells. *Cell. Signal.* 18, 336–348.

Roy, A. A., Nunn, C., Ming, H., Zou, M. X., Penninger, J., Kirshen- baum, L. A., Dixon, S. J., and Chidiac, P. (2006b). Up-regulation of endogenous RGS2 mediates cross-desensitization between Gs and Gq signaling in osteoblasts. *J. Biol. Chem.* 281, 32684–32693.

Roy, A. A., Lemberg, K. E., and Chidiac, P. (2003). Recruitment of RGS2 and RGS4 to the plasma membrane by G proteins and receptors reflects func- tional interactions. *Mol. Pharmacol.* 64, 587–593.

Sakamoto, S., Schuessler, R. B., Lee, A. M., Aziz, A., Lall, S. C., and Dami- ano, R. J. Jr. (2010). Vagal dener- vation and reinnervation after abla- tion of ganglionated plexi. *J. Thorac. Cardiovasc. Surg.* 139, 444–452.

Salim, S., Sinnarajah, S., Kehrl, J. H., and Dessauer, C. W. (2003). Identi- fication of RGS2 and type V adeny- lyl cyclase interaction sites. *J. Biol. Chem.* 278, 15842–15849.

Sarmast, F., Kolli, A., Zaitsev, A., Parisian, K., Dhamoon, A. S., Guha, P. K., Warren, M., Anumonwo, J. M., Taffet, S. M., Berenfeld, O., and Jalife, J. (2003). Cholinergic atrial fibrilla- tion: I(K,ACh) gradients determine unequal left/right atrial frequencies and rotor dynamics. *Cardiovasc. Res.* 59, 863–873.

Savelieva, I., and Camm, A. J. (2001). Clinical trends in atrial fibrillation at the turn of the millenium. *J. Intern. Med.* 250, 369–372.

Scherlag, B. J., Patterson, E., and Po, S. S. (2006). The neural basis of atrial fib- rillation. *J. Electrocardiol.* 39(Suppl. 4), S180–S183.

Schotten, U., Verheule, S., Kirchhof, P., and Goette, A. (2011). Pathophys- iological mechanisms of atrial fib- rillation: a translational appraisal. *Physiol. Rev.* 91, 265–325.

Shen, M. J., Choi, E. K., Tan, A. Y., Han, S., Shinohara, T., Maruyama, M., Chen, L. S., Shen, C., Hwang, C., Lin, S. F., and Chen, P. S. (2011). Patterns of baseline auto- nomic nerve activity and the devel- opment of pacing-induced sustained atrial fibrillation. *Heart Rhythm* 8, 583–589.

Shi, H., Wang, H., Yang, B., Xu, D., and Wang, Z. (2004). The M3 receptor-mediated K(+) cur- rent (IKM3), a G(q) protein-coupled K(+) channel. *J. Biol. Chem.* 279, 21774–21778.

Shi, H., Yang, B., Xu, D., Wang, H., and Wang, Z. (2003). Electrophysi- ological characterization of cardiac muscarinic acetylcholine receptors: different subtypes mediate differ- ent potassium currents. *Cell. Physiol. Biochem.* 13, 59–74.

Shiroshita-Takeshita, A., Sakabe, M., Haugan, K., Hennan, J. K., and Nattel, S. (2007). Model- dependent effects of the gap junction conduction-enhancing antiarrhythmic peptide rotigaptide (ZP123) on experimental atrial fibrillation in dogs. *Circulation* 115, 310–318.

Sinnarajah, S., Dessauer, C. W., Sriku- mar, D., Chen, J., Yuen, J., Yilma, S., Dennis, J. C., Morrison, E. E., Vodyanoy, V., and Kehrl, J. H. (2001). RGS2 regulates signal transduction in olfactory neurons by attenuat- ing activation of adenylyl cyclase III. *Nature* 409, 1051–1055.

Skanes, A. C., Mandapati, R., Beren- feld, O., Davidenko, J. M., and Jalife, J. (1998). Spatiotemporal periodic- ity during atrial fibrillation in the isolated sheep heart. *Circulation* 98, 1236–1248.

Souza, M. V., Duarte, M. M., Coeli, C. M., and Vaisman, M. (2012). Atrial fibrillation and hyperthy- roidism: relation between transoe- sophageal markers of a thrombo- genic milieu and clinical risk fac- tors for thromboembolism. *Clin. Endocrinol. (Oxf.)* 76, 448–453.

Tamargo, J., Caballero, R., Gomez, R., Valenzuela, C., and Delpon, E. (2004). Pharmacology of cardiac potassium channels. *Cardiovasc. Res.* 62, 9–33.

Tank, J., Obst, M., Diedrich, A., Brychta, R. J., Blumer, K. J., Heusser, K., Jordan, J., Luft, F. C., and Gross, V. (2007). Sympathetic nerve traffic and circulating norepinephrine lev- els in RGS2-deficient mice. *Auton. Neurosci.* 136, 52–57.

The Cardiac Arrhythmia Suppres- sion Trial (CAST) Investigators. (1989). Preliminary report: effect of encainide, and flecainide on mortal- ity in a randomized trial of arrhyth- mia suppression after myocardial infarction. *N. Engl. J Med.* 321, 406–412.

Thibodeau, I. L., Xu, J., Li, Q., Liu, G., Lam, K., Veinot, J. P., Birnie, D. H., Jones, D. L., Krahn, A. D., Lemery, R., Nicholson, B. J., and Gollob, M. H. (2010). Par- adigm of genetic mosaicism and lone atrial fibrillation: physiolog- ical characterization of a con- nexin 43-deletion mutant identified from atrial tissue. *Circulation* 122, 236–244.

Thijssen, V. L., Ausma, J., Liu, G. S., Allessie, M. A., van Eys, G. J., and Borgers, M. (2000). Structural changes of atrial myocardium dur- ing chronic atrial fibrillation. *Car- diovasc. Pathol.* 9, 17–28.

Tovey, S. C., and Willars, G. B. (2004). Single-cell imaging of intracellular Ca2+ and phospholipase C activ- ity reveals that RGS 2, 3, and 4 differentially regulate signaling via the Galphaq/11-linked muscarinic M3 receptor. *Mol. Pharmacol.* 66, 1453–1464.

Tsang, S., Woo, A. Y., Zhu, W., and Xiao, R. P. (2010). Deregulation of RGS2 in cardiovascular dis- eases. *Front. Biosci. (Schol. Ed.)* 2, 547–557.

Tseng, C. C., and Zhang, X. Y. (1998). Role of regulator of G protein signaling in desensitization of the glucose-dependent insulinotropic peptide receptor. *Endocrinology* 139, 4470–4475.

Tuomi, J. M., Chidiac, P., and Jones, D. L. (2010). Evidence for enhanced M3 muscarinic receptor function and sensitivity to atrial arrhythmia in the RGS2-deficient mouse. *Am. J. Physiol. Heart Circ. Physiol.* 298, H554–H561.

Tuomi, J. M., Tyml, K., and Jones, D. L. (2011). Atrial tachycar- dia/fibrillation in the connexin 43 G60S mutant (Oculodentodigital dysplasia) mouse. *Am. J. Physiol. Heart Circ. Physiol.* 300, H1402– H1411.

Vaquero, M., Calvo, D., and Jalife, J. (2008). Cardiac fibrillation: from ion channels to rotors in the human heart. *Heart Rhythm* 5, 872–879.

Voigt, N., Trausch, A., Knaut, M., Matschke, K., Varro, A., Van Wag- oner, D. R., Nattel, S., Ravens, U., and Dobrev, D. (2010). Left-to-right atrial inward rectifier potassium current gradients in patients with paroxysmal versus chronic atrial fib- rillation. *Circ. Arrhythm. Electro- physiol.* 3, 472–480.

Vulpain, A. (1874). Note sur les effets de la faradisation directe des ventricu- laes du coeur le chien. *Arch. Physiol.* i, 975.

Wakili, R., Voigt, N., Kaab, S., Dobrev, D., and Nattel, S. (2011). Recent advances in the molecular patho- physiology of atrial fibrillation. *J Clin. Invest.* 121, 2955–2968.

Wang, H., Lu, Y., and Wang, Z. (2007a). Function of cardiac M3 recep- tors. *Auton. Autacoid. Pharmacol.* 27, 1–11.

Wang, X., Zeng, W., Kim, M. S., Allen, P. B., Greengard, P., and Muallem, S. (2007b). Spinophilin/neurabin rec- iprocally regulate signaling inten- sity by G protein-coupled receptors. *EMBO J.* 26, 2768–2776.

Wang, T. L., Tseng, Y. Z., and Chang, H. (2000). Regulation of connexin 43 gene expression by cyclical mechanical stretch in neonatal rat cardiomyocytes. *Biochem. Biophys. Res. Commun.* 267, 551–557.

Wang, Z., Shi, H., and Wang, H. (2004). Functional M3 muscarinic acetylcholine receptors in mam- malian hearts. *Br. J. Pharmacol.* 142, 395–408.

Wieland, T., Lutz, S., and Chidiac, P. (2007). Regulators of G protein signalling: a spotlight on emerg- ing functions in the cardiovascular system. *Curr. Opin. Pharmacol.* 7, 201–207.

Yamada, S., Maruyama, S., Takagi, Y., Uchida, S., and Oki, T. (2006). In vivo demonstration of M3 mus- carinic receptor subtype selectivity of darifenacin in mice. *Life Sci.* 80, 127–132.

Yamazaki, M., Vaquero, L. M., Hou, L., Campbell, K., Zlochiver, S., Klos, M., Mironov, S., Berenfeld, O., Honjo, H., Kodama, I., Jalife, J., and Kalifa, J. (2009). Mechanisms of stretch- induced atrial fibrillation in the pres- ence and the absence of adreno- cholinergic stimulation: interplay between rotors and focal discharges. *Heart Rhythm* 6, 1009–1017.

Yan, G. X., and Kowey, P. R. (2011). *Management of Cardiac Arrhyth- mias.* New York: Humana Press.

Yeh, Y. H., Qi, X., Shiroshita-Takeshita, A., Liu, J., Maguy, A., Chartier, D., Hebert, T., Wang, Z., and Nat- tel, S. (2007). Atrial tachycardia induces remodelling of muscarinic receptors and their coupled potas- sium currents in canine left atrial and pulmonary vein cardiomy- ocytes. *Br. J. Pharmacol.* 152, 1021–1032.

Yue, P., Zhang, Y., Du, Z., Xiao, J., Pan, Z., Wang, N., Yu, H., Ma, W., Qin, H., Wang, W. H., Lin, D. H., and Yang, B. (2006). Ischemia impairs the association between connexin 43 and M3 subtype of acetylcholine muscarinic receptor (M3-mAChR) in ventricu- lar myocytes. *Cell. Physiol. Biochem.* 17, 129–136.

Zhang, W., Anger, T., Su, J., Hao, J., Xu, X., ZHU, M., Gach, A., Cui, L., Liao, R., and Mende, U. (2006). Selective loss of fine tun- ing of Gq/11 signaling by RGS2 protein exacerbates cardiomyocyte hypertrophy. *J. Biol. Chem.* 281, 5811–5820.

Zhao, Q., Huang, C., Jiang, H., Okello, E., Tang, Y. H., Wang, Z., and Wu, Z. (2008). M2 and M3-muscarinic acetylcholine receptors remodelling in patients with a dilated atrium. *Acta Cardiol* 63, 166–170.

Zipes, D. P. (1997). The seventh annual Gordon K. Moe Lecture. Atrial fibrillation: from cell t bed- side. *J. Cardiovasc. Electrophysiol.* 8, 927–938.

Zipes, D. P., Mihalick, M. J., and Robbins, G. T. (1974). Effects of selective vagal and stellate ganglion stimulation of atrial refractoriness. *Cardiovasc. Res.* 8, 647–655.

Zou, M. X., Roy, A. A., Zhao, Q., Kirshenbaum, L. A., Karmazyn, M., and Chidiac, P. (2006). RGS2 is upregulated by and attenuates the hypertrophic effect of alpha1- adrenergic activation in cultured ventricular myocytes. *Cell. Signal.* 18, 1655–1663.

19

Integrated mechanisms of CaMKII-dependent ventricular remodeling

Michael M. Kreusser*[1,2] *and Johannes Backs*[1,2]

[1] *Research Unit Cardiac Epigenetics, Department of Cardiology, University of Heidelberg, Heidelberg, Germany*
[2] *German Center for Cardiovascular Research (DZHK), Partner Site Heidelberg/Mannheim, Germany*

Correspondence:
Johannes Backs, Research Unit Cardiac Epigenetics, Department of Cardiology, University of Heidelberg and DZHK (German Centre for Cardiovascular Research), Im Neuenheimer Feld 410, 69120 Heidelberg, Germany
e-mail: johannes.backs@ med.uni-heidelberg.de

CaMKII has been shown to be activated during different cardiac pathological processes, and CaMKII-dependent mechanisms contribute to pathological cardiac remodeling, cardiac arrhythmias, and contractile dysfunction during heart failure. Activation of CaMKII during cardiac stress results in a broad number of biological effects such as, on the one hand, acute effects due to phosphorylation of distinct cellular proteins as ion channels and calcium handling proteins and, on the other hand, integrative mechanisms by changing gene expression. This review focuses on transcriptional and epigenetic effects of CaMKII activation during chronic cardiac remodeling. Multiple mechanisms have been described how CaMKII mediates changes in cardiac gene expression. CaMKII has been shown to directly phosphorylate components of the cardiac gene regulation machinery. CaMKII phosphorylates several transcription factors such as CREB that induces the activation of specific gene programs. CaMKII activates transcriptional regulators also indirectly by phosphorylating histone deacetylases, especially HDAC4, which in turn inhibits transcription factors that drive cardiac hypertrophy, fibrosis, and dysfunction. Recent studies demonstrate that CaMKII also phosphorylate directly histones, which may contribute to changes in gene expression. These findings of CaMKII-dependent gene regulation during cardiac remodeling processes suggest novel strategies for CaMKII-dependent "transcriptional or epigenetic therapies" to control cardiac gene expression and function. Manipulation of CaMKII-dependent signaling pathways in the settings of pathological cardiac growth, remodeling, and heart failure represents an auspicious therapeutic approach.

Keywords: CaMKII, epigenetics, transcription factors, HDAC4, remodeling

INTRODUCTION

Heart failure is the leading cause of death in developed countries and is characterized by adverse cardiac remodeling upon pathological stress situations such as arterial hypertension, ischemic injuries or due to genetic causes. Adverse left ventricular remodeling is usually described by a combination of myocardial hypertrophy, cell death, interstitial fibrosis and an activation of a so-called fetal gene program (Koitabashi and Kass, 2012). Calcium-dependent signaling pathways including Calcium/Calmodulin-dependent kinase II (CaMKII) signaling play pivotal roles in adverse cardiac remodeling (Heineke and Molkentin, 2006; Bers, 2008; Backs et al., 2009; Ling et al., 2009). Activation of CaMKII during cardiac stress results in a broad number of biological effects. On the one hand, CaMKII mediates immediate effects due to phosphorylation of cellular proteins such as ion channels and calcium handling proteins (Anderson et al., 2011). On the other hand, CaMKII affects structural features of the cardiac phenotype due to phosphorylation of proteins of the transcriptional machinery (Anderson et al., 2011). This review focuses on CaMKII-dependent transcriptional and epigenetic mechanisms that occur in cardiomyocytes during pathological and physiological processes. First, we will review the different CaMKII genes and splice variants that localize to different subcellular compartments.

CaMKII ISOFORMS AND SPLICE VARIANTS

In 2003, Colomer and colleagues observed an increased activity of Calcium/Calmodulin-dependent kinases upon pathological pressure overload due to transverse aortic constriction (TAC), and they described the expression patterns of the Calcium/Calmodulin-dependent kinases CaMKI, CaMKII, and CaMKIV (Colomer et al., 2003). They found CaMKI to be expressed in left ventricular tissue, but not up-regulated upon TAC. Whereas artificial overexpression of CaMKIV in a transgenic model was sufficient to induce cardiac hypertrophy in another study (Passier et al., 2000), in the model of Colomer, left ventricular CaMKIV was not detectable, and mice lacking CaMKIV did not display an altered response to TAC, indicating that CaMKIV is not required for cardiac hypertrophy. They convincingly demonstrated that CaMKII is the only multifunctional CaMK that is not only up-regulated on the expression level but also activated after TAC.

CaMKII consists of four different isoforms with distinct expression patterns. CaMKIIα and CaMKIIβ are enriched in neuronal tissue, and CaMKIIδ, and CaMKIIγ are expressed ubiquitously (Hudmon and Schulman, 2002). CaMKIIδ is the most abundant cardiac CaMKII isoform but CaMKIIγ is also expressed in the heart (Hoch et al., 1999; Colomer et al., 2003). The first *in vivo* studies establishing CaMKII as a potential target for cardiac arrhythmias and structural heart disease were conducted by the use of a pharmacological inhibitor such as KN-62 or KN-93 and a CaMKII inhibitory peptide (Zhang et al., 2005; Vila-Petroff et al., 2007; Liu et al., 2011). Due to the unclear role of the single CaMKII isoforms and potential unspecific effects of CaMKII inhibitors, isoform-specific genetic loss of function models were generated. Mice with a global deletion of CaMKIIδ were protected against adverse cardiac remodeling (Backs et al., 2009; Ling et al., 2009). CaMKIIδ global knockout mice produced by us were protected from cardiac fibrosis and hypertrophy 3 weeks after TAC surgery. CaMKIIδ global knockout model generated by Ling and colleagues were protected from fibrosis and dysfunction. These mice were not protected from cardiac hypertrophy 2 weeks but only 6 weeks after TAC. These seemingly different phenotypes with regard to cardiac hypertrophy may be explained by different surgery techniques, different genetic backgrounds, or different knockout strategies. With regard to the latter, in the first model, no residual protein was expressed (transcriptional null due to deletion of exon 1 and 2), whereas in the second model the possible existence of a truncated protein encoding a region before exon 8 was not ruled out (exons 9–11 were deleted). The specific role of cardiac CaMKIIγ and a potential redundancy with CaMKIIδ have not been investigated yet. In human and experimental heart failure, enhanced CaMKII activity was mainly attributed to an enhanced expression of the CaMKIIδ splice variants CaMKIIδB and CaMKIIIδC (Edman and Schulman, 1994; Hoch et al., 1999). From transgenic mouse models with artificial overexpression of these splice variants it was concluded that CaMKIIδB (localizes to the nucleus) promotes cardiac hypertrophy and CaMKIIδC (localizes to the cytosol) results in dilated cardiomyopathy, respectively (Zhang et al., 2002b, 2003). Moreover, CaMKIIδA (localizes to sarcolemmal and nuclear membranes) was implied as another splice variant that is regulated at least in a model of cardiac hypertrophy due to isoproterenol treatment in mice (Xu et al., 2005; Li et al., 2011). However, to our knowledge transgenic models of CaMKIIδA have not been generated so far. An overview of available genetic mouse models related to cardiac CaMKII is given in **Table 1**.

CaMKII AND TRANSCRIPTIONAL REGULATION

Effects of CaMKII on cardiac gene expression was first reported by the group of Joan Heller Brown when transient expression of CaMKIIδB in neonatal rat ventricular myocytes induced gene expression of atrial natriuretic factor (ANF) and resulted in enhanced transcriptional activation of an ANF-luciferase reporter gene (Ramirez et al., 1997). As we know now, CaMKII is involved in the regulation of many transcription factors such as the activation protein-1 (AP-1) (Antoine et al., 1996), activating transcription factor-1 (ATF-1) (Shimomura et al., 1996), serum response factor (SRF) (Fluck et al., 2000), cAMP-response element binding protein (CREB) (Sun et al., 1994), and myocyte enhancer factor 2 (MEF2). The latter is discussed in the next paragraph. An overview about the identified transcriptional regulators is given in **Figure 1**.

A well-known transcription factor in striated muscle biology is SRF, and Calcium/Calmodulin-dependent regulation of SRF via interaction with CaMKIV and histone deacetylase 4 (HDAC4), but not CaMKII, was demonstrated to be involved in the development of cardiac hypertrophy (Davis et al., 2003). A direct phosphorylation of SRF by CaMKII has been shown in skeletal muscle at Ser-103 and Thr-160 (Fluck et al., 2000), but its relevance in cardiomyocytes remains unclear. However, data from other cell types indicate that SRF-dependent gene transcription might depend on phosphorylation by CaMKII (Ely et al., 2011). As genetic animal models provide evidence for an important role for SRF in the induction and maintenance of the cardiac myogenic program (Lin et al., 1997; Parlakian et al., 2005; Backs et al., 2011), a better understanding of CaMKII-dependent SRF regulation is urgently needed.

AP-1 elements are a group of transcription factors composed of either homodimers of the Jun family (c-Jun, JunB, and JunD) or heterodimers of the Fos and Jun families (c-Fos, Fra-1, Fra-2, and FosB) (Mechta-Grigoriou et al., 2001). There is evidence for CaMKII-dependent transcriptional activity via AP-1 in non-cardiac tissues (Mishra et al., 2005; Zayzafoon et al., 2005). Recently, CaMKII-dependent upregulation of the sodium/calcium exchanger 1 (NCX1) has been shown to depend on AP-1 transcription factors c-Jun and JunB in cardiomyocytes (Mani et al., 2010). However, it remains unclear whether CaMKII phosphorylates AP-1 elements directly or indirectly.

Table 1 | Genetic mouse models for CaMKIIδ and γ.

Gene/splicing variant	Type	Strategy	Cardiac phenotype	Location	References
CaMKIIδ*B*	Gain of function	α*MHC*-driven transgene	Cardiac hypertrophy	Nucleus	Zhang et al., 2002b
CaMKIIδ*C*	Gain of function	α*MHC*-driven transgene	Dilated cardiomyopathy	Cytosol	Zhang et al., 2003
CaMKIIδ	Loss of function	Global knockout exons 9–11	Protection from fibrosis, dysfunction, and late hypertrophy	Nucleus/Cytosol	Ling et al., 2009
CaMKIIδ	Loss of function	Global knockout exons 1–2	Protection from early hypertrophy and fibrosis	Nucleus/Cytosol	Backs et al., 2009
CaMKIIγ	Loss of function	Global knockout exons 1–2	Not investigated	Nucleus/Cytosol	Backs et al., 2010

Cardiomyocyte-specific transgenic overexpression of CaMKIIδ (splice variants B and C) are driven by the αMHC promoter. Global knockout models for CaMKIIδ were generated by two labs. The second cardiac CaMKII isoform, CaMKIIγ, has so far not been investigated with regard to cardiac stress situations.

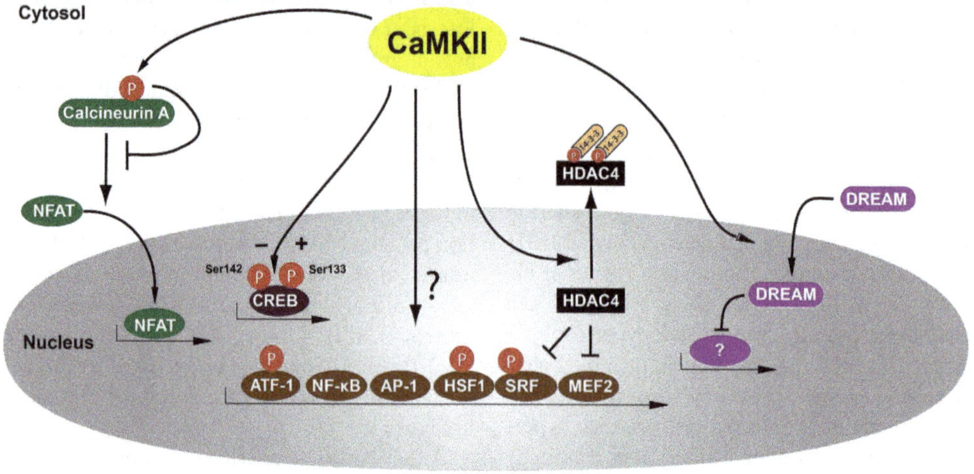

FIGURE 1 | Schematic of transcription factors and transcriptional repressors regulated by CaMKII in cardiomyocytes. CaMKII phosphorylates HDAC4 at Ser-467 and Ser-632, allowing binding of the chaperone protein 14-3-3, leading to nucleo-cytoplasmic shuttling of a phospho-HDAC4/14-3-3 complex out of the nucleus and resulting in derepression of transcription factors such as MEF2 that regulates genes responsible for adverse cardiac remodeling. Other transcription factors such as NF-κB or HSP-1 may play maladaptive or adaptive roles and these factors can be directly or indirectly regulated by CaMKII. Another transcription factor regulated after β-adrenergic stimulation is CREB that can be phosphorylated by CaMKII at two serine residues, Ser-133 and Ser-142, resulting in opposing effects in regard to activation of CREB. However, the functional effects of CREB/CaMKII interaction during cardiac remodeling remain unclear. Another recently recognized mechanism is translocation of the transcriptional repressor DREAM from the cytosol to the nucleus. Calcineurin/NFAT interaction may also be inhibited by direct phosphorylation by CaMKII at Ser-411, leading to decreased NFAT translocation to the nucleus and subsequent reduced transcriptional activity. AP-1 activation protein-1, ATF-1 activating transcription factor-1, CaMKII Calcium/Calmodulin-dependent kinase II, CREB cAMP-response element binding protein, DREAM downstream regulatory element agonist modulator, HDAC4 histone deacetylase 4, HSF-1 heat shock factor 1, MEF2 myocyte elongation factor, NFAT nuclear factor of activated T-cells, NF-κB nuclear factor κB, and SRF serum response factor.

As one of the well characterized transcription factors activated by G-protein coupled receptors, CREB has been shown to be phosphorylated by Calcium/Calmodulin-dependent kinases (Sheng et al., 1991). Several phosphorylation sites in CREB have been identified to regulate transcriptional activity and have been shown to be regulated by CaMKII in a dual way. Phosphorylation of CREB at Ser-133 by PKA and CaMKII is required for CREB activation, whereas phosphorylation of Ser-142 by CaMKII inhibits CREB activity by inhibition of CREB dimerization and protein/protein interactions that are necessary to form an active promoter complex (Wu and McMurray, 2001). *In vitro* studies using purified CaMKIV and CaMKII have demonstrated that CaMKIV phosphorylates CREB on Ser-133, whereas CaMKII has equal affinity for Ser-133 and Ser-142 (Sun et al., 1994). However, whereas nuclear calcium elevations increase CREB-dependent transcriptional activity (Kobrinsky et al., 2011), it remains unclear whether CaMKII-dependent CREB phosphorylation plays a significant role in cardiac remodeling processes (Li et al., 2006). Another member of the cAMP-responsive transcription factor family is ATF-1. ATF-1 is phosphorylated at Ser-63 by CaMKII, increasing its transcriptional activity (Shimomura et al., 1996), but the relevance of ATF-1 activity in cardiomyocytes is unknown.

Studies using KN-93, a CaMKII-inhibitory chemical compound, postulated CaMKII-dependent activation of transcription factor nuclear factor-κB (NF-κB) leading to cardiomyocyte hypertrophy (Kashiwase et al., 2005). In CaMKIIδ knockout mouse studies, NF-κB-dependent mechanisms and subsequent activation of inflammatory genes were found to play a maladaptive role in myocardial ischemia and ischemia/reperfusion injury in mice (Singh et al., 2009; Ling et al., 2013). Of note, the latter work conducted by the group of Mark Anderson was the first to perform gene expression profiling in a relevant animal model of cardiac stress, after myocardial infarction in mice. In this study, a CaMKII inhibitory peptide was used. Thus, potential off target effects need to be taken into account. For instance, it was shown that the CaMKII inhibitory peptide can also inhibit protein kinase D (PKD) (Backs et al., 2009). Gene expression arrays in genetic loss of function models might provide important additional information.

A possible physiological CaMKII-dependent transcriptional effect mediated by CaMKIIδB is the activation of heat shock factor 1 (HSF-1), a transcription factor responsible for inducible heat shock protein 70 (iHSP70) gene regulation. CaMKII is known to phosphorylate HSF-1 at Ser-230 (Holmberg et al., 2001), and Wei Peng and colleagues provided data suggesting that this might be a CaMKII-dependent antiapoptotic mechanism during cardiac ischemia and reperfusion (Peng et al., 2010). In this context, others could show that CaMKIIδB protects from doxorubicine-induced apoptosis, perhaps through GATA4-related expression of the antiapoptotic bcl-2 (B-cell lymphoma 2) gene (Little et al., 2009), although the mechanism how CaMKII induced GATA4-dependent gene expression was not shown. Taken the central role of GATA4 in cardiac hypertrophy and growth (Oka et al., 2006; Heineke et al., 2007), more data are warranted to clarify the role of GATA4 as a downstream target of CaMKII. Taken together, there are only sparse data available on how CaMKII directly interacts with transcription factors, and for most factors a direct binding and phosphorylation by CaMKII is not yet shown (See also **Table 2**).

In an interesting recent *in vitro* study, Jarkko Ronkainen et al. describe how CaMKII potentiates the translocation of the transcriptional repressor DREAM (downstream regulatory element agonist modulator) into the nucleus and thereby promotes DREAM-induced transcriptional repression. In their study, the authors could show that this mechanism is involved in CaMKII-dependent downregulation of the pore-forming α-subunit (Cav1.2) of the *L*-type calcium channel (LTCC) and postulate this to be a physiological feedback mechanism, which enables cardiomyocytes to adjust calcium influx through the LTCC to calcium-activated CaMKII activity (Ronkainen et al., 2011).

Another "indirect" transcriptional mechanism seems to be mediated by an interaction between CaMKII and calcineurin A. The phosphatase calcineurin A dephosphorylates nuclear factor of activated T-cells (NFAT), resulting in nuclear accumulation of NFAT and consequent activation of NFAT-dependent transcriptional programs and severe cardiac hypertrophy (Molkentin et al., 1998). In an elegant study, it was demonstrated that cytosolic CaMKIIδC phosphorylates calcineurin A within its calmodulin binding domain at Ser-411 and thereby inhibits its activity (MacDonnell et al., 2009). Although the relevance of these findings needs to be proven *in vivo*, this suggest that CaMKIIδC may act as a negative modulator of calcineurin/NFAT activity.

CaMKII AND EPIGENETIC REGULATION

Besides its direct effects on transcriptional regulators, CaMKII regulates gene expression also by phosphorylation of proteins of the epigenetic machinery, especially histone deacetylases (HDACs) and in particular class II HDACs. These interesting mechanisms were initially identified upon the observation that class II HDACs interact with the transcription factor MEF2. MEF2 was introduced to depend on CaMKI and CaMKIV more than 10 years ago by the group of Eric Olson and has been established as a critical transcription factor in cardiac remodeling processes (Passier et al., 2000). MEF2 is a common target for several hypertrophic pathways, although its precise function in cardiac remodeling and the cardiac genes that are modulated by this factor are still under investigation. MEF2 proteins are responsive to calcium-controlled signaling pathways, such as CaMKI, CaMKII, CaMKIV, and Calcineurin (Passier et al., 2000; McKinsey et al., 2002; Zhang et al., 2007). Class II HDACs are expressed in the heart and contain a MEF2 binding domain in the N-terminal region, which is not present in other HDACs. This N-terminal domain binds to the chaperone 14-3-3 and is then exported from the nucleus with the consequent de-repression of MEF2 (Backs and Olson, 2006; McKinsey, 2007; Ling et al.,

Table 2 | CaMKII-dependent regulators of cardiac transcription.

Name	Abbrev.	Type	Effect	Phosphorylation site	Kinase assay	References
cAMP-response element binding protein	CREB	Transcription factor	Unknown	Ser-133, Ser-142	Yes	Sun et al., 1994
Activating transcription factor 1	ATF-1	Transcription factor	Unknown	Ser-63	Yes	Shimomura et al., 1996
Myocyte elongation factor 2	MEF2	Transcription factor	Hypertrophy/remodeling	Unknown	/	Passier et al., 2000
Serum response factor	SRF	Transcription factor	Unknown	Ser-103, Thr-160	Yes	Fluck et al., 2000
Nuclear factor κB	NF-κB	Transcription factor	Hypertrophy/remodeling	Indirect via IκB kinase	/	Kashiwase et al., 2005; Ling et al., 2013
Histone deacetylase 4	HDAC4	Transcriptional repressor	Hypertrophy/remodeling	Ser-467, Ser-632	Yes	Backs et al., 2006
Histone deacetylase 5	HDAC5	Transcriptional repressor	Hypertrophy/remodeling	Unknown	/	Wu et al., 2006; Backs et al., 2008
GATA4	/	Transcription factor	Antiapoptotic	Unknown	/	Little et al., 2009
Activation protein 1	AP-1	Transcription factor	Calcium homeostasis	Unknown	/	Mani et al., 2010
Heat shock factor 1	HSF-1	Transcription factor	Antiapoptotic	Ser-230	Yes	Holmberg et al., 2001; Peng et al., 2010
Downstream regulatory element agonist modulator	DREAM	Transcriptional repressor	Calcium homeostasis	Unknown	/	Ronkainen et al., 2011
Histone H3	H3	Histone	Hypertrophy/remodeling	Ser-10	Yes	Awad et al., 2013

CaMKII interacts with various transcription factors, transcriptional repressors, and histone 3 and thereby influences cardiac gene expression. This interaction can be a direct phosphorylation of Ser/Thr residues by CaMKII, indirect via other proteins (other kinases or cardiac repressors) or by unknown mechanisms. Known phosphorylation site and proof of direct phosphorylation are indicated. CaMKII Calcium/Calmodulin-dependent kinase II.

2013). 14-3-3 binding depends on phosphorylation of HDACs by different kinases. For example, PKD phosphorylates all class II HDAC family members (HDAC4, HDAC5, HDAC7, HDAC9) (Vega et al., 2004; Harrison et al., 2006).

We found that CaMKII selectively signals to HDAC4 via binding to a unique docking site and phosphorylation of Ser-467 and Ser-632 (Backs et al., 2006) (See also **Figure 2**). These data were confirmed by others and phosphorylation of HDAC4 by CaMKII was suggested as a central mechanism in the development of cardiac hypertrophy and remodeling (Little et al., 2007; Zhang et al., 2007; Backs et al., 2009). HDAC5 does not bind to CaMKII and can therefore only be regulated by CaMKII when it is located in close proximity to HDAC4. When HDAC5 oligomerizes with HDAC4, it can be phosphorylated and exported in a complex with HDAC4 and CaMKII (Backs et al., 2008). Accordingly, HDAC5 has been shown to be regulated by CaMKII under certain conditions. The Bers lab demonstrated that calcium in the nuclear envelope is regulated independently from the global calcium transients that cause contraction at each heartbeat. Interestingly, calcium release from the nuclear envelope activates nuclear CaMKII, which triggers nuclear export of HDAC5 (Wu and Bers, 2006; Wu et al., 2006). Whereas nuclear CaMKIIδB and cytosolic CaMKIIδC exert different effects on the phosphorylation of calcium handling proteins as the ryanodine receptor or phospholamban and on calcium homeostasis (Zhang et al., 2007), both isoforms lead to cytosolic accumulation of HDAC4 and an increase in the activity of the transcription factor MEF2 (Backs et al., 2006). Nuclear CaMKIIδB phosphorylates HDAC4 in the nucleus, leading to nucleo-cytoplasmic shuttling of HDAC4. Activation of cytoplasmic CaMKIIδC phosphorylates HDAC4 in the cytosol and prevents the import of HDAC4 from the cytosol to the nucleus (Backs et al., 2006). Thus, cytoplasmic CaMKII is also capable to regulate transcription in addition to its effects on excitation-contraction coupling. These findings strongly suggested that CaMKII indirectly regulates MEF2 by dissociating HDAC4 and HDAC5. However, HDAC4 binds to many other proteins such as other transcription factors including SRF (Davis et al., 2003), co-repressors as CtBP (C-terminal-binding protein) (Zhang et al., 2001) but also to other chromatin modifying enzymes (Zhang et al., 2002a), opening the possibility that CaMKII exerts via cytosolic accumulation of HDAC4 broader effects than simply activating MEF2 (Lehmann et al., 2013).

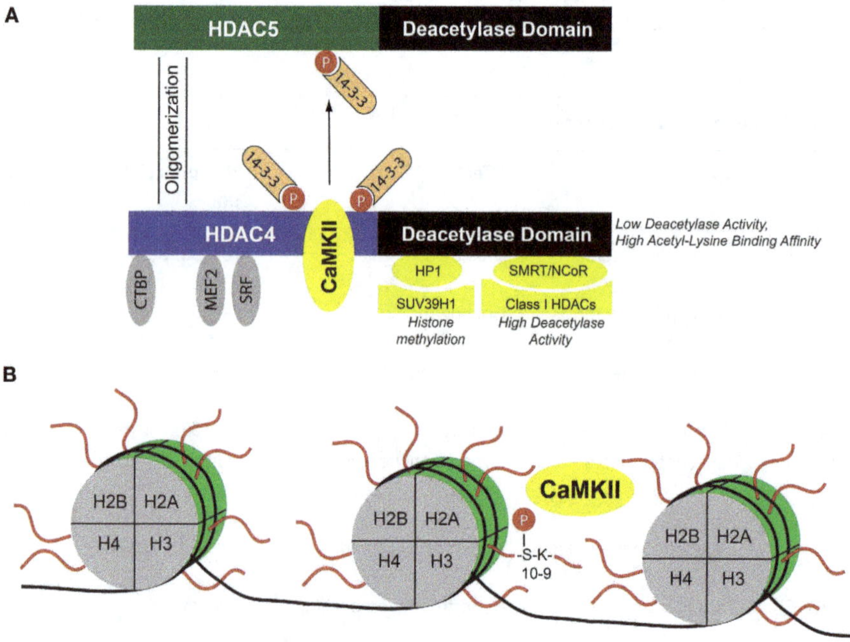

FIGURE 2 | Schematic of CaMKII-dependent epigenetic mechanisms. **(A)** HDAC4 as a nodal point for CaMKII-dependent epigenetic regulation. CaMKII binds to HDAC4 and phosphorylates HDAC4 at Ser-467 and Ser-632, leading to nucleo-cytoplasmic shuttling of HDAC4. When located in the nucleus, HDAC4 represses transcription factors such as MEF2, SRF, or the co-repressor CtBP. Binding to these transcriptional regulators directs HDAC4 to specific chromatin regions. HDAC4 recruits other chromatin modifying enzymes and direct them to the aforementioned specific chromatin regions. This results in CaMKII/HDAC4-dependent regulation of histone methylation (via interaction with HP1 and histone methyltransferase SUV39H1) and deacetylation (via interaction with SMRT/N-CoR and class I HDACs). Moreover, HDAC4 oligomerizes with HDAC5, and thereby induces 14-3-3 dependent nucleo-cytoplasmic shuttling of the HDAC4/HDAC5 complex, leading to de-repression of HDAC4/HDAC5-dependent transcription factors. Thus HDAC4 integrates CaMKII-dependent signals via epigenetic mechanisms. **(B)** Histones (H2A, H2B, H3, and H4) assemble with DNA to form nucleosomes. CaMKII directly phosphorylates Ser-10 in the N-terminal region of histone 3, which is located next to Lys-9, a major site for acetylation, and methylation. Phosphorylation at Ser-10 was suggested to result in cardiomyocyte hypertrophy and increased chromatin binding of CaMKII at specific gene loci reactivated during cardiac hypertrophy. CaMKII Calcium/Calmodulin-dependent kinase II, CtBP C-terminal binding protein, HDAC histone deacetylase, HP1 heterochromatin protein 1, MEF2 myocyte elongation factor, N-CoR nuclear receptor co-repressor, SMRT silencing mediator of retinoic acid and thyroid hormone receptor, and SRF serum response factor.

Histones are major components of chromatin and assemble with DNA to form nucleosomes, (Jenuwein and Allis, 2001). The N-terminal regions of histones are subjected to a variety of post-translational modifications, including acetylation, methylation, ubiquitination, SUMOylation, and phosphorylation (Kouzarides, 2007; Ruthenburg et al., 2007). **Figure 2** summarizes important interacting proteins of HDAC4 that direct HDAC4 to specific chromatin regions by binding to transcription factors. Of note, the deacetylase activity of class II HDACs is low but the binding affinity to acetylated lysines is high, suggesting that HDAC4 is mainly recruited to acetylated chromatin regions in close proximity to regions where MEF2 or SRF binds (Lahm et al., 2007). Although its deacetylase activity is low, HDAC4 binds indirectly via the co-repressors SMRT (silencing mediator of retinoic acid and thyroid hormone receptor) and N-CoR (nuclear receptor co-repressor) to class I HDACs with high deacetylase activity (Fischle et al., 2002) and via HP1 (heterochromatin protein 1) to histone methyltransferases (Zhang et al., 2002a). Thus it is tempting to speculate that CaMKII effects besides transcriptional activity of MEF2 and SRF also class I HDAC-dependent histone acetylation and histone methyltransferase-dependent histone methylation. Indeed, together with the Maack lab we could show that HDAC4 controls histone methylation in a CaMKII-dependent manner (Hohl et al., 2013). ANF and brain natriuretic peptide (BNP) expression in failing hearts was accompanied by demethylation of histone 3 at lysine 9 (H3K9) and dissociation of HP1 from the promoter regions of ANF and BNP, and this was controlled by HDAC4, possibly by forming a transcriptional repressor complex with the histone methyltransferase SUV39H1 that was disrupted by CaMKII-induced phosphorylation of HDAC4. The importance of the CaMKII/HDAC4/MEF2-pathway with regard to epigenetic mechanisms in cardiac remodeling was underscored by a recent study from the Condorelli lab (Papait et al., 2013). The authors performed chromatin immunoprecipitation combined with genomic sequencing (ChIP-Seq) and RNA sequencing in isolated cardiomyocytes after TAC surgery and found a specific epigenetic signature that regulated gene expression by governing the activity of promoters and enhancers related to cardiac hypertrophy. Interestingly, they found MEF2 to be the main transcription factor to orchestrate this hypertrophic gene program by regulating the activity of transcriptional enhancers.

With regard to epigenetic mechanisms, in cardiac biology most attention so far was paid to histone acetylation and methylation. Histone phosphorylation is thought to be important for cell cycle regulation and was thus not carefully studied in the adult heart (Walter et al., 2008; Baek, 2011). Recently, it was reported by the group of Coralie Poizat that nuclear CaMKII activates cardiac transcription by direct binding to the chromatin. CaMKII was shown to phosphorylate Ser-10 of histone 3 (H3S10) which is located next to Lys-9, a major site for acetylation and methylation (Awad et al., 2013). Phosphorylation of H3S10 was accompanied by hypertrophy of primary cultured cardiomcyocytes and with increased chromatin binding of CaMKII at specific gene loci reactivated during cardiac hypertrophy under control of the transcription factor MEF2. These findings represent an interesting new epigenetic mechanism governed by CaMKII. The possibility, that ventricular remodeling can be mediated by CaMKII-dependent chromatin modifications opens a new avenue of regulatory mechanisms. Important further studies are warranted. ChIP-Seq studies may identify direct target genes of CaMKII that are important for diseases processes.

SUMMARY AND OUTLOOK

CaMKII regulates not only immediate cellular functions but also chronic processes such as ventricular remodeling leading to heart failure. In particular, CaMKII integrates several cellular pathways by inducing gene programs that are not understood in detail. Here, we reviewed the yet known transcriptional and epigenetic mechanisms by which CaMKII regulates cardiac gene expression. However, the relative importance of the different downstream mechanisms still needs to be clarified. Unbiased gene expression analyses and epigenetic profiling are warranted to define the specific gene programs that contribute to phenotypic changes induced by CaMKII.

ACKNOWLEDGMENTS

We thank David Stanmore for editing the manuscript. Johannes Backs was supported by the DZHK (Deutsches Zentrum für Herz-Kreislauf-Forschung—German Center for Cardiovascular Research) and by the European Commission (FP7-Health-2010; MEDIA-261409). Michael M. Kreusser was supported by a research grant from the Ernst-und-Berta-Grimmke foundation and by the Young Investigator program of the University of Heidelberg.

REFERENCES

Anderson, M. E., Brown, J. H., and Bers, D. M. (2011). CaMKII in myocardial hypertrophy and heart failure. *J. Mol. Cell. Cardiol.* 51, 468–473. doi: 10.1016/j.yjmcc.2011.01.012

Antoine, M., Gaiddon, C., and Loeffler, J. P. (1996). Ca2+/calmodulin kinase types II and IV regulate c-fos transcription in the AtT20 corticotroph cell line. *Mol. Cell. Endocrinol.* 120, 1–8. doi: 10.1016/0303-7207(96)03806-3

Awad, S., Kunhi, M., Little, G. H., Bai, Y., An, W., Bers, D., et al. (2013). Nuclear CaMKII enhances histone H3 phosphorylation and remodels chromatin during cardiac hypertrophy. *Nucleic Acids Res.* 41, 7656–7672. doi: 10.1093/nar/gkt500

Backs, J., Backs, T., Bezprozvannaya, S., McKinsey, T. A., and Olson, E. N. (2008). Histone deacetylase 5 acquires calcium/calmodulin-dependent kinase II responsiveness by oligomerization with histone deacetylase 4. *Mol. Cell. Biol.* 28, 3437–3445. doi: 10.1128/MCB.01611-07

Backs, J., Backs, T., Neef, S., Kreusser, M. M., Lehmann, L. H., Patrick, D. M., et al. (2009). The delta isoform of CaM kinase II is required for pathological cardiac hypertrophy and remodeling after pressure overload. *Proc. Natl. Acad. Sci. U.S.A.* 106, 2342–2347. doi: 10.1073/pnas.0813013106

Backs, J., Stein, P., Backs, T., Duncan, F. E., Grueter, C. E., McAnally, J., et al. (2010). The gamma isoform of cam kinase ii controls mouse egg activation by regulating cell cycle resumption. *Proc. Natl. Acad. Sci. U.S.A.* 107, 81–86. doi: 10.1073/pnas.0912658106

Backs, J., and Olson, E. N. (2006). Control of cardiac growth by histone acetylation/deacetylation. *Circ. Res.* 98, 15–24. doi: 10.1161/01.RES.0000197782.21444.8f

Backs, J., Song, K., Bezprozvannaya, S., Chang, S., and Olson, E. N. (2006). CaM kinase II selectively signals to histone deacetylase 4 during cardiomyocyte hypertrophy. *J. Clin. Invest.* 116, 1853–1864. doi: 10.1172/JCI27438

Backs, J., Worst, B. C., Lehmann, L. H., Patrick, D. M., Jebessa, Z., Kreusser, M. M., et al. (2011). Selective repression of MEF2 activity by PKA-dependent proteolysis of HDAC4. *J. Cell Biol.* 195, 403–415. doi: 10.1083/jcb.201105063

Baek, S. H. (2011). When signaling kinases meet histones and histone modifiers in the nucleus. *Mol. Cell* 42, 274–284. doi: 10.1016/j.molcel.2011.03.022

Bers, D. M. (2008). Calcium cycling and signaling in cardiac myocytes. *Annu. Rev. Physiol.* 70, 23–49. doi: 10.1146/annurev.physiol.70.113006.100455

Colomer, J. M., Mao, L., Rockman, H. A., and Means, A. R. (2003). Pressure overload selectively up-regulates Ca2+/calmodulin-dependent protein kinase II *in vivo*. *Mol. Endocrinol.* 17, 183–192. doi: 10.1210/me.2002-0350

Davis, F. J., Gupta, M., Camoretti-Mercado, B., Schwartz, R. J., and Gupta, M. P. (2003). Calcium/calmodulin-dependent protein kinase activates serum response factor transcription activity by its dissociation from histone deacetylase, HDAC4. Implications in cardiac muscle gene regulation during hypertrophy. *J. Biol. Chem.* 278, 20047–20058. doi: 10.1074/jbc.M209998200

Edman, C. F., and Schulman, H. (1994). Identification and characterization of delta B-CaM kinase and delta C-CaM kinase from rat heart, two new multifunctional Ca2+/calmodulin-dependent protein kinase isoforms. *Biochim. Biophys. Acta* 1221, 89–101. doi: 10.1016/0167-4889(94)90221-6

Ely, H. A., Mellon, P. L., and Coss, D. (2011). GnRH induces the c-Fos gene via phosphorylation of SRF by the calcium/calmodulin kinase II pathway. *Mol. Endocrinol.* 25, 669–680. doi: 10.1210/me.2010-0437

Fischle, W., Dequiedt, F., Hendzel, M. J., Guenther, M. G., Lazar, M. A., Voelter, W., et al. (2002). Enzymatic activity associated with class II HDACs is dependent on a multiprotein complex containing HDAC3 and SMRT/N-CoR. *Mol. Cell* 9, 45–57. doi: 10.1016/S1097-2765(01)00429-4

Fluck, M., Booth, F. W., and Waxham, M. N. (2000). Skeletal muscle CaMKII enriches in nuclei and phosphorylates myogenic factor SRF at multiple sites. *Biochem. Biophys. Res. Commun.* 270, 488–494. doi: 10.1006/bbrc.2000.2457

Harrison, B. C., Kim, M. S., van Rooij, E., Plato, C. F., Papst, P. J., Vega, R. B., et al. (2006). Regulation of cardiac stress signaling by protein kinase d1. *Mol. Cell. Biol.* 26, 3875–3888. doi: 10.1128/MCB.26.10.3875-3888.2006

Heineke, J., Auger-Messier, M., Xu, J., Oka, T., Sargent, M. A., York, A., et al. (2007). Cardiomyocyte GATA4 functions as a stress-responsive regulator of angiogenesis in the murine heart. *J. Clin. Invest.* 117, 3198–3210. doi: 10.1172/JCI32573

Heineke, J., and Molkentin, J. D. (2006). Regulation of cardiac hypertrophy by intracellular signalling pathways. *Nat. Rev. Mol. Cell Biol.* 7, 589–600. doi: 10.1038/nrm1983

Hoch, B., Meyer, R., Hetzer, R., Krause, E. G., and Karczewski, P. (1999). Identification and expression of delta-isoforms of the multifunctional Ca2+/calmodulin-dependent protein kinase in failing and nonfailing human myocardium. *Circ. Res.* 84, 713–721. doi: 10.1161/01.RES.84.6.713

Hohl, M., Wagner, M., Reil, J. C., Muller, S. A., Tauchnitz, M., Zimmer, A. M., et al. (2013). HDAC4 controls histone methylation in response to elevated cardiac load. *J. Clin. Invest.* 123, 1359–1370. doi: 10.1172/JCI61084

Holmberg, C. I., Hietakangas, V., Mikhailov, A., Rantanen, J. O., Kallio, M., Meinander, A., et al. (2001). Phosphorylation of serine 230 promotes inducible transcriptional activity of heat shock factor 1. *EMBO J.* 20, 3800–3810. doi: 10.1093/emboj/20.14.3800

Hudmon, A., and Schulman, H. (2002). Neuronal CA2+/calmodulin-dependent protein kinase II: the role of structure and autoregulation in cellular function. *Annu. Rev. Biochem.* 71, 473–510. doi: 10.1146/annurev.biochem.71.110601.135410

Jenuwein, T., and Allis, C. D. (2001). Translating the histone code. *Science* 293, 1074–1080. doi: 10.1126/science.1063127

Kashiwase, K., Higuchi, Y., Hirotani, S., Yamaguchi, O., Hikoso, S., Takeda, T., et al. (2005). CaMKII activates ASK1 and NF-kappaB to induce cardiomyocyte hypertrophy. *Biochem. Biophys. Res. Commun.* 327, 136–142. doi: 10.1016/j.bbrc.2004.12.002

Kobrinsky, E., Duong, S. Q., Sheydina, A., and Soldatov, N. M. (2011). Microdomain organization and frequency-dependence of CREB-dependent transcriptional signaling in heart cells. *FASEB J.* 25, 1544–1555. doi: 10.1096/fj.10-176198

Koitabashi, N., and Kass, D. A. (2012). Reverse remodeling in heart failure–mechanisms and therapeutic opportunities. *Nat. Rev. Cardiol.* 9, 147–157. doi: 10.1038/nrcardio.2011.172

Kouzarides, T. (2007). Chromatin modifications and their function. *Cell* 128, 693–705. doi: 10.1016/j.cell.2007.02.005

Lahm, A., Paolini, C., Pallaoro, M., Nardi, M. C., Jones, P., Neddermann, P., et al. (2007). Unraveling the hidden catalytic activity of vertebrate class IIa histone deacetylases. *Proc. Natl. Acad. Sci. U.S.A.* 104, 17335–17340. doi: 10.1073/pnas.0706487104

Lehmann, L. H., Worst, B. C., Stanmore, D. A., and Backs, J. (2013). Histone deacetylase signaling in cardioprotection. *Cell. Mol. Life Sci.* doi: 10.1007/s00018-013-1516-9. [Epub ahead of print].

Li, B., Dedman, J. R., and Kaetzel, M. A. (2006). Nuclear Ca2+/calmodulin-dependent protein kinase II in the murine heart. *Biochim. Biophys. Acta* 1763, 1275–1281. doi: 10.1016/j.bbamcr.2006.09.029

Li, C., Cai, X., Sun, H., Bai, T., Zheng, X., Zhou, X. W., et al. (2011). The deltaA isoform of calmodulin kinase II mediates pathological cardiac hypertrophy by interfering with the HDAC4-MEF2 signaling pathway. *Biochem. Biophys. Res. Commun.* 409, 125–130. doi: 10.1016/j.bbrc.2011.04.128

Lin, Q., Schwarz, J., Bucana, C., and Olson, E. N. (1997). Control of mouse cardiac morphogenesis and myogenesis by transcription factor MEF2C. *Science* 276, 1404–1407. doi: 10.1126/science.276.5317.1404

Ling, H., Gray, C. B., Zambon, A. C., Grimm, M., Gu, Y., Dalton, N., et al. (2013). Ca2+/Calmodulin-dependent protein kinase II delta mediates myocardial ischemia/reperfusion injury through nuclear factor-kappaB. *Circ. Res.* 112, 935–944. doi: 10.1161/CIRCRESAHA.112.276915

Ling, H., Zhang, T., Pereira, L., Means, C. K., Cheng, H., Gu, Y., et al. (2009). Requirement for Ca2+/calmodulin-dependent kinase II in the transition from pressure overload-induced cardiac hypertrophy to heart failure in mice. *J. Clin. Invest.* 119, 1230–1240. doi: 10.1172/JCI38022

Little, G. H., Bai, Y., Williams, T., and Poizat, C. (2007). Nuclear calcium/calmodulin-dependent protein kinase IIdelta preferentially transmits signals to histone deacetylase 4 in cardiac cells. *J. Biol. Chem.* 282, 7219–7231. doi: 10.1074/jbc.M604281200

Little, G. H., Saw, A., Bai, Y., Dow, J., Marjoram, P., Simkhovich, B., et al. (2009). Critical role of nuclear calcium/calmodulin-dependent protein kinase IIdeltaB in cardiomyocyte survival in cardiomyopathy. *J. Biol. Chem.* 284, 24857–24868. doi: 10.1074/jbc.M109.003186

Liu, N., Ruan, Y., Denegri, M., Bachetti, T., Li, Y., Colombi, B., et al. (2011). Calmodulin kinase II inhibition prevents arrhythmias in RyR2(R4496C+/-) mice with catecholaminergic polymorphic ventricular tachycardia. *J. Mol. Cell. Cardiol.* 50, 214–222. doi: 10.1016/j.yjmcc.2010.10.001

MacDonnell, S. M., Weisser-Thomas, J., Kubo, H., Hanscome, M., Liu, Q., Jaleel, N., et al. (2009). CaMKII negatively regulates calcineurin-NFAT signaling in cardiac myocytes. *Circ. Res.* 105, 316–325. doi: 10.1161/CIRCRESAHA.109.194035

Mani, S. K., Egan, E. A., Addy, B. K., Grimm, M., Kasiganesan, H., Thiyagarajan, T., et al. (2010). beta-Adrenergic receptor stimulated Ncx1 upregulation is mediated via a CaMKII/AP-1 signaling pathway in adult cardiomyocytes. *J. Mol. Cell. Cardiol.* 48, 342–351. doi: 10.1016/j.yjmcc.2009.11.007

McKinsey, T. A. (2007). Derepression of pathological cardiac genes by members of the CaM kinase superfamily. *Cardiovasc. Res.* 73, 667–677. doi: 10.1016/j.cardiores.2006.11.036

McKinsey, T. A., Zhang, C. L., and Olson, E. N. (2002). MEF2: a calcium-dependent regulator of cell division, differentiation and death. *Trends Biochem. Sci.* 27, 40–47. doi: 10.1016/S0968-0004(01)02031-X

Mechta-Grigoriou, F., Gerald, D., and Yaniv, M. (2001). The mammalian Jun proteins: redundancy and specificity. *Oncogene* 20, 2378–2389. doi: 10.1038/sj.onc.1204381

Mishra, J. P., Mishra, S., Gee, K., and Kumar, A. (2005). Differential involvement of calmodulin-dependent protein kinase II-activated AP-1 and c-Jun N-terminal kinase-activated EGR-1 signaling pathways in tumor necrosis factor-alpha and lipopolysaccharide-induced CD44 expression in human monocytic cells. *J. Biol. Chem.* 280, 26825–26837. doi: 10.1074/jbc.M500244200

Molkentin, J. D., Lu, J. R., Antos, C. L., Markham, B., Richardson, J., Robbins, J., et al. (1998). A calcineurin-dependent transcriptional pathway for cardiac hypertrophy. *Cell* 93, 215–228. doi: 10.1016/S0092-8674(00)81573-1

Oka, T., Maillet, M., Watt, A. J., Schwartz, R. J., Aronow, B. J., Duncan, S. A., et al. (2006). Cardiac-specific deletion of Gata4 reveals its requirement for hypertrophy, compensation, and myocyte viability. *Circ. Res.* 98, 837–845. doi: 10.1161/01.RES.0000215985.18538.c4

Papait, R., Cattaneo, P., Kunderfranco, P., Greco, C., Carullo, P., Guffanti, A., et al. (2013). Genome-wide analysis of histone marks identifying an epigenetic signature of promoters and enhancers underlying cardiac hypertrophy. *Proc. Natl. Acad. Sci. U.S.A.* 110, 20164–20169. doi: 10.1073/pnas.1315155110

Parlakian, A., Charvet, C., Escoubet, B., Mericskay, M., Molkentin, J. D., Gary-Bobo, G., et al. (2005). Temporally controlled onset of dilated cardiomyopathy through disruption of the SRF gene in adult heart. *Circulation* 112, 2930–2939. doi: 10.1161/CIRCULATIONAHA.105.533778

Passier, R., Zeng, H., Frey, N., Naya, F. J., Nicol, R. L., McKinsey, T. A., et al. (2000). CaM kinase signaling induces cardiac hypertrophy and activates the MEF2 transcription factor *in vivo*. *J. Clin. Invest.* 105, 1395–1406. doi: 10.1172/JCI8551

Peng, W., Zhang, Y., Zheng, M., Cheng, H., Zhu, W., Cao, C. M., et al. (2010). Cardioprotection by CaMKII-deltaB is mediated by phosphorylation of heat shock factor 1 and subsequent expression of inducible heat shock protein 70. *Circ. Res.* 106, 102–110. doi: 10.1161/CIRCRESAHA.109.210914

Ramirez, M. T., Zhao, X. L., Schulman, H., and Brown, J. H. (1997). The nuclear deltaB isoform of Ca2+/calmodulin-dependent protein kinase II regulates atrial natriuretic factor gene expression in ventricular myocytes. *J. Biol. Chem.* 272, 31203–31208. doi: 10.1074/jbc.272.49.31203

Ronkainen, J. J., Hanninen, S. L., Korhonen, T., Koivumaki, J. T., Skoumal, R., Rautio, S., et al. (2011). Ca2+-calmodulin-dependent protein kinase II represses cardiac transcription of the L-type calcium channel alpha(1C)-subunit gene (Cacna1c) by DREAM translocation. *J. Physiol.* 589, 2669–2686. doi: 10.1113/jphysiol.2010.201400

Ruthenburg, A. J., Li, H., Patel, D. J., and Allis, C. D. (2007). Multivalent engagement of chromatin modifications by linked binding modules. *Nat. Rev. Mol. Cell Biol.* 8, 983–994. doi: 10.1038/nrm2298

Sheng, M., Thompson, M. A., and Greenberg, M. E. (1991). CREB: a Ca(2+)-regulated transcription factor phosphorylated by calmodulin-dependent kinases. *Science* 252, 1427–1430. doi: 10.1126/science.1646483

Shimomura, A., Ogawa, Y., Kitani, T., Fujisawa, H., and Hagiwara, M. (1996). Calmodulin-dependent protein kinase II potentiates transcriptional activation through activating transcription factor 1 but not cAMP response element-binding protein. *J. Biol. Chem.* 271, 17957–17960. doi: 10.1074/jbc.271.30.17957

Singh, M. V., Kapoun, A., Higgins, L., Kutschke, W., Thurman, J. M., Zhang, R., et al. (2009). Ca2+/calmodulin-dependent kinase II triggers cell membrane injury by inducing complement factor B gene expression in the mouse heart. *J. Clin. Invest.* 119, 986–996. doi: 10.1172/JCI35814

Sun, P., Enslen, H., Myung, P. S., and Maurer, R. A. (1994). Differential activation of CREB by Ca2+/calmodulin-dependent protein kinases type II and type IV involves phosphorylation of a site that negatively regulates activity. *Genes Dev.* 8, 2527–2539. doi: 10.1101/gad.8.21.2527

Vega, R. B., Harrison, B. C., Meadows, E., Roberts, C. R., Papst, P. J., Olson, E. N., et al. (2004). Protein kinases C and D mediate agonist-dependent cardiac hypertrophy through nuclear export of histone deacetylase 5. *Mol. Cell. Biol.* 24, 8374–8385. doi: 10.1128/MCB.24.19.8374-8385.2004

Vila-Petroff, M., Salas, M. A., Said, M., Valverde, C. A., Sapia, L., Portiansky, E., et al. (2007). CaMKII inhibition protects against necrosis and apoptosis in irreversible ischemia-reperfusion injury. *Cardiovasc. Res.* 73, 689–698. doi: 10.1016/j.cardiores.2006.12.003

Walter, W., Clynes, D., Tang, Y., Marmorstein, R., Mellor, J., and Berger, S. L. (2008). 14-3-3 interaction with histone H3 involves a dual modification pattern of phosphoacetylation. *Mol. Cell. Biol.* 28, 2840–2849. doi: 10.1128/MCB.01457-07

Wu, X., and Bers, D. M. (2006). Sarcoplasmic reticulum and nuclear envelope are one highly interconnected Ca2+ store throughout cardiac myocyte. *Circ. Res.* 99, 283–291. doi: 10.1161/01.RES.0000233386.02708.72

Wu, X., and McMurray, C. T. (2001). Calmodulin kinase II attenuation of gene transcription by preventing cAMP response element-binding protein (CREB) dimerization and binding of the CREB-binding protein. *J. Biol. Chem.* 276, 1735–1741. doi: 10.1074/jbc.M006727200

Wu, X., Zhang, T., Bossuyt, J., Li, X., McKinsey, T. A., Dedman, J. R., et al. (2006). Local InsP3-dependent perinuclear Ca2+ signaling in cardiac myocyte excitation-transcription coupling. *J. Clin. Invest.* 116, 675–682. doi: 10.1172/JCI27374

Xu, X., Yang, D., Ding, J. H., Wang, W., Chu, P. H., Dalton, N. D., et al. (2005). ASF/SF2-regulated CaMKIIdelta alternative splicing temporally reprograms excitation-contraction coupling in cardiac muscle. *Cell* 120, 59–72. doi: 10.1016/j.cell.2004.11.036

Zayzafoon, M., Fulzele, K., and McDonald, J. M. (2005). Calmodulin and calmodulin-dependent kinase IIalpha regulate osteoblast differentiation by controlling c-fos expression. *J. Biol. Chem.* 280, 7049–7059. doi: 10.1074/jbc.M412680200

Zhang, C. L., McKinsey, T. A., Lu, J. R., and Olson, E. N. (2001). Association of COOH-terminal-binding protein (CtBP) and MEF2-interacting transcription repressor (MITR) contributes to transcriptional repression of the MEF2 transcription factor. *J. Biol. Chem.* 276, 35–39. doi: 10.1074/jbc.M007364200

Zhang, C. L., McKinsey, T. A., and Olson, E. N. (2002a). Association of class II histone deacetylases with heterochromatin protein 1: potential role for histone methylation in control of muscle differentiation. *Mol. Cell. Biol.* 22, 7302–7312. doi: 10.1128/MCB.22.20.7302-7312.2002

Zhang, R., Khoo, M. S., Wu, Y., Yang, Y., Grueter, C. E., Ni, G., et al. (2005). Calmodulin kinase II inhibition protects against structural heart disease. *Nat. Med.* 11, 409–417. doi: 10.1038/nm1215

Zhang, T., Johnson, E. N., Gu, Y., Morissette, M. R., Sah, V. P., Gigena, M. S., et al. (2002b). The cardiac-specific nuclear delta(B) isoform of Ca2+/calmodulin-dependent protein kinase II induces hypertrophy and dilated cardiomyopathy associated with increased protein phosphatase 2A activity. *J. Biol. Chem.* 277, 1261–1267. doi: 10.1074/jbc.M108525200

Zhang, T., Kohlhaas, M., Backs, J., Mishra, S., Phillips, W., Dybkova, N., et al. (2007). CaMKIIdelta isoforms differentially affect calcium handling but similarly regulate HDAC/MEF2 transcriptional responses. *J. Biol. Chem.* 282, 35078–35087. doi: 10.1074/jbc.M707083200

Zhang, T., Maier, L. S., Dalton, N. D., Miyamoto, S., Ross, J. Jr., Bers, D. M., et al. (2003). The deltaC isoform of CaMKII is activated in cardiac hypertrophy and induces dilated cardiomyopathy and heart failure. *Circ. Res.* 92, 912–919. doi: 10.1161/01.RES.0000069686.31472.C5

20

Mouse models in arrhythmogenic right ventricular cardiomyopathy

Elisabeth M. Lodder[1]* and Stefania Rizzo[2]

[1] Department of Experimental Cardiology, Heart Failure Research Center, Academic Medical Center, University of Amsterdam, Amsterdam, Netherlands
[2] Department of Cardiac, Thoracic and Vascular Sciences, University of Padua, Padua, Italy

Correspondence:
Elisabeth M. Lodder, Department of Experimental Cardiology, Heart Failure Research Center, Academic Medical Center, University of Amsterdam, Meibergdreef 15, Room L2-107, PO Box 22660, 1100DD Amsterdam, Netherlands.
e-mail: e.m.lodder@amc.uva.nl

Arrhythmogenic right ventricular cardiomyopathy (ARVC) is a heart muscle disorder characterized by fibro-fatty replacement of cardiomyocytes. The cardinal manifestations are arrhythmias, sudden cardiac death, and seldom heart failure. Mutations in genes encoding desmosomal proteins and their interaction partners have been implicated in the pathogenesis of ARVC and it is now widely accepted that ARVC is a disease caused by abnormal cell–cell adhesion. The mechanism(s) by which mutations in desmosomal proteins lead to fibro-fatty replacement remains to be fully elucidated. To this aim over the last 10 years different transgenic and targeted mouse models have been developed, these models and what they have taught us will be discussed in this review.

Keywords: ARVC, animal models, sudden death, desmosomes

INTRODUCTION

Arrhythmogenic right ventricular cardiomyopathy (ARVC) is an important cause of ventricular arrhythmias and sudden cardiac death, especially in the young and in athletes (Marcus et al., 1982; Thiene et al., 1988; Basso et al., 2009). Mutations in one or more genes encoding desmosomal proteins are found in $\sim$50% of patients (McKoy et al., 2000; Rampazzo et al., 2002; Gerull et al., 2004; Pilichou et al., 2006; Syrris et al., 2006). Desmosomes are highly conserved structures that, together with adherens junctions and gap junctions, connect cardiac myocytes end to end at the level of the intercalated disks and thereby play a crucial role in maintaining proper myocardial function (Delmar and McKenna, 2010). Recent findings indicating the presence of mixed type junctions (the area composite; Franke et al., 2006) and crosstalk between protein complexes pertaining to the different types of junctions (Delmar, 2004; Meadows and Isom, 2005; Saffitz, 2005; Tavora et al., 2009; Li and Radice, 2010; Sato et al., 2011) have markedly changed the perception of the intercalated disk. Altered junctional organization, as the result of mutations, is thought to lead to myocardial damage and replacement fibrosis, the classical histopathologic pattern of ARVC (Basso et al., 2009). In advanced stages of the disease, focal scars cause electrical isolation of cardiomyocytes within non-conducting fibrous tissue, resulting in slow conduction and delayed activation, thus forming the substrate for re-entrant circuits and ventricular electrical instability. Over the years several mouse models have been developed to investigate the mechanisms of disease development in ARVC (Pilichou et al., 2011), focusing on four of the desmosomal proteins: Plakophilin-2, Plakoglobin (γ-catenin), Desmoplakin, and Desmoglein 2. All four will be discussed in detail below; an overview of all the models is given in **Table 1**.

PLAKOPHILIN-2 TARGETED DELETION

The first mouse model described that addresses disruption of one of the desmosomal proteins is the study by Grossmann et al. (2004) that describes the targeted deletion of plakophilin-2. The heterozygous mice carrying one wild type copy of plakophilin-2 were completely viable without any cardiac phenotype. Mouse homozygous for the deletion (Pkp2$^{-/-}$) died during embryonic development around day 11 post fertilization. Embryos at day 10.5 appeared pale with blood aggregates in the interperitoneal cavity indicating the presence of small holes in the endothelial layers lining the heart and vessels. It would be interesting to see if the Pkp2$^{\pm}$ mice develop an ARVC like phenotype upon exercise.

PLAKOGLOBIN TARGETED DELETION AND OVEREXPRESSION MODELS

The first papers on mouse models involving a desmosomal protein described the targeted deletion of *Plakoglobin* (*Pg*) by two independent groups in 1996 (models Pg1 and Pg2; Bierkamp et al., 1996; Ruiz et al., 1996). Homozygous targeted deletion of *Plakoglobin* leads to embryonic lethality between embryonic day 9.5 and 16 due to cardiac malformations: thin cardiac walls and less trabeculation and frequent burst of the epicardial wall; in addition mice showed a blistering skin phenotype. Heterozygous animals appeared healthy and fertile. However, closer inspection of these mice (model Pg2) after the link between ARVC and desmosomal proteins had become clear showed that Pg$^{\pm}$ mice at 10 months after birth had enlarged right ventricles, increased spontaneous ventricular arrhythmias and right ventricular conduction slowing. No replacement fibrosis and remodeling of the junctions was observed, Cx43 localization and distribution were normal on immunofluorescence microscopy. All observed changes were exacerbated and expedited when mice were subjected to exercise

Table 1 | Arrhythmogenic right ventricular cardiomyopathy mouse models.

Nr	Protein	Gene	Mutation/targeted exons	Model type	Reference
Pk1	Plakophilin-2	*Pkp2*	Exon 1-intron 1	Targeted deletion	Grossmann et al. (2004)
Pk2	Plakophilin-2	*Pkp2*	Exon 1-intron 1	Targeted deletion	Grossmann et al. (2004)
Pg1	Plakoglobin	*Jup*	Exon 2–5	Targeted deletion	Bierkamp et al. (1996)
Pg2–Pg4	Plakoglobin	*Jup*	Exon 34	Targeted deletion	Ruiz et al. (1996), Kirchhof et al. (2006), Fabritz et al. (2011)
Pg5	Plakoglobin	*Jup*	Exon 2–3	Inducible deletion; αMHCcre induced	Li et al. (2011)
Pg6	Plakoglobin β-catenin	*Jup* *Ctnnb1*	Exon 2–3 Exon 2–5	αMHC/MerCreMer tamoxifen induced double deletion	Swope et al. (2012)
Pg7	Plakoglobin	*Jup*	Wild type	Flag tagged transgene	Lombardi et al. (2011)
Pg8	Plakoglobin	*Jup*	23654Δ2 Truncated	Transgene	Lombardi et al. (2011)
Dp1	Desmoplakin	*Dsp*	Δ281–473	Targeted deletion with extra-embryonic rescue	Gallicano et al. (2001)
Dp2	Desmoplakin	*Dsp*	Exon 2	Inducible deletion; αMHCcre induced	Garcia-Gras et al. (2006), Gomes et al. (2012)
Dp3	Desmoplakin	*Dsp*	Wild type	Flag tagged transgene, αMHC promoter	Yang et al. (2006)
Dp4	Desmoplakin	*Dsp*	R2834H	Flag tagged transgene, αMHC promoter	Yang et al. (2006)
Dp5	Desmoplakin	*Dsp*	Q90R	Flag tagged transgene, αMHC promoter	Yang et al. (2006)
Dp6	Desmoplakin	*Dsp*	V30M	Flag tagged transgene, αMHC promoter	Yang et al. (2006)
Dg1	Desmoglein 2	*Dsg2*	Wild type	Flag tagged transgene, αMHC promoter	Pilichou et al. (2009)
Dg2	Desmoglein 2	*Dsg2*	N271S	Flag tagged transgene, αMHC promoter	Pilichou et al. (2009)
Dg3	Desmoglein 3	*Dsg2*	Exon 4–6	Targeted deletion	Krusche et al. (2011), Kant et al. (2012)

training (model Pg3; Kirchhof et al., 2006). Load reducing therapy is able to prevent these symptoms of ARVC in $Pg^{\pm}$ mice (model Pg4; Fabritz et al., 2011).

To circumvent the problem of neonatal lethality, a cardiac specific targeted deletion of Pg was developed under the control of αMHCcre. $Pg^{f/f}$ αMHCcre (model Pg5) mice have ~30% of the WT protein as measured by Western blot, no Pg was detectable by immunofluorescence on cardiac sections. Phenotypically these mice largely recapitulate the human ARVC phenotype: cardiac sudden death, progressive dilation, and fibrosis in the cardiac walls (both in the left and the right ventricle) from 2 month onward. No cardiac fat deposition was observed. With transmission electron microscopy the structure of the desmosomes seemed to be disrupted: other desmosomal proteins (e.g., Dsg2) appeared to be absent from the intercalated disk (Li et al., 2011). Cell death in the $Pg^{f/f}$ αMHCcre mice was at least partially through myocyte apoptosis in addition to myocyte necrosis in contrast to mice overexpressing N271S-Dsg2, which mainly showed myocyte necrosis (see below; Pilichou et al., 2006; Li et al., 2011). Interestingly, increased β-catenin staining was observed at the intercalated disk suggesting partial rescue by this close relative of Pg (γ-catenin). To test whether the lack of fast spontaneous death in these mice (model Pg5) was due to a partial rescue by β-catenin, double-targeted mice were created, carrying both a floxed Pg gene and a floxed β-catenin locus ($Pg^{f/f}$; β-$catenin^{f/f}$). Crossing with αMHC/MerCreMer mice and subsequent tamoxifen injections effected specific targeted deletion. Double-targeted mice (model Pg6) showed a strong arrhythmogenic phenotype, with 100% of the double-targeted animals dying of sudden cardiac death between 3 and 5 months after tamoxifen injections. In contrast to either single targeted deletion and wild type littermates of which 4–9% died within 6 months of tamoxifen injection (Swope et al., 2012).

Two lines overexpressing wild type (model Pg7) and mutant (model Pg8) Pg were generated (Lombardi et al., 2011); both showed similar levels of increased incidence of sudden cardiac death, an indication that even moderate levels of overexpression of *Pg* disturb the balance of the mechanical interaction and signaling functions of *Pg* independent of the introduced truncating mutation.

DESMOPLAKIN TARGETED DELETION AND OVEREXPRESSION MODELS

Desmoplakin (*Dsp*) targeted deletion mice $Dsp^{-/-}$ die at embryonic day 6.5 of malformations in the extra-embryonic tissue before assessment of a cardiac phenotype is possible (Gallicano et al., 1998). To overcome this problem the extra-embryonic phenotype was rescued by tetraploid aggregation (model Dp1). The resulting embryos die around embryonic day E11. At E10 they show severe cardiac malformation although desmosomal-like structures appear to be present by transmission electron microscopy. As these mice die well before birth they are obviously unsuitable as a proper model for ARVC (Gallicano et al., 2001). The embryonic lethality of the $Dsp^{-/-}$ mice is partially circumvented in the cardiac specific, αMHCcre induced, targeted deletion of *Dsp* (model Dp2; Garcia-Gras et al., 2006). The homozygous cardiac specific deletion of *Dsp* leads to embryonic growth arrest at day E10–E12 with embryos that appeared very pale, with no circulating red blood cells in organs. The heart was poorly formed with no chamber specification, 80% of $Dsp^{-/-}$ mice did not survive until delivery. Mice that did survive the embryonic period died within 6 weeks after birth. Heterozygous *Dsp*$^{\pm}$ mice developed normally, however adult *Dsp*$^{\pm}$ mice had thin ventricular walls, increased left ventricular diameters and reduced left ventricular ejection fraction. Spontaneous arrhythmias were observed on surface ECG and 4/5 mice developed ventricular arrhythmias after a single ventricular extra stimulus.

A more detailed study of these *Dsp*$^{\pm}$ mice at earlier stages of disease development, when no abnormalities at the surface ECGs could be detected and no evidence of replacement fibrosis could yet be found, showed a significant increase in the activation time and inducible arrhythmias in Langendorff perfused hearts. These results indicate the presence of electrophysiological abnormalities before the onset of overt structural changes (Gomes et al., 2012). However, no electron microscopy was done to exclude the presence of disrupted desmosomes at the ultrastructural level.

Transgenic mice with cardiac overexpression of flag tagged human *Dsp* cDNA both wild type (WT-Tg, model Dp3) and with a C-terminal mutation (R2834H-Tg, model Dp4) were generated by Yang et al. (2006). Overexpression of *Dsp* with N-terminal mutations, e.g., V30M (model Dp5) and Q90R (model Dp6) led to embryonic lethality after embryonic day 13.5 due to reduced ventricular wall thickness and ventricular dilatation. R2834H-Tg mice had an increased heart weight/body weight ratio compared to both wild type littermates and Wt-Tg mice. R2834H-Tg hearts showed increased apoptosis and fibrosis along with reduced ventricular function and dilatation of both right and left ventricles. Co-immunoprecipitation indicated the disruption of the interaction between Dsp and Pg. at the ultrastructural level widening of the intercalated disk was observed in Dp4 mice.

DESMOGLEIN OVEREXPRESSION MODELS

Transgenic mice with cardiac overexpression of flag tagged Dsg2 both wild type (Tg-WT, model Dg1) and N271S-Dsg2 mutant (Tg-NS, model Dg2) were generated; the murine N271S mutation is the mouse homolog of the human ARVC mutation DSG2–N266S. While mice overexpressing of wild type *Dsg2* were indistinguishable from their wild type littermates at 2 months of age, Tg-Ns mice developed spontaneous ventricular arrhythmias, conduction slowing, ventricular dilatation and aneurysms, and replacement fibrosis, leading to sudden cardiac death from a less than 2 weeks of age. The disease process was triggered by myocyte necrosis followed by calcification and fibrous tissue replacement (Pilichou et al., 2009). These findings are consistent with the results obtained in mice carrying a targeted deletion in the extracellular adhesion domain of Dsg2 (model Dg3). Approximately 30% of the mice homozygous for the mutation survived embryonic development. These mice develop left and right ventricular dilatation, fibrosis, calcification, and spontaneous death similar to the Tg-NS mice (Krusche et al., 2011). Detailed investigation of this model by transmission electron microscopy revealed a widening of the intercellular space at the intercalated disk and loss of desmosomal structure close to macroscopically visible lesions of the heart (Kant et al., 2012).

DISCUSSION AND CONCLUSION

The diverse mouse models discussed here recapitulate ARVC disease phenotype and have led to several new insights in the etiology of the cardiac phenotype in ARVC patients. The initial targeted deletion of single desmosomal genes, although embryonically lethal, gave fundamental insights in effects of desmosomal gene dysfunction on cardiac function. All the different models surviving embryonic development, recapitulate the human phenotype in the sense of the arrhythmogenicity, replacement fibrosis, and calcification. None of the models show the clear fatty infiltrations seen in human, this is most likely a reflection of the different composition of the extracellular matrix and non-cardiomyocytes interstitial cells in the wild type murine heart, which lacks a significant adipocyte population (Pilichou et al., 2009). In all described mouse models that survive the embryonic period, the disease process is triggered by cardiac cell death upon cardiac stress after birth. However, they are inconsistent considering the type of cell death occurring, with necrosis being the prominent feature in the Desmoglein 2 models (Dg2 and Dg3) and apoptosis (in addition to necrosis) in the plakoglobin models (Pg5 and Pg6). As a consequence of the myocyte death, calcification, and replacement fibrosis occurs leading to reduced cardiac function and ventricular dilatation. This scar formation also provides a substrate for the arrhythmogenic phenotype seen both in human patients and the ARVC mouse models. The study by Fabritz et al. (2011) shows the positive effect of load reducing therapy on disease progression, clearly underwriting the current disease management strategy of discouraging strenuous physical exercise in patients.

Knowledge of the early disease stages would help in designing more effective treatments (Basso et al., 2011). However, the earliest phase of the disease remains thus far elusive due to the early postnatal severe pathogenicity of the phenotype, precluding the effective dissection of the first pathological changes in the affected hearts. The recent study of Gomes et al. suggests the presence of an electrophysiological disturbance before the development of overt cardiomyopathic changes (Kaplan et al., 2004; Gomes et al., 2012). The proposal of electrical disturbances at this early stage of the disease is an attractive one in the light of the recent data showing cross talk between the mechanical junctions, the gap junctions and the Na^{+} channel complex (Sato et al., 2009, 2011) and the presence of arrhythmias early in the disease process in humans (Bauce et al., 2005). Unfortunately, this study fails to examine the desmosomal structure at this specific time point; it would be interesting to see whether there are ultrastructural changes present that cause the observed electrical changes. Furthermore, the electrophysiological data presented lacks sufficient detail (e.g., Na^{+}-current and action potential measurements) to be able to draw definitive conclusions on the nature of the observed early electrical disturbances.

In conclusion, since the discovery a little over a decade ago that the cause of ARVC lies within the cardiac desmosomal complex and its associated proteins, a wealth of knowledge has been build up on the etiology of the disease. The use of the murine transgenic and targeted models has played a pivotal role in this process. The quest to answer the many remaining questions on the first stages of the disease and the search for a good treatment will continue during the next decade, the developed mouse models will undoubtedly play an important role in this process.

ACKNOWLEDGMENTS

This project was funded by the Netherlands Heart Foundation (2008B051). During this investigation, Dr. S. Rizzo was a visiting researcher from the University of Padua at the Academic Medical Center, University of Amsterdam, supported by Cardio-Cerebro Vascular Pathology Registry, Veneto Region, Italy.

REFERENCES

Basso, C., Bauce, B., Corrado, D., and Thiene, G. (2011). Pathophysiology of arrhythmogenic cardiomyopathy. *Nat. Rev. Cardiol.* 9, 223–233.

Basso, C., Corrado, D., Marcus, F. I., Nava, A., and Thiene, G. (2009). Arrhythmogenic right ventricu- lar cardiomyopathy. *Lancet* 373, 1289–1300.

Bauce, B., Basso, C., Rampazzo, A., Beffagna, G., Daliento, L., Frigo, G., Malacrida, S., Settimo, L., Danieli, G., Thiene, G., and Nava, A. (2005). Clinical profile of four families with arrhythmogenic right ventricu- lar cardiomyopathy caused by dom- inant desmoplakin mutations. *Eur. Heart J.* 26, 1666–1675.

Bierkamp, C., Mclaughlin, K. J., Schwarz, H., Huber, O., and Kem- ler, R. (1996). Embryonic heart and skin defects in mice lack- ing plakoglobin. *Dev. Biol.* 180, 780–785.

Delmar, M. (2004). The intercalated disk as a single functional unit. *Heart Rhythm* 1, 12–13.

Delmar, M., and McKenna, W. J. (2010). The cardiac desmosome and arrhythmogenic cardiomyopathies: from gene to disease. *Circ. Res.* 107, 700–714.

Fabritz, L., Hoogendijk, M. G., Sci- cluna, B. P., Van Amersfoorth, S. C., Fortmueller, L., Wolf, S., Laakmann, S., Kreienkamp, N., Piccini, I., Bre- ithardt, G., Noppinger, P. R., Witt, H., Ebnet, K., Wichter, T., Levkau, B., Franke, W. W., Pieperhoff, S., De Bakker, J. M., Coronel, R., and Kirchhof, P. (2011). Load-reducing therapy prevents development of arrhythmogenic right ventricular cardiomyopathy in plakoglobin- deficient mice. *J. Am. Coll. Cardiol.* 57, 740–750.

Franke, W. W., Borrmann, C. M., Grund, C., and Pieperhoff, S. (2006). The area composita of adhering junctions connecting heart muscle cells of vertebrates. I. Molecular definition in intercalated disks of cardiomyocytes by immunoelectron microscopy of desmosomal pro- teins. *Eur. J. Cell Biol.* 85, 69–82.

Gallicano, G. I., Bauer, C., and Fuchs, E. (2001). Rescuing desmoplakin function in extra-embryonic ecto- derm reveals the importance of this protein in embryonic heart, neu- roepithelium, skin and vasculature. *Development* 128, 929–941.

Gallicano, G. I., Kouklis, P., Bauer, C., Yin, M., Vasioukhin, V., Degenstein, L., and Fuchs, E. (1998). Desmo- plakin is required early in develop- ment for assembly of desmosomes and cytoskeletal linkage. *J. Cell Biol.* 143, 2009–2022.

Garcia-Gras, E., Lombardi, R., Gio- condo, M. J., Willerson, J. T., Schnei- der, M. D., Khoury, D. S., and Mar- ian, A. J. (2006). Suppression of canonical Wnt/ beta-catenin signal- ing by nuclear plakoglobin recapitu- lates phenotype of arrhythmogenic right ventricular cardiomyopathy. *J. Clin. Invest.* 116, 2012–2021.

Gerull, B., Heuser, A., Wichter, T., Paul, M., Basson, C. T., Mcdermott, D. A., Lerman, B. B., Markowitz, S. M., Ellinor, P. T., Macrae, C. A., Peters, S., Grossmann, K. S., Drenckhahn, J., Michely, B., Sasse-Klaassen, S., Birchmeier, W., Dietz, R., Breithardt, G., Schulze-Bahr, E., and Thier- felder, L. (2004). Mutations in the desmosomal protein plakophilin- 2 are common in arrhythmogenic right ventricular cardiomyopathy. *Nat. Genet.* 36, 1162–1164.

Gomes, J., Finlay, M., Ahmed, A. K., Ciaccio, E. J., Asimaki, A., Saffitz, J. E., Quarta, G., Nobles, M., Syrris, P., Chaubey, S., Mckenna, W. J., Tin- ker, A., and Lambiase, P. D. (2012). Electrophysiological abnormalities precede overt structural changes in arrhythmogenic right ventricu- lar cardiomyopathy due to muta- tions in desmoplakin-A combined murine and human study. *Eur. Heart J.* doi: 10.1093/eurheartj/ehr472. [Epub ahead of print].

Grossmann, K., Grund, C., Huelsken, J., Behrend, M., Erdmann, B., Franke, W., and Birchmeier, W. (2004). Requirement of plakophilin 2 for heart morphogenesis and cardiac junction formation. *J. Cell Biol.* 167, 149–160.

Kant, S., Krull, P., Eisner, S., Leube, R. E., and Krusche, C. A. (2012). Histolog- ical and ultrastructural abnormali- ties in murine desmoglein 2-mutant hearts. *Cell Tissue Res.* 348, 249–259.

Kaplan, S. R., Gard, J. J., Protonotarios, N., Tsatsopoulou, A., Spiliopoulou, C., Anastasakis, A., Squarcioni, C. P., Mckenna, W. J., Thiene, G., Basso, C., Brousse, N., Fontaine, G., and Saffitz, J. E. (2004). Remodeling of myocyte gap junctions in arrhythmogenic right ventricular cardiomyopathy due to a deletion in plakoglobin (Naxos disease). *Heart Rhythm* 1, 3–11.

Kirchhof, P., Fabritz, L., Zwiener, M., Witt, H., Schafers, M., Zellerhoff, S., Paul, M., Athai, T., Hiller, K. H., Baba, H. A., Breithardt, G., Ruiz, P., Wichter, T., and Lev- kau, B. (2006). Age- and training- dependent development of arrhyth- mogenic right ventricular cardiomy- opathy in heterozygous plakoglobin- deficient mice. *Circulation* 114, 1799–1806.

Krusche, C. A., Holthofer, B., Hofe, V., Van De Sandt, A. M., Eshkind, L., Bockamp, E., Merx, M. W., Kant, S., Windoffer, R., and Leube, R. E. (2011). Desmoglein 2 mutant mice develop cardiac fibrosis and dilation. *Basic Res. Cardiol.* 106, 617–633.

Li, D., Liu, Y., Maruyama, M., Zhu, W., Chen, H., Zhang, W., Reuter, S., Lin, S. F., Haneline, L. S., Field, L. J., Chen, P. S., and Shou, W. (2011). Restrictive loss of plakoglobin in cardiomy- ocytes leads to arrhythmogenic car- diomyopathy. *Hum. Mol. Genet.* 20, 4582–4596.

Li, J., and Radice, G. L. (2010). A new perspective on intercalated disc organization: implications for heart disease. *Dermatol. Res. Pract.* 2010, 207835.

Lombardi, R., Da Graca Cabreira- Hansen, M., Bell, A., Fromm, R. R., Willerson, J. T., and Marian, A. J. (2011). Nuclear plakoglobin is essential for differentiation of car- diac progenitor cells to adipocytes in arrhythmogenic right ventricu- lar cardiomyopathy. *Circ. Res.* 109, 1342–1353.

Marcus, F. I., Fontaine, G. H., Guiraudon, G., Frank, R., Lau- renceau, J. L., Malergue, C., and Grosgogeat, Y. (1982). Right ven- tricular dysplasia: a report of 24 adult cases. *Circulation* 65, 384–398.

McKoy, G., Protonotarios, N., Crosby, A., Tsatsopoulou, A., Anastasakis, A., Coonar, A., Norman, M., Baboon- ian, C., Jeffery, S., and Mckenna, W. J. (2000). Identification of a dele- tion in plakoglobin in arrhythmo- genic right ventricular cardiomy- opathy with palmoplantar kerato- derma and woolly hair (Naxos dis- ease). *Lancet* 355, 2119–2124.

Meadows, L. S., and Isom, L. L. (2005). Sodium channels as macromol- ecular complexes: implications for inherited arrhythmia syn- dromes. *Cardiovasc. Res.* 67, 448–458.

Pilichou, K., Bezzina, C. R., Thiene, G., and Basso, C. (2011). Arrhyth- mogenic cardiomyopathy: trans- genic animal models provide novel insights into disease pathobiol- ogy. *Circ. Cardiovasc. Genet.* 4, 318–326.

Pilichou, K., Nava, A., Basso, C., Beffagna, G., Bauce, B., Lorenzon, A., Frigo, G., Vettori, A., Valente, M., Towbin, J., Thiene, G., Danieli, G. A., and Rampazzo, A. (2006). Mutations in desmoglein-2 gene are associated with arrhythmogenic right ventricu- lar cardiomyopathy. *Circulation* 113, 1171–1179.

Pilichou, K., Remme, C. A., Basso, C., Campian, M. E., Rizzo, S., Bar-nett, P., Scicluna, B. P., Bauce, B., Van Den Hoff, M. J., De Bakker, J. M., Tan, H. L., Valente, M., Nava, A., Wilde, A. A., Moorman, A. F., Thiene, G., and Bezzina, C. R. (2009). Myocyte necro- sis underlies progressive myocar- dial dystrophy in mouse dsg2-related arrhythmogenic right ventricular cardiomyopathy. *J. Exp. Med.* 206, 1787–1802.

Rampazzo, A., Nava, A., Malacrida, S., Beffagna, G., Bauce, B., Rossi, V., Zimbello, R., Simionati, B., Basso, C., Thiene, G., Towbin, J. A., and Danieli, G. A. (2002). Mutation in human desmoplakin domain binding to plakoglobin causes a dominant form of arrhyth- mogenic right ventricular cardiomy- opathy. *Am. J. Hum. Genet.* 71, 1200–1206.

Ruiz, P., Brinkmann, V., Ledermann, B., Behrend, M., Grund, C., Thal- hammer, C., Vogel, F., Birchmeier, C., Gunthert, U., Franke, W. W., and Birchmeier, W. (1996). Targeted mutation of plakoglobin in mice reveals essential functions of desmo- somes in the embryonic heart. *J. Cell Biol.* 135, 215–225.

Saffitz, J. E. (2005). Dependence of electrical coupling on mechani- cal coupling in cardiac myocytes: insights gained from cardiomy- opathies caused by defects in cell-cell connections. *Ann. N. Y. Acad. Sci.* 1047, 336–344.

Sato, P. Y., Coombs, W., Lin, X., Nekrasova, O., Green, K. J., Isom, L. L., Taffet, S. M., and Delmar, M. (2011). Interactions between ankyrin-G, plakophilin-2, and connexin43 at the cardiac intercalated disc. *Circ. Res.* 109, 193–201.

Sato, P. Y., Musa, H., Coombs, W., Guerrero-Serna, G., Patino, G. A., Taffet, S. M., Isom, L. L., and Del- mar, M. (2009). Loss of plakophilin-2 expression leads to decreased sodium current and slower con- duction velocity in cultured car- diac myocytes. *Circ. Res.* 105, 523–526.

Swope, D., Cheng, L., Gao, E., Li, J., and Radice, G. L. (2012). Loss of cadherin-binding proteins beta- catenin and plakoglobin in the heart leads to gap junction remodeling and arrhythmogenesis. *Mol. Cell. Biol.* 32, 1056–1067.

Syrris, P., Ward, D., Asimaki, A., Sen- Chowdhry, S., Ebrahim, H. Y., Evans, A., Hitomi, N., Norman, M., Pan-tazis, A., Shaw, A. L., Elliott, P. M., and Mckenna, W. J. (2006). Clinical expression of plakophilin- 2 mutations in familial arrhythmo- genic right ventricular cardiomy- opathy. *Circulation* 113, 356–364.

Tavora, F., Creswell, N., and Burke, A. P. (2009). Arrhythmogenic right ventricular cardiomyopathy. *N. Engl. J. Med.* 360, 2784. [author reply 2785–2786].

Thiene, G., Nava, A., Corrado, D., Rossi, L., and Pennelli, N. (1988). Right ventricular cardiomyopa- thy and sudden death in young people. *N. Engl. J. Med.* 318, 129–133.

Yang, Z., Bowles, N. E., Scherer, S. E.,

Taylor, M. D., Kearney, D. L., Ge, S., Nadvoretskiy, V. V., Defreitas, G., Carabello, B., Brandon, L. I., God- sel, L. M., Green, K. J., Saffitz, J. E.,

Li, H., Danieli, G. A., Calkins, H., Marcus, F., and Towbin, J. A. (2006). Desmosomal dysfunction due to mutations in desmoplakin causes arrhythmogenic right ventricular dysplasia/cardiomyopathy. *Circ. Res.* 99, 646–655.

21

CaMKII regulation of cardiac K channels

Julian Mustroph, Lars S. Maier and Stefan Wagner*

Department of Cardiology, University Medical Center Göttingen, Göttingen, Germany

***Correspondence:**
Stefan Wagner, Department of Cardiology, University Medical Center Göttingen, Robert-Koch-Strasse 40, 37075 Göttingen, Germany
e-mail: swagner@med.uni-goettingen.de

Cardiac K channels are critical determinants of cardiac excitability. In hypertrophied and failing myocardium, alterations in the expression and activity of voltage-gated K channels are frequently observed and contribute to the increased propensity for life-threatening arrhythmias. Thus, understanding the mechanisms of disturbed K channel regulation in heart failure (HF) is of critical importance. Amongst others, Ca/calmodulin-dependent protein kinase II (CaMKII) has been identified as an important regulator of K channel activity. In human HF but also various animal models, increased CaMKII expression and activity has been linked to deteriorated contractile function and arrhythmias. This review will discuss the current knowledge about CaMKII regulation of several K channels, its influence on action potential properties, dispersion of repolarization, and arrhythmias with special focus on HF.

Keywords: CaMKII, K channel, heart failure, action potential, arrhythmias

INTRODUCTION

Heart failure (HF) is a leading cause of death in western countries (United States and Europe), (Neumann et al., 2009; Go et al., 2012; Nichols et al., 2013) but also in developing countries like China (Hu et al., 2012). Morbidity in HF is characterized by contractile dysfunction and an increased propensity for arrhythmias (Luo and Anderson, 2013). Both are known consequences of the electromechanical remodeling of the cardiomyocyte. It is well established that reduced expression of K channels in hypertrophied and failing myocardium (Kääb et al., 1996) can lead to action potential (AP) prolongation, which is known to be pro-arrhythmogenic. Moreover, AP prolongation also leads to greater systolic Ca entry through voltage-gated L-type Ca channels ($Ca_V1.2$) and impairs the Ca export function of cardiac Na/Ca exchange (NCX, Bers, 2002a), which results in cytosolic Ca overload and dramatically impairs diastolic contractile function (**Figure 1**).

Thus, understanding the mechanisms that are involved in the regulation of cardiac K channel expression and function in HF could greatly improve patient treatment.

Ca/calmodulin-dependent protein kinase II (CaMKII) has been identified as an important regulator of ion channels and transporters involved in cardiac excitation–contraction coupling under physiological but also pathophysiological conditions (Maier and Bers, 2007). Increased CaMKII expression and function was found in HF and is linked to contractile dysfunction and arrhythmias. Interestingly, there is substantial evidence that CaMKII is also involved in K channel regulation (Nerbonne, 2011). This review will discuss CaMKII-dependent regulation of several cardiac potassium channels and its significance for arrhythmogenesis and contractile function in HF.

K CHANNELS ARE IMPORTANT REGULATORS OF CARDIAC EXCITABILITY

The cardiac AP is initiated by activation of voltage-gated Na channels ($Na_V1.5$). The resulting Na current (I_{Na}) leads to a rapid depolarization, i.e., the AP upstroke (phase 0; Bers, 2002b). The upstroke is limited by inactivation of I_{Na} and voltage-dependent activation of transient outward K channels ($K_V4.2$, $K_V4.3$, and $K_V1.4$ generating I_{to}). I_{to} activation results in an early repolarization (notch, phase 1), thus setting the voltage plateau of the AP. Activation of L-type Ca channels generates a depolarizing Ca current (I_{Ca}) that stabilizes the membrane potential during the plateau phase (phase 2). Repolarization in phase 3 is mainly caused by activation of delayed rectifying K channels [hERG (*KCNH2*), Kv7.1 (*KCNQ1*), and Kv1.5 (*KCNA5*) responsible for I_{Kr}, I_{Ks}, and I_{Kur}, respectively]. Additionally, activation of inward rectifying K channels (Kir2.x, generating I_{K1}) contributes to late phase repolarization. The resting membrane potential (phase 4) is stabilized by I_{K1}, but ion conductance in phase 4 is also influenced by the Na/K-ATPase and NCX.

In pacemaker cells, the absence of a stabilizing I_{K1} is responsible for a more positive resting membrane potential (Cho et al., 2003). The non-specific cation current I_f (channel protein HCN) can thus generate diastolic depolarization leading to the generation of APs (Bers, 2002b).

Several mechanisms of arrhythmogenesis involving K channels have been described. Reduced function of Kv7.1 and hERG are the hallmark of congential long QT syndrome 1 and 2, respectively (Brenyo et al., 2012). A smaller I_{Ks} and I_{Kr} results in prolonged repolarization that is associated with torsade de pointes and sudden cardiac death (Roden, 2008). The underlying arrhythmic mechanisms involve increased triggered activity due to early afterdepolarizations (EADs) or reentry due to increased spatial heterogeneities in repolarization (see below). Recently, a mutation of an ATP-sensitive K channel (Medeiros-Domingo et al., 2010) has been identified in a patient with early repolarization syndrome, which is characterized by a prominent J wave on the ECG (see below) and is associated with an increased risk of ventricular fibrillation (VF) and cardiac death (Tikkanen et al., 2009).

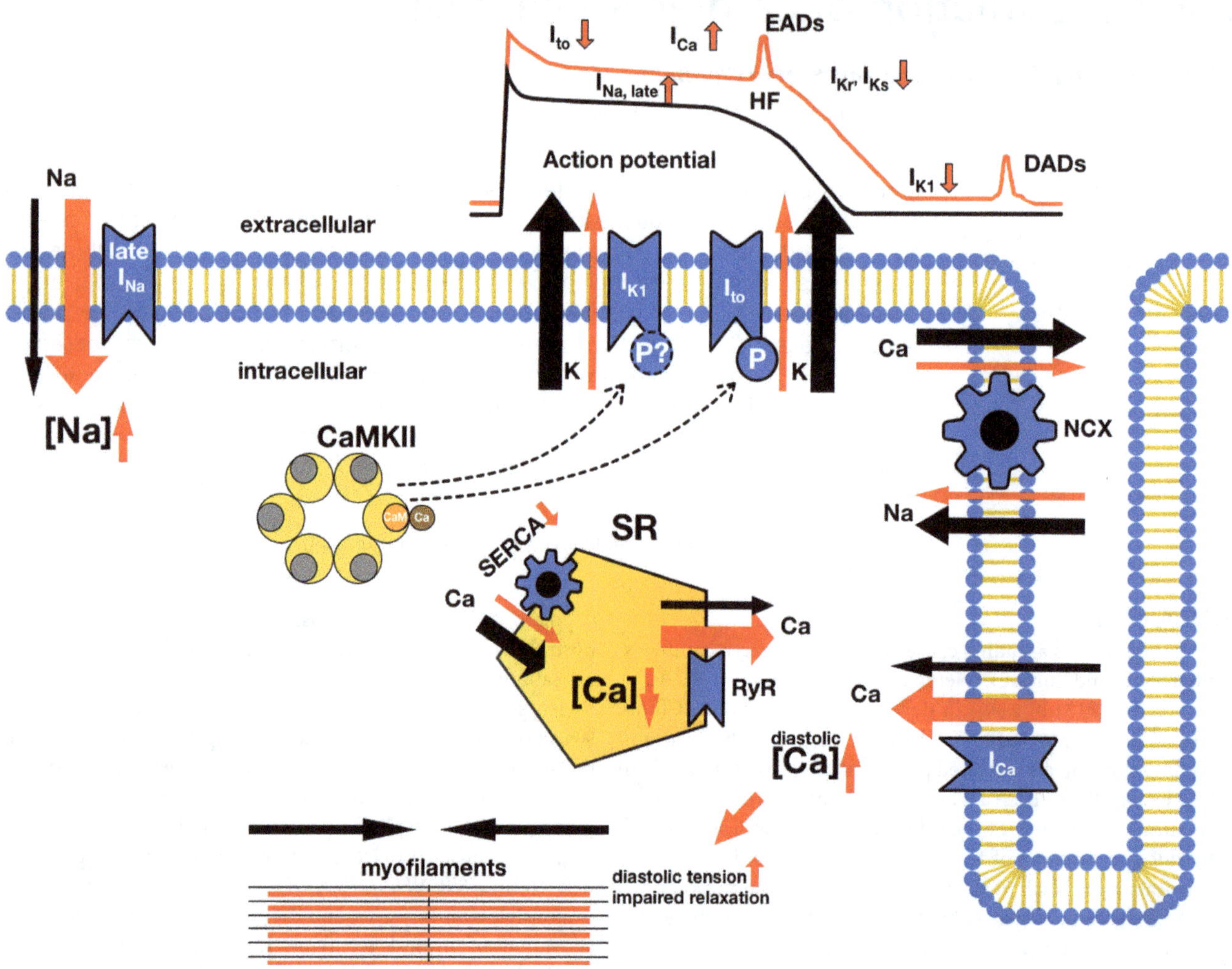

FIGURE 1 | Electro-mechanical remodeling in ventricular myocytes in HF. Normal currents are indicated by black arrows, while changes in HF are indicated by red arrows and changes in size to indicate an increase or decrease in current density. CaMKII effects on potassium currents are indicated by bar-headed lines (in this figure only CaMKII effects on K currents are shown, for a detailed review of CaMKII effects refer to Maier and Bers, 2007). Decreased expression and function of repolarizing K currents (I_{to}, I_{Kr}, I_{Ks}, I_{K1}), for instance due CaMKII-mediated effects leads to prolongation of the AP duration. This can result in greater systolic Ca entry through voltage-gated Ca channels, but also Na entry through increased late Na current (via voltage-gated Na channels, Shryock et al., 2013). Increased cytosolic Na concentrations, a feature also observed in HF (Pieske et al., 2002), together with prolonged AP duration also impairs the Ca export function of cardiac Na/Ca exchanger (Bers, 2002a), which further aggravates the net gain in cytosolic Ca. In the face of a reduced function of the sarcoplasmic reticulum (SR) Ca ATPase in HF **(SERCA; Hasenfuss, 1998)**, this Ca remains in the cytosol thereby dramatically impairing diastolic function. Moreover, increased depolarizing currents (Na and Ca currents) during the plateau phase of the AP could lead to early afterdepolarizations (EADs), while increased diastolic SR Ca leak through ryanodine-receptor 2 (RyR) facilitates delayed afterdepolarizations (DADs).

It was shown that this mutation results in gain of function in K_{ATP} (Medeiros-Domingo et al., 2010), consequently resulting in increased transmural heterogeneity of repolarization (see below).

Interestingly, besides rare congenital disease, altered K channel function has also been described for HF. It was shown that decreased I_{K1} and I_{to} density could lead to AP prolongation (Kaab et al., 1998).

Increased triggered activity is an important consequence of prolonged repolarization. The longer phase 2 of the AP results in reactivation of Ca channels that generate a depolarizing current possibly resulting in an EAD and ultimately leading to a triggered AP (Weiss et al., 2010). On the other hand, K channels have been also been shown to be involved in the generation of delayed afterdepolarizations (DADs) that are a consequence of cytosolic and sarcoplasmic reticulum (SR) Ca overload. The latter causes an increased propensity of spontaneous ryanodine-receptor (RyR) activation leading to a depolarizing inward NCX current (Kääb et al., 1996). Interestingly, this inward NCX current is more likely to induce DADs if I_{K1} is functionally downregulated, causing an unstable resting membrane potential (Dhamoon and Jalife, 2005).

Differential K channel expression across the ventricular wall is the basis for transmural dispersion of repolarization (TDR,

Antzelevitch and Fish, 2001). Physiologically, the endocardial myocyte has a smaller I_{to} amplitude compared to the epicardial myocyte. This, together with increased depolarizing currents, contributes to a more positive AP plateau and a longer AP duration in the endocardial compared to the epicardial myocyte. The result is a physiological TDR that also determines the positive T wave on the surface ECG. However, under pathophysiological conditions this fine balanced regional difference in K channel function can be substantially altered. A preferential shortening of the epicardial AP by enhanced I_{to}, for instance, together with a preferential prolongation of the endocardial AP by enhanced late I_{Na} and minor changes in the small I_{to} would increase the TDR. While a TDR increase in phase 1 and 2 of the AP results in the occurance of a J wave (positive deflection at the QRS-ST junction; Yan and Antzelevitch, 1996), increased TDR in phase 3 and 4 can cause abnormal T waves. If the increase in TDR in phase 3 and 4 reached a threshold, abnormal electrical activity would find excitable myocytes, resulting in reentry and leading to torsade de pointes (Yan and Antzelevitch, 1996). Computational modeling of a rabbit ventricular myocyte overexpressing CaMKII was used to investigate the importance of the expression level of I_{to} for AP duration (Grandi et al., 2007). If 100% I_{to} expression was used (= epicardial myocytes), CaMKII overexpression resulted in a shortening of the AP duration mainly due to a CaMKII-dependent enhancement of I_{to}. With 10% I_{to} expression (= endocardial myocytes), however, AP duration increased because CaMKII-enhanced late I_{Na} and L-type Ca current outweighed the effect on the smaller I_{to}. The mechanisms by which CaMKII alters potassium channel expression and function will be discussed in this review.

CaMKII AND HF

Calcium-Calmodulin-dependent kinase II is a serine/threonine kinase that can regulate multiple ion channels and transporters including K channels (see below). Currently, four isoforms and up to 30 splice-variants of the serine/threonine CaMKII have been identified, with CaMKIIδ as the predominant cardiac isoform (Maier and Bers, 2007). CaMKII contains an N-terminal catalytic kinase-domain with an ATP-binding site as well as substrate binding sites. Adjacent to the catalytic subunit, an autoregulatory domain with a calmodulin (CaM)-binding site and important regulatory threonine (T287, T306, T307) and methionine residues (M281/282) precedes the C-terminal association-domain, which is critical for the assembly of the holoenzyme. *In vivo*, self-association of CaMKII holoenzymes forms two ring-like CaMKII-hexamers which are stacked on top of each other (dodecameric configuration; Rellos et al., 2010). CaMKII is activated by binding of a Ca/CaM complex to its autoregulatory domain, resulting in conformational changes which expose the catalytic subunit, enabling ATP and substrate binding. An important substrate is the autoregulatory domain of an adjacent subunit, resulting in inter-subunit phosphorylation at T287 (auto-phosphorylation). The latter enables CaM-independent activity after the dissociation of Ca/CaM (Maier and Bers, 2007). Novel alternative activation pathways have also been described involving oxidation or glycosylation at M281/282, both of which result in Ca-independent activity similar to auto-phosphorylation (Erickson et al., 2008, 2013).

CaMKII has been associated with HF development. In human HF, expression and activity of CaMKII is increased (Hoch et al., 1999; Kirchhefer et al., 1999; Ai et al., 2005). Moreover, CaMKIIδ-transgenic mice develop HF with increased AP duration, disturbed Ca handling, and are prone to ventricular arrhythmias (Maier, 2003; Wagner et al., 2011). In contrast, transgenic CaMKII inhibition or CaMKII knockout prevents cardiac remodeling and HF development after myocardial infarction or increased afterload (Zhang et al., 2005; Backs et al., 2009; Ling et al., 2009).

TRANSIENT OUTWARD K CURRENT

I_{to} is generated by a pore-forming α-subunit with six transmembrane segments (S1–S6). Accessory β-subunits can associate with this α-subunit (**Figure 2A**, Niwa and Nerbonne, 2010). In their either homologous or heterologous tetrameric assembly, the subunits' S5 and S6 segments face each other to form the pore, while segment S4 senses voltage (Snyders, 1999; Niwa and Nerbonne, 2010). I_{to} is critical for the early repolarization ("notch") immediately following the upstroke in phase 0 of the cardiac AP. There are at least two components of I_{to} generated by different channel isoforms, that can be distinguished according to their recovery and inactivation kinetics (**Figure 2B**; Brahmajothi et al., 1999). The fast component ($I_{to,fast}$) inactivates and recovers with time constants (τ) of less than 100 ms, whereas the slow component ($I_{to,slow}$) inactivates with τ of about 200 ms and recovers with τ ranging from hundreds of milliseconds up to several seconds (Brahmajothi et al., 1999; Xu et al., 1999).

In human, rat, and canine tissue, I_{to} is generated mostly by the rapidly recovering channel population Kv4.3 (KCND3, Dixon et al., 1996). In a tachycardia-induced canine model of HF, a reduced ventricular Kv4.3 protein expression has been reported along with decreased I_{to} density (Zicha et al., 2004). It has also been shown that Kv4.3 expression is significantly reduced in human HF and that this is associated with a significant decrease in I_{to} density (Kaab et al., 1998; Zicha et al., 2004). Reduced I_{to} density is known to contribute to AP prolongation and prolonged QT intervals (Barry et al., 1998).

Despite this important role of Kv4.3 for I_{to} in human cardiac tissue, many animals species show a rather heterogeneous channel population comprised of Kv4.3, Kv1.4 (*KCNA4*), Kv4.2 (*KCND2*), and accessory KChIP subunits. In these species, I_{to} can be separated into the fast and slow component with varying relative contributions to total I_{to}. In rabbit and mouse cardiac myocytes, for instance, Kv1.4 has been shown to be responsible for the slow component while a complex of Kv4.2, Kv4.3, and KChIPs is responsible for the fast component (Niwa and Nerbonne, 2010). Similar to the dog model of HF, tachycardia-induced HF in rabbits showed reduced total I_{to} density while AP duration was prolonged (Rose, 2005). Interestingly, mRNA levels of Kv1.4 and Kv4.2, as well as KChIP2, were significantly reduced, while Kv4.3 mRNA was unchanged. Protein expression of Kv4.2 and KChIP2 was significantly reduced, though Kv4.3 and Kv1.4 were unchanged (Rose, 2005). In a TNF-α-overexpressing mouse model of HF, $I_{to,fast}$ density and Kv4.2 protein expression was significantly reduced (Petkova-Kirova, 2006). Other mouse models

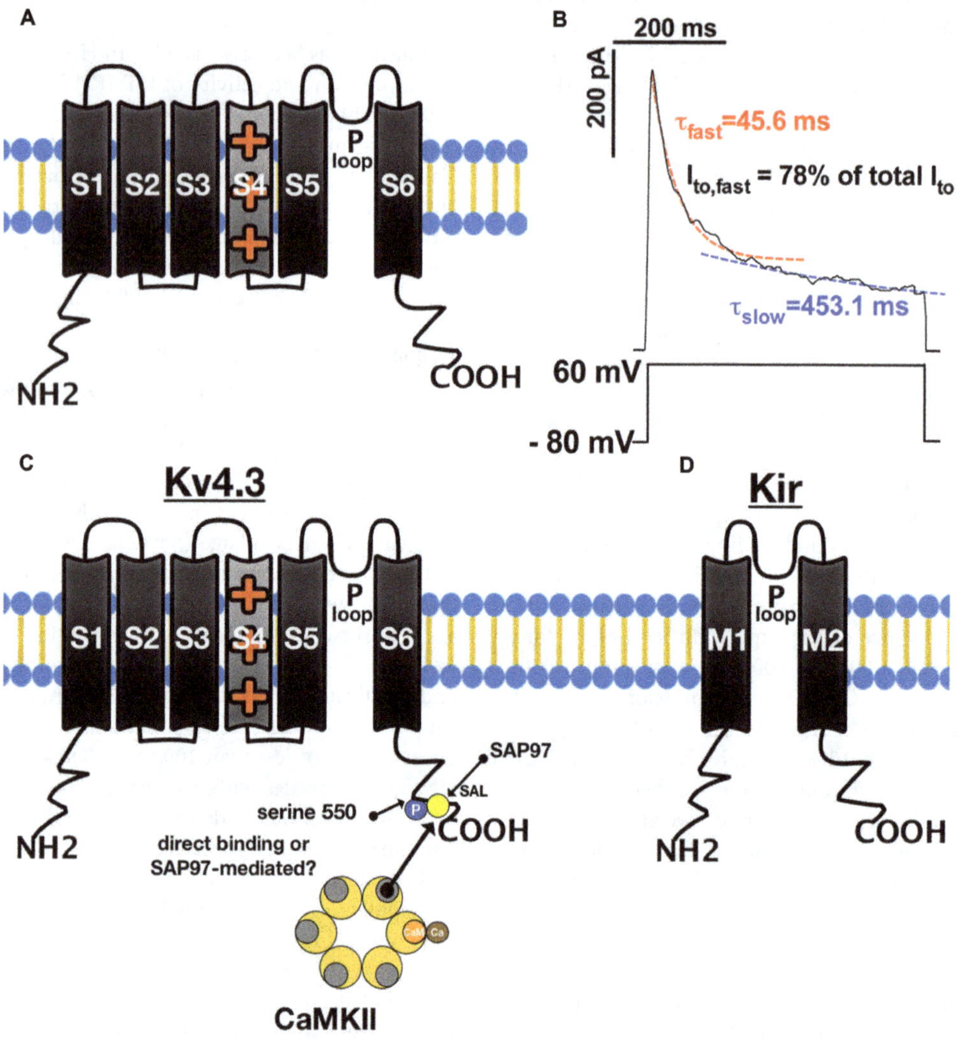

FIGURE 2 | Structure and function of K channels. (A) Structure of voltage-gated K channel α-sunbunit (Kv) with six transmembrane segments (S1–S6). The S5–S6 segments face each other to form the central pore. The P-loop between the S5 and S6 segments acts as an ion conductance pathway and its signature motif G(Y/F)G functions as a K ion selectivity filter. Segment S4 senses voltage and moves outward during cell membrane depolarization resulting in conformational changes which open the pore. **(B)** There are two current components of I_{to} generated that can be distinguished according to their inactivation kinetics. $I_{to,fast}$ inactivates with time constants (τ) of less than 100 ms, whereas the $I_{to,slow}$ inactivates with τ of about 200 ms. **(C)** CaMKII can bind to Kv4.3 and phosphorylate serine 550 of its C terminus, which leads to altered current kinetics. SAP97 can also bind to Kv4.3 [at its Ser-Ala-Leu (SAL) segment] and possibly mediates the CaMKII-Kv4.3 interaction. **(D)** Inward rectifying potassium channels are formed by four α-subunits containing only two transmembrane segments (M1–M2) with a central P-loop as ion conductance pathway.

of HF exhibited similar reductions in I_{to} density and increased AP duration (Knollmann et al., 2000; Mitarai, 2000).

The differential regulation in the expression and function of the various channel isoforms underlying I_{to} suggests that the two components $I_{to,fast}$ and $I_{to,slow}$ are functionally and structurally independent ion currents.

CaMKII-DEPENDENT REGULATION OF I_{to} EXPRESSION

CaMKII has been shown to influence the expression of channel isoforms underlying I_{to}. In mice overexpressing CaMKIIδ, it was shown that total I_{to} density is significantly reduced (Wagner et al., 2009). This reduction was secondary to a reduced expression of Kv4.2 with reduced $I_{to,fast}$ and accompanied by a prolongation of the cardiac AP (Wagner et al., 2009). In contrast, expression of Kv1.4 and $I_{to,slow}$ were increased but this increase could not fully compensate the reduction in $I_{to,fast}$ (Wagner et al., 2009). Interestingly, chronic CaMKII inhibition in mice by transgenic expression of the specific CaMKII inhibitory peptide AC3-I, a derivative of CaMKII substrate autocamtide-3, resulted in an increase in $I_{to,fast}$ and shorter AP duration. On the other hand, the increase in I_{to} density was absent in crossbred mice expressing AC3-I but lacking phospholamban (PLN; Li et al., 2006). Since mice overexpressing CaMKIIδ also develop HF and chronic CaMKII inhibition may also affect the SR, it is not clear whether these changes are CaMKII-specific or secondary to remodeling or interference with other pathways. This is supported by the fact that short-term overexpression of CaMKIIδ in rabbit myocytes increases I_{to} (Wagner et al., 2009). Similary, in silico experiments with simulated CaMKII overexpression in rabbit myocytes also led to an increase in I_{to} along with faster $I_{to,slow}$ recovery from inactivation (Grandi et al., 2007). Furthermore, Li et al. (2006) found no change in the expression of pore-forming subunits Kv4.2/Kv4.3 underlying increased I_{to} but only a downregulation of the accessory subunit KChIP2, suggesting that the regulation of I_{to} is complex, involving many interacting partners. In this respect it is not surprising that Kv4.3 and Kv4.2 form large macromolecular complexes with other proteins such as diaminopeptidyl transferase-like protein 6 (DPP6) and Eps15 homology domain-containing protein 4 (EHD4) (Marionneau et al., 2011). Recent evidence suggests that these proteins are important for endocytosis, vesicular recycling and trafficking (Cai et al., 2013). Perhaps more importantly, it has been shown that KChIP1 clamps two adjacent Kv4.3 α-subunits together via two contact interfaces that interact with the N-termini of Kv4.3 (Pioletti et al., 2006; Wang et al., 2006b). This stabilizes $K_V4.3$ tetramers and also exerts an influence on current kinetics with current density being increased, inactivation slowed, and recovery from inactivation enhanced (Wang et al., 2006b). In addition, KChIP1 has been shown to be essential for proper Kv4 trafficking to the membrane (Cui et al., 2008).

More evidence that the downregulation of Kv4 in HF after CaMKII overexpression may be secondary and not directly mediated by CaMKII is derived from experiments investigating the interaction of the MAGUK (membrane-associated guanylate kinase) protein SAP97 with Kv4.

In neurons, the interaction of the C-terminal Ser-Ala-Leu (SAL)-sequence of Kv4.2 with SAP97 has been shown to be crucial for trafficking of Kv4.2 to the synaptic membrane (Gardoni et al., 2007). Interestingly, this trafficking has been shown to be enhanced by CaMKII phosphorylation of SAP97 at Serin-39 (Gardoni et al., 2007). Furthermore, it was shown in cardiac myocytes that Kv4.2/Kv4.3 channels form complexes with SAP97 and CaMKII (El-Haou et al., 2009). In the same publication, suppression of SAP97 in rat atrial myocytes via shRNA led to a decrease in I_{to}, whereas SAP97 overexpression resulted in enhanced I_{to}. Moreover, expression of Kv4.3 lacking the C-terminal SAL-sequence or SAP97 silencing via shRNA abolished the co-precipitation with CaMKII (El-Haou et al., 2009). Also, inhibition of CaMKII with autocamtide-2 related inhibitory peptide (AIP) resulted in reduced I_{to} and the inhibition was more pronounced after SAP97 overexpression (El-Haou et al., 2009). Interestingly, recent evidence suggests that SAP97 is downregulated in patients with dilated cardiomyopathy (Szuts et al., 2013).

CaMKII-DEPENDENT REGULATION OF I_{to} GATING

The first evidence for a CaMKII-dependent regulation of cardiac potassium channel gating came from a study investigating human atrial myocytes (Tessier et al., 1999). The myocytes were isolated from donors with either chronic atrial dilation or chronic atrial fibrillation (AF). Patch–clamp experiments showed that inactivation of I_{to} was accelerated by CaMKII inhibition with either KN-93 or AIP (Tessier et al., 1999). Moreover, Tessier et al. (1999) also showed an increased expression level of CaMKII in the atrium of donors with chronic atrial dilation or chronic AF. More evidence for CaMKII regulating I_{to} came from experiments using transgenic mice overexpressing CaMKIIδ$_c$ and also short-term CaMKIIδ$_c$ overexpression in rabbit myocytes. It was shown that the recovery from inactivation of $I_{to,fast}$ and $I_{to,slow}$ was enhanced by CaMKII overexpression (Wagner et al., 2009). This enhancement could be blocked by acute CaMKII inhibition suggesting that this was not secondary to HF development (Wagner et al., 2009). The underlying mechanism of CaMKII-dependent regulation of I_{to} may involve direct CaMKII-dependent phosphorylation of Kv4.2 at serine 438/459, and of Kv1.4 at serine 123 (Roeper, 1997; Varga, 2004). Patch-clamp experiments in HEK-293 cells transfected with Kv4.3 showed that addition of autothiophosphorylated (pre-activated) CaMKII slowed I_{to} inactivation consistent with the results obtained by Tessier et al. (1999) and enhanced recovery from inactivation (Sergeant, 2005). Conversely, HEK cells treated with CaMKII-inhibitor KN-93 or CaMKII-inhibitory-peptide displayed significantly accelerated current inactivation and slowed recovery from inactivation (Sergeant, 2005). Moreover, if the C-terminal Kv4.3 mutant (serine 550 to alanine) was expressed, I_{to} inactivation was enhanced and I_{to} recovery was slowed (Sergeant, 2005). Neither addition of autothiophosphorylated CaMKII nor dialysis of CaMKII inhibitors could affect I_{to} recovery in HEK cells expressing this Kv4.3 S550A mutant (Sergeant, 2005), supporting the concept that the C-terminus of Kv4.3 is a hotspot for CaMKII-dependent association and regulation of $I_{to,fast}$ (**Figure 2C**). Further evidence for a direct regulation of $I_{to,fast}$ by CaMKII comes from studies in rat ventricular myocyte lysates showing that CaMKII co-immunoprecipitates with both Kv4.3 and Kv4.2 (Colinas, 2006), and inhibition of CaMKII with KN-93 resulted in a significant acceleration of I_{to} inactivation even through recovery from inactivation was unaffected (Colinas, 2006).

Interestingly, this CaMKII-dependent enhancement of I_{to} may also be important for reactive oxygen-species (ROS) induced arrhythmogenesis. ROS are known to oxidize and activate CaMKII (Erickson et al., 2008; Wagner et al., 2011) and ROS-induced arrhythmias are known to be CaMKII-dependent (Wagner et al., 2011). Recently, it was proposed that ROS-dependent activation of I_{to} favors EADs by facilitating I_{Ca} reactivation (Zhao et al., 2012).

Thus, CaMKIIδ$_c$ appears to regulate both channel expression and/or trafficking, but also acutely regulates channel gating properties. In both cases, acute regulation results in an enhancement of I_{to}. In contrast to this, chronic CaMKII overexpression that leads to HF development results in a reduction of I_{to} but this appears to be a secondary effect.

Kv4.3 AS AN IMPORTANT REGULATOR OF CaMKII ACTIVITY

While Kv4.3 is an important target for CaMKII, it may also influence CaMKII localization and activity. Recently, in HEK-293 cells transfected with Kv4.3 and His-tagged CaMKII, it was shown that Kv4.3 binds to CaM-dissociated CaMKII competitively at its CaM binding site (residues 301 and 307; Keskanokwong et al., 2010). This binding was independent from the auto-phosphorylation status of CaMKII, since both constitutively active (T-287D) or inactive (T-287A) CaMKII-mutants could also bind to Kv4.3 (Keskanokwong et al., 2010).

Since the CaMKII inhibitor KN93 also binds CaMKII at the CaM binding site (Sumi, 1991), it is conceivable that KN-93 disturbs the interaction of CaMKII and Kv4.3. Consistent with this idea, Keskanokwong et al. showed that co-purification of Kv4.3 and CaMKII is abolished upon addition of KN-93. Furthermore, it was shown that application of the Kv4.3 blocker 4-aminopyridine (4-AP) disturbes the co-purification of CaMKII and Kv4.3 in HEK-293 cells, while CaMKII auto-phosphorylation is increased (Keskanokwong et al., 2010). Similarly, increased CaMKII activity was found in guinea pig ventricular myocytes treated with 4-AP (Wang et al., 2006a). Moreover, 4-AP-induced blockade of Kv4.3 in HEK-293 cells has been shown to result in increased apoptosis and enhanced CaMKII-auto-phosphorylation, while the authors were able to prevent apoptosis by inhibition of CaMKII with KN-93 (Zhang et al., 2012).

This suggests that Kv4.3 may function as a reservoir for inactive CaMKII-units and exert an influence on CaMKII activation levels (**Figure 2C**). In accordance with this hypothesis, *in vivo* overexpression of Kv4.3 in mouse ventricular myocardium via multiple-site virus injection decreased the level of phosphorylated CaMKII, while CaMKII expression was not affected. CaMKII bound to Kv4.3 was also shown to be protected from activation by systolic Ca transients (Keskanokwong et al., 2010). The Kv4.3-CaMKII interaction may also be important for the regulation of other CaMKII target proteins. For instance, it was shown that blockade of Kv4.3 with 4-AP results in increased I_{Ca} that could be blocked by buffering cytosolic Ca with BAPTA or application of AIP (Wang et al., 2006a).

As previously mentioned, Kv4.3 is downregulated in HF (Kaab et al., 1998) while CaMKII is upregulated (Hoch et al., 1999). The CaMKII-Kv4.3 interaction may thus be severely altered in HF, contributing to higher CaMKII activity. In this context, the previously mentioned role for SAP97 in the regulation of Kv4.3 expression and Kv4.3-CaMKII interaction may be important. Downregulation of SAP97 in HF (Szuts et al., 2013) may underlie reduced Kv4.3 and may contribute to increased CaMKII activity.

INWARDLY RECTIFYING CURRENT I_{K1}

In contrast to the voltage-gated K channels, inwardly rectifying potassium channels [Kir2.1 (*KCNJ2*), Kir2.2 (*KCNJ12*), Kir2.3 (*KCNJ4*), and Kir2.4 (*KCNJ14*)] are formed by four α-subunits containing only two transmembrane segments (M1–M2) with a central P-loop but without a voltage-sensor (**Figure 2D**; Hibino et al., 2010). The main characteristic of this class of potassium channels is inward rectification, which features a strong potassium conductance during hyperpolarization, but a decrease in ion conductance upon depolarization due to blockade of the pore by Mg, Ca and cell membrane polyamines (Matsuda et al., 1987; Matsuda and Cruz, 1993; Hibino et al., 2010).

This peculiar inward rectifying property of the Kir2.x channels that generate I_{K1} renders these channels important stabilizers of the resting membrane potential by neutralizing resting influx of positive ions (Fauconnier et al., 2005). In addition, Kir2.x channels also contribute to late-phase (phase 4) repolarization (Dhamoon, 2004; Dhamoon and Jalife, 2005; Fauconnier et al., 2005).

In sinoatrial myocytes, the expression of channels forming I_{K1} is notably reduced, which allows for an unstable resting membrane potential that can be depolarized by I_f, thus inducing diastolic depolarization (Bers, 2002b).

There is evidence that Kir2.x isoforms can assemble as homo- or heterotetrameres (Zobel et al., 2003). The functional characteristics of I_{K1} depend very much on the Kir isoforms that comprise I_{K1} (Panama et al., 2010), since rectification of current at depolarized membrane potentials (> -30 mV) is complete for Kir2.1 and Kir2.2, but incomplete for Kir2.3 (Dhamoon, 2004). There is great variability in the expression of these isoforms between left and right ventricle (Warren et al., 2003) but also atrium and ventricle (Gaborit et al., 2007). Similar to channel subunits generating I_{to}, expression of the Kir isoforms appears to be strongly species-dependent (Jost et al., 2013).

Ca OR CaMKII-DEPENDENT REGULATION OF I_{K1}

I_{K1} functional expression also seems to be regulated differently under pathophysiological conditions. It was shown that I_{K1} density is reduced in failing rat ventricular myocytes (Fauconnier et al., 2005). Interestingly, this reduction was attenuated in the presence of high EGTA (10 mmol/L) and abolished if intracellular Ca was buffered with BAPTA (20 mM; Fauconnier et al., 2005). Moreover, activation of RyR by application of ryanodine or FK506 led to a similar reduction of I_{K1} density in non-failing wild-type rat ventricular cells and this effect could be blocked by Ca-buffering with BAPTA (Fauconnier et al., 2005). Whether this reduction occurs via direct Ca-dependent blockade of I_{K1} via the mechanism described (Matsuda and Cruz, 1993) or mechanisms involving altered expression/trafficking of the underlying Kir isoforms is, however, completely unknown. Fauconnier et al. (2005) also suggested the involvement of protein kinase C (PKC), since the PKC inhibitor staurosporine antagonized the effect of ryanodine on I_{K1}. PKC has been shown to phosphorylate Kir2.1 at serine 64 and threonine 353, leading to reduced I_{K1} in human atrial myocytes (Karle, 2002). On the other hand, opposite results have recently been shown in canine ventricular myocytes. Addition of 900 nmol/L Ca in the patch pipette significantly increased I_{K1} current compared to measurements with 160 nM Ca (Nagy et al., 2013). Therefore, the effect of Ca on I_{K1} may be species-dependent. Supporting evidence comes from intact field-stimulated (1 Hz) canine right ventricular papillary muscle. Increasing extracellular Ca from 2 to 4 mmol/L, resulted in increased Ca transient amplitude and significantly shortened AP duration. This Ca-dependent AP shortening could be prevented by inhibition of I_{K1} using $BaCl_2$. Moreover, $BaCl_2$ preferentially prolonged AP duration at 4 mM $[Ca]_o$ vs. 2 mM $[Ca]_o$. The authors conclude that Ca-dependent enhancement of I_{K1}, at least in canine myocytes, may be an important contributor to repolarization reserve and an endogenous negative feedback mechanism inhibiting the generation of DADs due to high Ca levels (Nagy et al., 2013). Moreover, Nagy et al. (2013) also showed that CaMKII inhibition with KN-93 abolished the Ca-induced activation of I_{K1}, suggesting that CaMKII is also involved in I_{K1} regulation. Supporting evidence for a CaMKII-dependent activation of I_{K1} also comes from rabbit ventricular myocytes. Acute overexpression of CaMKIIδ by adenovirus-mediated gene transfer resulted in a significant increase in I_{K1} density that could be blocked by addition of CaMKII-inhibitory peptide AIP to the pipette (Wagner et al., 2009). In the same, study, transgenic CaMKIIδ overexpression in mice that develop HF, however, resulted in a reduced I_{K1} density and reduced expression of Kir2.1 (Wagner et al., 2009). Thus, the discrepancy between the studies showing either increased or decreased I_{K1} may be due to species-differences but this remains speculative. In accordance, mouse ventricular myocytes with transgenic inhibition of CaMKII showed an increased I_{K1} and a shorter AP duration without a significant change in Kir2.1 and Kir2.2 expression levels (Li et al., 2006).

Aside from the species, it could also be relevant if the studied model results in HF. It was shown that SAP97 co-immunoprecipitates with Kir2.2 in rat hearts (Leonoudakis et al., 2004). Interestingly, in human dilated cardiomyopathy, the co-localization of SAP97 with Kir2.x was shown to be disturbed (Szuts et al., 2013). This suggests that a mechanism similar to the above mentioned Kv4.x-SAP97 interaction may be present. Therefore, further studies are greatly needed to clarify the importance of Ca and CaMKII for the regulation of I_{K1} in different animal models and in human disease (**Table 1**).

I_{K1} AND ARRHYTHMIAS

I_{K1} is generally regarded as anti-arrhythmic by stabilizing resting membrane potential. In a canine model of tachycardia-induced HF, reduced I_{K1} has been shown to increase the propensity for sudden cardiac death and ventricular tachycardia (Kääb et al., 1996). Also, loss of function mutations in *KCNJ2* have been associated with long QT syndrome (LQT7), in which increased AP duration and increased propensity for arrhythmias can be observed (Tsuboi and Antzelevitch, 2006).

On the other hand, contrasting results have been shown for wild-type Kir2.1 overexpressing mice that have an increased propensity for ventricular arrhythmias (Noujaim et al., 2006; Piao et al., 2007) or AF (Li, 2004). Kir2.1 knock-down in mice was associated with longer AP duration and a reduced incidence of premature ventricular contractions before and after AV node ablation, reduced arrhythmias due to extracellular hypokalemia, and a reduced incidence of halothane-induced ventricular tachycardia (Piao et al., 2007).

This discrepancy may be solved by the fact that both increase or decrease of I_{K1} can be pro-arrhythmic if there is a substantial spatial heterogeneity in the functional expression profile (Sekar et al., 2009). In accordance with this, gain-of-function mutations in *KCNJ2* can result in short QT syndrome (SQT3), which is also pro-arrhythmogenic (Brenyo et al., 2012).

DELAYED RECTIFYING K CHANNELS

The three channels Kv1.5 (*KCNA5*), hERG (*KCNH2*), and Kv7.1 (*KCNQ1*) comprise the group of the delayed rectifying K channels. They generate I_{Kur} (ultra rapid), I_{Kr} (rapid), and I_{Ks} (slow), respectively. Together, they are important currents for phase 3 repolarization.

I_{Kur} is only present in atrial myocardium. In chronic human AF, it was shown that AP duration is reduced, possibly contributing to the arrhythmogenic mechanisms (Wettwer, 2004). Evidence for a role of Kv1.5 in AF came from a study investigating pharmacological Kv1.5 inhibition in a canine model of AF (Regan et al., 2007). They could show that AF terminates if Kv1.5 is inhibited. Furthermore, SAP97 was reported to co-immunoprecipitate with Kv1.5 (Murata et al., 2001) resulting in increased I_{Kur} (Godreau et al., 2002; Eldstrom et al., 2003).

Since SAP97 and CaMKII have been shown to interact (El-Haou et al., 2009), CaMKII expression is increased in AF (Tessier et al., 1999; Neef et al., 2010), and given the similarities between SAP97-dependent Kv4.3 and Kv1.5 regulation (Tessier et al., 1999; Godreau et al., 2002; El-Haou et al., 2009), it seems tempting to speculate that CaMKII could also regulate Kv1.5. Interestingly, in human atrial myocytes it was shown that CaMKIIδ is especially localized at intercalated disks, the region where Kv1.5 is also located (Tessier et al., 1999). Furthermore, Tessier et al. (1999) showed that selective inhibition of CaMKII with KN-93 or AIP reduced the amplitude of the sustained component of outward K current (I_{sus}), whereas inhibition of phosphatases with okadaic acid increased I_{sus} (Tessier et al., 1999; Tessier, 2001). This I_{sus} is regarded as mainly generated by Kv1.5 (Fedida et al., 1993), suggesting that CaMKII, possibly by phosphorylation, regulates Kv1.5 (Tessier et al., 1999).

Besides I_{Kur}, other K currents may also be involved in AF. I_{K1}, for instance, has been shown to be upregulated in AF possibly contributing to shortening of AP duration (Dobrev and Ravens, 2003).

I_{Ks} is comprised of the pore-forming α-subunit Kv7.1, but also the auxiliary β-subunit KCNE1 (Ruscic et al., 2013). Loss-of-function mutations in *KCNQ1* are linked to an increase in AP duration associated with long QT-syndrome type I, whereas gain-of-function mutations in *KCNQ1* are associated with short QT-syndrome (SQT2) (Brenyo et al., 2012) and familial AF (Chen et al., 2003). Additionally, loss-of-function mutations in *KCNE1* have been associated with long QT-syndrome 5 (Splawski et al., 1997), which points out the important role of KCNE1 for the generation of I_{Ks}. Indeed it has been shown that KCNE1 is important in slowing down the movement of the voltage-sensor S4 of Kv7.1 upon depolarization, thus explaining the slow activation kinetics of I_{Ks} (Ruscic et al., 2013). Similar mechanisms may very well regulate other voltage-gated channels and underlie their distinct activation kinetics.

Interestingly, co-immunoprecipitation experiments in yeast cells expressing wild-type Kv7.1 or mutated Kv7.1 with truncated α-helices showed that calmodulin can bind to the C-terminus of Kv7.1 (Shamgar, 2006). This IQ-motif appears to be a hot spot for mutations: yeast 2-hybrid experiments indicated that *KCNQ1* mutations A371T and S373P, which are associated with LQTS, lose their calmodulin-Kv7.1 interaction.

Moreover, agarose-pulldown assays in HEK-293 cells revealed that LQTS-associated Kv7.1 mutants W392R, S373P, and A371T bound significantly less calmodulin than wild-type Kv7.1 (Shamgar, 2006). This disturbed calmodulin- Kv7.1 interaction may be important for channel expression. Cell surface expression experiments with biotinylated channel proteins showed that mutants with impaired CaM-binding are significantly less expressed than wild-type Kv7.1 (Shamgar, 2006). Interestingly, overexpression of calmodulin in HEK-293 cells either expressing wild-type Kv7.1 or mutant S373P showed significant increases in Kv7.1 (5x) as well as S373P (100x) cell surface and protein expression, which highlights

Table 1 | Synopsis of studies investigating I_{K1} and arrhythmias.

Species	Model	I_{K1} Current	Phenotype	Reference
Rat ventricular myocytes	Myocardial infarction	↓		Fauconnier et al. (2005)
Canine ventricular myocytes	High intracellular calcium	↑		Nagy et al. (2013)
Rabbit ventricular myocytes	Adenoviral CaMKII overexpression	↑		Wagner et al. (2009)
Mouse ventricular myocytes	Transgenic CaMKII overexpression	↓	Polymorphic and monomorphic VTs	Wagner et al. (2006, 2009)
Mouse ventricular myocytes	Transgenic CaMKII inhibition (AC3-I expression)	↑		Li et al. (2006)
Mouse ventricular myocytes	Acute CaMKII inhibition by AC3-I dialysis	→		Li et al. (2006)
Mouse ventricular myocytes	Kir2.1 knock-down	↓	Less ventricular arrhythmias	Piao et al. (2007)
Mouse ventricular myocytes	Kir2.1 overexpression	↑	More ventricular arrhythmias	Piao et al. (2007)
Kir2.1-overexpressing [ESC]-derived myocytes	Transplantation of ESC-derived myocytes into mouse ventricles after MI	↑	Less spontaneous VTs, less inducible VTs	Liao et al. (2013)
Rabbit ventricular myocytes	Tachycardia-induced HF			Rose (2005)
Mouse ventricular myocytes	Calsequestrin-overexpression-induced HF	↓	QRS and QTc prolongation	Knollmann et al. (2000)
Mouse ventricular myocytes	Gαq-overexpression-induced hypertrophy	↓		Mitarai (2000)
Mouse ventricular myocytes	Calcineurin overexpression	→		Petrashevskaya et al. (2002)
Mouse ventricular myocytes	Dominant-negative Kv4.2 expression - induced HF	↓		Wickenden et al. (1999)
Mouse ventricular myocytes	Dominant-negative Kv4.2 expression	↓	QRS and QTc prolongation	McLerie (2003)
Mouse ventricular myocytes	Kir2.1 overexpression	↑	More inducible, more stable VTs	Noujaim et al. (2006)
Mouse ventricular myocytes	Kir2.1 overexpression	↑	Bradycardia, AF, AV-Block, PVC, short QT	Li (2004)
Guinea pig ventricular myocytes	Kir2.1 overexpression	↑	QTc shortening	Miake et al. (2003)
Guinea pig ventricular myocytes	Dominant-negative Kir2.1 expression (downregulation)	↓	QTc prolongation	Miake et al. (2003)
Human ventricular myocytes	Dilated or ischemic cardiomyopathy	↓	APD prolongation	Beuckelmann et al. (1993)
Canine ventricular myocytes	Tachycardia-induced HF	↓	APD prolongation, QTc prolongation, more VTs	Kääb et al. (1996), Pak et al. (1997)
Monolayers of cultured neo-natal rat ventricular myocytes	Homogeneous Kir2.1 overexpression	↑	No reentry arrhythmias inducible	Sekar et al. (2009)
Monolayers of cultured neo-natal rat ventricular myocytes	Heterogeneous Kir2.1 overexpression	↑	Inducible reentry arrhythmias	Sekar et al. (2009)
Monolayers of cultured neo-natal rat ventricular myocytes	Homogeneous Kir2.1 suppression	↓	No reentry arrhythmias inducible	Sekar et al. (2009)
Monolayers of cultured neo-natal rat ventricular myocytes	Heterogeneous Kir2.1 suppression	↓	Inducible reentry arrhythmias	Sekar et al. (2009)
Canine atrial myocytes	Tachycardia-induced HF	→	Inducible atrial fibrillation (AF)	Li et al. (2002)

the important role of calmodulin for I_{Ks} assembly and cell surface expression (Shamgar, 2006).

In addition, the CaM- Kv7.1 interaction may also be relevant for the regulation of I_{Ks} gating. Patch-clamp experiments of inside-out membrane from *Xenopus* oocytes showed that application of calmodulin antagonist W7 significantly reduced current density of Kv7.1/KCNE1, while an increase in Ca significantly shifted voltage-dependence of channel activation toward more hyperpolarized membrane potentials (Shamgar, 2006).

Thus, the interaction of calmodulin and Kv7.1 appears to be critical for expression and function of I_{Ks}, with the intriguing possibility that regulatory mechanisms could also involve some form of CaMKII interaction with calmodulin and Kv7.1 or KCNE1.

ATP-SENSITIVE POTASSIUM CURRENT K_{ATP}

The ATP-sensitive potassium current K_{ATP}, comprising of Kir6.1 (*KCNJ8*) and Kir6.2 (*KCNJ11*) α-subunits, plays an important role in ischemic preconditioning (Li et al., 2007). K_{ATP} can be a substrate for CaMKII: in mice expressing CaMKII-inhibitory peptide AC3-I, an increased K_{ATP} current density has been shown along with an increase in the sarcolemmal Kir6.2 membrane surface expression (Li et al., 2007). Also, recent evidence from pancreatic β-cells suggests that Kir6.2 can be phosphorylated by CaMKII at threonine 224 (Kline et al., 2013). Co-expression of CaMKII and Kir6.2 in COS-cells resulted in a decreased K_{ATP} current.

The significance of K_{ATP} in HF and arrhythmogenesis is still largely unknown. There is evidence suggesting that K_{ATP}-channel opening with cromakalim produces more stable ventricular arrhythmias (Quintanilla et al., 2013). In addition, Langendorff-perfused canine failing hearts with induced VF showed an increased rate of spontaneous VF termination, if K_{ATP} was blocked with glibenclamide (Taylor et al., 2012). Also, recently, a mutation in cardiac Kir6.1 that is associated with gain of function has been identified in a patient with early repolarization syndrome (see above; Medeiros-Domingo et al., 2010).

On the other hand, K_{ATP}-blockade with glibenclamide in non-failing canine hearts with induced VF delayed the termination of VF (Taylor et al., 2012). Thus, the role of cardiac K_{ATP} and its regulation by CaMKII has yet to be evaluated.

SUMMARY

While there is increasing evidence for an involvement of CaMKII in the regulation of K channels, many discrepancies are not yet understood. These discrepancies result from the great variability in the expression profile of K channels in different species and disease models. The greatest evidence so far exists for CaMKII-dependent regulation of Kv4.x expression, trafficking and function. Most intriguingly, the Kv4.x macromolecular complex appears to serve as a hotspot and reservoir for CaMKII, which may have profound impact on the regulation of various other CaMKII targets like Ca channels. CaMKII expression and activity has been shown to be increased in many animal models of HF, but also in human HF. Increased CaMKII activity has been shown to induce contractile dysfunction and arrhythmias. Therefore, a more detailed understanding of the mechanisms of K channel regulation by CaMKII is warranted.

ACKNOWLEDGMENTS

Stefan Wagner and Lars S. Maier are funded by Deutsche Forschungsgemeinschaft (DFG) through an International Research Training Group GRK 1816. Lars S. Maier is funded by DFG grant MA 1982/4-2 and TPA03 SFB 1002. Lars S. Maier is also funded by the Fondation Leducq Transatlantic Network on "Redox and Nitrosative Regulation of Cardiac Remodeling." Lars S. Maier, and Stefan Wagner, are funded by the DZHK (Deutsches Zentrum für Herz-Kreislauf-Forschung – German Centre for Cardiovascular Research). We acknowledge support by the German Research Foundation and the Open Access Publication Funds of the Göttingen University.

REFERENCES

Ai, X., Curran, J. W., Shannon, T. R., Bers, D. M., and Pogwizd, S. M. (2005). Ca2+/calmodulin–dependent protein kinase modulates cardiac ryanodine receptor phosphorylation and sarcoplasmic reticulum Ca2+ leak in heart failure. *Circ. Res.* 97, 1314–1322. doi: 10.1161/01.RES.0000194329.41863.89

Antzelevitch, C., and Fish, J. (2001). Electrical heterogeneity within the ventricular wall. *Basic Res. Cardiol.* 96, 517–527. doi: 10.1007/s003950170002

Backs, J., Backs, T., Neef, S., Kreusser, M. M., Lehmann, L. H., Patrick, D. M., et al. (2009). The δ isoform of CaM kinase II is required for pathological cardiac hypertrophy and remodeling after pressure overload. *Proc. Natl. Acad. Sci. U.S.A.* 106, 2342–2347. doi: 10.1073/pnas.0813013106

Barry, D. M., Xu, H., Schuessler, R. B., and Nerbonne, J. M. (1998). Functional knockout of the transient outward current, long-QT syndrome, and cardiac remodeling in mice expressing a dominant-negative Kv4 subunit. *Circ. Res.* 83, 560–567. doi: 10.1161/01.RES.83.5.560

Bers, D. M. (2002a). Cardiac excitation-contraction coupling. *Nature* 415, 198–205. doi: 10.1038/415198a

Bers, D. M. (2002b). *Excitation-Contraction Coupling and Cardiac Contractile Force*, ed. D. M. Bers (Boston, MA: Kluwer Academic Publishers), 39–62.

Beuckelmann, D. J., Nabauer, M., and Erdmann, E. (1993). Alterations of K+ currents in isolated human ventricular myocytes from patients with terminal heart failure. *Circ. Res.* 73, 379–385. doi: 10.1161/01.RES.73.2.379

Brahmajothi, M. V., Campbell, D. L., Rasmusson, R. L., Morales, M. J., Trimmer, J. S., Nerbonne, J. M., et al. (1999). Distinct transient outward potassium current (Ito) phenotypes and distribution of fast-inactivating potassium channel alpha subunits in ferret left ventricular myocytes. *J. Gen. Physiol.* 113, 581–600. doi: 10.1085/jgp.113.4.581

Brenyo, A. J., Huang, D. T., and Aktas, M. K. (2012). Congenital long and short QT syndromes. *Cardiology* 122, 237–247. doi: 10.1159/000339537

Cai, B., Giridharan, S. S. P., Zhang, J., Saxena, S., Bahl, K., Schmidt, J. A., et al. (2013). Differential roles of C-terminal Eps15 homology domain proteins as vesiculators and tubulators of recycling endosomes. *J. Biol. Chem.* 288, 30172–30180. doi: 10.1074/jbc.M113.488627

Chen, Y.-H., Xu, S.-J., Bendahhou, S., Wang, X.-L., Wang, Y., Xu, W.-Y., et al. (2003). KCNQ1 gain-of-function mutation in familial atrial fibrillation. *Science* 299, 251–254. doi: 10.1126/science.1077771

Cho, H.-S., Takano, M., and Noma, A. (2003). The electrophysiological properties of spontaneously beating pacemaker cells isolated from mouse sinoatrial node. *J. Physiol.* 550, 169–180. doi: 10.1113/jphysiol.2003.040501

Colinas, O. (2006). Differential modulation of Kv4.2 *and Kv*4.3 channels by calmodulin-dependent protein kinase II in rat cardiac myocytes. *Am. J. Physiol. Heart Circ. Physiol.* 291, H1978–H1987. doi: 10.1152/ajpheart.01373.2005

Cui, Y. Y., Liang, P., and Wang, K. W. (2008). Enhanced trafficking of tetrameric Kv4.3 channels by KChIP1 clamping. *Neurochem. Res.* 33, 2078–2084. doi: 10.1007/s11064-008-9688-7

Dhamoon, A. S. (2004). Unique Kir2.x properties determine regional and species differences in the cardiac inward rectifier K+ current. *Circ. Res.* 94, 1332–1339. doi: 10.1161/01.RES.0000128408.66946.67

Dhamoon, A. S., and Jalife, J. (2005). The inward rectifier current (IK1) controls cardiac excitability and is involved in arrhythmogenesis. *Heart Rhythm* 2, 316–324. doi: 10.1016/j.hrthm.2004.11.012

Dixon, J. E., Shi, W., Wang, H.-S., McDonald, C., Yu, H., Wymore, R. S., et al. (1996). Role of the Kv4.3 K+ channel in ventricular muscle: a molecular correlate for the transient outward current. *Circ. Res.* 79, 659–668. doi: 10.1161/01.RES.79.4.659

Dobrev, D., and Ravens, U. (2003). Remodeling of cardiomyocyte ion channels in human atrial fibrillation. *Basic Res. Cardiol.* 98, 137–148. doi: 10.1007/s00395-003-0409-8

Eldstrom, J., Choi, W. S., Steele, D. F., and Fedida, D. (2003). SAP97 increases Kv1.5 currents through an indirect N-terminal mechanism. *FEBS Lett.* 547, 205–211. doi: 10.1016/S0014-5793(03)00668-9

El-Haou, S., Balse, E., Neyroud, N., Dilanian, G., Gavillet, B., Abriel, H., et al. (2009). Kv4 potassium channels form a tripartite complex with the anchoring protein SAP97 and CaMKII in cardiac myocytes. *Circ. Res.* 104, 758–769. doi: 10.1161/CIRCRESAHA.108.191007

Erickson, J. R., Joiner, M. A., Guan, X., Kutschke, W., Yang, J., Oddis, C. V., et al. (2008). A dynamic pathway for calcium-independent activation of CaMKII by methionine oxidation. *Cell* 133, 462–474. doi: 10.1016/j.cell.2008.02.048

Erickson, J. R., Pereira, L., Wang, L., Han, G., Ferguson, A., Dao, K., et al. (2013). Diabetic hyperglycemia activates CaMKII and arrhythmias by O-linked glycosylation. *Nature* 502, 372–376. doi: 10.1038/nature12537

Fauconnier, J., Lacampagne, A., Rauzier, J., Vassort, G., and Richard, S. (2005). Ca-dependent reduction of I in rat ventricular cells: a novel paradigm for arrhythmia in heart failure? *Cardiovasc. Res.* 68, 204–212. doi: 10.1016/j.cardiores.2005.05.024

Fedida, D., Wible, B., Wang, Z., Fermini, B., Faust, F., Nattel, S., et al. (1993). Identity of a novel delayed rectifier current from human heart with a cloned K+ channel current. *Circ. Res.* 73, 210–216. doi: 10.1161/01.RES.73.1.210

Gaborit, N., Le Bouter, S., Szuts, V., Varro, A., Escande, D., Nattel, S., et al. (2007). Regional and tissue specific transcript signatures of ion channel genes in the non-diseased human heart. *J. Physiol.* 582, 675–693. doi: 10.1113/jphysiol.2006.126714

Gardoni, F., Mauceri, D., Marcello, E., Sala, C., Di Luca, M., and Jeromin, A. (2007). SAP97 directs the localization of Kv4.2 to spines in hippocampal neurons: regulation by CaMKII. *J. Biol. Chem.* 282, 28691–28699. doi: 10.1074/jbc.M701899200

Go, A. S., Mozaffarian, D., Roger, V. L., Benjamin, E. J., Berry, J. D., Borden, W. B., et al. (2012). Heart disease and stroke statistics–2013 update: a report from the american heart association. *Circulation* 127, e6–e245. doi: 10.1161/CIR.0b013e31828124ad

Godreau, D., Vranckx, R., Maguy, A., Rücker-Martin, C., Goyenvalle, C., Abdelshafy, S., et al. (2002). Expression, regulation and role of the MAGUK protein SAP-97 in human atrial myocardium. *Cardiovasc. Res.* 56, 433–442. doi: 10.1016/S0008-6363(02)00602-8

Grandi, E., Puglisi, J. L., Wagner, S., Maier, L. S., Severi, S., and Bers, D. M. (2007). Simulation of Ca-calmodulin-dependent protein kinase II on rabbit ventricular myocyte Ion currents and action potentials. *Biophys. J.* 93, 3835–3847. doi: 10.1529/biophysj.107.114868

Hasenfuss, G. (1998). Alterations of calcium-regulatory proteins in heart failure. *Cardiovasc. Res.* 37, 279–289. doi: 10.1016/S0008-6363(97)00277-0

Hibino, H., Inanobe, A., Furutani, K., Murakami, S., Findlay, I., and Kurachi, Y. (2010). Inwardly rectifying potassium channels: their structure, function, and physiological roles. *Physiol. Rev.* 90, 291–366. doi: 10.1152/physrev.00021.2009

Hoch, B., Meyer, R., Hetzer, R., Krause, E.-G., and Karczewski, P. (1999). Identification and expression of -isoforms of the multifunctional Ca2+/calmodulin-dependent protein kinase in failing and nonfailing human myocardium. *Circ. Res.* 84, 713–721. doi: 10.1161/01.RES.84.6.713

Hu, S. S., Kong, L. Z., Gao, R. L., Zhu, M. L., Wang, W., Wang, Y. J., et al. (2012). Outline of the report on cardiovascular disease in China, 2010. *Biomed. Environ. Sci.* 25, 251–256.

Jost, N., Virag, L., Comtois, P., Ordög, B., Szuts, V., Seprenyi, G., et al. (2013). Ionic mechanisms limiting cardiac repolarization reserve in humans compared to dogs. *J. Physiol.* 591, 4189–4206. doi: 10.1113/jphysiol.2013.261198

Kaab, S., Dixon, J., Duc, J., Ashen, D., Nabauer, M., Beuckelmann, D. J., et al. (1998). Molecular basis of transient outward potassium current downregulation in human heart failure: a decrease in Kv4.3 mRNA correlates with a reduction in current density. *Circulation* 98, 1383–1393. doi: 10.1161/01.CIR.98.14.1383

Kääb, S., Nuss, H. B., Chiamvimonvat, N., O'Rourke, B., Pak, P. H., Kass, D. A., et al. (1996). Ionic mechanism of action potential prolongation in ventricular myocytes from dogs with pacing-induced heart failure. *Circ. Res.* 78, 262–273. doi: 10.1161/01.RES.78.2.262

Karle, C. A. (2002). Human cardiac inwardly-rectifying K+ channel Kir2.1b is inhibited by direct protein kinase C-dependent regulation in human isolated cardiomyocytes and in an expression system. *Circulation* 106, 1493–1499. doi: 10.1161/01.CIR.0000029747.53262.5C

Keskanokwong, T., Lim, H. J., Zhang, P., Cheng, J., Xu, L., Lai, D., et al. (2010). Dynamic Kv4.3-CaMKII unit in heart: an intrinsic negative regulator for CaMKII activation. *Eur. Heart J.* 32, 305–315. doi: 10.1093/eurheartj/ehq469

Kirchhefer, U., Schmitz, W., Scholz, H., and Neumann, J. (1999). Activity of cAMP-dependent protein kinase and Ca2+/calmodulin-dependent protein kinase in failing and nonfailing human hearts. *Cardiovasc. Res.* 42, 254–261. doi: 10.1016/S0008-6363(98)00296-X

Kline, C. F., Wright, P. J., Koval, O. M., Zmuda, E. J., Johnson, B. L., Anderson, M. E., et al. (2013). IV-Spectrin and CaMKII facilitate Kir6.2 regulation in pancreatic beta cells. *Proc. Natl. Acad. Sci. U.S.A.* 110, 17576–17581. doi: 10.1073/pnas.1314195110

Knollmann, B. C., Knollmann-Ritschel, B. E., Weissman, N. J., Jones, L. R., and Morad, M. (2000). Remodelling of ionic currents in hypertrophied and failing hearts of transgenic mice overexpressing calsequestrin. *J. Physiol.* 525, 483–498. doi: 10.1111/j.1469-7793.2000.t01-1-00483.x

Leonoudakis, D., Conti, L. R., Radeke, C. M., McGuire, L. M. M., and Vandenberg, C. A. (2004). A multiprotein trafficking complex composed of SAP97, CASK, Veli, and Mint1 is associated with inward rectifier Kir2 potassium channels. *J. Biol. Chem.* 279, 19051–19063. doi: 10.1074/jbc.M400284200

Li, J. (2004). Transgenic upregulation of IK1 in the mouse heart leads to multiple abnormalities of cardiac excitability. *Am. J. Physiol. Heart Circ. Physiol.* 287, H2790–H2802. doi: 10.1152/ajpheart.00114.2004

Li, J., Marionneau, C., Koval, O., Zingman, L., Mohler, P. J., Nerbonne, J. M., et al. (2007). Calmodulin kinase II inhibition enhances ischemic preconditioning by augmenting ATP-sensitive K+ current. *Channels* 1, 387–394.

Li, J., Marionneau, C., Zhang, R., Shah, V., Hell, J. W., Nerbonne, J. M., et al. (2006). Calmodulin kinase II Inhibition shortens action potential duration by upregulation of K+ currents. *Circ. Res.* 99, 1092–1099. doi: 10.1161/01.RES.0000249369.71709.5c

Li, Y., Kranias, E. G., Mignery, G. A., and Bers, D. M. (2002). Protein kinase A phosphorylation of the ryanodine receptor does not affect calcium sparks in mouse ventricular myocytes. *Circ. Res.* 90, 309–316. doi: 10.1161/hh0302.105660

Liao, S.-Y., Tse, H.-F., Chan, Y.-C., Mei-Chu Yip, P., Zhang, Y., Liu, Y., et al. (2013). Overexpression of Kir2.1 channel in embryonic stem cell-derived cardiomyocytes attenuates posttransplantation proarrhythmic risk in myocardial infarction. *Heart Rhythm* 10, 273–282. doi: 10.1016/j.hrthm.2012.10.008

Ling, H., Zhang, T., Pereira, L., Means, C. K., Cheng, H., Gu, Y., et al. (2009). Requirement for Ca2+/calmodulin–dependent kinase II in the transition from pressure overload–induced cardiac hypertrophy to heart failure in mice. *J. Clin. Invest.* 119, 1230–1240. doi: 10.1172/JCI38022

Luo, M., and Anderson, M. E. (2013). Mechanisms of altered Ca2+ handling in heart failure. *Circ. Res.* 113, 690–708. doi: 10.1161/CIRCRESAHA.113.301651

Maier, L., and Bers, D. (2007). Role of Ca2+/calmodulin-dependent protein kinase (CaMK) in excitation–contraction coupling in the heart. *Cardiovasc. Res.* 73, 631–640. doi: 10.1016/j.cardiores.2006.11.005

Maier, L. S. (2003). Transgenic CaMKIIdeltaC overexpression uniquely alters cardiac myocyte Ca2+ handling: reduced SR Ca2+ load and activated SR Ca2+ release. *Circ. Res.* 92, 904–911. doi: 10.1161/01.RES.0000069685.20258.F1

Marionneau, C., Townsend, R. R., and Nerbonne, J. M. (2011). Proteomic analysis highlights the molecular complexities of native Kv4 channel macromolecular complexes. *Semin. Cell Dev. Biol.* 22, 145–152. doi: 10.1016/j.semcdb.2010.10.004

Matsuda, H., and Cruz, J. D. S. (1993). Voltage-dependent block by internal Ca2+ ions of inwardly rectifying K+ channels in guinea-pig ventricular cells. *J. Physiol.* 470, 295–311.

Matsuda, H., Saigusa, A., and Irisawa, H. (1987). Ohmic conductance through the inwardly rectifying K channel and blocking by internal Mg2+. *Nature* 325, 156–159. doi: 10.1038/325156a0

McLerie, M. (2003). Dominant-negative suppression of I(K1) in the mouse heart leads to altered cardiac excitability. *J. Mol. Cell. Cardiol.* 35, 367–378. doi: 10.1016/S0022-2828(03)00014-2

Medeiros-Domingo, A., Tan, B.-H., Crotti, L., Tester, D. J., Eckhardt, L., Cuoretti, A., et al. (2010). Gain-of-function mutation S422L in the KCNJ8-encoded cardiac KATP channel Kir6.1 as a pathogenic substrate for J-wave syndromes. *Heart Rhythm* 7, 1466–1471. doi: 10.1016/j.hrthm.2010.06.016

Miake, J., Marbán, E., and Nuss, H. B. (2003). Functional role of inward rectifier current in heart probed by Kir2.1 overexpression and dominant-negative suppression. *J. Clin. Invest.* 111, 1529–1536. doi: 10.1172/JCI200317959

Mitarai, S. (2000). Changes in ionic currents and beta-adrenergic receptor signaling in hypertrophied myocytes overexpressing Gaq. *Am. J. Physiol. Heart Circ. Physiol.* H139–H148. doi: 10.1016/S0008-6363(02)00403-0

Murata, M., Buckett, P. D., Zhou, J., Brunner, M., Folco, E., and Koren, G. (2001). SAP97 interacts with Kv1. 5 in heterologous expression systems. *Am. J. Physiol. Heart Circ. Physiol.* 281, H2575–H2584.

Nagy, N., Acsai, K., Kormos, A., Sebők, Z., Farkas, A. S., Jost, N., et al. (2013). [Ca2+]i-induced augmentation of the inward rectifier potassium current (IK1) in canine and human ventricular myocardium. *Pflügers Arch. Eur. J. Physiol.* Available at: http://link.springer.com/10.1007/s00424-013-1309-x (accessed August 29, 2013).

Neef, S., Dybkova, N., Sossalla, S., Ort, K. R., Fluschnik, N., Neumann, K., et al. (2010). CaMKII-dependent diastolic SR Ca2+ leak and elevated diastolic Ca2+ levels in right atrial myocardium of patients with atrial fibrillation. *Circ. Res.* 106, 1134–1144. doi: 10.1161/CIRCRESAHA.109.203836

Nerbonne, J. M. (2011). Repolarizing cardiac potassium channels: multiple sites and mechanisms for CaMKII-mediated regulation. *Heart Rhythm* 8, 938–941. doi: 10.1016/j.hrthm.2011.01.018

Neumann, T., Biermann, J., Neumann, A., Wasem, J., Ertl, G., Dietz, R., et al. (2009). Herzinsuffizienz: Häufigster Grund für Krankenhausaufenthalte. *Dtsch. Ärztebl.* 106, 269–275.

Nichols, M., Townsend, N., Scarborough, P., and Rayner, M. (2013). Cardiovascular disease in Europe: epidemiological update. *Eur. Heart J.* 34, 3028–3034. doi: 10.1093/eurheartj/eht356

Niwa, N., and Nerbonne, J. M. (2010). Molecular determinants of cardiac transient outward potassium current (Ito) expression and regulation. *J. Mol. Cell. Cardiol.* 48, 12–25. doi: 10.1016/j.yjmcc.2009.07.013

Noujaim, S. F., Pandit, S. V., Berenfeld, O., Vikstrom, K., Cerrone, M., Mironov, S., et al. (2006). Up-regulation of the inward rectifier K+ current (IK1) in the mouse heart accelerates and stabilizes rotors. *J. Physiol.* 578, 315–326. doi: 10.1113/jphysiol.2006.121475

Pak, P. H., Nuss, H. B., Tunin, R. S., Kääb, S., Tomaselli, G. F., Marban, E., et al. (1997). Repolarization abnormalities, arrhythmia and sudden death in canine tachycardia-induced cardiomyopathy. *J. Am. Coll. Cardiol.* 30, 576–584. doi: 10.1016/S0735-1097(97)00193-9

Panama, B. K., McLerie, M., and Lopatin, A. N. (2010). Functional consequences of Kir2.1/Kir2.2 subunit heteromerization. *Pflügers Arch. Eur. J. Physiol.* 460, 839–849. doi: 10.1007/s00424-010-0864-7

Petkova-Kirova, P. S. (2006). Electrical remodeling of cardiac myocytes from mice with heart failure due to the overexpression of tumor necrosis factor-alpha. *Am. J. Physiol. Heart Circ. Physiol.* 290, H2098–H2107. doi: 10.1152/ajpheart.00097.2005

Petrashevskaya, N. N., Bodi, I., Rubio, M., Molkentin, J. D., and Schwartz, A. (2002). Cardiac function and electrical remodeling of the calcineurin-overexpressed transgenic mouse. *Cardiovasc. Res.* 54, 117–132. doi: 10.1016/S0008-6363(02)00241-9

Piao, L., Li, J., McLerie, M., and Lopatin, A. N. (2007). Transgenic upregulation of IK1 in the mouse heart is proarrhythmic. *Basic Res. Cardiol.* 102, 416–428. doi: 10.1007/s00395-007-0659-y

Pieske, B., Maier, L. S., Piacentino, V., Weisser, J., Hasenfuss, G., and Houser, S. (2002). Rate Dependence of [Na+]i and contractility in non-failing and failing human myocardium. *Circulation* 106, 447–453. doi: 10.1161/01.CIR.0000023042.50192.F4

Pioletti, M., Findeisen, F., Hura, G. L., and Minor., D. L. (2006). Three-dimensional structure of the KChIP1–Kv4.3 T1 complex reveals a cross-shaped octamer. *Nat. Struct. Mol. Biol.* 13, 987–995. doi: 10.1038/nsmb1164

Quintanilla, J. G., Moreno, J., Archondo, T., Chin, A., Pérez-Castellano, N., Usandizaga, E., et al. (2013). KATP channel opening accelerates and stabilizes rotors in a swine heart model of ventricular fibrillation. *Cardiovasc. Res.* 99, 576–585. doi: 10.1093/cvr/cvt093

Regan, C. P., Kiss, L., Stump, G. L., McIntyre, C. J., Beshore, D. C., Liverton, N. J., et al. (2007). Atrial antifibrillatory effects of structurally distinct IKur blockers 3-[(dimethylamino)methyl]-6-methoxy-2-methyl-4-phenylisoquinolin-1(2H)-one and 2-Phenyl-1,1-dipyridin-3-yl-2-pyrrolidin-1-yl-ethanol in dogs with underlying heart failure. *J. Pharmacol. Exp. Ther.* 324, 322–330. doi: 10.1124/jpet.107.127654

Rellos, P., Pike, A. C. W., Niesen, F. H., Salah, E., Lee, W. H., Von Delft, F., et al. (2010). Structure of the CaMKII delta calmodulin complex reveals the molecular mechanism of CaMKII kinase activation. *PLoS Biol.* 8:e1000426. doi: 10.1371/journal.pbio.1000426

Roden, D. M. (2008). Long-QT Syndrome. *N. Engl. J. Med.* 358, 169–176. doi: 10.1056/NEJMcp0706513

Roeper, J. (1997). Frequency-dependent inactivation of mammalian A-type K channel KV1.4 regulated by Ca2/calmodulin- dependent protein kinase. *J. Neurosci.* 3379–3391.

Rose, J. (2005). Molecular correlates of altered expression of potassium currents in failing rabbit myocardium. *Am. J. Physiol. Heart Circ. Physiol.* 288, H2077–H2087. doi: 10.1152/ajpheart.00526.2003

Ruscic, K. J., Miceli, F., Villalba-Galea, C. A., Dai, H., Mishina, Y., Bezanilla, F., et al. (2013). PNAS Plus: IKs channels open slowly because KCNE1 accessory subunits slow the movement of S4 voltage sensors in KCNQ1 pore-forming subunits. *Proc. Natl. Acad. Sci. U.S.A.* 110, E559–E566. doi: 10.1073/pnas.1222616110

Sekar, R. B., Kizana, E., Cho, H. C., Molitoris, J. M., Hesketh, G. G., Eaton, B. P., et al. (2009). IK1 heterogeneity affects genesis and stability of spiral waves in cardiac myocyte monolayers. *Circ. Res.* 104, 355–364. doi: 10.1161/CIRCRESAHA.108.178335

Sergeant, G. P. (2005). Regulation of Kv4.3 currents by Ca2+/calmodulin-dependent protein kinase II. *Am. J. Physiol. Cell Physiol.* 288, C304–C313. doi: 10.1152/ajpcell.00293.2004

Shamgar, L. (2006). Calmodulin is essential for cardiac IKS channel gating and assembly: impaired function in long-QT mutations. *Circ. Res.* 98, 1055–1063. doi: 10.1161/01.RES.0000218979.40770.69

Shryock, J. C., Song, Y., Rajamani, S., Antzelevitch, C., and Belardinelli, L. (2013). The arrhythmogenic consequences of increasing late INa in the cardiomyocyte. *Cardiovasc. Res.* Available at: http://cardiovascres.oxfordjournals.org/content/early/2013/07/01/cvr.cvt145.abstract (accessed December 12, 2013).

Snyders, D. J. (1999). Structure and function of cardiac potassium channels. *Cardiovasc. Res.* 42, 377–390. doi: 10.1016/S0008-6363(99)00071-1

Splawski, I., Tristani-Firouzi, M., Lehmann, M. H., Sanguinetti, M. C., and Keating, M. T. (1997). Mutations in the hminK gene cause long QT syndrome and suppress IKs function. *Nat. Genet.* 17, 338–340. doi: 10.1038/ng1197-338

Sumi. (1991). The newly synthesized selective Ca2+/calmodulin dependent protein kinase II inhibitor KN-93 reduces dopamine contents in PC12h cells. *Biochem. Biophys. Res. Commun.* 181, 968–975. doi: 10.1016/0006-291X(91)92031-E

Szuts, V., Ménesi, D., Varga-Orvos, Z., Zvara, Á., Houshmand, N., Bitay, M., et al. (2013). Altered expression of genes for Kir ion channels in dilated cardiomyopathy1. *Can. J. Physiol. Pharmacol.* 91, 648–656. doi: 10.1139/cjpp-2012-0413

Taylor, T. G., Venable, P. W., Shibayama, J., Warren, M., and Zaitsev, A. V. (2012). Role of KATP channel in electrical depression and asystole during long-duration ventricular fibrillation in ex vivo canine heart. *Am. J. Physiol. Heart Circ. Physiol.* 302, H2396–H2409. doi: 10.1152/ajpheart.00752.2011

Tessier, S. (2001). Cumulative inactivation of the outward potassium current: a likely mechanism underlying electrical memory in human atrial myocytes. *J. Mol. Cell. Cardiol.* 33, 755–767. doi: 10.1006/jmcc.2001.1345

Tessier, S., Karczewski, P., Krause, E.-G., Pansard, Y., Acar, C., Lang-Lazdunski, M., et al. (1999). Regulation of the transient outward K+ current by Ca2+/calmodulin-dependent protein kinases II in human atrial myocytes. *Circ. Res.* 85, 810–819. doi: 10.1161/01.RES.85.9.810

Tikkanen, J. T., Anttonen, O., Junttila, M. J., Aro, A. L., Kerola, T., Rissanen, H. A., et al. (2009). Long-term outcome associated with early repolarization on electrocardiography. *N. Engl. J. Med.* 361, 2529–2537. doi: 10.1056/NEJMoa0907589

Tsuboi, M., and Antzelevitch, C. (2006). Cellular basis for electrocardiographic and arrhythmic manifestations of Andersen-Tawil syndrome (LQT7). *Heart Rhythm* 3, 328–335. doi: 10.1016/j.hrthm.2005.11.026

Varga, A. W. (2004). Calcium-calmodulin-dependent kinase II modulates Kv4.2 channel expression and upregulates neuronal A-type potassium currents. *J. Neurosci.* 24, 3643–3654. doi: 10.1523/JNEUROSCI.0154-04.2004

Wagner, S., Dybkova, N., Rasenack, E. C., Jacobshagen, C., Fabritz, L., Kirchhof, P., et al. (2006). Ca/Calmodulin-dependent protein kinase II regulates cardiac Na^{+} channels. *J. Clin. Invest.* 116, 3127–3138. doi: 10.1172/JCI26620

Wagner, S., Hacker, E., Grandi, E., Weber, S. L., Dybkova, N., Sossalla, S., et al. (2009). Ca/calmodulin kinase II differentially modulates potassium currents. *Circ. Arrhythm. Electrophysiol.* 2, 285–294. doi: 10.1161/CIRCEP.108.842799

Wagner, S., Ruff, H. M., Weber, S. L., Bellmann, S., Sowa, T., Schulte, T., et al. (2011). Reactive oxygen species–activated Ca/calmodulin kinase IIδ is required for late INa augmentation leading to cellular Na and Ca overload. *Circ. Res.* 108, 555–565. doi: 10.1161/CIRCRESAHA.110.221911

Wang, Y., Cheng, J., Tandan, S., Jiang, M., McClosey, D. T., and Hill, J. A. (2006a). Transient-outward K+ channel inhibition facilitates L-type Ca2+ current in heart. *J. Cardiovasc. Electrophysiol.* 17, 298–304. doi: 10.1111/j.1540-8167.2006.00362.x

Wang, H., Yan, Y., Liu, Q., Huang, Y., Shen, Y., Chen, L., et al. (2006b). Structural basis for modulation of Kv4 K+ channels by auxiliary KChIP subunits. *Nat. Neurosci.* 10, 32–39. doi: 10.1038/nn1822

Warren, M., Guha, P. K., Berenfeld, O., Zaitsev, A., Anumonwo, J. M. B., Dhamoon, A. S., et al. (2003). Blockade of the inward rectifying potassium current terminates ventricular fibrillation in the guinea pig heart. *J. Cardiovasc. Electrophysiol.* 14, 621–631. doi: 10.1046/j.1540-8167.2003.03006.x

Weiss, J. N., Garfinkel, A., Karagueuzian, H. S., Chen, P.-S., and Qu, Z. (2010). Early afterdepolarizations and cardiac arrhythmias. *Heart Rhythm* 7, 1891–1899. doi: 10.1016/j.hrthm.2010.09.017

Wettwer, E. (2004). Role of IKur in controlling action potential shape and contractility in the human atrium: influence of chronic atrial fibrillation. *Circulation* 110, 2299–2306. doi: 10.1161/01.CIR.0000145155.60288.71

Wickenden, A. D., Lee, P., Sah, R., Huang, Q., Fishman, G. I., and Backx, P. H. (1999). Targeted expression of a dominant-negative Kv4.2 K+ channel subunit in the mouse heart. *Circ. Res.* 85, 1067–1076. doi: 10.1161/01.RES.85.11.1067

Xu, H., Guo, W., and Nerbonne, J. M. (1999). Four kinetically distinct depolarization-activated K+ currents in adult mouse ventricular myocytes. *J. Gen. Physiol.* 113, 661–678. doi: 10.1085/jgp.113.5.661

Yan, G.-X., and Antzelevitch, C. (1996). Cellular basis for the electrocardiographic J wave. *Circulation* 93, 372–379. doi: 10.1161/01.CIR.93.2.372

Zhang, R., Khoo, M. S. C., Wu, Y., Yang, Y., Grueter, C. E., Ni, G., et al. (2005). Calmodulin kinase II inhibition protects against structural heart disease. *Nat. Med.* 11, 409–417. doi: 10.1038/nm1215

Zhang, X., Szeto, C., Gao, E., Tang, M., Jin, J., Fu, Q., et al. (2012). Cardiotoxic and cardioprotective features of chronic -adrenergic signaling. *Circ. Res.* 112, 498–509. doi: 10.1161/CIRCRESAHA.112.273896

Zhao, Z., Xie, Y., Wen, H., Xiao, D., Allen, C., Fefelova, N., et al. (2012). Role of the transient outward potassium current in the genesis of early afterdepolarizations in cardiac cells. *Cardiovasc. Res.* 95, 308–316. doi: 10.1093/cvr/cvs183

Zicha, S., Xiao, L., Stafford, S., Cha, T. J., Han, W., Varro, A., et al. (2004). Transmural expression of transient outward potassium current subunits in normal and failing canine and human hearts. *J. Physiol.* 561, 735–748. doi: 10.1113/jphysiol.2004.075861

Zobel, C., Cho, H. C., Nguyen, T.-T., Pekhletski, R., Diaz, R. J., Wilson, G. J., et al. (2003). Molecular dissection of the inward rectifier potassium current (IK1) in rabbit cardiomyocytes: evidence for heteromeric co-assembly of Kir2.1 and Kir2.2. *J. Physiol.* 550, 365–372. doi: 10.1113/jphysiol.2002.036400

22

An introduction to murine models of atrial fibrillation

Genna Riley[1], Fahima Syeda[1], Paulus Kirchhof[1,2] and Larissa Fabritz[1,2]*

[1] *Centre for Cardiovascular Sciences, School of Clinical and Experimental Medicine, University of Birmingham, Birmingham, UK*
[2] *Department of Cardiology and Angiology, University Hospital Münster, Münster, Germany*

Correspondence:
Larissa Fabritz, Centre for Cardiovascular Sciences, School of Clinical and Experimental Medicine, College of Medical and Dental Sciences, University of Birmingham, Edgbaston, Birmingham B15 2TT, UK.
e-mail: l.fabritz@bham.ac.uk

Understanding the mechanism of re-entrant arrhythmias in the past 30 years has allowed the development of almost curative therapies for many rhythm disturbances. The complex, polymorphic arrhythmias of atrial fibrillation (AF) and sudden death are, unfortunately, not yet well understood, and hence still in need of adequate therapy. AF contributes markedly to morbidity and mortality in aging Western populations. In the past decade, many genetically altered murine models have been described and characterized. Here, we review genetically altered murine models of AF; powerful tools that will enable a better understanding of the mechanisms of AF and the assessment of novel therapeutic interventions.

Keywords: atrial fibrillation, atrial tachycardia, cardiac function, electrocardiogram, electrophysiology, mouse heart, murine model, sick sinus syndrome

INTRODUCTION

Atrial fibrillation (AF) affects 1–2% of the population in Europe, and this number is expected to increase twofold to threefold in the next decade, due to both an age-dependent increase in AF and an increased incidence of the arrhythmia (Camm et al., 2010). Even when treated according to best current knowledge, AF remains associated with high residual morbidity and an excess mortality (Camm et al., 2010) that calls for better understanding, diagnosis, and therapy of the arrhythmia rather than the management of symptoms alone. The considered use of animal models has facilitated the characterization of at least four positive feedback loops that contribute to the development of AF (Schotten et al., 2011). Two of these loops augment Ca^{2+} loading and alter ion channel dynamics, which result in the shortening of atrial action potential duration (APD) and focal ectopic activity. Both can be treated with anti-arrhythmic drugs and catheter ablation (Kirchhof et al., 2009) and these techniques can help prevent AF recurrence in selected patients, but the overall recurrence rate of AF remains high.

Unfortunately, some patients with AF are predisposed to recurrent arrhythmias even on such therapy. The changes that predispose the atria toward recurrence of AF have been broadly summarized as "structural remodeling". Better characterization of these processes are required to enable the identification of patients at risk of recurrence and to develop new therapies for the arrhythmia (Schotten et al., 2011; Wakili et al., 2011).

OF MICE AND MEN

There is no doubt that the best model in which to study human disease mechanisms is the patient. However, many of the molecular changes that confer AF are more pronounced in left atrial tissue (Kahr et al., 2011), which is not readily accessible in patients. Furthermore, the polygenic and multi-factorial processes that govern AF render genetically modified models attractive tools in which to dissect the molecular mechanisms of arrhythmia. Models facilitate the control of confounding factors, enable demonstration of causation rather than association and offer opportunities to validate new therapies in an experimental setting. In recent years, owing to its small size, short gestation period, rapid maturation, and the relative ease with which genetic alterations can be achieved, the mouse has become an attractive mammalian model in which to investigate a number of human conditions. Inbred murine models reduce genetic and environmental variability, enabling disease progression and the effect of genetic modifiers including gender, diet, and physical activity on pathology, to be studied in a closed, complex physiological system. Historically, cardiac arrhythmias were studied in larger mammals such as the goat, pig, or dog, as it was believed that arrhythmia did not occur in mice due to their lack of critical cardiac mass (Janse and Rosen, 2006). Furthermore, the hearts of larger mammals such as non-human primates and dogs are more akin to the human heart than rabbits or smaller rodent species (Russell and Proctor, 2006). However, the seminal and relatively recent demonstrations, disproving the theory of critical cardiac mass (Vaidya et al., 1999), have promoted the use of mice in the study of cardiac arrhythmias. There is considerable genetic homology between humans and mice and this is reflected in the conservation of cardiac developmental pathways, morphological structure, and signaling pathways. There are however, inevitable differences between the murine and human heart: the murine heart rate is up to 10 times faster than that of the human heart and the murine APD is shorter and lacks the typical plateau phase (Fabritz et al., 2003). Yet the relationship between electrical diastole and APD in the mouse is comparable with that of humans. In summary, whilst the mouse provides an excellent model system for primary investigation, molecular underpinnings, and proof of principle strategies, all findings need to be confirmed in other animal models and *in vitro* systems prior to considering clinical application.

MURINE MODELS OF ATRIAL FIBRILLATION

In terms of cardiac assessment, the pipelines of large-scale phenotyping consortia are usually limited to the analysis of blood chemistry, the assessment of heart weight relative to tibial length and the assessment of left ventricular function which, whilst good indicators of cardiac dysfunction, will no doubt often fail to identify an arrhythmic phenotype. Electrocardiograms (ECGs) in lightly sedated and freely roaming mice can be used to diagnose atrial arrhythmias. To study electrophysiological mechanisms of atrial arrhythmias, the use of isolated, beating, perfused hearts have been invaluable. These can be subjected to catheter-based recording of electrograms and action potentials; to electrical stimulation and other arrhythmia provocation techniques, and can be used in conjunction with optical mapping to visualize membrane potential and calcium transients (Eloff et al., 2001; Mathur et al., 2009). These techniques, first developed to study ventricular arrhythmias in mice, have more recently been adapted to study atrial arrhythmias as well (de Diego et al., 2008; Lang et al., 2011). There has been a recent increase in the number of murine models reported to harbor atrial arrhythmias, some of which have been reviewed before (Schotten et al., 2011; Wakili et al., 2011). In this review, murine models were grouped according to the molecular signaling pathway with which they have been most associated as follows: alterations in: G-protein coupled receptor (GPCR) signaling; ion channel dynamics, anchoring, and junctional complexes, calcium homeostasis; transcriptional, post transcriptional, and epigenetic regulation; cytokines and growth factors. In this review we have provided a simplified schematic depicting the position of these murine models both within the context of previously established molecular signaling pathways of atrial arrhythmia and subcellular compartment (**Figure 1**). We have also generated a tabulated list of murine models in which AF or a surrogate parameter was reported (**Table 1**). The table indicates whether structural atrial changes were found and gives an idea of whether AF occurred spontaneously under free roaming conditions, under anesthesia, or was provoked during programmed stimulation.

In the following text we will highlight several of these models to exemplify the complex and divergent changes that can result in

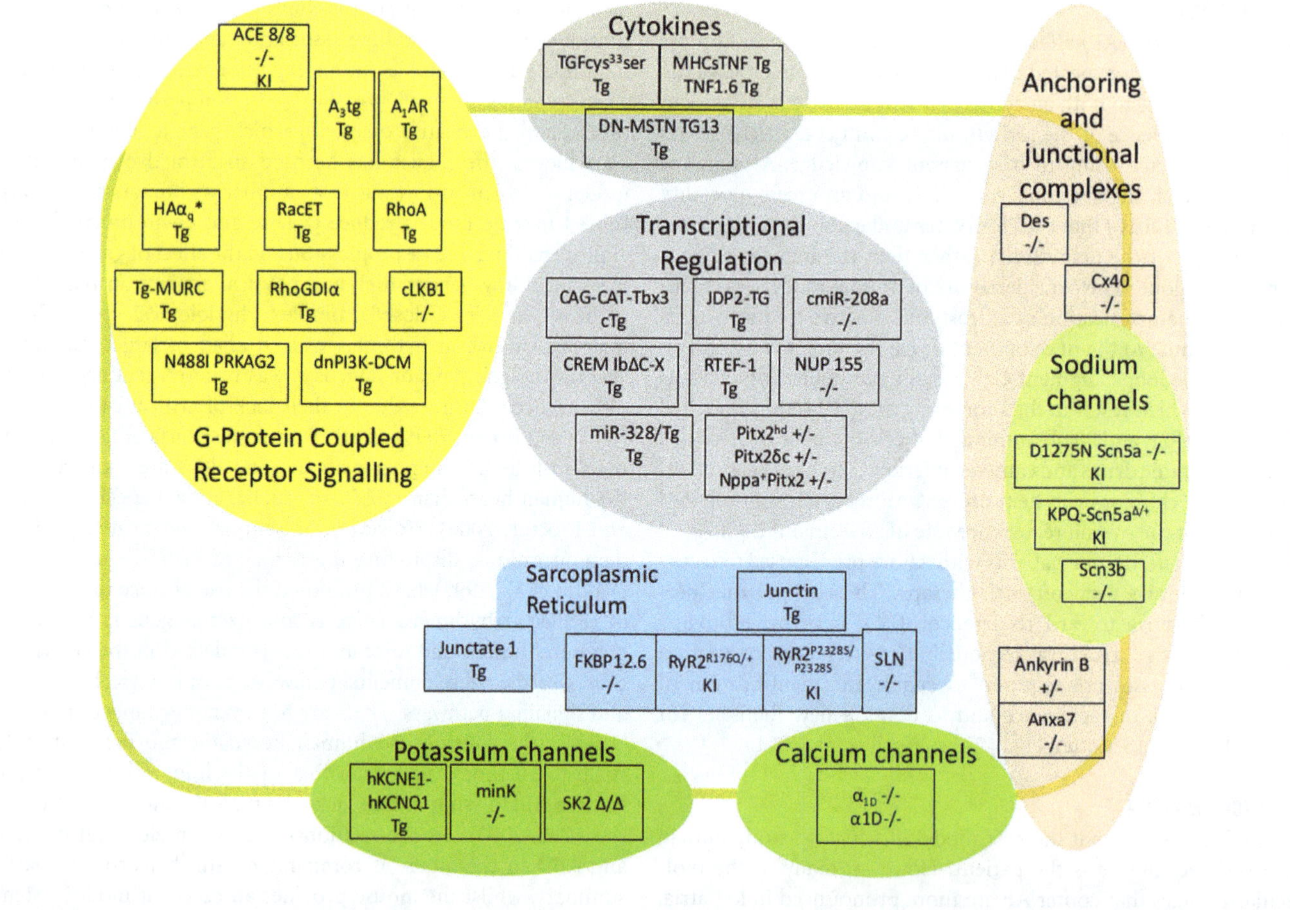

FIGURE 1 | Murine Models of Atrial Fibrillation. Schematic diagram depicting murine models of atrial arrhythmia within the context of arrhythmic signaling pathway and subcellular localization. Models were subdivided into altered G-Protein Coupled Receptor signaling; altered ion channels dynamics, anchoring, and junctional complexes; altered calcium homeostasis; altered transcriptional, post transcriptional, and epigenetic regulators; and cytokines and growth factors. The genotype of knockout models associated with atrial fibrillation is provided; knockin models are followed by the suffix (KI), and transgenic models by the suffix (Tg). A brief description of each model, the experimental circumstances used to elicit AF and references can be found within **Table 1**.

Table 1 | Murine Models of Atrial Fibrillation.

Mouse mutant	Description of transgenic (promoter)	Increased AT/AF telemetric ECG	Increased AT/AF in sedated mice	Increased AT/AF in EP study	AVB	Conduction	A APD	A ERP	Contractile function	Atrial dilation	Atrial thrombi	Atrial fibrosis	Reference
ALTERED G-PROTEIN COUPLED RECEPTOR SIGNALING													
ACE 8/8$^{-/-}$ (KI)	Knockin mutant of α*Mhc* promoter at angiotensin I converting enzyme locus (α*Mhc*)	✓			✓				V=	✓		✓	Xiao et al. (2004)
A_1AR (Tg)	Transgenic mutant overexpressing adenosine A1 receptor (α*Mhc*)			✓	✓		=		=	×			Matherne et al. (1997), Kirchhof et al. (2003)
A_3tg (Tg)	Transgenic mutant overexpressing adenosine A3 receptor (α*Mhc*)			✓	✓				↓	✓		✓	Black et al. (2002), Fabritz et al. (2004)
HAα_q*(Tg)	Transgenic mutant overexpressing constitutively active Gαq (α*Mhc*)	✓	✓	✓	✓	✓	↑		↓	✓	✓	✓	Mende et al. (1998), Hirose et al. (2009), Laakmann et al. (2010)
RhoA (Tg)	Transgenic mutant overexpressing constitutively active Rho A (α*Mhc*)		✓		✓				↓	✓		✓	Sah et al. (1999)
RhoGDIα (Tg)	Transgenic mutant overexpressing bovine Rho GDP dissociation inhibitor α (α*Mhc*)		✓		✓			↑	**V**=	✓		×	Wei et al. (2004)
RacET (Tg)	Transgenic mutant overexpressing constitutively active Rac1 (α*Mhc*)		✓	✓	✓	✓	=	=	↓	✓		✓	Sussman et al. (2000), Adam et al. (2007), Reil et al. (2010)
cLKB1$^{-/-}$	Conditional knockout of serine/threonine kinase 11 using α*Mhc-cre.*		✓						↓	✓	✓	✓	Bardeesy et al. (2002), Ikeda et al. (2009)
Tg-MURC (Tg)	Transgenic mutant overexpressing muscle-related coiled-coil protein (α*Mhc*)		✓		✓				↓	✓	✓	✓	Ogata et al. (2008)
N488I PRKAG2 (Tg)	Transgenic mutant overexpressing human protein kinase AMP-activated gamma 2 subunit carrying N488I mutation (α*Mhc*)	✓			×	×			V↓	✓			Arad et al. (2003)
dnPI3K-DCM (Tg)	Double transgenic mutant overexpressing dominant negative phosphatidyl inositol 3 kinase lacking kinase activity and overexpression of macrophage stimulating 1 (both α*Mhc*)	✓	✓		✓				↓	✓	✓	✓	Pretorius et al. (2009)
ALTERED ION CHANNEL DYNAMICS, ANCHORING, AND JUNCTIONAL COMPLEXES AND CALCIUM HOMEOSTASIS													
Potassium channels													
minK$^{-/-}$	Systemic knockout of the KCNE1 (minK) potassium channel	✓		✓		✓	↓		=				Kupershmidt et al. (1999), Temple et al. (2005)
SK2 $^{\Delta/\Delta}$	Systemic knockout of the SK2 potassium channel			✓	✓		↑	=	=				Bond et al. (2004), Li et al. (2009)
hKCNE1-hKCNQ1 (Tg)	Transgenic mutant overexpressing hKCNE1-hKCNQ1 fusion protein (α*Mhc*)			✓		=	↓	=	=				Marx et al. (2002), Chiello Tracy et al. (2003), Sampson et al. (2008)

(Continued)

Table 1 | Continued

Mouse mutant	Description of transgenic (promoter)	Increased AT/AF telemetric ECG	Increased AT/AF in sedated mice	Increased AT/AF in EP study	AVB	Conduction	A APD	A ERP	Contractile function	Atrial dilation	Atrial thrombi	Atrial fibrosis	Reference
Sodium channels													
Scn5a$^{\Delta/+}$ (KI)	Knockin mutant expressing Scn5a sodium channel subunit with 1505-KPQ-1507 deletion			✓	✓	✓	↑	↑	=	✓	×	×	Nuyens et al. (2001), Dautova et al. (2009), Guzadhur et al. (2010), Blana et al. (2010)
Scn3b$^{-/-}$	Systemic knockout of Scn3b sodium channel subunit			✓	✓		↓						Hakim et al. (2008), Hakim et al. (2010)
D1275N Scn5a$^{-/-}$ (KI)	Knockin mutant expressing Scn5a sodium channel subunit with D1275N mutation		✓		✓	✓	↑		V↓				Watanabe et al. (2011)
Anchoring and junctional complexes													
Des$^{-/-}$	Systemic knockout of desmin			✓	=	✓		↓				✓	Li et al. (1996), Milner et al. (1996), Schrickel et al. (2010)
Cx40$^{-/-}$	Systemic knockout of connexin40			✓	✓	↓		↑					Kirchhoff et al. (1998), Hagendorff et al. (1999), Verheule (1999)
Ankyrin$_B$±	Systemic knockout of ankyrin2			✓			↓						Scotland et al. (1998), Cunha et al. (2011)
Altered calcium homeostasis													
α1D$^{-/-}$	Systemic knockout of the α1D subunit of the L-type Ca^{2+} channel		✓	✓	✓	↓	=			×			Platzer et al. (2000), Mancarella et al. (2008)
$\alpha_{1D}{}^{-/-}$	Systemic knockout of the α1D subunit of the L-type Ca^{2+} channel			✓	✓		↑	=					Namkung et al. (2001), Zhang et al. (2002a), Zhang et al. (2005)
SLN$^{-/-}$	Systemic knockout of sarcolipin		✓				↑		A/V↑			✓	Babu et al. (2007a), Xie et al. (2012)
RyR2$^{R176Q/+}$ (KI)	Knockin mutant expressing ryanodine receptor 2 carrying R176Q mutation			✓		=	=	=		×		×	Chelu et al. (2009)
RyR2$^{P2328S/P2328S}$ (KI)	Knockin mutant expressing Ryanodine Receptor 2 carrying P2328S mutation			✓		=	=	=					Goddard et al. (2008), Zhang et al. (2011)
FKBP12.6$^{-/-}$	Systemic knockout of FK506 binding protein 12.6			✓		=		=		×		×	Wehrens et al. (2003), Sood et al. (2008), Li et al. (2012)
Junctate 1 (Tg)	Transgenic mutant overexpressing Junctate 1 (α*Mhc*)		✓						↓	✓	✓	✓	Hong et al. (2008)
Junctin (Tg)	Transgenic mutant overexpressing canine junctin (α*Mhc*)		✓				↑		↓	✓	✓	✓	Hong et al. (2002), Kirchhefer et al. (2004)
Anxa7$^{-/-}$	Systemic knockout of annexin Aa7			✓	✓			=	=				Herr et al. (2001), Schrickel et al. (2007)

(Continued)

Table 1 | Continued

Mouse mutant	Description of transgenic (promoter)	Increased AT/AF telemetric ECG	Increased AT/AF in sedated mice	Increased AT/AF in EP study	AVB	Conduction	A APD	A ERP	Contractile function	Atrial dilation	Atrial thrombi	Atrial fibrosis	Reference
ALTERED TRANSCRIPTIONAL, POST TRANSCRIPTIONAL, AND EPIGENETIC REGULATORS													
CREM-IbΔC-X (Tg)	Transgenic mutant expressing human cardiac CREM isoform (α*Mhc*)	✓	✓	✓	✓		↑		V ↑ A ↓	✓	✓		Müller et al. (2005), Kirchhof et al. (2011a)
miR-328/Tg (Tg)	Transgenic mutant overexpressing premiR-328 (α*Mhc*)		✓				↓				✓		Lu et al. (2010)
cmiR-208a$^{-/-}$	Conditional knockout of miR-208a using β*Actn-cre*		✓						↓				Callis et al. (2009)
Pitx2 δc$^{+/-}$	Systemic knockout of Pitx2c isoform			✓	=		↓		=	×			Liu et al. (2002), Kirchhof et al. (2011b)
Pitx2$^{hd+/-}$	Systemic knockout of Pitx2			✓									Lu et al. (1999), Wang et al. (2010)
Nppa^{+} Pitx2$^{-/-}$	Conditional knockout of Pitx2 using *Nppa-cre*									✓			Gage et al. (1999), Chinchilla et al. (2011)
cTg-CAG-CAT-Tbx3 (Tg)	Conditional transgenic overexpressing human T-box 3 crossed to *Nppa-cre*		✓		✓							✓	Hoogaars et al. (2007)
NUP155$^{+/-}$	Systemic knockout of nucleoporin 155	✓								×			Zhang et al. (2008)
JDP-Tg (Tet-JDP2/α-MHC-tTA)$^{+/-}$	Tetracycline-regulated overexpression of Jun dimerization protein 2 using α*Mhc-tTA*		✓		✓	↓			=	✓		×	Kehat et al. (2006)
RTEF-1 (Tg)	Transgenic mutant overexpressing human TEA domain family member 4 (α*Mhc*)	✓	✓	✓	✓	↓				✓	✓		Chen et al. (2004)
Cytokines/Growth Factors													
MHC-TGFcys^{33}ser (Tg)	Transgenic mutant overexpressing human TGF-beta 1 carrying C33S mutation (α*Mhc*)			✓	✓		=	=		×		✓	Nakajima et al. (2000), Verheule et al. (2004), Choi et al. (2012)
MHCsTNF (Tg)	Transgenic mutant overexpressing tumor necrosis factor (α*Mhc*)		✓	✓	✓			↑		✓			Li et al. (2000), Sivasubramanian et al. (2001), Sawaya et al. (2007)
TNF1.6 (Tg)	Transgenic mutant overexpressing tumor necrosis factor (α*Mhc*)	✓		✓	✓		=		A ↓	✓	✓	✓	Kubota et al. (1997), Saba et al. (2005)
DN-MSTN TG13 (Tg)	Transgenic mutant overexpressing inhibitory N-terminal pro-peptide (α*Mhc*)		✓	✓	✓				=/↑	✓		✓	Rosenberg et al. (2012)

Murine models of AF were divided into five categories: Altered G-Protein Coupled signaling; altered ion channel dynamics, anchoring, and junctional complexes, altered calcium homeostasis; altered transcriptional, post transcriptional, and epigenetic regulators; cytokines and growth factors. Models were identified via a publication search on Pubmed using the terms "mouse atrial arrhythmia." This returned a total of 351 hits all which were then individually screened for relevance in terms of: spontaneous atrial tachycardia and/or fibrillation (AT/AF) during telemetric or sedated analysis; increased induced occurrence of atrial tachycardia and/or fibrillation (AT/AF) in electrophysiology (EP) studies; atrial ventricular block (AVB) including PQ/PR prolongation as AVBI; effect on atrial conduction (direct and indirect); effect on atrial action potential duration (APD); effect on atrial effective refractory period (ERP); effect on contractile function refractory period, ERP; contractile function (V-ventricular, A-atrial); presence of atrial dilation; atrial thrombi, and atrial fibrosis. ✓ indicates presence of that condition, × indicates absence of the condition, unticked boxes do not necessarily mean that a condition has been completely ruled out for a given model, only that there is no evidence as yet. =, unaltered. References are shown in the right hand column. The first reference for each model describes the generation of that model.

murine AF. We hope that understanding mechanisms of arrhythmia in such models will further our understanding and treatment of AF in humans.

MODELS OF AF WITH ALTERED G-PROTEIN COUPLED RECEPTOR SIGNALING

Systemically, GPCRs are involved in extracellular-intracellular signaling and underpin a wide variety of biological responses (Neer, 1994; Park et al., 2004). The most commonly studied GPCRs in the heart include the adrenergic, angiotensin, endothelin, and adenosine receptors (Salazar et al., 2007).

ANGIOTENSIN II

The role of renin-angiotensin signaling within cardiac pathological states, particularly in regard to blood pressure, is well documented. However, there is increasing evidence that angiotensin II exerts a more local stimulatory effect on heart function (Sancho et al., 1976; Lindpaintner et al., 1988; De Mello and Frohlich, 2011). Furthermore, atrial angiotensin II expression levels are increased in patients with AF (Boldt et al., 2003; Cong et al., 2010; De Jong et al., 2011). *In vitro*, rapid pacing of atrial myocytes increased the paracrine secretion of angiotensin II (Tsai et al., 2011), suggesting that fibrillation promotes angiotensin II production and therefore signaling. Cardiac-specific overexpression of angiotensin I converting enzyme (ACE), a peptidase that converts angiotensin I to its biologically active counterpart, angiotensin II, in mice, resulted in atrial dilation, fibrosis, and spontaneous AF under free roaming conditions (Xiao et al., 2004), suggesting that increased angiotensin II signaling promotes the development of AF. Yet, cardiac-specific overexpression of the angiotensin receptor AT_{1a} caused marked atrial enlargement, bradycardia, and abnormal atrio-ventricular (AV) conduction, but failed to increase AF susceptibility in neonatal mice (Hein et al., 1997).

ADENOSINE RECEPTORS

Adenosine receptors are a type of purinergic G-Protein coupled receptor, activated by adenosine, that have an inhibitory effect on adenlyl cyclase signaling (and therefore cAMP levels) and voltage-gated ion channels, whilst concomitantly activating potassium channels (Priori et al., 1993; Headrick et al., 2011). Short-term adenosine A1 receptor (A_1AR) stimulation induces bradycardia and AV block in humans (DiMarco et al., 1983). Transgenic models of adenosine A1 and A3 receptors were developed primarily to evaluate the protective effect of receptor overexpression on myocardial ischemia (Matherne et al., 1997). However, enhanced expression of either A1 or A3 adenosine receptors also provoked atrial bradycardia and AV block and increased susceptibility to AF dependent on the degree of bradycardia ("tachycardia-bradycardia syndrome"; Kirchhof et al., 2003; Fabritz et al., 2004), that could potentially lead to bradycardiomyopathy (Fabritz et al., 2004). Therefore, increased cAMP levels (as shown by this model and that of ACE overexpression) appear to contribute to the development of AF.

GALPHA Q

Heterotrimeric G-proteins are membrane-associated complexes that comprise an alpha, beta, and gamma subunit and are the intracellular effectors of GPCRs (Neer, 1994; Park et al., 2004; Salazar et al., 2007). In the heart, Gαq associates with alpha1-adrenergic, endothelin (ET_A), and angiotensin II type I (AT_1) receptors. Following ligand activation, Gαq is phosphorylated which results in the activation of numerous downstream effectors including phospholipase C (PLC), protein kinase C (PKC), thymoma viral protein-oncogene (Akt), and Ras homologous (Rho; Salazar et al., 2007; Filtz et al., 2009; Ben-Ami et al., 2011; Pfreimer et al., 2012). To investigate the putative role of Gαq in cardiac hypertrophy, two transgenic mouse lines overexpressing endogenous and a constitutively active *Gαq* subunit under the control of the *αMhc* promoter were independently generated (D'Angelo et al., 1997; Mende et al., 1998). Both models developed cardiac hypertrophy in the absence of myocyte disarray or necrosis, followed by diffuse atrial and ventricular fibrosis and heart failure (D'Angelo et al., 1997; Mende et al., 1998; Hirose et al., 2009). A number of these mice developed left atrial thrombi, another pathological characteristic associated with AF (Mende et al., 1998; Laakmann et al., 2010), and indeed, AF was recorded as occurring spontaneously under roaming conditions (Hirose et al., 2009). Similar to the Ras homolog gene family member A (*RhoA*) overexpression model discussed below, there is recent evidence to suggest that in this model, AF may be a primary pathology within its own right that does not occur secondary to ventricular remodeling (Sah et al., 1999; Laakmann et al., 2010).

RAS HOMOLOG GENE FAMILY MEMBER A

Initially identified for its role within hypertrophic signaling pathways (Sah et al., 1996), RHOA is a small membrane-associated GTPase involved in actin cytoskeleton organization (Ridley and Hall, 1992). Mice overexpressing either wild type RHOA or an activated form of RHOA under the control of the cardiac-specific *αMhc* promoter died prematurely and developed cardiac enlargement, cellular hypertrophy, interstitial fibrosis, and heart failure (Sah et al., 1999). Atrial enlargement was more pronounced than ventricular enlargement, suggesting atrial dilation preceded ventricular dilation, which is consistent with the reported temporal cardiac expression profile of *αMhc* (Chizzonite et al., 1982; Sweeney et al., 1985; Bouvagnet et al., 1987; Colbert et al., 1997). Electrocardiography (ECG) performed under anesthesia was indicative of AF and AV block (Sah et al., 1999).

More recently overexpression of RhoGDIα, an endogenous specific GDP dissociation inhibitor for all Rho family proteins, led to atrial arrhythmias and mild ventricular hypertrophy (Wei et al., 2004). ECG and intracardiac electrophysiological analysis showed these mice developed bradycardia, AV block, and atrial arrhythmias concomitant with reduced expression of the gap junction protein, connexin 40, before the onset of cardiac hypertrophy and heart failure (Wei et al., 2004). Taken together these murine models suggest that altered expression levels of Rho family proteins can propagate a pro-arrhythmic environment.

Rac1

Rat sarcoma (RAS)-related C3 botulinum toxin substrate 1 (Rac1) has long been recognized for its role in actin cytoskeleton organization, and is a plasma membrane-associated GTPase belonging to the RAS superfamily (Ridley and Hall, 1992; Sussman et al., 2000). Homozygous mice overexpressing constitutively active *Rac1* under the control of the *αMhc* promoter were found to be viable

(Chizzonite et al., 1982). However, a proportion of progeny died within 2 weeks of birth owing to increased postnatal α*Mhc* promoter activity as a result of increased circulating levels of thyroid hormone (Chizzonite et al., 1982; Sussman et al., 2000). Mice surviving this initial vulnerable period achieved survival comparable with that of wild type (Sussman et al., 2000), but by 2 months of age, mutants developed atrial enlargement and atrial wall thinning juxtaposed to ventricular wall thickening and reduced ventricular chamber size (Sussman et al., 2000). Interstitial fibrosis and systolic heart failure progressively developed and 75% of the transgenic mice developed spontaneous AF under anesthesia (Adam et al., 2007).

OTHER MODELS OF ALTERED GPCR SIGNALING

Several other murine models of AF have been generated by the genetic manipulation of other proteins within GPCR signaling cascades using α*Mhc* promoter-driven expression. Briefly, models reported to develop spontaneous AF under anesthesia include a knockout of serine/threonine kinase 11 (Stk11/Lkb1; Bardeesy et al., 2002; Ikeda et al., 2009; Pretorius et al., 2009); a transgenic mouse overexpressing Muscle-Related Coiled-Coil protein (MURC1; Ogata et al., 2008) and a transgenic mouse overexpressing human protein kinase AMP-activated gamma 2 subunit (PRKAG2) carrying the N488I mutation (Arad et al., 2003). A double transgenic mutant overexpressing dominant negative phosphatidyl inositol 3 kinase and macrophage stimulating 1 (Mst1) was also reported to develop spontaneous AF during telemetry (Pretorius et al., 2009).

MODELS OF AF WITH ALTERED ION CHANNEL DYNAMICS, ANCHORING, AND JUNCTIONAL COMPLEXES AND CALCIUM HOMEOSTASIS

ION CHANNEL DYNAMICS

Potassium channels

Potassium ion channels remove K^+ from the cell defining the repolarization phase of the action potential. Therefore, any genetic modification that alters the expression levels or gating of potassium channels has the potential to alter the cardiac action potential and thereby act as an arrhythmic substrate. Models include: the systemic knockout of the small conductance calcium-activated potassium channel (SK2) which increased susceptibility to AF induction (Bond et al., 2004; Li et al., 2009), and the systemic knockout of the voltage-gated subfamily E member 1 potassium channel (KCNE1) which resulted in spontaneous AF under telemetry (Kupershmidt et al., 1999; Temple et al., 2005).

Sodium channels

SCN5A. Sodium currents are responsible for the rapid depolarization of myocytes and are important for conduction, repolarization, and refractoriness. Similar to potassium channel disruption, several animal models in which sodium channel dynamics have been altered develop AF. *SCN5A* encodes the alpha subunit of the cardiac voltage-gated sodium channel (Nav1.5; Gellens et al., 1992). Mutations within *SCN5A* underlie a number of clinically defined arrhythmias including long QT syndrome type 3 (LQT3), Brugada syndrome, progressive conduction disease, and AF (Ruan et al., 2010; Wilde and Brugada, 2011) and many of these diseases harbor a propensity for atrial arrhythmias (Eckardt et al., 2001; Zellerhoff et al., 2009).

Systemic targeted disruption of *Scn5a* results in homozygous lethality whilst heterozygotes display a 50% reduction in sodium conductance (Papadatos et al., 2002). A knockin murine model, Scn5a Δ1505-1507 KPQ (ΔKPQ-Scn5a), of a human mutation in which three amino acids within the inactivation domain of Nav1.5 were deleted, resulted in a persistent inward Na^+ current thus delaying the repolarization of the action potential and causing longer QT intervals (Wang et al., 1996; Nuyens et al., 2001; Head et al., 2005). ECG recorded by telemetry and under anesthesia revealed that heterozygous mice mimic the long QT syndrome 3 phenotype found in patients (Nuyens et al., 2001). More recently, atrial electrophysiology was assessed in ΔKPQ-Scn5a mutant mice. Concurrent with ventricular action potentials, atrial action potentials were also prolonged (Dautova et al., 2009; Blana et al., 2010). ΔKPQ-Scn5a mice were more susceptible to atrial arrhythmias induced by maneuvers known to provoke torsades de pointes, namely short-long-short stimulation sequences (Blana et al., 2010). Aged ΔKPQ-Scn5a mice were reported to be more susceptible to atrial arrhythmias induced by programmed stimulation (Guzadhur et al., 2010), and have altered sinoatrial node function and intra-atrial conduction (Head et al., 2005; Wu et al., 2012).

Analysis of another knockin murine model, homozygous for the human D1275N mutation (Groenewegen et al., 2003; Remme et al., 2006), reported slowed conduction, atrial arrhythmias, sinus node dysfunction, and progressive AV block, that culminated in sudden death at around 12 weeks of age (Watanabe et al., 2011). Mutations within other accessory subunits of the cardiac sodium channel also affect channel dynamics; homozygous deletion of the beta subunit, *SCN3B*, led to conduction disturbances, bradycardia, and an increased susceptibility to induced atrial arrhythmias (Hakim et al., 2008, 2010; Olesen et al., 2011).

ANCHORING AND JUNCTIONAL COMPLEXES

Connexins

The cardiac voltage sodium channel, Nav1.5, was shown to colocalize with Connexin 43 within the intercalated disk of ventricular cardiomyocytes (Maier et al., 2002). The gap junction proteins Connexin 40 (Cx40, GJA5) and Connexin 43 (Cx43, GJA1) function to electrically couple cardiomyocytes, facilitating syncytial contraction. Cx40 and Cx43 are expressed at equal levels in atria however, only Cx43 is expressed in the ventricles (Lin et al., 2010). Both mutations in *CX40* and *CX43* have been reported in patients with idiopathic AF (Gollob et al., 2006; Thibodeau et al., 2010). Cardiac-specific loss of Cx43 and overexpression of a dominant negative mutant of Cx43 led to the development of spontaneous ventricular arrhythmias (Hong et al., 2008; Sood et al., 2008; Li et al., 2012), consistent with a predominating ventricular role in the mouse. However, systemic loss of Cx40 (or GJA5) in the mouse resulted in an increased propensity to induced atrial arrhythmias and reduced conduction velocity (Kirchhoff et al., 1998; Hagendorff et al., 1999; Verheule, 1999). Furthermore, loss/redistribution of Cx40 appears to be a common feature of other murine models of AF including overexpression of RHOA, overexpression of constitutively active RAC1, cardiac-specific overexpression of ACE, overexpression of Tumor necrosis factor (TNF), and cardiac overexpression of cAMP Response element modulator (CREM; Sah et al., 1999; Kasi et al., 2007; Sawaya et al., 2007; Adam et al., 2010; Kirchhof et al., 2011a; see **Table 1** and **Figure 1** for further details).

Recent evidence suggests that in the heart of higher vertebrates, the protein complexes that traditionally comprise the cell–cell junctions of the adherens junctions and desmosomes of epithelial cells, actually coordinate to form a single heterogeneous junction referred to as the area composita (Borrmann et al., 2006; Franke et al., 2006). Loss of desmin, an intermediate filament that selectively associates with desmosomal complexes, has been reported to lead to atrial fibrosis and increased susceptibility to AF induction (Li et al., 1996; Milner et al., 1996; Schrickel et al., 2010). Hence, disrupted cell–cell mechanical coupling may also act as a substrate for AF.

Ankyrin B

The ankyrin family are membrane-associated adaptor proteins that serve to link membrane-associated proteins with the cytoskeleton (Bennett and Gilligan, 1993; Li et al., 1993). Loss of function of Ankyrin B (ANK2) is associated with long QT syndrome and sudden cardiac death in humans and mice (Mohler et al., 2003). Previously, ankyrin B was shown to regulate cardiac sodium channels dynamics (Chauhan et al., 2000), Na/K ATPase, Na/Ca exchanger 1, and inositol triphosphate (InsP3; Mohler et al., 2005). Loss of ankyrin B was reported to increase cardiac Na^{+} channel opening times, increasing APD (Chauhan et al., 2000). Recent evidence suggests that disrupted ankyrin B function is a predisposing factor for the development of atrial arrhythmias in humans (Cunha et al., 2011). Mice heterozygous for ankyrin B were reported to develop spontaneous atrial arrhythmias under telemetry and ECG studies showed increased susceptibility to AF induction by pacing (Cunha et al., 2011). In the same work, ankyrin B was shown to bind to the alpha 1C subunit of the L-type Ca^{2+} channel (Cav1.2) and loss of ankyrin B resulted in reduced inward Ca^{2+} current and a shortened APD (Cunha et al., 2011). Hence, it would appear that ankyrin B regulates both Na^{+} and Ca^{2+} currents and that disruption of ankyrin B perturbed these currents and lead to spontaneous AF.

CALCIUM HOMEOSTASIS

The voltage-dependent L-type Ca^{2+} channel contributes to the late depolarizing currents of the cardiac action potential. Comprising five subunits in total, the alpha subunit of the L-type Ca^{2+} channel is the transmembrane spanning subunit. In the heart, the alpha 1d subunit (Cav1.3) is exclusively expressed in the atria (Zhang et al., 2005), where it plays an important role in the spontaneous diastolic depolarization of pacemaker cells (Zhang et al., 2002a). Systemic deletion of Cav1.3 rendered mice susceptible to AF induction (Zhang et al., 2005; Mancarella et al., 2008).

Calcium homeostasis is important in the maintenance of normal sinus rhythm and contraction: Ca^{2+} induced Ca^{2+} release is the mainstay of mechanoelectrical coupling, clearance of Ca^{2+} from the cytosol significantly contributes to the late depolarizing currents of the cardiac action potential and Ca^{2+} acts as a secondary messenger within many intracellular signaling pathways. Therefore, any genetic modification that alters the expression levels or gating of calcium channels; or modifies signaling cascades in which Ca^{2+} features as a secondary messenger, has the potential to act as an arrhythmogenic substrate. Previous reviews of AF models have focused on calcium homeostasis therefore, we will only mention them briefly (Schotten et al., 2011; Wakili et al., 2011).

Murine models with mutations in the ryanodine receptor and associated proteins are reported to be susceptible to AF (see **Table 1**). Models include: mice carrying the human mutation, R176Q, within the outward Ca^{2+} channel of the sarcoplasmic reticulum, ryanodine receptor 2 (RyR2; Chelu et al., 2009); mice carrying the human mutation, P2328S, within RyR2 (Goddard et al., 2008; Zhang et al., 2011); systemic deletion of the RyR2 binding protein, FKBP12.6 (Wehrens et al., 2003; Sood et al., 2008; Li et al., 2012); cardiac-specific overexpression of the Ca^{2+} binding protein, junctate 1 (Hong et al., 2002, 2008); cardiac-specific overexpression of the sarcoplasmic transmembrane protein, junctin (Hong et al., 2002; Kirchhof et al., 2007), and systemic deletion of the Ca^{2+}- and GTP-dependent membrane-associated protein, annexin Aa7 (Anxa7; Herr et al., 2001; Schrickel et al., 2007). Of note, spontaneous AF was observed in mice with a 29-fold overexpression of junctin, whereas mice with 10-fold overexpression showed only reduced adaption of heart rate to stress (Hong et al., 2002; Kirchhof et al., 2007).

Sarcolipin (SLN) is a transmembrane protein located within the sarcoplasmic reticulum that like phospholamban, is a key regulator of sarcoplasmic reticulum Ca^{2+} ATPase (SERCA) function (Odermatt et al., 1998; Asahi et al., 2003; Minamisawa et al., 2003; Babu et al., 2007a; Bhupathy et al., 2009). However, unlike phospholamban, SLN activity is mediated by calcium-calmodulin dependent protein kinase II (CaMKII), not protein kinase A (PKA; Bhupathy et al., 2009). At low Ca^{2+} concentrations, SLN inhibits SERCA, reducing its affinity for Ca^{2+} which has the effect of slowing Ca^{2+} uptake into the sarcoplasmic reticulum, reducing contractility (reduced force generation and speed of relaxation; Tupling et al., 2002). Reduced levels of SLN mRNA and protein expression are associated with chronic AF in humans (Uemura et al., 2004; Shanmugam et al., 2011). Aged homozygous SLN knockout mice (Babu et al., 2007b) were reported to develop atrial fibrosis and spontaneous AF under anesthesia (Xie et al., 2012), suggesting that increased SERCA function promotes AF.

MODELS OF AF WITH ALTERED TRANSCRIPTIONAL, POST TRANSCRIPTIONAL, AND EPIGENETIC REGULATION

Dysregulation of GPCR signaling, ion channel dynamics, and calcium homeostasis have long been associated with the development and maintenance of AF however, the net effect of these pathways upon transcription and the contribution of transcriptional, post transcriptional, and epigenetic dysregulation to AF are less well understood. This represents a rapidly expanding area of AF research and it is here, within this category, the majority of the more recently described animal models of AF reside.

cAMP RESPONSE ELEMENT MODULATOR

cAMP Response element modulator belongs to the cAMP response element binding (CREB)/activating transcription factors (ATF) family of transcription factors and is a phosphorylation target of PKA. Cardiac-directed expression of CREM-IbΔC-X, a human cardiac CREM repressor isoform, resulted in both atrial and ventricular enlargement, atrial wall thinning, atrial thrombus formation, disturbed myocyte architecture, and increased basal left ventricular function (Müller et al., 2005). Echocardiography analysis revealed that atrial chamber dilation preceded the development of AF (Kirchhof et al., 2011a). In addition to reduced wall thickness, atrial myocytes were elongated and atrial weight increased, while neither cellular hypertrophy nor fibrosis were found (Kirchhof et al., 2011a). Telemetric ECG indicated that mutants suffered from atrial ectopies, the occurrence of which increased with age until mice entered an almost constant state of atrial tachycardia (Kirchhof et al., 2011a). Reduced phosphorylation of CREM (due to overexpression of CREM-IbΔC-X) was associated with altered Ca^{2+} homeostasis concurrent with spontaneous Ca^{2+} release and reduced gap junction protein expression (CX40; Kirchhof et al., 2011a). CREM transcription factors bind to the cAMP response element found within several promoters (Foulkes et al., 1991). Whilst many of the genetic targets of CREM involved in spermatogenesis have been identified (Kosir et al., 2012), cardiac-specific gene targets remain largely unknown and are subject to current studies.

PITX2c

The paired-like homeodomain transcription factor 2 (Pitx2) is a downstream target of Nodal within the transforming growth factor beta (TGFβ) signaling pathway and was primarily recognized as having a role in establishing left-right asymmetry during embryonic development (Meno et al., 1998; Ryan et al., 1998). The highest Pitx2 isoform expressed in the murine and human heart is Pitx2c (Kitamura et al., 1999; Schweickert et al., 2000). Systemic loss of Pitx2c in mice lead to embryonic lethality and resulted in a number of phenotypes including abnormal cardiac morphogenesis (Gage et al., 1999). During embryogenesis, Pitx2c was shown to synergistically drive expression of natriuretic peptide A (*Nppa*) in the presence of the homeobox transcription factor, *Nkx2.5* (Ganga et al., 2003) which in turn, suppressed the expression of the pacemaker channel gene, *Hcn4*, and the T-box transcription factor (*Tbx3*), gene, thus delineating contractile atrial myocardium from the sinoatrial node (Hoogaars et al., 2007; Mommersteeg et al., 2007).

Genome-wide association studies (GWAS) identified sequence variation within 4q25 as conferring increased susceptibility to AF (Schott et al., 1995; Gudbjartsson et al., 2007; Kääb et al., 2009). Hence, owing to its genomic location within this candidate region, *PITX2* was considered a prime candidate gene for the development of atrial arrhythmias in man. Indeed, expression analysis confirmed that *PITX2C* was also expressed in adult left atrial tissue, further supporting a biological function beyond that of embryonic left-right patterning (Wang et al., 2010; Kirchhof et al., 2011b). In mice carrying a hypomorphic allele of *Pitx2c*, sedation and pacing revealed an increased tendency of atrial flutter and tachycardia in heterozygous mutants (Wang et al., 2010). Isolated, beating hearts carrying a heterozygous *Pitx2c*-deletion had a reduced APD and were also susceptible to AF (Kirchhof et al., 2011b). Echocardiography suggested there were no apparent morphological defects (Kirchhof et al., 2011b). In contrast, homozygous deletion of *Pitx2c* in the heart, appeared to provoke structural changes later in life as well as changes in ion channel expression (Chinchilla et al., 2011), which could also offer mechanistic insight into the observed arrhythmic phenotype.

Given its role in suppressing "pacemaker" genes and defining the contractile myocardium, it has been proposed that loss of Pitx2c results in a "less left" atrial phenotype promoting ectopic left atrial activity however, how this is achieved in fully differentiated, adult myocardium is unclear at present.

T-BOX TRANSCRIPTION FACTOR 3

Similar to loss of Pitx2c, mice over expressing Tbx3, another gene implicated in the specification of pacemaker cells, in a cardiac-specific manner, developed atrial ectopic beats (Hoogaars et al., 2007).

RTEF-1

Transcription enhancer factor-1-related factor (RTEF-1) is a transcriptional target of alpha1-adrenergic signaling (Stewart et al., 1998; Ueyama et al., 2000). Cardiac-specific overexpression of human RTEF-1 in mice led to the development of spontaneous AF under telemetry, an increased tendency to AF induction by burst pacing in younger mice and the development of sustained AF in older (12 months) transgenic founder mice (Chen et al., 2004). Atrial dilation and thrombi were reported in this transgenic model however, there was no evidence of fibrosis. Owing to reduced atrial conduction velocity, the expression levels of phosphorylated compared to dephosphorylated Cx40 were assessed: The levels of phosphorylated Cx40 were found to be reduced concomitant with an increase in dephosphorylated Cx40 suggesting that gap junction complexes were compromised in this model of AF (Chen et al., 2004).

JUN DIMERIZATION PROTEIN 2

c-Jun dimerization protein 2 (JDP2) is a transcriptional repressor belonging to the basic leucine zipper (bZIP) family of transcription factors (Aronheim et al., 1997; Jin et al., 2001). Tetracycline-regulated cardiac-specific overexpression of JDP2 resulted in atrial dilatation and atrial myocyte hypertrophy and reduced conduction velocity (Kehat et al., 2006). Furthermore, spontaneous AF under anesthesia was reported in a "small number" of mice (Kehat et al., 2006). Cx40 protein levels were also perturbed in this model (reduced expression level of total Cx40), which was indicative of the inhibitory effect of JDP2 on Cx40 promoter activity (Kehat et al., 2006). Hence loss of Cx40 may also be an attributing factor to the observed conduction defects and the development of AF in this model.

NUCLEOPORIN 155

Nucleoporin 155 (NUP155) is a major component of the nuclear pore complex within the nuclear envelope that facilitates the transport of DNA and mRNA from the nucleus to the cytoplasm (Zhang et al., 2002b). Systemic heterozygous deletion of NUP155 in mice, reportedly lead to spontaneous AF under roaming conditions (Zhang et al., 2008). More importantly, a single nucleotide polymorphism that evokes a missense mutation within NUP155 has been identified as contributing to AF in patients (Zhang et al., 2008). *In vitro* analysis showed that this mutation impaired nuclear permeability to *Nup155* gene products (Zhang et al., 2008). NUP155 was recently shown to interact with histone deacetylase 4 (HDAC4), hence this arrhythmic phenotype may also be the consequence of altered transcriptional activity (Kehat et al., 2011).

MICRORNAs

In recent years a number of microRNAs (miRNA), endogenous non-coding ~22mer RNA molecules that regulate gene expression by gene silencing, have been increasingly implicated in cardiac pathology (Wakili et al., 2011; Wang et al., 2011). This highlights the potential role of post transcriptional regulation alongside other such control mechanisms as transcriptional regulation, translational regulation, and post-translational modification.

miR-328

miR-223, miR-328, and miR-664 were found to be upregulated in a canine model of AF (Yue et al., 1997; Lu et al., 2010). The generation of a transgenic mouse overexpressing miR-328 under the control of the α*Mhc* promoter, resulted in the development of spontaneous AF under anesthesia (Lu et al., 2010). Furthermore loss of miR-328 protected against AF induction via pacing following muscarinic acetylcholine receptor stimulation (Lu et al., 2010). The alpha 1c and beta 1 subunits of the L-type Ca^{2+} channel were identified as targets of miR-328, and the expression levels of the L-type Ca^{2+} channel protein subunits encoded by these genes, Cav1.2 and Cavβ1, were also reduced, suggesting that the observed shorter APD in this model is the result of reduced L-type Ca^{2+} currents (Lu et al., 2010).

miR-208

Transgenic mice overexpressing miR-208a displayed reduced cardiac function by 3 months of age and went on to develop first and second degree AV block (Callis et al., 2009). Conversely, loss of miR-208a in a murine knockout model had a protective effect on cardiac remodeling following thoracic aortic banding (van Rooij et al., 2007). Despite the seemingly positive effect of reducing miR-208a on cardiac pathology, miR-208a knockout mice also developed spontaneous AF under anesthesia (Callis et al., 2009). The effect of miR-208b on cardiac conduction has yet to be investigated but it differed from miR-208a by only 3 bp and shared identical seed regions (Callis et al., 2009), hence it seems likely that miR-208b regulates the same targets as miR-208a (Callis et al., 2009) and that both feature within arrhythmogenic signaling pathways. miR-208a and miR-208b are encoded within intron 27 of the α*Mhc* and β*Mhc* genes respectively (van Rooij et al., 2007) and regulatory targets of miR-208a include thyroid hormone associated protein 1 and myostatin (see next paragraph; Callis et al., 2009).

CYTOKINES AND GROWTH FACTORS

MYOSTATIN

Myostatin was among the first proteins to be identified as a negative regulator of hypertrophy (McPherron et al., 1997). Very recently, cardiac-specific expression of the inhibitory N-terminus of myostatin pro-peptide was shown to increase susceptibility to AF induction in mice (Rosenberg et al., 2012). Taken together, these results suggest that loss of myostatin expression can act as a substrate for AF. Preliminary data has shown the voltage-gated potassium channel Kv1.4 (KCNA4) to be upregulated in this model, although the impact of this on APD has yet to be determined (Callis et al., 2009; Rosenberg et al., 2012).

TRANSFORMING GROWTH FACTOR BETA 1

Transforming growth factor beta 1 (TGFß1) is a cytokine that regulates numerous cellular processes including growth, differentiation, adhesion, migration, and apoptosis. However, in the adult heart, TGFß1 is a key regulator of fibrosis. Enhanced fibrosis reduces the electrical coupling of cardiomyocytes (Shaw and Rudy, 1997; Allessie et al., 2005). The atria have been shown to be more susceptible to fibrotic remodeling (Burstein et al., 2008) and pacing of cultured atrial-derived myocytes was shown to increase expression of TGFβ1 (Yeh et al., 2011). In patients, increased expression levels of TGFß1 are associated with chronic AF, valvular heart disease, atherosclerosis, and pressure overload (Lamirault et al., 2006; Xu et al., 2010; Creemers and Pinto, 2011). In mice, cardiac-specific overexpression of constitutively active TGFß1 caused atrial fibrosis, atrial conduction disturbances, and AF (Verheule et al., 2004). Recent data suggested that triggered activity arising due to reduced APD and spontaneous Ca^{2+} release, contribute to the development of AF in this murine model (Choi et al., 2012). Increased levels of angiotensin II and reactive oxygen species were shown to increase the promoter activity of *Tgfβ1*, connective tissue growth factor (*Ctgf*), and collagen in fibroblasts thus perpetuating a profibrotic environment that could promote conduction defects (Hao et al., 2011; Tsai et al., 2011).

TUMOR NECROSIS FACTOR

Tumor necrosis factor (formerly referred to as TNFα) is another inflammatory cytokine implicated in the development and pathology of AF in humans (Cao et al., 2011; Deng et al., 2011). Cardiac-specific overexpression of TNFα in mice resulted in atrial dilation, fibrosis, thrombi development, and spontaneous AF under roaming conditions (Kubota et al., 1997; Saba et al., 2005). In a second TNF overexpression model, downregulation of the gap junction protein Connexin 40 was also reported (Sawaya et al., 2007).

CONCLUSION

A long list of murine models that confer increased susceptibility to atrial arrhythmias, further substantiates the value of genetically altered murine models in advancing our understanding of the processes that initiate and propagate AF. In this review, models were grouped into signaling pathways already associated with AF. However, this is not to say that the proteins they encode are restricted to any single pathway. Each "pathway" most likely represents a small component of a much larger, more complex, pro-arrhythmic pathway.

In the vast majority of models, atrial arrhythmia was reported to be induced in a non-physiological setting such as anesthesia or pacing (more than three quarters of mouse mutants reported in **Table 1**). The relationship between anesthesia and AF is still of clinical relevance (Laakmann et al., 2010). However pacing induced arrhythmia suggests that whilst there is a substrate for atrial arrhythmia, this can be well tolerated and undetected in the absence of a triggering factor. Reported cases of spontaneous atrial arrhythmias in freely roaming mice were relatively rare (less than a quarter of the mouse mutants reported in **Table 1**) and almost always accompanied by atrial enlargement and/or fibrosis. We were intrigued to find that the majority of models reported to develop spontaneous AF without anesthesia or interventions were transgenic overexpression mutants. High levels of overexpression may have a toxic effect on the cell that also contributes to atrial phenotype, whereby overexpression leads to structural changes beyond those observed during "normal" pathophysiology. It is also possible that such expression levels may actually trigger a common final pathological pathway that mimics human pathology. Indeed the majority of the mutant models discussed in this review displayed dose dependent phenotypes that arose due to the heterozygous or homozygous expression and/or the positional effect of transgene integration (D'Angelo et al., 1997; Mende et al., 1998; Sussman et al., 2000; Fabritz et al., 2004; Kasi et al., 2007). The differential onset of α*Mhc* promoter expression during embryogenesis in the atria and at birth in the ventricles (Chizzonite et al., 1982; Sweeney et al., 1985; Bouvagnet et al., 1987; Colbert et al., 1997; Hein et al., 1997; Wei et al., 2004) might also mitigate a gene dosage effect across the heart.

Atrial fibrillation is a complex arrhythmia, and is likely to depend on multiple intertwined mechanisms. While the principal dysregulations in ion channel function and intracellular calcium homeostasis have been characterized, more recent genetic findings suggest that dysregulation of gene transcription and an imbalance in major regulatory pathways of cell function may contribute to the complex genesis of AF. Future challenges include the identification and investigation of the downstream components of these pathways and henceforth, the identification of therapeutic targets. The use of GWAS will lead to the development of new models of AF that better mimic human pathology from a different perspective. The differences between man and mice notwithstanding, murine models offer unique opportunities to investigate the functional and biochemical consequences of such complex regulatory changes, and to integrate these domains into our understanding of the genesis of AF.

ACKNOWLEDGMENTS

Supported by funds from DFG FA 413/3-1(LF) "Molecular mechanisms of atrial arrhythmia development," SFB656 Mobil A8 (Larissa Fabritz, Paulus Kirchhof); University of Birmingham starter grant (Paulus Kirchhof, Larissa Fabritz) and preliminary data award (Larissa Fabritz) of Research Development Fund, University of Birmingham, as well as international consortiums investigating atrial fibrillation mechanisms ENAFRA and EUTRAF.

REFERENCES

Adam, O., Frost, G., Custodis, F., Suss- man, M. A., Schäfers, H. J., Böhm, M., and Laufs, U. (2007). Role of Rac1 GTPase activation in atrial fib- rillation. *J. Am. Coll. Cardiol.* 50, 359–367.

Adam, O., Lavall, D., Theobald, K., Hohl, M., Grube, M., Ameling, S., Sussman, M. A., Rosenkranz, S., Kroe- mer, H. K., Schäfers, H. J., Böhm,M., and Laufs, U. (2010). Rac1- induced connective tissue growth factor regulates connexin 43 and N-cadherin expression in atrial fib- rillation. *J. Am. Coll. Cardiol.* 55, 469–480.

Allessie, M., Schotten, U., Verheule, S., and Harks, E. (2005). Gene therapy for repair of cardiac fibrosis: a long way to Tipperary. *Circulation* 111, 391–393.

Arad, M., Moskowitz, I. P., Patel, V. V., Ahmad, F., Perez-Atayde, A. R., Sawyer, D. B., Walter, M., Li, G. H., Burgon, P. G., Maguire, C. T., Stapleton, D., Schmitt, J. P., Guo, X. X., Pizard, A., Kuper- shmidt, S., Roden, D. M., Berul, C. I., Seidman, C. E., and Seid- man, J. G. (2003). Transgenic mice overexpressing mutant PRKAG2 define the cause of Wolff-Parkinson- White syndrome in glycogen storage cardiomyopathy. *Circulation* 107, 2850–2856.

Aronheim, A., Zandi, E., Hennemann, H., Elledge, S. J., and Karin, M. (1997). Isolation of an AP-1 repres- sor by a novel method for detecting protein-protein interactions. *Mol. Cell. Biol.* 17, 3094–3102.

Asahi, M., Nakayama, H., Tada, M., and Otsu, K. (2003). Regula- tion of sarco(endo)plasmic reticu- lum Ca2+ adenosine triphosphatase by phospholamban and sarcolipin: implication for cardiac hypertrophy and failure. *Trends Cardiovasc. Med.* 13, 152–157.

Babu, G. J., Bhupathy, P., Carnes, C. A., Billman, G. E., and Periasamy, M. (2007a). Differential expression of sarcolipin protein during mus- cle development and cardiac patho- physiology. *J. Mol. Cell. Cardiol.* 43, 215–222.

Babu, G. J., Bhupathy, P., Timofeyev, V., Petrashevskaya, N. N., Reiser, P. J., Chiamvimonvat, N., and Peri- asamy, M. (2007b). Ablation of sar- colipin enhances sarcoplasmic retic- ulum calcium transport and atrial contractility. *Proc. Natl. Acad. Sci. U.S.A.* 104, 17867–17872.

Bardeesy, N., Sinha, M., Hezel, A. F., Sig- noretti, S., Hathaway, N. A., Sharpless, N. E., Loda, M., Carrasco, D. R., and DePinho, R. A. (2002). Loss of the Lkb1 tumour suppressor pro- vokes intestinal polyposis but resis- tance to transformation. *Nature* 419, 162–167.

Ben-Ami, I., Yao, Z., Naor, Z., and Seger, R. (2011). Gq protein-induced apoptosis is mediated by AKT kinase inhibition that leads to protein kinase C-induced c-Jun N-terminal kinase activation. *J. Biol. Chem.* 286, 31022–31031.

Bennett, V., and Gilligan, D. M. (1993). The spectrin-based mem- brane skeleton and micron-scale organization of the plasma mem- brane. *Annu. Rev. Cell Biol.* 9, 27–66.

Bhupathy, P., Babu, G. J., Ito, M., and Periasamy, M. (2009). Threonine-5 at the N-terminus can modu- late sarcolipin function in cardiac myocytes. *J. Mol. Cell. Cardiol.* 47, 723–729.

Black, R. G. Jr., Guo, Y., Ge, Z. D., Mur- phree, S. S., Prabhu, S. D., Jones, W. K., Bolli, R., and Auchampach, J. A. (2002). Gene dosage-dependent effects of cardiac-specific overex- pression of the A3 adenosine recep- tor. *Circ. Res.* 91, 165–172.

Blana, A., Kaese, S., Fortmüller, L., Laak-mann, S., Damke, D., van Bragt, K., Eckstein, J., Piccini, I., Kirchhefer, U., Nattel, S., Breithardt, G., Carmeliet, P., Carmeliet, E., Schotten, U., Ver- heule, S., Kirchhof, P., and Fabritz, L. (2010). Knock-in gain-of-function sodium channel mutation prolongs atrial action potentials and alters atrial vulnerability. *Heart Rhythm* 7, 1862–1869.

Boldt, A., Wetzel, U., Weigl, J., Gar- bade, J., Lauschke, J., Hindricks, G., Kottkamp, H., Gummert, J. F., and Dhein, S. (2003). Expres- sion of angiotensin II receptors in human left and right atrial tis- sue in atrial fibrillation with and without underlying mitral valve disease. *J. Am. Coll. Cardiol.* 42, 1785–1792.

Bond, C. T., Herson, P. S., Strassmaier, T., Hammond, R., Stackman, R., Maylie, J., and Adelman, J. P. (2004). Small conductance Ca2+-activated K+ channel knock-out mice reveal the identity of calcium-dependent afterhyperpolarization currents. *J. Neurosci.* 24, 5301–5306.

Borrmann, C. M., Grund, C., Kuhn, C., Hofmann, I., Pieperhoff, S., and Franke, W. W. (2006). The area com- posita of adhering junctions con- necting heart muscle cells of verte- brates. II. Colocalizations of desmo- somal and fascia adhaerens mole- cules in the intercalated disk. *Eur. J. Cell Biol.* 85, 469–485.

Bouvagnet, P., Neveu, S., Montoya, M., and Leger, J. J. (1987). Development changes in the human cardiac isomyosin distribution: an immunohistochemical study using mono- clonal antibodies. *Circ. Res.* 61, 329–336.

Burstein, B., Libby, E., Calderone, A., and Nattel, S. (2008). Dif- ferential behaviors of atrial ver- sus ventricular fibroblasts: a poten- tial role for platelet-derived growth factor in atrial-ventricular remod- eling differences. *Circulation* 117, 1630–1641.

Callis, T. E., Pandya, K., Seok, H. Y., Tang, R. H., Tatsuguchi, M., Huang, Z. P., Chen, J. F., Deng, Z., Gunn, B., Shu- mate, J., Willis, M. S., Selzman, C. H., and Wang, D. Z. (2009). MicroRNA- 208a is a regulator of cardiac hypertrophy and conduction in mice. *J. Clin. Invest.* 119, 2772–2786.

Camm, A. J., Kirchhof, P., Lip, G. Y., Schotten, U., Savelieva, I., Ernst, S., Van Gelder, I. C., Al-Attar, N., Hin- dricks, G., Prendergast, B., Heid- buchel, H., Alfieri, O., Angelini, A., Atar, D., Colonna, P., De Caterina, R., De Sutter, J., Goette, A., Gorenek, B., Heldal, M., Hohloser, S. H., Kolh, P., Le Heuzey, J. Y., Ponikowski, P., and Rutten, F. H. (2010). Guide- lines for the management of atrial fibrillation: the Task Force for the Management of Atrial Fibrillation of the European Society of Cardiology (ESC). *Eur. Heart J.* 31, 2369–2429.

Cao, Y., Zhang, J., Meng, X., and Wang, D. (2011). TNF-alpha induces early growth response gene-1 expression via ERK1/2 activation in endothelial cells. *Acta Diabetol.*

Chauhan, V. S., Tuvia, S., Buhusi, M., Bennett, V., and Grant, A. O. (2000). Abnormal cardiac Na(+) channel properties and QT heart rate adapta- tion in neonatal ankyrin(B) knock- out mice. *Circ. Res.* 86, 441–447.

Chelu, M. G., Sarma, S., Sood, S., Wang, S., van Oort, R. J., Skapura, D. G., Li, N., Santonastasi, M., Müller, F. U., Schmitz, W., Schotten, U., Anderson, M. E., Valderrábano, M., Dobrev, D., and Wehrens, X. H. (2009). Calmodulin kinase II-mediated sarcoplas- mic reticulum Ca2+ leak promotes atrial fibrillation in mice. *J. Clin. Invest.* 119, 1940–1951.

Chen, H. H., Baty, C. J., Maeda, T., Brooks, S., Baker, L. C., Ueyama, T., Gursoy, E., Saba, S., Salama, G., London, B., and Stewart, A. F. (2004). Transcription enhancer factor-1-related factor-transgenic mice develop cardiac conduction defects associated with altered con- nexin phosphorylation. *Circulation* 110, 2980–2987.

Chiello Tracy, C., Cabo, C., Coromilas, J., Kurokawa, J., Kass, R. S., and Wit, A. L. (2003). Electrophysiological con- sequences of human IKs channel expression in adult murine heart. *Am. J. Physiol. Heart Circ. Physiol.* 284, H168–H175.

Chinchilla, A., Daimi, H., Lozano- Velasco, E., Dominguez, J. N., Caballero, R., Delpón, E., Tamargo, J., Cinca, J., Hove-Madsen, L., Aranega, A. E., and Franco, D. (2011). PITX2 insufficiency leads to atrial electrical and structural remodeling linked to arrhythmo- genesis. *Circ. Cardiovasc. Genet.* 4, 269–279.

Chizzonite, R. A., Everett, A. W., Clark, A., Jakovcic, S., Rabinowitz, M., and Zak, R. (1982). Isolation and characterization of two molecular variants of myosin heavy chain from rabbit ventricle. Change in their con- tent during normal growth and after treatment with thyroid hormone. *J. Biol. Chem.* 257, 2056–2065.

Choi, E. K., Chang, P. C., Lee, Y. S., Lin, S. F., Zhu, W., Maruyama, M., Fish- bein, M. C., Chen, Z., Rubart-von der Lohe, M., Field, L. J., and Chen, P. (2012). Triggered firing and atrial fibrillation in transgenic mice with selective atrial fibrosis induced by overexpression of TGF-beta1. *Circ. J.* 76, 1354–1362.

Colbert, M. C., Hall, D. G., Kimball, R., Witt, S. A., Lorenz, J. N., Kirby, M. L., Hewett, T. E., Klevit- sky, R., and Robbins, J. (1997). Car- diac compartment-specific overex- pression of a modified retinoic acid receptor produces dilated cardiomy- opathy and congestive heart failure in transgenic mice. *J. Clin. Invest.* 100, 1958–1968.

Cong, H., Li, X., Ma, L., Jiang, H., Mao, Y., and Xu, M. (2010). Angiotensin II receptor type 1 is upregulated in atrial tissue of patients with rheumatic valvular disease with atrial fibrillation. *J. Thorac. Cardio- vasc. Surg.* 140, 298–304.

Creemers, E. E., and Pinto, Y. M. (2011). Molecular mechanisms that control interstitial fibrosis in the pressure- overloaded heart. *Cardiovasc. Res.* 89, 265–272.

Cunha, S. R., Hund, T. J., Hashemi, S., Voigt, N., Li, N., Wright, P., Koval, O., Li, J., Gudmundsson, H., Gumina, R. J., Karck, M., Schott, J. J., Probst, V., Le Marec, H., Ander- son, M. E., Dobrev, D., Wehrens, H., and Mohler, P. J. (2011). Defects in ankyrin-based membrane protein targeting pathways under- lie atrial fibrillation. *Circulation* 124, 1212–1222.

D'Angelo, D. D., Sakata, Y., Lorenz, J. N., Boivin, G. P., Walsh, R. A., Liggett, S. B., and Dorn, G. W. II. (1997). Transgenic Galphaq overexpression induces cardiac contractile failure in mice. *Proc. Natl. Acad. Sci. U.S.A.* 94, 8121–8126.

Dautova, Y., Zhang, Y., Sabir, I., Grace, A. A., and Huang, C. L. (2009). Atrial arrhythmogenesis in wild-type and Scn5a+/delta murine hearts model- ling LQT3 syndrome. *Pflugers Arch.* 458, 443–457.

de Diego, C., Chen, F., Xie, L. H., Dave, A. S., Thu, M., Rongey, C., Weiss, J. N., and Valderrábano, M. (2008). Car- diac alternans in embryonic mouse ventricles. *Am. J. Physiol. Heart Circ. Physiol.* 294, H433–H440.

De Jong, A. M., Maass, A. H., Oberdorf- Maass, S. U., Van Veldhuisen, D. J., Van Gilst, W. H., and Van Gelder, I. C. (2011). Mechanisms of atrial structural changes caused by stretch occurring before and during early atrial fibrillation. *Cardiovasc. Res.* 89, 754–765.

De Mello, W. C., and Frohlich, E. D. (2011). On the local cardiac renin angiotensin system. Basic and clinical implications. *Peptides* 32, 1774–1779.

Deng, Y. H., Alex, D., Huang, H. Q., Wang, N., Yu, N., Wang, Y. T., Leung, G. P., and Lee, S. M. (2011). Inhibition of TNF- alpha-mediated endothelial cell- monocyte cell adhesion and adhe- sion molecules expression by the resveratrol derivative, trans-3,5,4[1] - trimethoxystilbene. *Phytother. Res.* 25, 451–457.

DiMarco, J. P., Sellers, T. D., Berne, R. M., West, G. A., and Belardinelli, L. (1983). Adenosine: electrophysio- logic effects and therapeutic use for terminating paroxysmal supraven- tricular tachycardia. *Circulation* 68, 1254–1263.

Eckardt, L., Kirchhof, P., Loh, P., Schulze-Bahr, E., Johna, R., Wichter, T., Breithardt, G., Haverkamp, W., and Borggrefe, M. (2001). Bru- gada syndrome and supraventricular tachyarrhythmias: a novel associa- tion? *J. Cardiovasc. Electrophysiol.* 12, 680–685.

Eloff, B. C., Lerner, D. L., Yamada, K. A., Schuessler, R. B., Saffitz, J. E., and Rosenbaum, D. S. (2001). High resolution optical mapping reveals conduction slowing in connexin43 deficient mice. *Cardiovasc. Res.* 51, 681–690.

Fabritz, L., Kirchhof, P., Fortmüller, L., Auchampach, J. A., Baba, H. A., Breithardt, G., Neumann, J., Boknik, P., and Schmitz, W. (2004). Gene dose-dependent atrial arrhythmias, heart block, and brady-cardiomyopathy in mice overexpressing A(3) adeno- sine receptors. *Cardiovasc. Res.* 62, 500–508.

Fabritz, L., Kirchhof, P., Franz, M. R., Eckardt, L., Mönnig, G., Milberg, P., Breithardt, G., and Haverkamp, W. (2003). Prolonged action potential durations, increased dispersion of repolarization, and polymorphic ventricular tachycardia in a mouse model of proarrhythmia. *Basic Res. Cardiol.* 98, 25–32.

Filtz, T. M., Grubb, D. R., McLeod- Dryden, T. J., Luo, J., and Woodcock, E. A. (2009). Gq-initiated cardiomy- ocyte hypertrophy is mediated by phospholipase Cbeta1b. *FASEB J.* 23, 3564–3570.

Foulkes, N. S., Borrelli, E., and Sassone- Corsi, P. (1991). CREM gene: use of alternative DNA-binding domains generates multiple antagonists of cAMP-induced transcription. *Cell* 64, 739–749.

Franke, W. W., Borrmann, C. M., Grund, C., and Pieperhoff, S. (2006). The area composita of adhering junctions connecting heart muscle cells of vertebrates. I. Molecular definition in intercalated disks of cardiomyocytes by immunoelectron microscopy of desmosomal pro- teins. *Eur. J. Cell Biol.* 85, 69–82.

Gage, P. J., Suh, H., and Camper, S. A. (1999). Dosage requirement of Pitx2 for development of multiple organs. *Development* 126, 4643–4651.

Ganga, M., Espinoza, H. M., Cox, C. J., Morton, L., Hjalt, T. A., Lee, Y., and Amendt, B. A. (2003). PITX2 isoform-specific regulation of atrial natriuretic factor expression: syner- gism and repression with Nkx2.5. *J. Biol. Chem.* 278, 22437–22445.

Gellens, M. E., George, A. L. Jr., Chen, L. Q., Chahine, M., Horn, R., Barchi, R. L., and Kallen, R. G. (1992). Primary structure and functional expression of the human cardiac tetrodotoxin-insensitive voltage- dependent sodium channel. *Proc. Natl. Acad. Sci. U.S.A.* 89, 554–558.

Goddard, C. A., Ghais, N. S., Zhang, Y., Williams, A. J., Colledge, W. H., Grace, A. A., and Huang, C. L. (2008). Physiological consequences of the P2328S mutation in the ryan- odine receptor (RyR2) gene in genet- ically modified murine hearts. *Acta Physiol. (Oxf.)* 194, 123–140.

Gollob, M. H., Jones, D. L., Krahn, A. D., Danis, L., Gong, X. Q., Shao, Q., Liu, X., Veinot, J. P., Tang, A. S., Stewart, A. F., Tesson, F., Klein, G. J., Yee, R., Skanes, A. C., Guiraudon, G. M., Ebi- hara, L., and Bai, D. (2006). Somatic mutations in the connexin 40 gene (GJA5) in atrial fibrillation. *N. Engl. J. Med.* 354, 2677–2688.

Groenewegen, W. A., Firouzi, M., Bezzina, C. R., Vliex, S., van Langen, I. M., Sandkuijl, L., Smits, J. P., Huls- beek, M., Rook, M. B., Jongsma, H. J., and Wilde, A. A. (2003). A cardiac sodium channel mutation cosegre- gates with a rare connexin40 geno- type in familial atrial standstill. *Circ. Res.* 92, 14–22.

Gudbjartsson, D. F., Arnar, D. O., Hel- gadottir, A., Gretarsdottir, S., Holm, H., Sigurdsson, A., Jonasdottir, A., Baker, A., Thorleifsson, G., Krist- jansson, K., Palsson, A., Blondal, T., Sulem, P., Backman, V. M., Hardar- son, G. A., Palsdottir, E., Helgason, A., Sigurjonsdottir, R., Sverrisson, J. T., Kostulas, K., Ng, M. C., Baum, L., So, W. Y., Wong, K. S., Chan, J. C., Furie, K. L., Greenberg, S. M., Sale, M., Kelly, P., MacRae, C. A., Smith, E. E., Rosand, J., Hillert, J., Ma, R. C., Ellinor, P. T., Thorgeirs- son, G., Gulcher, J. R., Kong, A., Thorsteinsdottir, U., and Stefansson, K. (2007). Variants conferring risk of atrial fibrillation on chromosome 4q25. *Nature* 448, 353–357.

Guzadhur, L., Pearcey, S. M., Duehmke, R. M., Jeevaratnam, K., Hohmann, A. F., Zhang, Y., Grace, A. A., Lei, M., and Huang, C. L. (2010). Atrial arrhythmogenicity in aged Scn5a+/deltaKPQ mice modeling long QT type 3 syndrome and its relationship to Na+ channel expression and cardiac conduction. *Pflugers Arch.* 460, 593–601.

Hagendorff, A., Schumacher, B., Kirch-hoff, S., Lüderitz, B., and Willecke, K. (1999). Conduction disturbances and increased atrial vulnerability in Connexin40-deficient mice analyzed by transesophageal stimulation. *Circulation* 99, 1508–1515.

Hakim, P., Brice, N., Thresher, R., Lawrence, J., Zhang, Y., Jackson, A. P., Grace, A. A., and Huang, C. L. (2010). Scn3b knockout mice exhibit abnormal sino-atrial and cardiac conduction properties. *Acta Physiol. (Oxf.)* 198, 47–59.

Hakim, P., Gurung, I. S., Pedersen, T. H., Thresher, R., Brice, N., Lawrence, J., Grace, A. A., and Huang, C. L. (2008). Scn3b knockout mice exhibit abnormal ventricular electrophysi- ological properties. *Prog. Biophys. Mol. Biol.* 98, 251–266.

Hao, X., Zhang, Y., Zhang, X., Nirmalan, M., Davies, L., Konstantinou, D., Yin, F., Dobrzynski, H., Wang, X., Grace, A., Zhang, H., Boyett, M., Huang, C. L., and Lei, M. (2011). TGF-beta1- mediated fibrosis and ion channel remodeling are key mechanisms in producing the sinus node dysfunc- tion associated with SCN5A defi- ciency and aging. *Circ. Arrhythm. Electrophysiol.* 4, 397–406.

Head, C. E., Balasubramaniam, R., Thomas, G., Goddard, C. A., Lei, M., Colledge, W. H., Grace, A. A., and Huang, C. L. (2005). Paced electrogram fractionation analysis of arrhythmogenic tendency in DeltaKPQ Scn5a mice. *J. Cardiovasc. Electrophysiol.* 16, 1329–1340.

Headrick, J. P., Peart, J. N., Reichelt, M. E., and Haseler, L. J. (2011). Adeno- sine and its receptors in the heart: regulation, retaliation and adapta- tion. *Biochim. Biophys. Acta* 1808, 1413–1428.

Hein, L., Stevens, M. E., Barsh, G. S., Pratt, R. E., Kobilka, B. K., and Dzau, V. J. (1997). Overexpression of angiotensin AT1 receptor trans- gene in the mouse myocardium pro- duces a lethal phenotype associated with myocyte hyperplasia and heart block. *Proc. Natl. Acad. Sci. U.S.A.* 94, 6391–6396.

Herr, C., Smyth, N., Ullrich, S., Yun, F., Sasse, P., Hescheler, J., Fleis- chmann, B., Lasek, K., Brixius, K., Schwinger, R. H., Fässler, R., Schröder, R., and Noegel, A. A. (2001). Loss of annexin A7 leads to alterations in frequency-induced shortening of isolated murine car- diomyocytes. *Mol. Cell. Biol.* 21, 4119–4128.

Hirose, M., Takeishi, Y., Niizeki, T., Shimojo, H., Nakada, T., Kub- ota, I., Nakayama, J., Mende, U., and Yamada, M. (2009). Diacylglyc- erol kinase zeta inhibits G(alpha)q- induced atrial remodeling in trans- genic mice. *Heart Rhythm* 6, 78–84. Hong, C. S., Cho, M. C., Kwak, Y. G., Song, C. H., Lee, Y. H., Lim, J. S., Kwon, Y. K., Chae, S. W., and Kim, D. H. (2002). Cardiac remodeling and atrial fibrillation in transgenic mice overexpressing junctin. *FASEB J.* 16, 1310–1312.

Hong, C. S., Kwon, S. J., Cho, M. C., Kwak, Y. G., Ha, K. C., Hong, B., Li, H., Chae, S. W., Chai, O. H., Song, C. H., Li,Y., Kim, J. C., Woo, S. H., Lee, S. Y., Lee, C. O., and Kim do, H. (2008). Overexpression of junctate induces cardiac hypertrophy and arrhythmia via altered calcium handling. *J. Mol. Cell. Cardiol.* 44, 672–682.

Hoogaars, W. M., Engel, A., Brons, J. F., Verkerk, A. O., de Lange, F. J., Wong, L. Y., Bakker, M. L., Clout, D. E., Wakker, V., Barnett, P., Ravesloot, J. H., Moorman, A. F., Verheijck, E. E., and Christoffels, V. M. (2007). Tbx3 controls the sinoatrial node gene program and imposes pace- maker function on the atria. *Genes Dev.* 21, 1098–1112.

Ikeda, Y., Sato, K., Pimentel, D. R., Sam, F., Shaw, R. J., Dyck, J. R., and Walsh, K. (2009). Cardiac-specific deletion of LKB1 leads to hypertro- phy and dysfunction. *J. Biol. Chem.* 284, 35839–35849.

Janse, M. J., and Rosen, M. R. (2006). History of arrhythmias. *Handb. Exp. Pharmacol.* 171, 1–39.

Jin, C., Ugai, H., Song, J., Murata, T., Nili, F., Sun, K., Horikoshi, M., and Yokoyama, K. K. (2001). Identifica- tion of mouse Jun dimerization pro- tein 2 as a novel repressor of ATF-2. *FEBS Lett.* 489, 34–41.

Kääb, S., Darbar, D., van Noord, C., Dupuis, J., Pfeufer, A., Newton- Cheh, C., Schnabel, R., Makino, S., Sinner, M. F., Kannankeril, P. J., Beckmann, B. M., Choudry, S., Don- ahue, B. S., Heeringa, J., Perz, S., Lunetta, K. L., Larson, M. G., Levy, D., MacRae, C. A., Ruskin, J. N., Wacker, A., Schömig, A., Wichmann, H. E., Steinbeck, G., Meitinger, T., Uitterlinden, A. G., Witteman, J. C., Roden, D. M., Benjamin, E. J., and Ellinor, P. T. (2009). Large scale repli- cation and meta-analysis of vari- ants on chromosome 4q25 asso- ciated with atrial fibrillation. *Eur. Heart J.* 30, 813–819.

Kahr, P. C., Piccini, I., Fabritz, L., Greber, B., Schöler, H., Scheld, H. H., Hoffmeier, A., Brown, N. A., and Kirchhof, P. (2011). Systematic analysis of gene expres- sion differences between left and right atria in different mouse strains and in human atrial tissue. *PLoS ONE* 6, e26389. doi:10.1371/journal.pone.0026389

Kasi, V. S., Xiao, H. D., Shang, L. L., Iravanian, S., Langberg, J., Witham, E. A., Jiao, Z., Gallego, C. J., Bernstein, K. E., and Dudley, S. C. Jr. (2007). Cardiac-restricted angiotensin-converting enzyme overexpression causes conduction defects and connexin dysregulation. *Am. J. Physiol. Heart Circ. Physiol.* 293, H182–H192.

Kehat, I., Accornero, F., Aronow, B. J., and Molkentin, J. D. (2011). Mod- ulation of chromatin position and gene expression by HDAC4 interac- tion with nucleoporins. *J. Cell Biol.* 193, 21–29.

Kehat, I., Heinrich, R., Ben-Izhak, O., Miyazaki, H., Gutkind, J. S., and Aronheim, A. (2006). Inhibition of basic leucine zipper transcription is a major mediator of atrial dilatation. *Cardiovasc. Res.* 70, 543–554.

Kirchhefer, U., Baba, H. A., Hanske, G., Jones, L. R., Kirchhof, P., Schmitz, W., and Neumann, J. (2004). Age- dependent biochemical and contrac- tile properties in atrium of trans- genic mice overexpressing junctin. *Am. J. Physiol. Heart Circ. Physiol.* 287, H2216–H2225.

Kirchhof, P., Bax, J., Blomstrom- Lundquist, C., Calkins, H., Camm, A. J., Cappato, R., Cosio, F., Crijns, H., Diener, H. C., Goette, A., Israel, C. W., Kuck, K. H., Lip, G. Y., Nattel, S., Page, R. L., Ravens, U., Schot- ten, U., Steinbeck, G., Vardas, P., Waldo, A., Wegscheider, K., Willems, S., and Breithardt, G. (2009). Early and comprehensive management of atrial fibrillation: executive sum- mary of the proceedings from the 2nd AFNET-EHRA consensus con- ference"research perspectives in AF." *Eur. Heart J.* 30, 2969–2977c.

Kirchhof, P., Fabritz, L., Fortmuller, L., Matherne, G. P., Lankford, A., Baba, H. A., Schmitz, W., Breithardt, G., Neumann, J., and Boknik, P. (2003). Altered sinus nodal and atrioventric- ular nodal function in freely moving mice overexpressing the A1 adeno- sine receptor. *Am. J. Physiol. Heart Circ. Physiol.* 285, H145–H153.

Kirchhof, P., Klimas, J., Fabritz, L., Zwiener, M., Jones, L. R., Schäfers, M., Hermann, S., Boknik, P., Schmitz, W., Breithardt, G., Kirch- hefer, U., and Neumann, J. (2007). Stress and high heart rate pro- voke ventricular tachycardia in mice expressing triadin. *J. Mol. Cell. Car- diol.* 42, 962–971.

Kirchhof, P., Marijon, E., Fabritz, L., Li, N., Wang, W., Wang, T., Schulte, K., Hanstein, J., Schulte, J. S., Vogel, M., Mougenot, N., Laakmann, S., Fortmueller, L., Eckstein, J., Ver- heule, S., Kaese, S., Staab, A., Grote-Wessels, S., Schotten, U., Moubarak, G., Wehrens, X. H., Schmitz, W., Hatem, S., and Müller, F. U. (2011a). Overexpression of cAMP-response element modulator causes abnor- mal growth and development of the atrial myocardium resulting in a substrate for sustained atrial fibril- lation in mice. *Int. J. Cardiol.* PMID: 22093963. [Epub ahead of print].

Kirchhof, P., Kahr, P. C., Kaese, S., Piccini, I., Vokshi, I., Scheld, H. H., Rotering, H., Fortmueller, L., Laakmann, S., Verheule, S., Schot- ten, U., Fabritz, L., and Brown, N. A. (2011b). PITX2c is expressed in the adult left atrium, and reducing Pitx2c expression promotes atrial fibrillation inducibility and complex changes in gene expression. *Circ. Cardiovasc. Genet.* 4, 123–133.

Kirchhoff, S., Nelles, E., Hagendorff, A., Krüger, O., Traub, O., and Willecke, K. (1998). Reduced cardiac conduction velocity and predisposition to arrhythmias in connexin40-deficient mice. *Curr. Biol.* 8, 299–302.

Kitamura, K., Miura, H., Miyagawa- Tomita, S., Yanazawa, M., Katoh- Fukui, Y., Suzuki, R., Ohuchi, H., Suehiro, A., Motegi, Y., Nakahara, Y., Kondo, S., and Yokoyama, M. (1999). Mouse Pitx2 deficiency leads to anomalies of the ventral body wall, heart, extra- and peri- ocular mesoderm and right pul- monary isomerism. *Development* 126, 5749–5758.

Kosir, R., Juvan, P., Perse, M., Budefeld, T., Majdic, G., Fink, M., Sassone- Corsi, P., and Rozman, D. (2012). Novel insights into the downstream pathways and targets controlled by transcription factors CREM in the testis. *PLoS ONE* 7, e31798. doi:10.1371/journal.pone.0031798

Kubota, T., McTiernan, C. F., Frye, C. S., Slawson, S. E., Lemster, B. H., Koretsky, A. P., Demetris, A. J., and Feldman, A. M. (1997). Dilated cardiomyopathy in transgenic mice with cardiac-specific overexpression of tumor necrosis factor-alpha. *Circ. Res.* 81, 627–635.

Kupershmidt, S., Yang, T., Anderson, M. E., Wessels, A., Niswender, K. D., Magnuson, M. A., and Roden, D. M. (1999). Replacement by homol- ogous recombination of the minK gene with lacZ reveals restriction of minK expression to the mouse car- diac conduction system. *Circ. Res.* 84, 146–152.

Laakmann, S., Fortmüller, L., Stümpel, F., Kirchhefer, U., Müller, F. U., Lutz, S., Wieland, T., Mende, U., Kirchhof, P., and Fabritz, L. (2010). Develop- ment of paroxysmal and periopera- tive atrial fibrillation and left atrial thrombi in Galphaq overexpressing mice. *Clin. Res. Cardiol.* 2010(99 Suppl. 1), 728.

Lamirault, G., Gaborit, N., Le Meur, N., Chevalier, C., Lande, G., Demolombe, S., Escande, D., Nattel, S., Léger, J. J., and Steenman, M. (2006). Gene expression profile associated with chronic atrial fibril- lation and underlying valvular heart disease in man. *J. Mol. Cell. Cardiol.* 40, 173–184.

Lang, D., Sulkin, M., Lou, Q., and Efi- mov, I. R. (2011). Optical mapping of action potentials and calcium transients in the mouse heart. *J. Vis. Exp.* 55, 3275.

Li, N., Timofeyev, V., Tuteja, D., Xu, D., Lu, L., Zhang, Q., Zhang, Z., Sin- gapuri, A., Albert, T. R., Rajagopal, A. V., Bond, C. T., Periasamy, M., Adelman, J., and Chiamvimonvat, N. (2009). Ablation of a Ca2+- activated K+ channel (SK2 channel) results in action potential prolon- gation in atrial myocytes and atrial fibrillation. *J. Physiol. (Lond.)* 587(Pt 5), 1087–1100.

Li, N., Wang, T., Wang, W., Cutler, M. J., Wang, Q., Voigt, N., Rosenbaum, D. S., Dobrev, D., and Wehrens, X. H. (2012). Inhibition of CaMKII phosphorylation of RyR2 prevents induction of atrial fibrillation in FKBP12.6 knockout mice. *Circ. Res.* 110, 465–470.

Li, X., Moody, M. R., Engel, D., Walker, S., Clubb, F. J. Jr., Siva- subramanian, N., Mann, D. L., and Reid, M. B. (2000). Cardiac-specific overexpression of tumor necro- sis factor-alpha causes oxidative stress and contractile dysfunction in mouse diaphragm. *Circulation* 102, 1690–1696.

Li, Z., Colucci-Guyon, E., Pinçon- Raymond, M., Mericskay, M., Pournin, S., Paulin, D., and Babinet, (1996). Cardiovascular lesions and skeletal myopathy in mice lacking desmin. *Dev. Biol.* 175, 362–366.

Li, Z. P., Burke, E. P., Frank, J. S., Bennett, V., and Philipson, K. (1993). The cardiac Na+-Ca2+ exchanger binds to the cytoskeletal protein ankyrin. *J. Biol. Chem.* 268, 11489–11491.

Lin, X., Gemel, J., Glass, A., Zemlin, C. W., Beyer, E. C., and Veenstra, R. D. (2010). Connexin40 and con- nexin43 determine gating properties of atrial gap junction channels. *J. Mol. Cell. Cardiol.* 48, 238–245.

Lindpaintner, K., Jin, M., Wilhelm, M. J., Suzuki, F., Linz, W., Schoelkens, B. A., and Ganten, D. (1988). Intracar- diac generation of angiotensin and its physiologic role. *Circulation* 77(6 Pt 2), I18–I23.

Liu, C., Liu, W., Palie, J., Lu, M. F., Brown, N. A., and Martin, J. F. (2002). Pitx2c patterns anterior myocardium and aortic arch vessels and is required for local cell move- ment into atrioventricular cushions. *Development* 129, 5081–5091.

Lu, M. F., Pressman, C., Dyer, R., Johnson, R. L., and Martin, J. F. (1999). Function of Rieger syndrome gene in left-right asymmetry and cran- iofacial development. *Nature* 401, 276–278.

Lu, Y., Zhang, Y., Wang, N., Pan, Z., Gao, X., Zhang, F., Zhang, Y., Shan, H., Luo, X., Bai, Y., Sun, L., Song, W., Xu, C., Wang, Z., and Yang, B. (2010). MicroRNA-328 contributes to adverse electrical remodeling in atrial fibrillation. *Circulation* 122, 2378–2387.

Maier, S. K., Westenbroek, R. E., Schenkman, K. A., Feigl, E. O., Scheuer, T., and Catterall, W. A. (2002). An unexpected role for brain-type sodium channels in cou- pling of cell surface depolarization to contraction in the heart. *Proc. Natl. Acad. Sci. U.S.A.* 99, 4073–4078.

Mancarella, S., Yue, Y., Karnabi, E., Qu, Y., El-Sherif, N., and Boutjdir, M. (2008). Impaired Ca2+ homeostasis is associated with atrial fibrillation in the alpha1D L-type Ca2+ chan- nel KO mouse. *Am. J. Physiol. Heart Circ. Physiol.* 295, H2017–H2024.

Marx, S. O., Kurokawa, J., Reiken, S., Motoike, H., D'Armiento, J., Marks, A. R., and Kass, R. S. (2002). Requirement of a macromolecular signaling complex for beta adren- ergic receptor modulation of the KCNQ1-KCNE1 potassium chan- nel. *Science* 295, 496–499.

Matherne, G. P., Linden, J., Byford, A. M., Gauthier, N. S., and Headrick, J. P. (1997). Transgenic A1 adenosine receptor overexpression increases myocardial resistance to ischemia. *Proc. Natl. Acad. Sci. U.S.A.* 94, 6541–6546.

Mathur, N., Sood, S., Wang, S., van Oort, R. J., Sarma, S., Li, N., Skapura, D. G., Bayle, J. H., Valderrábano, M., and Wehrens, X. H. (2009). Sudden infant death syndrome in mice with an inherited mutation in RyR2. *Circ. Arrhythm. Electrophysiol.* 2, 677–685.

McPherron, A. C., Lawler, A. M., and Lee, S. J. (1997). Regulation of skeletal muscle mass in mice by a new TGF-beta superfamily member. *Nature* 387, 83–90.

Mende, U., Kagen, A., Cohen, A., Aramburu, J., Schoen, F. J., and Neer, E. J. (1998). Transient car- diac expression of constitutively active Galphaq leads to hypertro- phy and dilated cardiomyopathy by calcineurin-dependent and inde- pendent pathways. *Proc. Natl. Acad. Sci. U.S.A.* 95, 13893–13898.

Meno, C., Shimono, A., Saijoh, Y., Yashiro, K., Mochida, K., Ohishi, S., Noji, S., Kondoh, H., and Hamada, H. (1998). lefty-1 is required for left- right determination as a regulator of lefty-2 and nodal. *Cell* 94, 287–297. Milner, D. J., Weitzer, G., Tran, D., Bradley, A., and Capetanaki, Y. (1996). Disruption of muscle archi- tecture and myocardial degeneration in mice lacking desmin. *J. Cell Biol.* 134, 1255–1270.

Minamisawa, S., Wang, Y., Chen, J., Ishikawa, Y., Chien, K. R., and Mat- suoka, R. (2003). Atrial chamber- specific expression of sarcolipin is regulated during development and hypertrophic remodeling. *J. Biol. Chem.* 278, 9570–9575.

Mohler, P. J., Davis, J. Q., and Bennett, V. (2005). Ankyrin-B coordi- nates the Na/K ATPase, Na/Ca exchanger, and InsP3 recep- tor in a cardiac T-tubule/SR microdomain. *PLoS Biol.* 3, e423. doi:10.1371/journal.pbio.0030423

Mohler, P. J., Schott, J. J., Gramolini, A. O., Dilly, K. W., Guatimosim, S., duBell, W. H., Song, L. S., Haurogné, K., Kyndt, F., Ali, M. E., Rogers, T. B., Lederer, W. J., Escande, D., Le Marec, H., and Bennett, V. (2003). Ankyrin-B mutation causes type 4 long-QT cardiac arrhythmia and sudden cardiac death. *Nature* 421, 634–639.

Mommersteeg, M. T., Brown, N. A., Prall, O. W., de Gier-de Vries, C., Harvey, R. P., Moorman, A. F., and Christoffels, V. M. (2007). Pitx2c and Nkx2-5 are required for the formation and identity of the pul- monary myocardium. *Circ. Res.* 101, 902–909.

Müller, F. U., Lewin, G., Baba, H. A., Bokník, P., Fabritz, L., Kirch- hefer, U., Kirchhof, P., Loser, K., Matus, M., Neumann, J., Rie- mann, B., and Schmitz, W. (2005). Heart-directed expression of a human cardiac isoform of cAMP-response element modulator in transgenic mice. *J. Biol. Chem.* 280, 6906–6914.

Nakajima, Y., Yamagishi, T., Hokari, S., and Nakamura, H. (2000). Mech- anisms involved in valvuloseptal endocardial cushion formation in early cardiogenesis: roles of trans- forming growth factor (TGF)-beta and bone morphogenetic protein (BMP). *Anat. Rec.* 258, 119–127.

Namkung, Y., Skrypnyk, N., Jeong, M. J., Lee, T., Lee, M. S., Kim, H. L., Chin, H., Suh, P. G., Kim, S. S., and Shin, H. S. (2001). Requirement for the L-type Ca(2+) channel alpha(1D) subunit in postnatal pancreatic beta cell generation. *J. Clin. Invest.* 108, 1015–1022.

Neer, E. J. (1994). G proteins: critical control points for transmembrane signals. *Protein Sci.* 3, 3–14.

Nuyens, D., Stengl, M., Dugarmaa, S., Rossenbacker, T., Compernolle, V., Rudy, Y., Smits, J. F., Flameng, W., Clancy, C. E., Moons, L., Vos, M. A., Dewerchin, M., Benndorf, K., Collen, D., Carmeliet, E., and Carmeliet, P. (2001). Abrupt rate accelerations or premature beats cause life-threatening arrhythmias in mice with long-QT3 syndrome. *Nat. Med.* 7, 1021–1027.

Odermatt, A., Becker, S., Khanna, V. K., Kurzydlowski, K., Leisner, E., Pette, D., and MacLennan, D. H. (1998). Sarcolipin regulates the activity of SERCA1, the fast-twitch skeletal muscle sarcoplasmic retic- ulum Ca2+-ATPase. *J. Biol. Chem.* 273, 12360–12369.

Ogata, T., Ueyama, T., Isodono, K., Tagawa, M., Takehara, N., Kawashima, T., Harada, K., Taka- hashi, T., Shioi, T., Matsubara, H., and Oh, H. (2008). MURC, a muscle-restricted coiled-coil pro- tein that modulates the Rho/ ROCK pathway, induces cardiac dysfunc- tion and conduction disturbance. *Mol. Cell. Biol.* 28, 3424–3436.

Olesen, M. S., Jespersen, T., Nielsen, J. B., Liang, B., Møller, D. V., Hedley, P., Christiansen, M., Varró, A., Ole- sen, S. P., Haunsø, S., Schmitt, N., and Svendsen, J. H. (2011). Muta- tions in sodium channel beta sub- unit SCN3B are associated with early onset lone atrial fibrillation. *Cardio- vasc. Res.* 89, 786–793.

Papadatos, G. A., Wallerstein, P. M., Head, C. E., Ratcliff, R., Brady, P. A., Benndorf, K., Saumarez, R. C., Trezise, A. E., Huang, C. L., Vanden- berg, J. I., Colledge, W. H., and Grace, A. A. (2002). Slowed conduction and ventricular tachycardia after targeted disruption of the cardiac sodium channel gene Scn5a. *Proc. Natl. Acad. Sci. U.S.A.* 99, 6210–6215.

Park, P. S., Filipek, S., Wells, J. W., and Palczewski, K. (2004). Oligomeriza- tion of G protein-coupled receptors: past, present, and future. *Biochem- istry* 43, 15643–15656.

Pfreimer, M., Vatter, P., Langer, T., Wieland, T., Gierschik, P., and Moepps, B. (2012). LARG links histamine-H1-receptor-activated Gq to Rho-GTPase-dependent signaling pathways. *Cell. Signal.* 24, 652–663.

Platzer, J., Engel, J., Schrott-Fischer, A., Stephan, K., Bova, S., Chen, H., Zheng, H., and Striessnig, J. (2000). Congenital deafness and sinoatrial node dysfunction in mice lacking class D L-type Ca2+ channels. *Cell* 102, 89–97.

Pretorius, L., Du, X. J., Woodcock, E. A., Kiriazis, H., Lin, R. C., Marasco, S., Medcalf, R. L., Ming, Z., Head, G. A., Tan, J. W., Cemerlang, N., Sadoshima, J., Shioi, T., Izumo, S., Lukoshkova, E. V., Dart, A. M., Jennings, G. L., and McMullen, J. R. (2009). Reduced phosphoinosi- tide 3-kinase (p110alpha) activa- tion increases the susceptibility to atrial fibrillation. *Am. J. Pathol.* 175, 998–1009.

Priori, S. G., Napolitano, C., and Schwartz, P. J. (1993). Cardiac recep- tor activation and arrhythmogene- sis. *Eur. Heart J.* 14(Suppl. E), 20–26. Reil, J. C., Hohl, M., Oberhofer, M., Kazakov, A., Kaestner, L., Mueller, P., Adam, O., Maack, C., Lipp, P., Mewis, C., Allessie, M., Laufs, U., Böhm, M., and Neuberger, H. R. (2010). Cardiac Rac1 overexpression in mice creates a substrate for atrial arrhythmias characterized by struc- tural remodelling. *Cardiovasc. Res.* 87, 485–493.

Remme, C. A., Verkerk, A. O., Nuyens, D., van Ginneken, A. C., van Brun- schot, S., Belterman, C. N., Wilders, R., van Roon, M. A., Tan, H. L., Wilde, A. A., Carmeliet, P., de Bakker, J. M., Veldkamp, M. W., and Bezzina, C. R. (2006). Overlap syndrome of cardiac sodium channel disease in mice carrying the equivalent muta- tion of human SCN5A-1795insD. *Circulation* 114, 2584–2594.

Ridley, A. J., and Hall, A. (1992). Dis-tinct patterns of actin organiza- tion regulated by the small GTP- binding proteins Rac and Rho. *Cold Spring Harb. Symp. Quant. Biol.* 57, 661–671.

Rosenberg, M. A., Das, S., Quintero Pinzon, P., Knight, A., Sosnovik, D., Ellinor, P. T., and Rosenzweig, A. (2012). A novel transgenic mouse model of cardiac hypertrophy and atrial fibrillation. *J. Atr. Fibrillation* 2.

Ruan, Y., Denegri, M., Liu, N., Bachetti, T., Seregni, M., Morotti, S., Sev- eri, S., Napolitano, C., and Pri- ori, S. G. (2010). Trafficking defects and gating abnormalities of a novel SCN5A mutation question gene- specific therapy in long QT syn- drome type 3. *Circ. Res.* 106, 1374–1383.

Russell, J. C., and Proctor, S. D. (2006). Small animal models of car- diovascular disease: tools for the study of the roles of metabolic syndrome, dyslipidemia, and ath- erosclerosis. *Cardiovasc. Pathol.* 15, 318–330.

Ryan, A. K., Blumberg, B., Rodriguez- Esteban, C., Yonei-Tamura, S., Tamura, K., Tsukui, T., de la Peña, J., Sabbagh, W., Greenwald, J., Choe, S., Norris, D. P., Robertson, E. J., Evans, R. M., Rosenfeld, M. G., and Izpisúa Belmonte, J. C. (1998). Pitx2 determines left-right asymmetry of internal organs in vertebrates. *Nature* 394, 545–551.

Saba, S., Janczewski, A. M., Baker, L. C., Shusterman, V., Gursoy, E. C., Feldman, A. M., Salama, G., McTier- nan, C. F., and London, B. (2005).

Atrial contractile dysfunction, fibro- sis, and arrhythmias in a mouse model of cardiomyopathy secondary to cardiac-specific overexpression of tumor necrosis factor-{alpha}. *Am. J. Physiol. Heart Circ. Physiol.* 289, H1456–H1467.

Sah, V. P., Hoshijima, M., Chien, K. R., and Brown, J. H. (1996). Rho is required for Galphaq and alpha1- adrenergic receptor signaling in car- diomyocytes. Dissociation of Ras and Rho pathways. *J. Biol. Chem.* 271, 31185–31190.

Sah, V. P., Minamisawa, S., Tam, S. P., Wu, T. H., Dorn, G. W. II, Ross, J. Jr., Chien, K. R., and Brown, J. H. (1999). Cardiac-specific overexpres- sion of RhoA results in sinus and atrioventricular nodal dysfunction and contractile failure. *J. Clin. Invest.* 103, 1627–1634.

Salazar, N. C., Chen, J., and Rock- man, H. A. (2007). Cardiac GPCRs: GPCR signaling in healthy and fail- ing hearts. *Biochim. Biophys. Acta* 1768, 1006–1018.

Sampson, K. J., Terrenoire, C., Cer- vantes, D. O., Kaba, R. A., Peters, N. S., and Kass, R. S. (2008). Adrenergic regulation of a key cardiac potas- sium channel can contribute to atrial fibrillation: evidence from an I Ks transgenic mouse. *J. Physiol. (Lond.)* 586, 627–637.

Sancho, J., Re, R., Burton, J., Barger, A. C., and Haber, E. (1976). The role of the renin-angiotensin- aldosterone system in cardiovascu- lar homeostasis in normal human subjects. *Circulation* 53, 400–405.

Sawaya, S. E., Rajawat, Y. S., Rami, T. G., Szalai, G., Price, R. L., Sivasubramanian, N., Mann, D. L., and Khoury, D. S. (2007). Downregula- tion of connexin40 and increased prevalence of atrial arrhythmias in transgenic mice with cardiac- restricted overexpression of tumor necrosis factor. *Am. J. Physiol. Heart Circ. Physiol.* 292, H1561–H1567.

Schott, J. J., Charpentier, F., Peltier, S., Foley, P., Drouin, E., Bouhour, J. B., Donnelly, P., Vergnaud, G., Bachner, L., Moisan, J. P., Le Marec, H., and Pascal, O. (1995). Mapping of a gene for long QT syndrome to chromo- some 4q25-27. *Am. J. Hum. Genet.* 57, 1114–1122.

Schotten, U., Verheule, S., Kirchhof, P., and Goette, A. (2011). Pathophysiological mechanisms of atrial fib- rillation: a translational appraisal. *Physiol. Rev.* 91, 265–325.

Schrickel, J. W., Brixius, K., Herr, C., Clemen, C. S., Sasse, P., Reetz, K., Grohé, C., Meyer, R., Tiemann, K., Schröder, R., Bloch, W., Nickenig, G., Fleischmann, B. K., Noegel, A. A., Schwinger, R. H., and Lewal- ter, T. (2007). Enhanced heterogene- ity of myocardial conduction and severe cardiac electrical instability in annexin A7-deficient mice. *Cardio- vasc. Res.* 76, 257–268.

Schrickel, J. W., Stöckigt, F., Krzyzak, W., Paulin, D., Li, Z., Lübkemeier, I., Fleischmann, B., Sasse, P., Linhart, M., Lewalter, T., Nickenig, G., Lickfett, L., Schröder, R., and Clemen, C. S. (2010). Cardiac conduction disturbances and differential effects on atrial and ventricular electrophysiological properties in desmin defi- cient mice. *J. Interv. Card. Electro- physiol.* 28, 71–80.

Schweickert, A., Campione1, M., Stein- beisser, H., and Blum, M. (2000). Pitx2 isoforms: involvement of Pitx2c but not Pitx2a or Pitx2b in vertebrate left-right asymmetry. *Mech. Dev.* 90, 41–51. Scotland, P., Zhou, D., Benveniste, H., and Bennett, V. (1998). Nervous sys- tem defects of AnkyrinB (–/–) mice suggest functional overlap between the cell adhesion molecule L1 and 440-kD AnkyrinB in premyelinated axons. *J. Cell Biol.* 143, 1305–1315.

Shanmugam, M., Molina, C. E., Gao, S., Severac-Bastide, R., Fischmeister, R., and Babu, G. J. (2011). Decreased sarcolipin protein expression and enhanced sarco(endo)plasmic retic- ulum Ca2+ uptake in human atrial fibrillation. *Biochem. Biophys. Res. Commun.* 410, 97–101.

Shaw, R. M., and Rudy, Y. (1997). Ionic mechanisms of propagation in car- diac tissue. Roles of the sodium and L-type calcium currents during reduced excitability and decreased gap junction coupling. *Circ. Res.* 81, 727–741.

Sivasubramanian, N., Coker, M. L., Kur- relmeyer, K. M., MacLellan, W. R., DeMayo, F. J., Spinale, F. G., and Mann, D. L. (2001). Left ventricular remodeling in transgenic mice with cardiac restricted overexpression of tumor necrosis factor. *Circulation* 104, 826–831.

Sood, S., Chelu, M. G., van Oort, R. J., Skapura, D., Santonastasi, M., Dobrev, D., and Wehrens, X. H. (2008). Intracellular calcium leak due to FKBP12.6 deficiency in mice facilitates the inducibility of atrial fibrillation. *Heart Rhythm* 5, 1047–1054.

Stewart, A. F., Suzow, J., Kubota, T., Ueyama, T., and Chen, H. H. (1998). Transcription factor RTEF-1 medi- ates alpha1-adrenergic reactivation of the fetal gene program in cardiac myocytes. *Circ. Res.* 83, 43–49.

Sussman, M. A., Welch, S., Walker, A., Klevitsky, R., Hewett, T. E., Price, R. L., Schaefer, E., and Yager, K. (2000). Altered focal adhesion reg- ulation correlates with cardiomy- opathy in mice expressing constitu- tively active rac1. *J. Clin. Invest.* 105, 875–886.

Sweeney, L. J., Nag, A. C., Eisenberg, B., Manasek, F. J., and Zak, R. (1985). Developmental aspects of cardiac contractile proteins. *Basic Res. Car- diol.* 80(Suppl. 2), 123–127.

Temple, J., Frias, P., Rottman, J., Yang, T., Wu, Y., Verheijck, E. E., Zhang, W., Siprachanh, C., Kanki, H., Atkin- son, J. B., King, P., Anderson, M. E., Kupershmidt, S., and Roden, D. M. (2005). Atrial fibrillation in KCNE1- null mice. *Circ. Res.* 97, 62–69.

Thibodeau, I. L., Xu, J., Li, Q., Liu, G., Lam, K., Veinot, J. P., Birnie, D. H., Jones, D. L., Krahn, A. D., Lemery, R., Nicholson, B. J., and Gollob, M. H. (2010). Paradigm of genetic mosaicism and lone atrial fibrillation: physiological character- ization of a connexin 43-deletion mutant identified from atrial tissue. *Circulation* 122, 236–244.

Tsai, C. T., Tseng, C. D., Hwang, J. J., Wu, C. K., Yu, C. C., Wang, Y. ., Chen, W. P., Lai, L. P., Chiang, F. T., and Lin, J. L. (2011). Tachy- cardia of atrial myocytes induces collagen expression in atrial fibrob- lasts through transforming growth factor beta1. *Cardiovasc. Res.* 89, 805–815.

Tupling, A. R., Asahi, M., and MacLen- nan, D. H. (2002). Sarcolipin overexpression in rat slow twitch mus- cle inhibits sarcoplasmic reticulum Ca2+ uptake and impairs contrac- tile function. *J. Biol. Chem.* 277, 44740–44746.

Uemura, N., Ohkusa, T., Hamano, K., Nakagome, M., Hori, H., Shimizu, M., Matsuzaki, M., Mochizuki, S., Minamisawa, S., and Ishikawa, Y. (2004). Down-regulation of sarcol- ipin mRNA expression in chronic atrial fibrillation. *Eur. J. Clin. Invest.* 34, 723–730.

Ueyama, T., Zhu, C., Valenzuela, Y. M., Suzow, J. G., and Stewart, A. F. (2000). Identification of the func- tional domain in the transcription factor RTEF-1 that mediates alpha 1-adrenergic signaling in hypertro- phied cardiac myocytes. *J. Biol. Chem.* 275, 17476–17480.

Vaidya, D., Morley, G. E., Samie, F. H., and Jalife, J. (1999). Reentry and fibrillation in the mouse heart. A chal- lenge to the critical mass hypothesis. *Circ. Res.* 85, 174–181.

van Rooij, E., Sutherland, L. B., Qi, X., Richardson, J. A., Hill, J., and Olson, E. N. (2007). Control of stress- dependent cardiac growth and gene expression by a microRNA. *Science* 316, 575–579.

Verheule, S. (1999). Cardiac conduc- tion abnormalities in mice lack- ing the gap junction protein con- nexin40. *J. Cardiovasc. Electrophys- iol.* 10, 1380–1389.

Verheule, S., Sato, T., Everett, T. IV, Engle, S. K., Otten, D., Rubart-von der Lohe, M., Nakajima, H. O., Naka- jima, H., Field, L. J., and Olgin, J. E. (2004). Increased vulnerabil- ity to atrial fibrillation in transgenic mice with selective atrial fibrosis caused by overexpression of TGF- beta1. *Circ. Res.* 94, 1458–1465.

Wakili, R., Voigt, N., Kääb, S., Dobrev, ., and Nattel, S. (2011). Recent advances in the molecular patho- physiology of atrial fibrillation. *J. Clin. Invest.* 121, 2955–2968.

Wang, D. W., Yazawa, K., George, A. L. Jr., and Bennett, P. B. (1996). Characterization of human car- diac Na+ channel mutations in the congenital long QT syndrome. *Proc. Natl. Acad. Sci. U.S.A.* 93, 13200–13205.

Wang, J., Klysik, E., Sood, S., Johnson, R. L., Wehrens, X. H., and Martin, J. F. (2010). Pitx2 prevents susceptibil- ity to atrial arrhythmias by inhibit- ing left-sided pacemaker specifica- tion. *Proc. Natl. Acad. Sci. U.S.A.* 107, 9753–9758.

Wang, Z., Lu, Y., and Yang, B. (2011). MicroRNAs and atrial fibrillation: new fundamentals. *Cardiovasc. Res.* 89, 710–721.

Watanabe, H., Yang, T., Stroud, D. M., Lowe, J. S., Harris, L., Atack, T. C., Wang, D. W., Hipkens, S. B., Leake, B., Hall, L., Kupershmidt, S., Chopra, N., Magnuson, M. A., Tanabe, N., Knollmann, B. C., George, A. L. Jr., and Roden, D. M. (2011). Strik- ing in vivo phenotype of a disease- associated human SCN5A mutation producing minimal changes in vitro. *Circulation* 124, 1001–1011.

Wehrens, X. H., Lehnart, S. E., Huang, F., Vest, J. A., Reiken, S. R., Mohler, P. J., Sun, J., Guatimosim, S., Song, L. S., Rosemblit, N., D'Armiento, J. M., Napolitano, C., Memmi, M., Priori, S. G., Lederer, W. J., and Marks, A. R. (2003). FKBP12.6 deficiency and defective calcium release channel (ryanodine receptor) function linked to exercise-induced sudden cardiac death. *Cell* 113, 829–840.

Wei, L., Taffet, G. E., Khoury, D. S., Bo, J., Li, Y., Yatani, A., Delaughter, M. C., Klevitsky, R., Hewett, T. E., Robbins, J., Michael, L. H., Schneider, M. D., Entman, M. L., and Schwartz, R. J. (2004). Disruption of Rho signaling results in progressive atrioventric- ular conduction defects while ventricular function remains preserved. *FASEB J.* 18, 857–859.

Wilde, A. A., and Brugada, R. (2011). Phenotypical manifestations of mutations in the genes encoding subunits of the cardiac sodium channel. *Circ. Res.* 108, 884–897.

Wu, J., Zhang, Y., Zhang, X., Cheng, L., Lammers, W. J., Grace, A. A., Fraser, J. A., Zhang, H., Huang, C. L., and Lei, M. (2012). Altered sinoatrial node function and intra-atrial con- duction in murine gain-of-function Scn5a+/ deltaKPQ hearts suggest an overlap syndrome. *Am. J. Physiol. Heart Circ. Physiol.* 302, H1510– H1523.

Xiao, H. D., Fuchs, S., Campbell, D. J., Lewis, W., Dudley, S. C. Jr., Kasi, V. S., Hoit, B. D., Keshelava, G., Zhao, H., Capecchi, M. R., and Bernstein, K. E. (2004). Mice with cardiac-restricted angiotensin- converting enzyme (ACE) have atrial enlargement, cardiac arrhythmia, and sudden death. *Am. J. Pathol.* 165, 1019–1032.

Xie, L. H., Shanmugam, M., Park, J. Y., Zhao, Z., Wen, H., Tian, B., Peri-asamy, M., and Babu, G. J. (2012). Ablation of sarcolipin results in atrial remodeling. *Am. J. Physiol. Cell Phys- iol.* 302, 1762–1771.

Xu, S., Liu, A. C., and Gotlieb, A. I. (2010). Common pathogenic features of atherosclerosis and calcific aortic stenosis: role of transforming growth factor- beta. *Cardiovasc. Pathol.* 19, 236–247.

Yeh, Y. H., Kuo, C. T., Chan, T. H., Chang, G. J., Qi, X. Y., Tsai, F., Nattel, S., and Chen, W. J. (2011). Transforming growth factor- beta and oxidative stress mediate tachycardia-induced cellular remod- elling in cultured atrial-derived myocytes. *Cardiovasc. Res.* 91, 62–70.

Yue, L., Feng, J., Gaspo, R., Li, G. R., Wang, Z., and Nattel, S. (1997). Ionic remodeling underlying action potential changes in a canine model of atrial fibrillation. *Circ. Res.* 81, 512–525.

Zellerhoff, S., Pistulli, R., Mönnig, G., Hinterseer, M., Beckmann, B. M., Köbe, J., Steinbeck, G., Kääb, S., Haverkamp, W., Fabritz, L., Gradaus, R., Breithardt, G., Schulze-Bahr, E., Böcker, D., and Kirchhof, P. (2009). Atrial arrhythmias in long QT syn- drome – a nested case control study. *J. Cardiovasc. Electrophysiol.* 20, 401–407.

Zhang, X., Chen, S., Yoo, S., Chakrabarti, S., Zhang, T., Ke, T., Oberti, C., Yong, S. L., Fang, F., Li, L., de la Fuente, R., Wang, L., Chen, Q., and Wang, Q. K. (2008). Mutation in nuclear pore component NUP155 leads to atrial fibrillation and early sudden cardiac death. *Cell* 135, 1017–1027.

Zhang, Y., Fraser, J. A., Jeevaratnam, K., Hao, X., Hothi, S. S., Grace, A. A., Lei, M., and Huang, C. L. (2011). Acute atrial arrhyth- mogenicity and altered Ca(2+) homeostasis in murine RyR2- P2328S hearts. *Cardiovasc. Res.* 89, 794–804.

Zhang, Z., He, Y., Tuteja, D., Xu, D., Timofeyev, V., Zhang, Q., Glatter, K. A., Xu, Y., Shin, H. S., Low, R., and Chiamvimonvat, N. (2005). Func- tional roles of Cav1.3(alpha1D) calcium channels in atria: insights gained from gene-targeted null mutant mice. *Circulation* 112, 1936–1944.

Zhang, Z., Xu, Y., Song, H., Rodriguez, J., Tuteja, D., Namkung, Y., Shin, H. S., and Chiamvimonvat, N. (2002a). Functional roles of Ca(v)1.3 (alpha(1D)) calcium channel in sinoatrial nodes: insight gained using gene-targeted null mutant mice. *Circ. Res.* 90, 981–987.

Zhang, X., Yang, H., Yu, J., Chen, C., Zhang, G., Bao, J., Du, Y., Kibukawa, M., Li, Z., Wang, J., Hu, S., Dong, W., Wang, J., Gregersen, N., Niebuhr, E., and Bolund, L. (2002b). Genomic organization, transcript variants and comparative analysis of the human nucleoporin 155 (NUP155) gene. *Gene* 288, 9–18.

Permissions

All chapters in this book were first published by Frontiers; hereby published with permission under the Creative Commons Attribution License or equivalent. Every chapter published in this book has been scrutinized by our experts. Their significance has been extensively debated. The topics covered herein carry significant findings which will fuel the growth of the discipline. They may even be implemented as practical applications or may be referred to as a beginning point for another development.

The contributors of this book come from diverse backgrounds, making this book a truly international effort. This book will bring forth new frontiers with its revolutionizing research information and detailed analysis of the nascent developments around the world.

We would like to thank all the contributing authors for lending their expertise to make the book truly unique. They have played a crucial role in the development of this book. Without their invaluable contributions this book wouldn't have been possible. They have made vital efforts to compile up to date information on the varied aspects of this subject to make this book a valuable addition to the collection of many professionals and students.

This book was conceptualized with the vision of imparting up-to-date information and advanced data in this field. To ensure the same, a matchless editorial board was set up. Every individual on the board went through rigorous rounds of assessment to prove their worth. After which they invested a large part of their time researching and compiling the most relevant data for our readers.

The editorial board has been involved in producing this book since its inception. They have spent rigorous hours researching and exploring the diverse topics which have resulted in the successful publishing of this book. They have passed on their knowledge of decades through this book. To expedite this challenging task, the publisher supported the team at every step. A small team of assistant editors was also appointed to further simplify the editing procedure and attain best results for the readers.

Apart from the editorial board, the designing team has also invested a significant amount of their time in understanding the subject and creating the most relevant covers. They scrutinized every image to scout for the most suitable representation of the subject and create an appropriate cover for the book.

The publishing team has been an ardent support to the editorial, designing and production team. Their endless efforts to recruit the best for this project, has resulted in the accomplishment of this book. They are a veteran in the field of academics and their pool of knowledge is as vast as their experience in printing. Their expertise and guidance has proved useful at every step. Their uncompromising quality standards have made this book an exceptional effort. Their encouragement from time to time has been an inspiration for everyone.

The publisher and the editorial board hope that this book will prove to be a valuable piece of knowledge for researchers, students, practitioners and scholars across the globe.

List of Contributors

Sathya D. Unudurthi
Department of Biomedical Engineering, College of Engineering, The Ohio State University, Columbus, OH, USA
The Dorothy M. Davis Heart and Lung Research Institute, The Ohio State University Wexner Medical Center, Columbus, OH, USA

Roseanne M. Wolf
Department of Mathematics, The University of Dubuque, Dubuque, IA, USA

Thomas J. Hund
Department of Biomedical Engineering, College of Engineering, The Ohio State University, Columbus, OH, USA
The Dorothy M. Davis Heart and Lung Research Institute, The Ohio State University Wexner Medical Center, Columbus, OH, USA
Division of Cardiovascular Medicine, Department of Internal Medicine, The Ohio State University Wexner Medical Center, Columbus, OH, USA

Natalia A. Trayanova, Patrick M. Boyle, Hermenegild J. Arevalo and Sohail Zahid
Department of Biomedical Engineering, Institute for Computational Medicine, Johns Hopkins University, Baltimore, MD, USA

Carlos L. del Rio
Department of Physiology and Cell Biology, The Ohio State University, Columbus, OH, USA
Department of Electrical and Computer Engineering, The Ohio State University, Columbus, OH, USA
Safety Pharmacology, QTest Labs, Columbus, OH, USA

Bradley D. Clymer
Department of Electrical and Computer Engineering, The Ohio State University, Columbus, OH, USA
Biomedical Engineering, The Ohio State University, Columbus, OH, USA

George E. Billman
Department of Physiology and Cell Biology, The Ohio State University, Columbus, OH, USA
Davis Heart and Lung Research Institute, The Ohio State University, Columbus, OH, USA

Elise L. Kessler, Harold V. M. van Rijen, Marc A. Vos and Toon A. B. van Veen
Division of Heart and Lungs, Department of Medical Physiology, University Medical Center Utrecht, Utrecht, Netherlands

Mohamed Boulaksil
Division of Heart and Lungs, Department of Medical Physiology, University Medical Center Utrecht, Utrecht, Netherlands
Department of Cardiology, Radboud University Medical Center, Nijmegen, Netherlands

Yael Yaniv
Biomedical Engineering Faculty, Technion- Israel Institute of Technology, Haifa, Israel

Kenta Tsutsui and Edward G. Lakatta
Laboratory of Cardiovascular Science, Biomedical Research Center, Intramural Research Program, National Institute on Aging, National Institutes of Health, Baltimore, MD, USA

Candido Cabo
Department of Computer Systems, New York City College of Technology, City University of New York, New York, NY, USA
Doctoral Program in Computer Science, Graduate Center, City University of New York, New York, NY, USA

Stefan Dhein, Martin Kostelka and Friedrich-Wilhelm Mohr
Clinic for Cardiac Surgery, Heart Center Leipzig, University Leipzig, Leipzig, Germany

Thomas Seidel
Nora Eccles Harrison Cardiovascular Research and Training Institute, University of Utah, Salt Lake City, UT, USA

Aida Salameh
Clinic for Pediatric Cardiology, Heart Center Leipzig, University Leipzig, Leipzig, Germany

Joanna Jozwiak and Gerd Hindrick
Clinic for Cardiology, Heart Center Leipzig, University Leipzig, Leipzig, Germany

Anja Hagen
Hospital for Children and Adolescents, University of Leipzig, Leipzig, Germany

Thomas A. Csepe, Anuradha Kalyanasundaram, Brian J. Hansen and Vadim V. Fedorov
Department of Physiology and Cell Biology, Davis Heart and Lung Research Institute, The Ohio State University Wexner Medical Center, Columbus, OH, USA

Jichao Zhao
Auckland Bioengineering Institute, The University of Auckland, Auckland, New Zealand

Andre G. Kleber and Jeffrey E. Saffitz
Department of Pathology, Beth Israel Medical Center, Harvard Medical School, Boston, MA, USA

Jussi T. Koivumäki and Mary M. C. Maleckar
Simula Research Laboratory, Center for Biomedical Computing and Center for Cardiological Innovation, Oslo, Norway

Robert B. Clark, Darrell Belke, Colleen Kondo and Wayne R. Giles
Faculty of Kinesiology, University of Calgary, Calgary, AB, Canada

Paul W. M. Fedak
Division of Cardiothoracic Surgery, Department of Cardiac Sciences, University of Calgary, Calgary, AB, Canada

Nicoline W. Smit
Department of Clinical and Experimental Cardiology, Heart Centre, Academic Medical Centre, University of Amsterdam, Amsterdam, Netherlands

Ruben Coronel
Department of Clinical and Experimental Cardiology, Heart Centre, Academic Medical Centre, University of Amsterdam, Amsterdam, Netherlands
L' Institut de RYthmologie et modélisation Cardiaque, Université Bordeaux Segalen, Bordeaux, France

Richard Ang and Aaisha Opel
Centre for Clinical Pharmacology, Division of Medicine, University College London, London, UK

Andrew Tinker
William Harvey Heart Centre, Barts and The London School of Medicine and Dentistry, London, UK

Mickael Derangeon, Jérôme Montnach, Isabelle Baró and Flavien Charpentier
INSERM, UMR1087, l'Institut du Thorax, Nantes, France
CNRS, UMR 6291, l'Institut du Thorax, Nantes, France
Université de Nantes, Nantes, France

Burcu Duygu, Ella M. Poels and Paula A. da Costa Martins
Department of Cardiology, CARIM School for Cardiovascular Diseases, Maastricht University, Maastricht, Netherlands

Diego Franco, Ana Chinchilla and Amelia E. Aránega
Department of Experimental Biology, University of Jaen, Jaen, Spain

Kai Friedrichs
Department of Electrophysiology, Cardiovascular Research Center, University Heart Center Hamburg, Hamburg, Germany

Stephan Baldus and Anna Klinke
Department of General and Interventional Cardiology, Cardiovascular Research Center, University Heart Center Hamburg, Hamburg, Germany

Maaike Hoekstra, Arthur A. M. Wilde and Connie R. Bezzina
Department of Clinical and Experimental Cardiology, Heart Failure Research Center, Academic Medical Center, University of Amsterdam, Amsterdam, Netherlands

Christine L. Mummery
Department of Anatomy and Embryology, Leiden University Medical Center, Leiden, Netherlands

Arie O. Verkerk
Department of Anatomy, Embryology, and Physiology, Heart Failure Research Center, Academic Medical Center, University of Amsterdam, Amsterdam, Netherlands

Jari M. Tuomi and Peter Chidiac
Department of Physiology and Pharmacology, The University of Western Ontario, London, ON, Canada

Douglas L. Jones
Department of Physiology and Pharmacology, The University of Western Ontario, London, ON, Canada
Department of Medicine, The University of Western Ontario, London, ON, Canada
Cardiovascular Group, Lawson Health Research Institute, London Health Sciences Center, London, ON, Canada
Canadian Surgical Technologies and Advance Robotics, Lawson Health Research Institute, London Health Sciences Center, London, ON, Canada

Michael M. Kreusser and Johannes Backs
Research Unit Cardiac Epigenetics, Department of Cardiology, University of Heidelberg, Heidelberg, Germany
German Center for Cardiovascular Research (DZHK), Partner Site Heidelberg/ Mannheim, Germany

Elisabeth M. Lodder and Stefania Rizzo
Department of Experimental Cardiology, Heart Failure Research Center, Academic Medical Center, University of Amsterdam, Amsterdam, Netherlands
Department of Cardiac, Thoracic and Vascular Sciences, University of Padua, Padua, Italy

Julian Mustroph, Lars S. Maier and Stefan Wagner
Department of Cardiology, University Medical Center Göttingen, Göttingen, Germany

Genna Riley and Fahima Syeda
Centre for Cardiovascular Sciences, School of Clinical and Experimental Medicine, University of Birmingham, Birmingham, UK

Paulus Kirchhof and Larissa Fabritz
Centre for Cardiovascular Sciences, School of Clinical and Experimental Medicine, University of Birmingham, Birmingham, UK
Department of Cardiology and Angiology, University Hospital Münster, Münster, Germany

Index